ADVANCES IN

DRUG RESEARCH

VOLUME 17

ADVANCES IN

DRUG RESEARCH

Edited by

BERNARD TESTA

School of Pharmacy, University of Lausanne, Lausanne, Switzerland

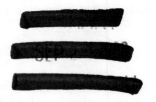

VOLUME 17

1988

ACADEMIC PRESS

Harcourt Brace Jovanovich, Publishers

LONDON   SAN DIEGO   NEW YORK   BOSTON
SYDNEY   TOKYO   TORONTO

ACADEMIC PRESS LIMITED
24/28 Oval Road
London NW1 7DX

United States Edition published by
ACADEMIC PRESS INC.
San Diego, CA 92101

British Library Cataloguing in Publication Data
Advances in drug research. —
Vol. 17 (1988)
1. Drugs – Serials
615'.1'05

ISBN 0–12–013317–2

Typeset by Paston Press, Loddon, Norfolk and printed in Great Britain by
St Edmundsbury Press, Bury St Edmunds, Suffolk

CONTENTS

Recent Advances in the Search for Selective Antiviral Agents

E. DE CLERCQ

Recent Developments in the Field of Cephem Antibiotics

W. DÜRCKHEIMER, F. ADAM, G. FISCHER AND R. KIRRSTETTER

Recent Experimental and Conceptual Advances in Drug Receptor Research in the Cardiovascular System

R. R. RUFFOLO, JR. AND A. J. NICHOLS

The Pharmacology and Therapeutic Potential of Serotonin Receptor Agonists and Antagonists

R. W. FULLER

Recent Advances in GABA Agonists, Antagonists and Uptake Inhibitors: Structure–Activity Relationships and Therapeutic Potential

P. KROGSGAARD-LARSEN, H. HJEDS, E. FALCH, F. S. JØRGENSEN AND L. NIELSEN

CONTRIBUTORS

F. ADAM, *Pharma-Synthese, Hoechst AG, Frankfurt/Main 80, FGR*

E. DE CLERCQ, *Rega Institute for Medical Research, Katholieke Universiteit Leuven, Leuven, Belgium*

W. DÜRCKHEIMER, *Pharma-Synthese, Hoechst AG, Frankfurt/Main 80, FRG*

E. FALCH, *Department of Chemistry, The Royal Danish School of Pharmacy, Copenhagen, Denmark*

G. FISCHER, *Pharma-Synthese, Hoechst AG, Frankfurt/Main 80, FRG*

R. W. FULLER, *Lilly Research Laboratories, Eli Lilly and Company, Lilly Corporate Center, Indianapolis, Indiana, USA*

H. HJEDS, *Department of Chemistry, The Royal Danish School of Pharmacy, Copenhagen, Denmark*

F. S. JØRGENSEN, *Department of Chemistry, The Royal Danish School of Pharmacy, Copenhagen, Denmark*

R. KIRRSTETTER, *Pharma-Synthese, Hoechst AG, Frankfurt/Main 80, FRG*

P. KROGSGAARD-LARSEN, *Department of Chemistry, The Royal Danish School of Pharmacy, Copenhagen, Denmark*

A. J. NICHOLS, *Department of Pharmacology, Smith Kline and French Laboratories, King of Prussia, Pennsylvania, USA*

L. NIELSEN, *Department of Chemistry, The Royal Danish School of Pharmacy, Copenhagen, Denmark*

R. R. RUFFOLO, JR., *Department of Pharmacology, Smith Kline and French Laboratories, King of Prussia, Pennsylvania, USA*

PREFACE:
TEXT AND CONTEXT

No research paper is adequately communicative and informative without an introductory part outlining the scientific context of the reported work, and a conclusion placing its findings in a broader context. Many of us certainly remember trying to grasp the meaning and significance of publications which, due to lack of explicit introduction and conclusion, should best be considered as technical reports written for the benefit of insiders. In other words, research papers are meaningful only within the frame of their scientific context.

Major review articles such as the chapters featured in this volume differ from research papers by more than their length and type of content. By definition, the contextual frame of reviews is much broader than that of research papers since they summarize findings and concepts originally presented in a number of original publications. Yet the essential difference lies elsewhere. By integrating many findings and concepts, reviews enlarge and explicate the scientific context of research papers both recent and future. Reviews as well as books are thus *context makers*, and as such fulfil a function essential to the advance of science.

These thoughts occurred to me while reading the scientific testament of Gregory Bateson (1980), a book in which this great anthropologist and epistemologist offers some enlightening sentences about context (or "pattern through time"), about "contexts which confer meaning because there is classification of contexts", and about "patterns which connect patterns".

To integrate the contexts of innumerable studies, and to offer a higher-order context giving sense and import to current research efforts, such are the goals and achievements of the texts making up this volume. Different as they may be in form and content, all five chapters have necessitated considerable dedication from their authors, as well as a readiness to fit into the approach and wise by which *Advances in Drug Research* in turn aim at becoming a "pattern connecting patterns".

The volume opens with two chapters dealing with chemotherapeutic agents, continues with a more general chapter on drug receptors in the cardiovascular system, and closes with two neuropharmacological chapters. The first chapter by De Clercq is an account of the latest findings in the search for selective antiviral agents. As one of the best world experts in this fast expanding field, De Clercq has prepared a text that is both highly readable and systematic, rationalizing present data and pointing to directions for future research. The second chapter covers recent developments in the field of cephems, a group of β-lactam antibiotics which is attracting much attention. It is the merit of Dürckheimer and colleagues to combine the synthetic chemistry, structure–activity relationships and disposition of cephem antibiotics into an encyclopaedic treatment which may well remain unequalled for many years.

These two chapters are followed by a monumental work on the cardiovascular system and its receptor regulations, a jigsaw puzzle whose complexity defies our understanding. The chapter by Ruffolo and Nichols reviews the pieces of the puzzle with clarity and depth only to transcend the analytical level and render this complexity discernible to the reader. This is followed by a short and dense chapter on serotonin receptor agonists and antagonists in which Fuller summarizes recent breakthroughs and critically evaluates some of their therapeutic potentials.

The last chapter by Krogsgaard-Larsen and co-workers is another testimony to scientific achievement and communicative skill. This team has successfully pioneered synthetic and pharmacological research on GABA agonists, antagonists and uptake inhibitors, and here offers a text of particular richness and impact.

Editing this volume has been a lasting source of fun and much enrichment. May the same feeling be felt by the reader, with whom the contributors share their knowledge, insight and enthusiasm. It was the inspired Bateson again who wrote that "at present, there is no existing science whose special interest is the combining of pieces of information" (Bateson, 1980). This statement is certainly valid, yet we may wonder whether the writing and study of texts such as those offered here are not endeavours pregnant with the unborn science of context making.

BERNARD TESTA

Reference

Bateson, G. (1980). "Mind and Nature—A Necessary Unity". Fontana Paperbacks, London.

Recent Advances in the Search for Selective Antiviral Agents

ERIK DE CLERCQ

Rega Institute for Medical Research, Katholieke Universiteit Leuven, Leuven, Belgium

1 Introduction

Antiviral chemotherapy has now definitely come of age. While almost 25 years have elapsed since the first antiviral agent (idoxuridine, IDU, 5-iodo-2'-deoxyuridine) was marketed, the clinical use of antiviral agents has gained renewed interest due to the successful introduction of acyclovir [ACV, 9-(2-hydroxyethoxymethyl)guanine] in medical practice (De Clercq, 1988a). The search for new antiviral agents has been further boosted by the advent of AIDS (acquired immune deficiency syndrome) and the identification of a retrovirus, now termed human immunodeficiency virus (HIV), as the causative agent of the disease. For recent reviews on the subject of antiviral chemotherapy, see Dolin (1985), De Clercq (1985a, 1986a,

ADVANCES IN DRUG RESEARCH, VOL. 17
ISBN 0-12-013317-2

2 E. DE CLERCQ

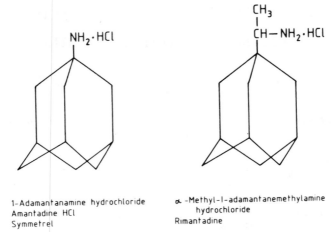

1-Adamantanamine hydrochloride
Amantadine HCl
Symmetrel

α-Methyl-1-adamantanemethylamine
hydrochloride
Rimantadine

FIG. 1. Amantadine and rimantadine.

1987b,c,d,e) and De Clercq and Walker (1986). The current armamentarium of antiviral drugs which have been licensed for clinical use consists of amantadine, rimantadine (Fig. 1), idoxuridine, trifluridine (Fig. 2), vidarabine (Fig. 3), acyclovir (Fig. 4), ribavirin (Fig. 5) and retrovir (Fig. 6). Amantadine and rimantadine are useful in the prophylaxis and early therapy of influenza A virus infections. Idoxuridine, trifluridine, vidarabine and acyclovir are used in the topical treatment of herpetic keratitis. Acyclovir is used for the systemic (intravenous or peroral) treatment of herpes simplex virus (HSV) and varicella-zoster virus (VZV) infections. ACV is particularly useful in the treatment of primary genital herpes and herpetic encephalitis, where it is superior to vidarabine. ACV can also be recommended for the prophylaxis of recurrent genital herpes, the therapy and prophylaxis of HSV infections in immunosuppressed patients and the treatment of VZV infections in immunosuppressed patients, where again it is superior to vidarabine. Ribavirin has been licensed for topical (aerosol) treatment of respiratory syncytial virus (RSV) infection in infants, and retrovir has recently become available for the treatment of patients with AIDS and ARC (AIDS-related complex).

While the availability of some antiviral compounds for some virus infections by no means suggests that no further search towards new and more potent or selective drugs for these diseases is warranted, there are many other viral diseases that are in great need of an effective antiviral

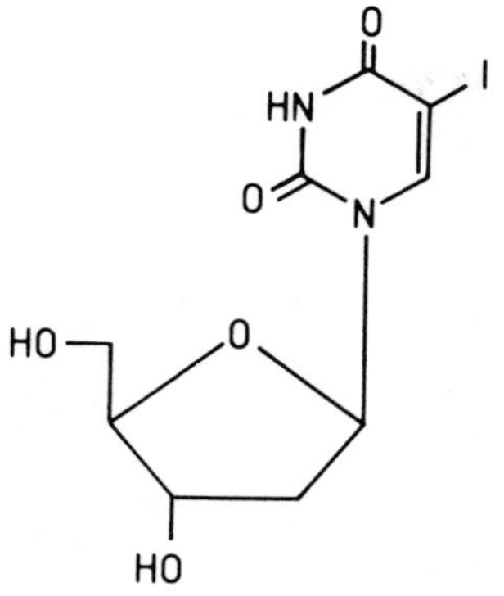

5-Iodo-2'-deoxyuridine
Idoxuridine
IDU

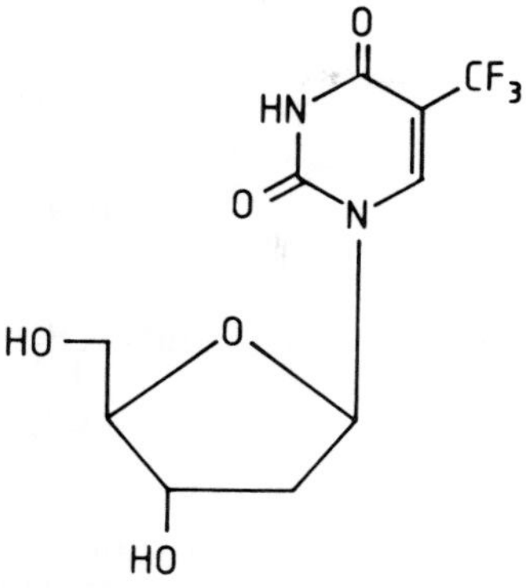

5-Trifluoro-2'-deoxythymidine
Trifluridine
TFT

FIG. 2. Idoxuridine and trifluridine.

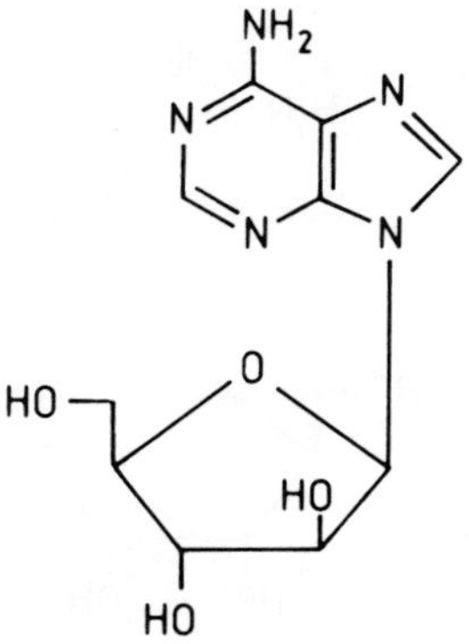

9-β-D-Arabinofuranosyladenine (Ara-A)
Adenine arabinoside
Vidarabine
Vira-A

FIG. 3. Vidarabine.

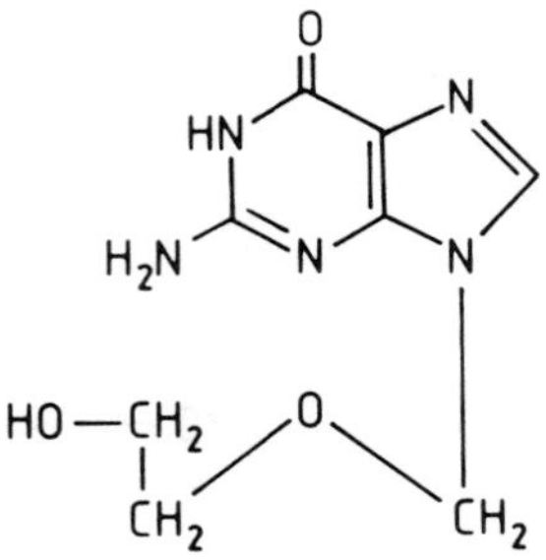

9-(2-Hydroxyethoxymethyl)guanine
Acycloguanosine
Acyclovir, aciclovir (ACV)
Zovirax

Fig. 4. Acyclovir.

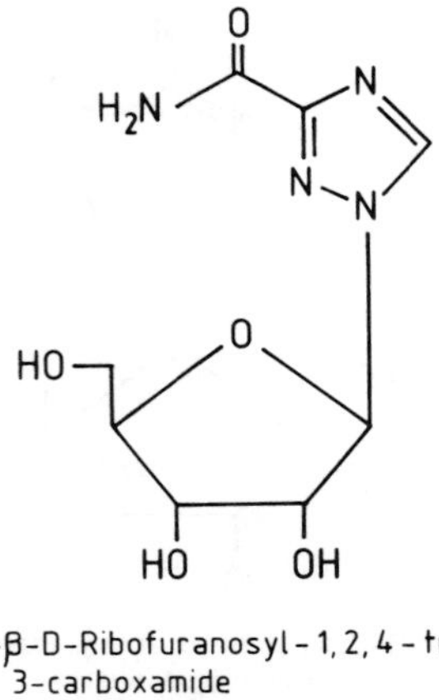

1-β-D-Ribofuranosyl-1,2,4-triazole-
3-carboxamide
Ribavirin
Virazole

Fig. 5. Ribavirin.

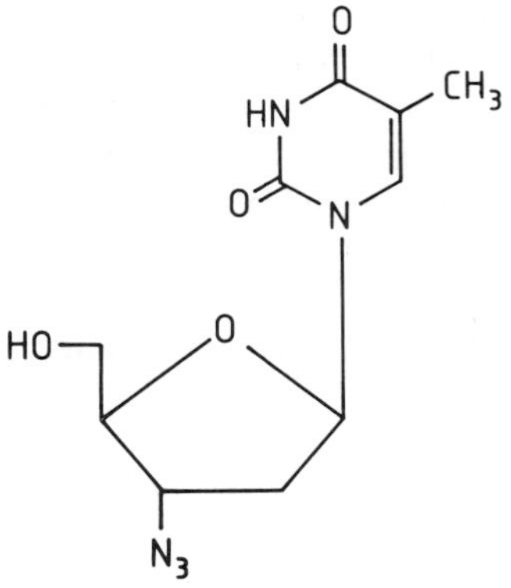

3'-Azido-2', 3'- dideoxythymidine (AzddThd)
Azidothymidine (AZT)
Retrovir
Zidovudine

FIG. 6. Retrovir.

chemotherapy. These include, among others, the members of the herpes-virus family, such as cytomegalovirus (CMV), which often leads to life-threatening complications in immunosuppressed patients, and Epstein-Barr virus (EBV), which is associated with various B-cell lymphoproliferative disorders; adenovirus infections, which again may be occasionally fatal in immunocompromised patients; papillomaviruses which are etiologically linked to warts, condylomata acuminata, genital carcinomas and other malignant tumours; rhinoviruses and other respiratory tract viruses, which can be considered as the infectious pathogens with the greatest socioeconomic impact; rotaviruses, which have been recognized as the single most important causative agents of acute diarrhoea, which, in turn, ranks among the leading causes of morbidity and mortality in infants and young children, particularly in developing countries; haemorrhagic fever viruses (i.e. Lassa, Junin, Machupo, Rift Valley) which rank among the most deadly pathogens, and, although confined to some areas of the world, are difficult to control by vaccination; and hepatitis B virus, which counts 200 million carriers in the world of which 40 million may die from cirrhosis and another 10 million from hepatocarcinoma (Hilleman, 1987).

It is clear, therefore, that the need for treatment of viral diseases has remained enormous, as the currently available drugs barely scratch the surface (Galasso, 1988). Science, politics and public apprehension about

AIDS have fuelled antiviral drug development, and the resulting burst of efforts has already generated a wealth of compounds which hold promise for the treatment of AIDS. This momentum in antiviral research should not only be nurtured and maintained, but accelerated and expanded to other viral diseases in urgent need of antivirals.

2 Herpesvirus Infections

2.1 ACYCLOVIR

Acyclovir (Fig. 4) has acquired an established position in the chemotherapy of HSV infections (Table 1). Oral acyclovir is the treatment of choice for first episodes of genital herpes (Mindel *et al.*, 1987); it is of slight benefit in the treatment of recurrent genital herpes, but when given prophylactically it prevents reactivation of symptomatic recurrences of genital herpes (Straus

TABLE 1

Major indications for the clinical use of acyclovir

Dosage (duration)	Route of administration[a]	Indication
		Therapy
3% eye ointment	top.	Herpetic keratitis
5% cream or ointment (up to 10 days)	top.	Primary genital herpes
15 mg/kg/day (5–10 days)	p.o., i.v.	Primary genital herpes
15 mg/kg/day (7 days)	i.v., p.o.	HSV infection in immuno-compromised patients
30 mg/kg/day (10 days)	i.v.	Herpes simplex encephalitis
30 mg/kg/day (7 days)	i.v.	Varicella or zoster in immuno-compromised patients
15–30 mg/kg/day	i.v.	Neonatal herpes
60 mg/kg/day (7 days)	p.o.	Zoster
		Prophylaxis
15 mg/kg/day	p.o.	HSV infection in bone marrow transplant recipients Recurrent genital herpes

[a]Top., topically; p.o., perorally; i.v., intravenously.

et al., 1984). For the latter indication the use of acyclovir is at present limited to a 6-month course in patients with frequent recurrences (Corey and Spear, 1986). In immunosuppressed patients with mucocutaneous HSV infections, intravenous or oral acyclovir relieves pain and accelerates healing of both symptomatic first and recurrent episodes, and, in addition, intravenous or oral acyclovir taken daily prevents recurrences during high-risk periods, i.e. immediately after bone marrow transplantation. In the treatment of recurrent herpes labialis, topical acyclovir (5% cream) is of no clinical benefit (Shaw *et al.*, 1985), and oral acyclovir has not been studied. In the treatment of herpes simplex encephalitis, acyclovir is clearly superior to vidarabine (Sköldenberg *et al.*, 1984; Whitley *et al.*, 1986). Acyclovir is also superior to vidarabine in the treatment of VZV infections in immunocompromised patients (Shepp *et al.*, 1986). For acyclovir to afford a beneficial effect in the treatment of varicella or zoster, it has to be administered at higher doses than for the treatment of HSV infections, i.e. 2 g/day i.v., or even 4 g/day p.o. (Kendrick *et al.*, 1986). Only with an oral dosage regimen of 0.8 g acyclovir 4-hourly are mean steady state peak and trough plasma drug concentrations achieved that are in excess of the median effective dose for most VZV strains (Kendrick *et al.*, 1986). The clinical usefulness of acyclovir is limited to HSV and VZV infections. It is of little, if any, avail in the treatment of CMV infections, and, although acyclovir inhibits oropharyngeal excretion of EBV in patients with acute infectious mononucleosis (Ernberg and Andersson, 1986), it remains to be seen whether this reduction in virus burden is reflected by an alleviation of the clinical symptoms.

The mechanism of action of acyclovir (Fig. 7) is fairly well established. The compound is preferentially recognized as substrate by the virus-induced 2'-deoxythymidine (dThd) kinase (Fyfe *et al.*, 1978). It is actually the 2'-deoxycytidine (dCyd) kinase activity associated with the viral dThd kinase which is responsible for the phosphorylation of acyclovir to its monophosphate (De Clercq, 1982). Acyclovir monophosphate (ACVMP) is then phosphorylated by the cellular GMP kinase (Miller and Miller, 1980) to acyclovir diphosphate (ACVDP), which in turn is phosphorylated to acyclovir triphosphate (ACVTP) by nucleoside diphosphate kinase or other cellular enzymes (Miller and Miller, 1982). The antivirally active form of acyclovir corresponds to its triphosphate. ACVTP is strongly inhibitory to HSV DNA polymerase and, to a lesser extent, cellular DNA polymerases (Furman *et al.*, 1979; St. Clair *et al.*, 1980) and this inhibition is competitive with respect to the natural substrate dGTP; but, in addition, ACVTP can also be incorporated into DNA at its 3'-terminal, and, as the 3'-terminal ACVMP residues cannot be excised by the DNA polymerase-associated 3',5'-exonuclease (Derse *et al.*, 1981), they prevent further chain elongation and thus act as DNA chain terminators. This explains the occurrence of

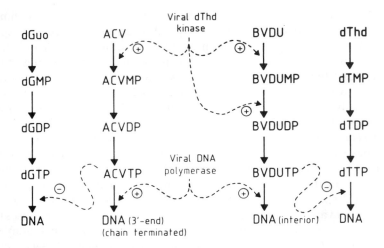

FIG. 7. Mechanism of action of acyclovir (ACV) and bromovinyldeoxyuridine (BVDU) against herpes simplex virus (HSV).

short DNA fragments in HSV-infected cells exposed to acyclovir (McGuirt *et al.*, 1984).

2.2 ACYCLOVIR DERIVATIVES

Acyclovir suffers from a number of drawbacks such as (i) poor solubility in water (about 0.2% at 25°C), (ii) low oral absorption (about 20% following administration of 200 mg) and (iii) limited activity spectrum, essentially confined to HSV and VZV and excluding such important pathogens as CMV. Because of its poor aqueous solubility, acyclovir cannot be given as eyedrops in the topical treatment of herpetic keratitis, or as intramuscular injections in the systemic treatment of HSV and VZV infections. To overcome this problem, water-soluble esters of acyclovir, i.e. *2'-O-glycylacyclovir* (Fig. 8), have been prepared (Colla *et al.*, 1983); and 2'-O-glycylacyclovir has proved efficacious in the treatment of herpetic keratitis when administered as a 1% eyedrop formulation to rabbits (Maudgal *et al.*, 1984). Attempts to find a prodrug of acyclovir which would be better absorbed after oral administration yielded *6-deoxyacyclovir* (Fig. 9). 6-Deoxyacyclovir is readily absorbed when administered p.o. and extensively converted to acyclovir by xanthine oxidase (Krenitsky *et al.*, 1984). Acyclovir concentrations achieved in the plasma following oral administration of 50 mg 6-deoxyacyclovir are comparable to those produced after

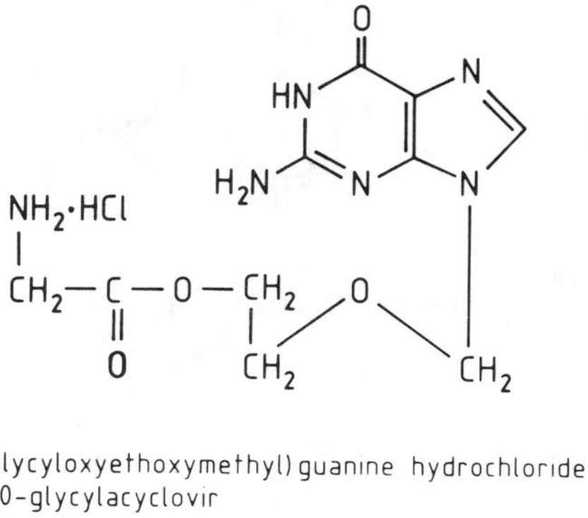
O
HN
N
H2N
N
N
NH2·HCl
CH2—C—O—CH2
O
O
CH2
CH2
9-(2-Glycyloxyethoxymethyl) guanine hydrochloride
2'-O-glycylacyclovir

FIG. 8. 2'-O-Glycylacyclovir.

400 mg acyclovir (Selby *et al.*, 1984; Whiteman *et al.*, 1984). The plasma acyclovir concentrations achieved by oral 6-deoxyacyclovir should bring less sensitive viruses such as VZV within the reach of an effective oral chemotherapy, pending, of course, the safety of this new prodrug.

In attempts to improve upon the activity spectrum of acyclovir, various acyclic guanosine analogues similar to acyclovir, but more closely resembling the natural nucleoside in structure, have been synthesized. Foremost among these acyclic nucleoside analogues are *DHPG* (also referred to as *2'NDG*, *BIOLF-62*, *BW B759U* and *ganciclovir*) (Fig. 10) and its racemic linear isomer, "iso"-NDG (iNDG) (Fig. 11). Of the two enantiomers (*R*)- and (*S*)-iNDG, (*S*)-iNDG is the most active (Ashton *et al.*, 1985; Karkas *et*

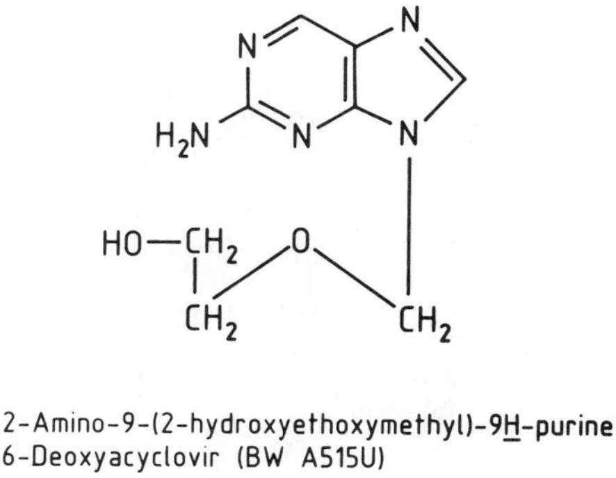
N
N
H2N
N
N
HO—CH2
O
CH2
CH2
2-Amino-9-(2-hydroxyethoxymethyl)-9H-purine
6-Deoxyacyclovir (BW A515U)

FIG. 9. 6-Deoxyacyclovir.

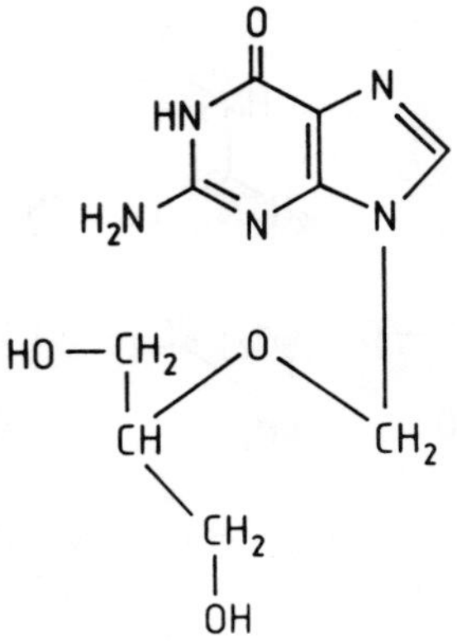

9-(1,3-Dihydroxy-2-propoxymethyl) guanine (DHPG)
9-[2-Hydroxy-1-(hydroxymethyl)ethoxymethyl] guanine (HHEMG)
2'-Nor-2'-deoxyguanosine (2'NDG)
BIOLF-62 ,   BW B759U ,   Ganciclovir

Fig. 10. Ganciclovir (DHPG, 2'NDG).

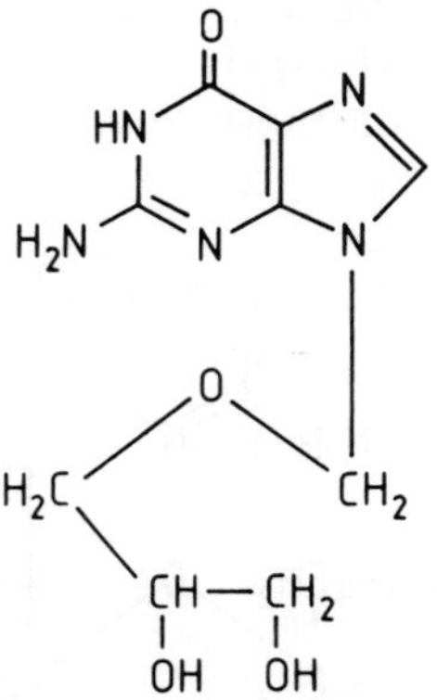

(S)-9-(2,3-Dihydroxy-1-propoxymethyl) guanine
(S)-iNDG

Fig. 11. (S)-iNDG.

al., 1986). Its *in vitro* activity against HSV is comparable to that of ACV and 2'NDG. From the first reports on DHPG (Smith *et al.*, 1982; Ashton *et al.*, 1982; Martin *et al.*, 1983; Smee *et al.*, 1983; Cheng *et al.*, 1983b; Field *et al.*, 1983), two advantages over acyclovir became immediately evident: (i) the higher activity against CMV *in vitro* and (ii) the greater efficacy against HSV *in vivo*. The superiority of DHPG over ACV has been demonstrated in various animal model infections, including herpetic keratitis in rabbits (Davies *et al.*, 1987; Shiota *et al.*, 1987). The most important asset of DHPG, however, is its activity against CMV (Mar *et al.*, 1983; Tocci *et al.*, 1984; Freitas *et al.*, 1985), at concentrations (0.1–1 μg/ml) which should be readily achievable upon intravenous administration of the drug at 7.5–15 mg/kg/day. Consequently, DHPG has been introduced in the clinic for the treatment of severe CMV infections in patients with AIDS or other immunodeficiencies (Shepp *et al.*, 1985; Felsenstein *et al.*, 1985; Bach *et al.*, 1985; Collaborative DHPG treatment study group, 1986; Laskin *et al.*, 1987). As a rule, AIDS patients with CMV retinitis or colitis stabilized or improved, whereas patients with CMV pneumonia responded poorly. However, most of the patients who improved while under DHPG, developed recrudescences after therapy had been discontinued, which means that long-term treatment may be required to control CMV infection in AIDS patients. DHPG has also been shown to exert a more potent and more prolonged inhibitory effect than ACV on the replication of EBV *in vitro* (Lin *et al.*, 1984); but this has not yet led to clinical trials with DHPG in patients with EBV infections.

The mechanism of action of DHPG is quite similar to that of ACV, the main difference being that DHPG is phosphorylated more rapidly to its mono-, di- and triphosphates than is ACV and that DHPG triphosphate persists for a much longer time upon drug removal than does ACVTP (Germershausen *et al.*, 1983; Smee *et al.*, 1985). Like ACVTP, DHPG triphosphate is more inhibitory to HSV DNA polymerase than cellular DNA polymerases (St. Clair *et al.*, 1984). Unlike ACVTP, however, which invariably acts as a chain terminator if incorporated into DNA, DHPG triphosphate would not solely act as a chain terminator but would also be able to enter internal linkages (Cheng *et al.*, 1983a; Frank *et al.*, 1984). That DHPG is a more potent inhibitor of CMV than ACV seems to be related to differences in the extent of phosphorylation of these drugs to their triphosphate by the CMV-infected cells (30-fold higher for DHPG) rather than to the affinity of the triphosphates for CMV DNA polymerase (5-fold lower for DHPG triphosphate) (Biron *et al.*, 1985). It is unclear whether the preferential phosphorylation of DHPG in CMV-infected cells results from the activity of an unidentified virus-encoded enzyme or from a virus-induced increase or alteration of a host enzyme; yet, the isolation of a DHPG-

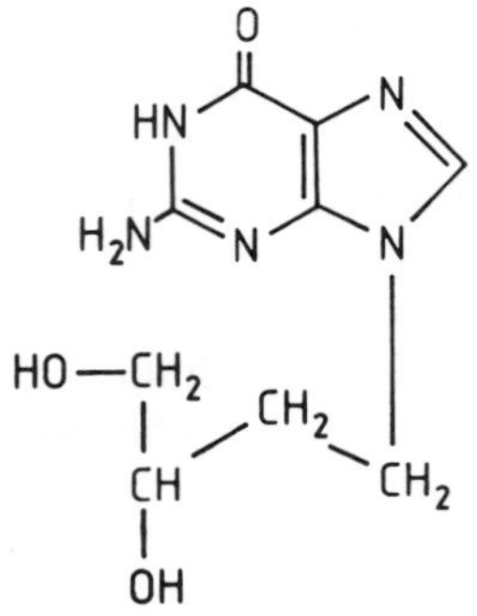

(R)-9-(3,4-Dihydroxybutyl) guanine
R-DHBG
Buciclovir (BCV).

FIG. 12. Buciclovir.

resistant CMV mutant which hampers the phosphorylation of DHPG points to the possibility that a CMV-encoded enzyme may be involved in the phosphorylation of DHPG (Biron *et al.*, 1986).

Buciclovir (*BCV*, Fig. 12) which corresponds to the (*R*)-enantiomer of DHBG, has an activity spectrum and mode of action that is quite similar to that of acyclovir. Its selective anti-HSV activity, like that of acyclovir, depends on a preferential phosphorylation by the virus-encoded dThd kinase (Larsson *et al.*, 1983; Ericson *et al.*, 1985). As for acyclovir, the antivirally active form of BCV has been shown to be its triphosphate, BCVTP. The latter is a potent inhibitor of HSV DNA polymerase, albeit less potent than ACVTP (Larsson *et al.*, 1986). In contrast with ACVTP, however, BCVTP would not be incorporated into DNA (Stenberg *et al.*, 1986). BCVTP, and even more so ACVTP, are also strongly inhibitory to CMV DNA polymerase (Wahren *et al.*, 1987), yet both ACV and BCV are poorly active against CMV DNA synthesis in intact cells. Evidently, the phosphorylation of ACV and BCV to their triphosphates is the rate-limiting process in the anti-CMV activity of these compounds. ACVTP and BCVTP are either not formed in sufficient amounts or decay too rapidly in CMV-infected cells to sustain an inhibitory effect at the DNA polymerase level. Conversely, with DHPG sufficiently high levels of DHPG triphosphate are generated and maintained in the CMV-infected cell to result in an appreciable inhibition of viral DNA synthesis.

2.3 VIDARABINE DERIVATIVES

For several years vidarabine was considered the drug of choice for the treatment of herpes simplex encephalitis (Whitley *et al.*, 1977, 1981) and herpes zoster in immunosuppressed patients (Whitley *et al.*, 1976, 1982). For both indications acyclovir is now the preferred drug, however (Sköldenberg *et al.*, 1984; Whitley *et al.*, 1986; Shepp *et al.*, 1986). The major drawbacks that impede the clinical usefulness of vidarabine are its poor solubility in water (not more than 0.05% at 25°C) and its rapid deamination to 9-β-D-arabinofuranosylhypoxanthine (Ara-Hx, which is markedly less active against HSV than the parent compound) by the ubiquitous adenosine deaminase. The first problem can be circumvented by using the more water-soluble 5'-monophosphate derivative (Ara-AMP). Yet, Ara-AMP has received scant attention as a therapeutic modality for the systemic treatment of HSV or VZV infections (Vilde *et al.*, 1983), and it is of no benefit in the topical treatment of recurrent herpes simplex labialis (Spruance *et al.*, 1979). The other liability in the effectiveness of Ara-A, namely its rapid deamination to Ara-Hx, can be overcome by using the carbocyclic derivative of Ara-A, *cyclaradine* (Fig. 13). Cyclaradine is resistant to adenosine deaminase (Vince and Daluge, 1977), less toxic than Ara-A

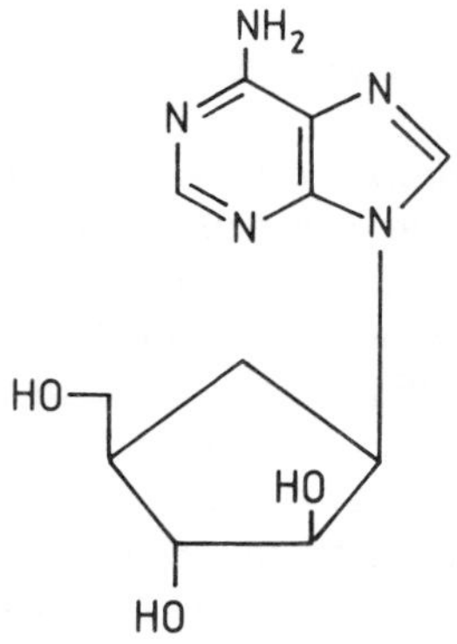

(±)-9-[cis-2, trans-3-Dihydroxy-4-(hydroxymethyl)cyclo-
pentyl] adenine
Carbocyclic arabinosyladenine (C-Ara-A)
Cyclaradine

FIG. 13. Cyclaradine.

(Shannon *et al.*, 1983), and as effective as acyclovir in the topical treatment of genital herpes in the guinea pig model (Vince *et al.*, 1983; Schwartz *et al.*, 1987). As cyclaradine, like Ara-A, does not depend for its antiviral activity on phosphorylation by the viral dThd kinase, it is active against dThd kinase-deficient (TK$^-$) acyclovir-resistant mutants of HSV (Schwartz *et al.*, 1987). This property is shared by other, more distantly related, analogues of vidarabine, such as xylotubercidin (De Clercq *et al.*, 1987a; De Clercq and Robins, 1986). Xylotubercidin holds particular promise for the topical and systemic treatment of HSV-2 infections. As to the mechanism of action of cyclaradine and xylotubercidin, very little is known. For Ara-A several targets of action have been identified, i.e. S-adenosylhomocysteine (SAH) hydrolase, ribonucleotide reductase and DNA polymerase. Ara-A is also incorporated internally into DNA, but this incorporation is not mandatory for its anti-HSV activity (Pelling *et al.*, 1981). More likely the inhibitory activity of Ara-A against HSV replication results from an inhibitory effect at the viral DNA polymerase level, as is also the case for ACV, DHPG and their congeners, and it is tempting to speculate that cyclaradine and xylotubercidin also act at the viral DNA polymerase level. This implies that the compounds are first phosphorylated to their 5′-triphosphates. Which enzymes are responsible for this phosphorylation and at which level cyclaradine and xylotubercidin acquire their selectivity as antiviral agents are intriguing questions requiring further investigation.

2.4 SUBSTITUTED 2′-DEOXYURIDINES

Among the various antiviral compounds, *ethyldeoxyuridine* (*EDU*) (Fig. 14) takes a place apart. The therapeutic potential of this compound has been known for more than two decades (see De Clercq and Shugar, 1975), and in contrast with its predecessors, idoxuridine and trifluridine, which have been in clinical use for almost 25 years despite their well-established mutagenicity (Cassiman *et al.*, 1983), EDU is non-mutagenic. Recent investigations with animal models have revealed that EDU is as effective as, if not more so than, acyclovir in the topical treatment of mucocutaneous HSV-1 and HSV-2 infections in guinea pigs (Spruance *et al.*, 1985; Schinazi *et al.*, 1985). The compound has been marketed (as Aedurid) for the topical treatment of herpetic keratitis, and controlled double-blind clinical trials have recently been initiated to assess its value in the topical treatment of genital herpes. From a mechanistic viewpoint it is now clear that HSV-infected cells phosphorylate EDU to a much greater extent than uninfected cells and that, within the HSV-1-infected cell, EDU is incorporated to a much greater extent into viral DNA than cellular DNA (De Clercq and Bernaerts, 1987).

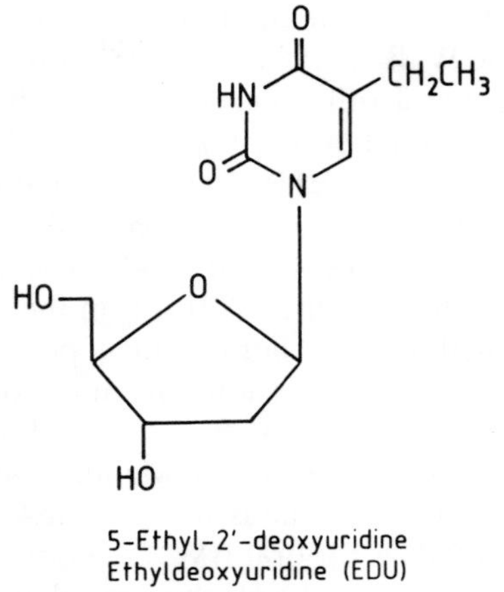

5-Ethyl-2'-deoxyuridine
Ethyldeoxyuridine (EDU)

FIG. 14. Ethyldeoxyuridine.

In fact, the incorporation of EDU into viral DNA is closely correlated with the inhibition of viral DNA synthesis and inhibition of virus progeny formation. One might infer from these data that the antiviral activity of EDU is causally linked to its incorporation into viral DNA.

Following EDU, numerous new 5-substituted 2'-deoxyuridines were synthesized (Goodchild *et al.*, 1983; De Clercq, 1985b), from which *bromovinyldeoxyuridine (BVDU)* (Fig. 15) and its iodovinyl analogue

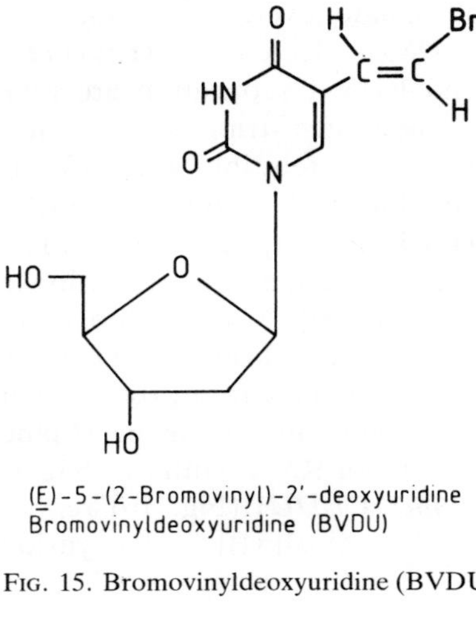

(E)-5-(2-Bromovinyl)-2'-deoxyuridine
Bromovinyldeoxyuridine (BVDU)

FIG. 15. Bromovinyldeoxyuridine (BVDU).

IVDU emerged as the most potent and most selective inhibitors of HSV-1 and VZV (De Clercq and Walker, 1984). The antiviral activity spectrum also extends to EBV and several other herpesviruses which are primarily of veterinary interest, i.e. suid herpesvirus type 1 (SHV-1, pseudorabies virus), bovid herpesvirus type 1 (BHV-1, infectious bovine rhinotracheitis virus), simian varicella virus (SVV), herpesvirus platyrrhinae (HVP), but not equid herpesvirus type 1 (EHV-1) or phocid herpesvirus type 1 (PHV-1) (De Clercq, 1986b; Osterhaus et al., 1987). From the clinical side, BVDU has been mainly pursued for its therapeutical potential in the peroral treatment of HSV-1 and VZV infections in immunosuppressed patients (Wildiers and De Clercq, 1984; Benoit et al., 1985; Tricot et al., 1986) and topical treatment of herpetic eye infections (Maudgal and De Clercq, 1987). The recommended treatment regimens are 7.5 mg/kg/day (adults) to 15 mg/kg/day (children) for 5 days for oral BVDU and 0.1% BVDU eyedrops 5–9 times per day for (up to) 7 weeks for the topical eye treatment. BVDU offers interesting perspectives for the treatment of VZV infections, as it can be administered orally at low doses and is about 1000-fold more active against VZV than is ACV. The selectivity indexes of BVDU against VZV and HSV-1 attain values of 10 000 to 100 000 in vitro. BVDU owes this remarkable selectivity to a highly preferential phosphorylation by the virus-encoded dThd kinase which converts BVDU successively to its 5'-monophosphate (BVDUMP) and 5'-diphosphate (BVDUDP) (Fig. 7), as is assumed to be the case for the dThd kinases specified by HSV-1 and VZV. The HSV-2-encoded dThd kinase converts BVDU to BVDUMP but not further onto BVDUDP (Descamps and De Clercq, 1981; Fyfe, 1982; Ayisi et al., 1984). Thus, in HSV-2-infected cells the phosphorylation of BVDU stops at the 5'-monophosphate level, and so does the phosphorylation of BVDU and IVDU in EHV-1-infected cells (Kit et al., 1987a,b). This may explain why HSV-2 and EHV-1 replication are relatively insensitive to BVDU. Once it has reached the 5'-triphosphate stage, BVDU may either inhibit the DNA polymerase [thereby inhibiting HSV-1 DNA polymerase to a greater extent than the cellular DNA polymerases (Allaudeen et al., 1981)] or serve as substrate of the DNA polymerase and be incorporated into DNA [via an internucleotide linkage and preferentially in viral DNA (Allaudeen et al., 1982a; Mancini et al., 1983)]. As noted above for EDU, the incorporation of BVDU into viral DNA is closely correlated with the inhibition of virus replication; this inhibition may result from either increased susceptibility of the DNA to single-strand breakage (Mancini et al., 1983) or diminished template activity for RNA synthesis (Sági et al., 1982), or both.

  Chloroethyldeoxyuridine (CEDU) (Fig. 16) represents a new class of 5-substituted [namely 5-(2)-haloalkyl)] 2'-deoxyuridines which could be

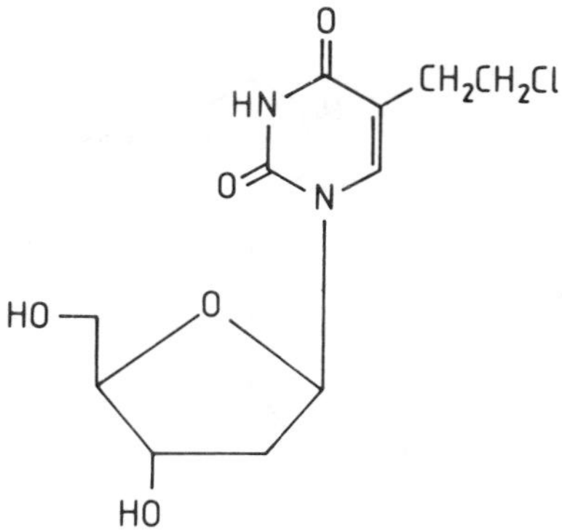

5-(2-Chloroethyl)-2'-deoxyuridine
Chloroethyldeoxyuridine (CEDU)

FIG. 16. Chloroethyldeoxyuridine.

viewed as BVDU derivatives in which the vinyl (ethenyl) side chain has been saturated to ethyl. Like BVDU, the 5-(2-haloalkyl)-2'-deoxyuridines are potent and selective inhibitors of HSV-1 (Griengl *et al.*, 1985). While 10-fold less active than BVDU *in vitro*, CEDU is as active as BVDU when applied topically, i.e. as 0.1% eyedrops in the treatment of herpes simplex keratitis (Maudgal and De Clercq, 1985), and active at a 5- to 15-fold lower dose than either BVDU or acyclovir when administered perorally in the treatment of systemic HSV-1 infection in mice (De Clercq and Rosenwirth, 1985; Rosenwirth *et al.*, 1985). However, the clinical perspectives of CEDU seem to be compounded by the mutagenic potential of the compound. This differentiates CEDU from BVDU, which has proved negative in several mutagenicity tests (Marquardt *et al.*, 1985).

A general characteristic of most, if not all, 5-substituted 2'-deoxyuridines is their propensity to serve as substrate for pyrimidine nucleoside phosphorylases, i.e. dThd phosphorylase (Desgranges *et al.*, 1983). As a consequence, 5-substituted 2'-deoxyuridines such as IDU, EDU, BVDU and CEDU are rapidly cleared from the bloodstream following systemic administration to rats (Desgranges *et al.*, 1984, 1986). EDU, BVDU and CEDU are converted to their bases following cleavage of the N-glycosidic linkage by the pyrimidine nucleoside phosphorylases. However, the active compounds can be generated again from their bases upon administration of an appropriate deoxyribosyl donor such as dThd or dUrd (Desgranges *et al.*, 1984, 1986). Resistance to phosphorolytic degradation can also be built in by modification of the deoxyribosyl moiety to a cyclopentyl, thus converting the

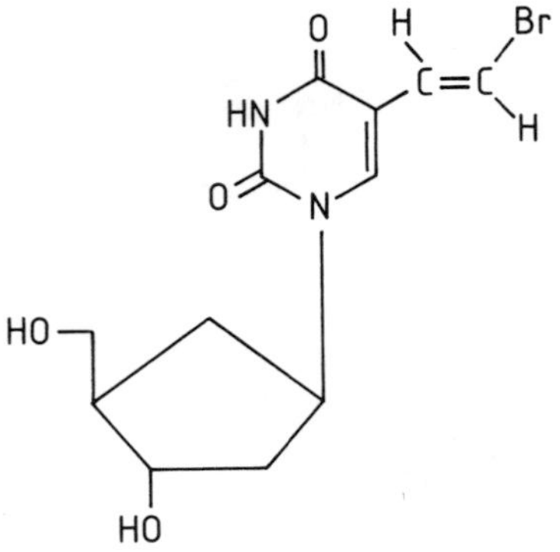

E. DE CLERCQ

(±)-1-[trans-3-Hydroxy-4-(hydroxymethyl)cyclopentyl]-
(E)-5-(2-bromovinyl)-1H-uracil
Carbocyclic bromovinyldeoxyuridine (C-BVDU)

FIG. 17. Carbocyclic BVDU (C-BVDU).

nucleosides into their carbocyclic analogues. Hence, the carbocyclic analogues of IDU (Shealy *et al.*, 1983), EDU (Shealy *et al.*, 1986), BVDU and IVDU (Herdewijn *et al.*, 1985; Cookson *et al.*, 1985) were synthesized and found to be efficient and selective inhibitors of HSV-1 replication. Sure enough, carbocyclic BVDU (*C-BVDU*) (Fig. 17) is not a substrate for dThd phosphorylase (De Clercq *et al.*, 1985c). Yet, C-BVDU and C-IVDU are as good, if not better, substrates for the HSV-1-encoded dThd kinase than BVDU and IVDU (De Clercq *et al.*, 1985a). C-BVDU and C-IVDU are effectively phosphorylated by HSV-1-infected, but not uninfected, cells. They can be incorporated into both viral and cellular DNA of HSV-1-infected cells (De Clercq *et al.*, 1985b). The extent of incorporation is low, however, since C-BVDUTP is not incorporated for more than 3.6% into a synthetic DNA [poly(dA.dT)] (Sági *et al.*, 1987). Sági *et al.* (1987) also found C-BVDUTP to be a potent inhibitor of DNA polymerase, leaving it to be ascertained whether the marked antiviral activity of C-BVDU is due to the inhibition of viral DNA polymerase rather than its incorporation into viral DNA.

In addition to C-BVDU, various other BVDU analogues, i.e. *bromovinyl*ara*uracil* (*BVaraU*) (Fig. 18) and the 3'-amino derivative of BVDU (De Clercq *et al.*, 1983), have been synthesized which are completely resistant to phosphorolytic cleavage by dThd phosphorylase (De Clercq *et al.*, 1985c). Otherwise, the potency, selectivity and activity spectra of these BVDU derivatives are quite similar to those of BVDU itself. Like BVDU,

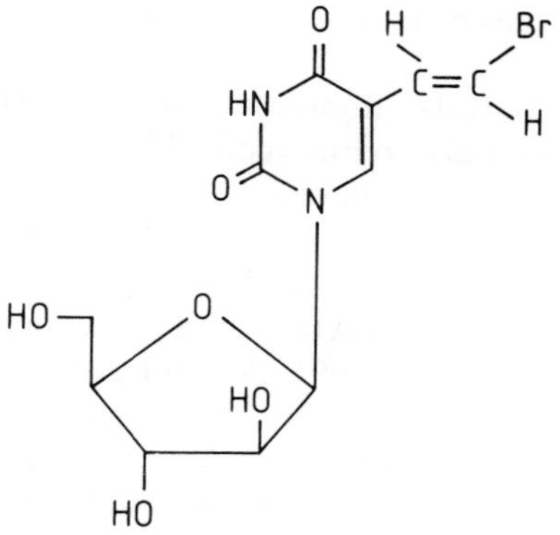

(E)-5-(2-Bromovinyl)-1-β-D-arabinofuranosyluracil
Bromovinyluracil arabinoside
Bromovinyl ara uracil (BV araU, BVAU)

FIG. 18. Bromovinyl*ara*uracil (BVaraU).

BVaraU depends for its activation on the virus-induced dThd kinase which converts BVaraU successively to its 5′-mono- and 5′-diphosphate (Ayisi *et al.*, 1987). Unlike BVDUTP, however, BVaraUTP does not appear to be internally incorporated into DNA; instead, it may act as a chain terminator in the DNA polymerization reaction (Ruth and Cheng, 1981; Descamps *et al.*, 1982). Whereas BVDU is exquisitely inhibitory to the proliferation of murine mammary carcinoma (FM3A) cells which have been transformed with the HSV-1 dThd kinase gene, BVaraU is not at all inhibitory to these cells (Balzarini *et al.*, 1985). Provided that BVDU and BVaraU are equally well phosphorylated by these cells, their differences in cytostatic activity may be related to their differential interaction with DNA. If, as presumed, BVaraUTP is incorporated at the DNA 3′-terminal, this incorporation may be reversible since 3′→5′ exonucleases could easily remove such 3′-terminal nucleotides. BVaraU is equally, if not more, potent against VZV than BVDU (Shigeta *et al.*, 1983; Machida, 1986). For BVaraU, Machida (1986) noted a minimum antiviral concentration of 0.08 ng/ml against VZV, a value which has never been reached with any compound against any virus. Thus, based on their *in vitro* potency against VZV, BVaraU and BVDU offer great potential for the therapy of VZV infections, and this contention is further corroborated by the efficacy of BVDU (Soike *et al.*, 1981) and BVaraU (Soike *et al.*, 1984) in the treatment of simian varicella virus infection in monkeys, a model that in many aspects is reminiscent of generalized varicella or zoster in humans.

2.5 2'-FLUOROARABINOSYLPYRIMIDINE NUCLEOSIDES

Following the original report that fluoroiodo*ara*cytosine (*FIAC*) (Fig. 19) is a potent and selective anti-herpesvirus agent (Watanabe *et al.*, 1979; Lopez *et al.*, 1980), a large variety of 2'-fluorinated arabinofuranosylpyrimidines have been synthesized, i.e. fluoroiodo*ara*uracil (*FIAU*) (Fig. 19), fluromethyl*ara*uracil (*FMAU*), fluoroethyl*ara*uracil (*FEAU*) (Fig. 20), fluorobromovinyl*ara*uracil (FBVAU) and fluorochloroethyl*ara*uracil (FCEAU) (Watanabe *et al.*, 1983, 1984; Perlman *et al.*, 1985; Su *et al.*, 1986; Mansuri *et al.*, 1987; Griengl *et al.*, 1987; Rosenwirth *et al.*, 1987). On the whole, these compounds show high potency against HSV-1, HSV-2, VZV and CMV, and their antiviral activity has been demonstrated both *in vitro* and *in vivo*. With a 50% antiviral effective dose of approximately 0.1 μg/ml (Mar *et al.*, 1984; Colacino and Lopez, 1985), FIAC and its congeners rank among the most potent inhibitors of EBV. They are also inhibitory to the replication of EBV; in contrast to the reversibility of EBV inhibition by acyclovir, FIAC and FMAU, as well as BVDU and DHPG (Lin *et al.*, 1984), have a prolonged suppressive effect on EBV replication which persists for several weeks after removal of the drugs from the cell culture medium (Lin *et al.*, 1983). When compared for their efficacy and selectivity as inhibitors of EBV, the order of (decreasing) potency was FIAC = FIAU > FMAU > DHPG > BVDU > ACV, whereas the order of (decreasing) selectivity was

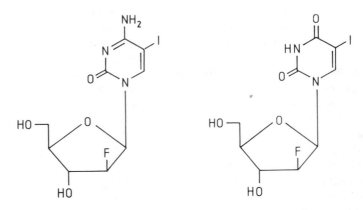

1-β-D-(2-Deoxy-2-fluoro-
arabinofuranosyl)-5-iodocytosine
Fluoroiodo ara cytosine (FIAC)

1-β-D-(2-Deoxy-2-fluoro-
arabinofuranosyl)-5-iodouracil
Fluoroiodo ara uracil (FIAU)

FIG. 19. Fluoroiodo*ara*cytosine (FIAC) and fluoroiodo*ara*uracil (FIAU).

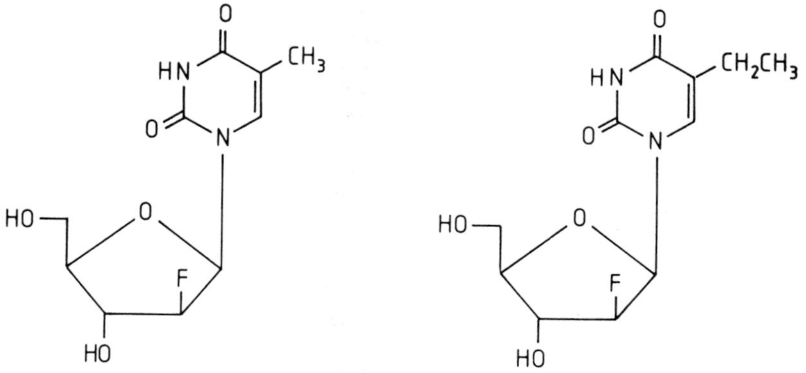

1-β-D-(2-Deoxy-2-fluoro-
arabinofuranosyl)-5-methyluracil
Fluoromethyl ara uracil (FMAU)

1-β-D-(2-Deoxy-2-fluoro-
arabinofuranosyl)-5-ethyluracil
Fluoroethyl ara uracil (FEAU)

FIG. 20. Fluoromethyl*ara*uracil (FMAU) and fluoroethyl*ara*uracil (FEAU).

BVDU > DHPG > FIAC > ACV > FIAU > FMAU. The 2'-fluorinated arabinosylpyrimidines, and in particular FMAU, are rather toxic compounds, and this has hampered their clinical development (McLaren *et al.*, 1985a), despite the excellent antiviral activity in animal models (Schinazi *et al.*, 1983) and the encouraging results from initial trials. The promising results obtained with FIAC in the treatment of VZV infections in immunocompromised patients (Young *et al.*, 1983) are in keeping with the efficacy of FIAU (the deaminated product of FIAC) against simian varicella virus infection in monkeys (Soike *et al.*, 1986). According to a recent report (Mansuri *et al.*, 1987), FEAU may be the most selective anti-HSV agent among the FIAC congeners. It would owe its selectivity, as do all other anti-HSV agents discussed above, to a specific phosphorylation by the virus-encoded dThd kinase. Likewise, a preferential phosphorylation by the virus-specified dThd kinase would explain the selectivity observed with FIAC and FMAU, although FIAC behaves metabolically as its dUrd derivative FIAU in HSV-1-infected cells (Chou *et al.*, 1984), which means that it is readily deaminated in these cells. As was noted for ACV, DHPG, BVDU and all the others, the active forms of FIAC, FIAU, FMAU and FEAU would correspond to their 5'-triphosphates. In this form they would primarily act as inhibitors of the DNA polymerase reaction, and thereby inhibit viral DNA polymerase to a larger extent than the host DNA polymerases (Ruth and Cheng, 1981; Allaudeen *et al.*, 1982b). In addition, the 5'-triphosphates of FIAC and its congeners may act as alternate substrates, at least for the viral DNA polymerase, and thus be incorporated into DNA. To what extent this incorporation may occur and to what degree it may contribute to the antiviral activity of the compounds has not been assessed.

3 DNA Virus Infections in General

3.1 PHOSPHONOFORMATE

Acyclovir-resistant HSV mutants have occasionally been isolated from immunosuppressed patients treated with acyclovir for an intercurrent HSV-1 infection (Crumpacker et al., 1982; Burns et al., 1982; Sibrack et al., 1982; Wade et al., 1983; MacLaren et al., 1985b; Schinazi et al., 1986). Most of these ACV-resistant HSV isolates proved to be dThd kinase-deficient (TK⁻). Another possible locus for virus-drug resistance is the viral DNA polymerase gene (Coen et al., 1984; Larder and Darby, 1984), but drug-resistant mutants based on a mutation in the DNA polymerase locus have not yet been isolated from patients. TK⁻ HSV mutants are generally assumed to be less pathogenic than their wild-type TK⁺ counterparts and, therefore, the belief prevails that if such drug-resistant HSV mutants were to emerge in clinical settings, they may be associated with diminished virulence (Sibrack et al., 1982), and thus pose little, if any, clinical problem. According to our own experience, this is not always so. We recently described the case of a chronic lymphocytic leukaemia (CLL) patient who had been treated with ACV for an orofacial HSV-1 infection. The virus developed resistance to the drug following a single treatment course. Despite successive therapeutic attempts with BVDU, DHPG and Ara-A, the clinical condition of the patient deteriorated. Virus was isolated from his oral lesions on several occasions and proved to be TK⁻. The HSV lesions finally healed following systemic (i.v.) treatment with phosphonoformate (Vinckier et al., 1987; De Clercq, 1987g). Thus, TK⁻ HSV mutants may present a clinical problem sometimes, and it would obviously seem important to have antiviral drugs at hand which are effective against such TK⁻ HSV strains. *Phosphonoformate (foscarnet, PFA)* (Fig. 21) is such a drug (Öberg, 1983). Foscarnet is effective against a broad variety of DNA viruses including herpesviruses (HSV-1, HSV-2, VZV, CMV, EBV), but also hepadnaviruses [hepatitis B virus (HBV)] and even retroviruses. It is directly targeted at the DNA polymerase, thus not requiring any previous activation. As an antiviral agent, PFA is not very potent (minimum antiviral concentration ∼20 μg/ml), but upon topical application to the skin it is more effective against cutaneous HSV infection in guinea pigs than could be

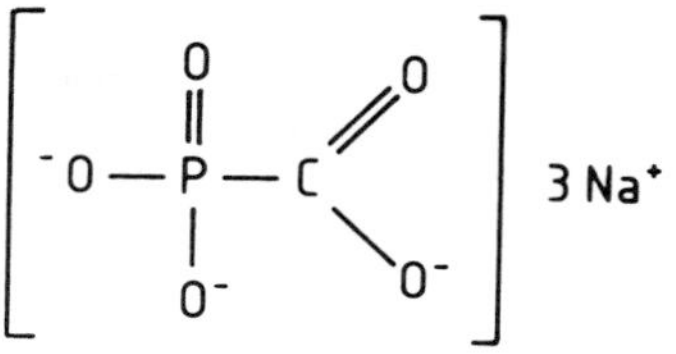

Phosphonoformate (PFA) trisodium salt
Foscarnet
Foscavir

FIG. 21. Foscarnet.

expected from its *in vitro* activity (Alenius *et al.*, 1982; Spruance *et al.*, 1986). Of direct clinical relevance are the results obtained with 0.3% foscarnet cream in the topical treatment of recurrent genital herpes (Wallin *et al.*, 1985): it caused a slight reduction in time to healing. As the clinical benefit obtained with foscarnet in several other studies was considered too minimal, it is no longer pursued in the topical treatment of recurrent herpes (Öberg *et al.*, 1988). Instead, foscarnet has gained more attention as an alternative to DHPG for the treatment of CMV infections in immunosuppressed patients (Klintmalm *et al.*, 1985). To this end the drug has to be given as a continuous i.v. infusion at a dose of up to 15 g/day for 2 weeks. Upon treatment of AIDS patients with i.v. foscarnet for CMV infections, stabilization or improvement of the disease has been noted, but relapses are common (Öberg *et al.*, 1988). As already mentioned above, foscarnet encompasses hepadnaviruses in its activity spectrum. Foscarnet has proved efficacious in reducing the replication of duck hepatitis B virus in chronically infected ducks (Sherker *et al.*, 1986). This opens interesting perspectives for the clinical use of the drug in the treatment of HBV infections.

3.2 2′-NOR-CGMP

From DHPG (2′NDG), a cyclic phosphate termed *2′-nor-cGMP* (Fig. 22) has been derived (Tolman *et al.*, 1985; Prisbe *et al.*, 1986). Prisbe *et al.* (1986) also synthesized the phosphate esters of DHPG as well as the 5′-homophosphonate form of DHPG. The phosphate esters showed comparable activity to DHPG against HSV-1, HSV-2 and CMV, and thus probably acted as prodrugs of DHPG. The phosphonate, however, was only active against CMV. The diphosphoryl derivative of this compound also proved inhibitory to CMV DNA polymerase (Duke *et al.*, 1986). While conversion of DHPG

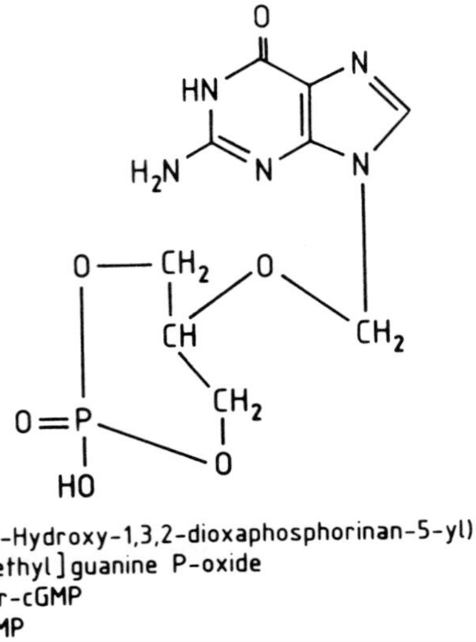

9-[(2-Hydroxy-1,3,2-dioxaphosphorinan-5-yl)
oxymethyl]guanine P-oxide
2'-Nor-cGMP
cNDGMP

FIG. 22. 2'-Nor-cGMP.

to its phosphonate derivative narrowed the activity spectrum essentially to CMV, the cyclic phosphate of DHPG (2'-nor-cGMP) acquired a significantly broadened activity spectrum extending to TK⁻ HSV mutants, poxviruses (i.e. vaccinia), papillomaviruses (i.e. SV₄₀ and bovine papilloma virus type 1) and adenoviruses (Tolman et al., 1985). The activity of 2'-nor-cGMP against TK⁻ HSV-1 has been confirmed by animal protection studies (Field et al., 1986). Obviously, this protective activity extends to TK⁺ HSV-1 and HSV-2 infections as well. The mechanism of action of 2'-nor-cGMP has been partially resolved (Germershausen et al., 1986): 2'-nor-cGMP is taken up by the cells essentially intact, after which it can be opened to the acyclic monophosphate and phosphorylated further to the triphosphate, bypassing the viral dThd kinase step necessary for the activation of 2'NDG. The possibility that 2'NDG was formed from 2'nor-cGMP on its way to the triphosphate was considered and disproved. Thus, 2'-nor-cGMP does not require viral dThd kinase for the formation of its active form (2'NDG triphosphate), and this explains its activity against a broad spectrum of DNA viruses, some of which do not induce a specific TK. Whether 2'NDG triphosphate is the sole active form of 2'-nor-cGMP is not certain, however. Germershausen et al. (1986) suggest that 2'-nor-cGMP may have an additional mode of action unrelated to the presence of 2'NDG triphosphate.

3.3 PHOSPHONYLMETHOXYPROPYLPURINE AND -PYRIMIDINE DERIVATIVES

Recently, a new class of compounds, with as prototypes (S)-HPMPA (Fig. 23) and PMEA (Fig. 24), has been found, which exhibits a potent and selective activity against a broad spectrum of DNA viruses, including herpesviruses (HSV-1, HSV-2, TK⁻ HSV-1, VZV, CMV, EBV, SHV-1, BHV-1, EHV-1, PHV-1, SVV, HVP), iridoviruses (African swine fever virus), poxviruses (vaccinia virus) and adenoviruses, as well as retroviruses (De Clercq et al., 1986b; Baba et al., 1987a,b; Osterhaus et al., 1987; Lin et al., 1987; Gil-Fernández and De Clercq, 1987). The potency and selectivity of (S)-HPMPA as an antiviral agent is illustrated by its activity against VZV: it inhibits the replication of this virus within the concentration range of 0.63–5.7 ng/ml (mean: 1.8 ng/ml), that is at a concentration which is 29 000-fold lower than that required for inhibition of host cell DNA synthesis (Baba et al., 1987a). In vivo, (S)-HPMPA has proved to be effective in a number of animal models, including TK⁻ HSV-1 keratitis in rabbits, where (S)-HPMPA exerted a prompt healing effect under conditions where BVDU and CEDU had no effect whatsoever (Maudgal et al., 1987). In addition to (S)-HPMPA and PMEA, various other phosphonylmethoxy-propyl derivatives have been shown to inhibit the replication of HSV-1, HSV-2, TK⁻ HSV-1, VZV, CMV, vaccinia virus and adenoviruses: i.e. the cyclic phosphonate of (S)-HPMPA which is about as active as (S)-HPMPA

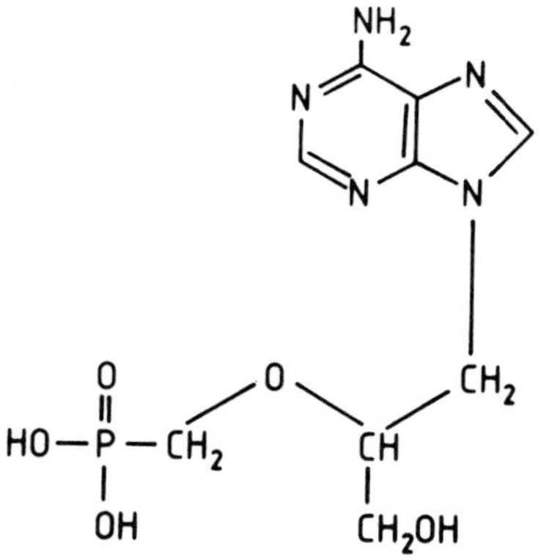

(S)-9-(3-Hydroxy-2-phosphonylmethoxypropyl) adenine
(S)-HPMPA

FIG. 23. (S)-HPMPA.

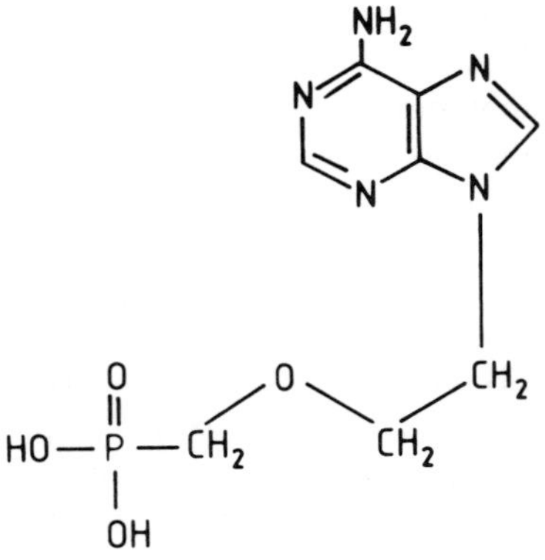

9-(2-Phosphonylmethoxyethyl) adenine
PMEA

Fig. 24. PMEA.

in all virus systems studied and probably acts as a prodrug of (S)-HPMPA; the 2,6-diaminopurine counterparts of (S)-HPMPA and PMEA, which are about as active as (S)-HPMPA and PMEA against HSV-1, HSV-2 and TK⁻ HSV-1; and (S)-HPMPC (Fig. 25), which, with a 50% effective dose of 0.08 μg/ml and a selectivity index of 625, is the most potent and most selective *in vitro* inhibitor of CMV replication described to date (De Clercq *et al.*,

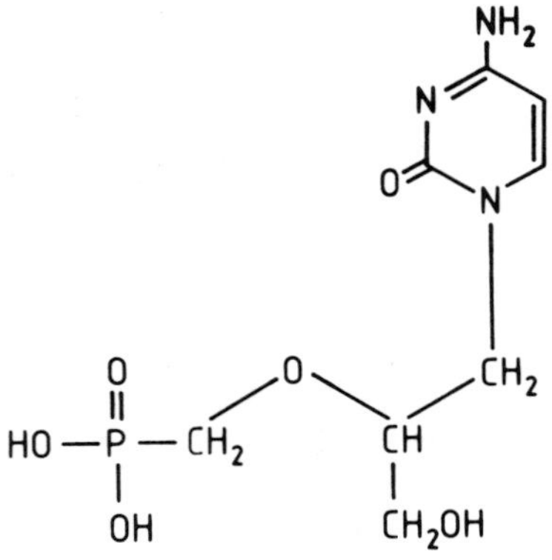

(S)-1-(3-Hydroxy-2-phosphonylmethoxypropyl) cytosine
(S)-HPMPC

Fig. 25. (S)-HPMPC.

1987b). As an inhibitor of CMV, (S)-HPMPC surpasses DHPG in both potency and selectivity. Only (S)-HPMPA has so far been the subject of studies aimed at elucidating its mechanism of action (Votruba *et al.*, 1987). The compound is taken up by the cells intact and is subsequently converted to its monophosphoryl and diphosphoryl derivatives. This phosphorylation occurs equally well in virus-infected and uninfected cells and thus must be accomplished by cellular enzymes, independently from any virus-induced kinase. (S)-HPMPA inhibits viral DNA synthesis at a concentration which is by several orders of magnitude lower than the concentration required for inhibition of cellular DNA synthesis, as has been demonstrated with both HSV-infected cells (Votruba *et al.*, 1987) and EBV-infected cells (Lin *et al.*, 1987). Whether the diphosphoryl derivative of (S)-HPMPA is responsible for the selective inhibition of viral DNA synthesis and how this selective inhibition is realized are intriguing questions that remain to be resolved.

4 RNA Virus Infections in General

4.1 ACYCLIC AND CARBOCYCLIC ADENOSINE ANALOGUES

(S)-HPMPA can be regarded as a phosphonate derivative of the aliphatic nucleoside analogue (S)-*DHPA* (Fig. 26). Substitution of the 2-hydroxyl group of (S)-DHPA by a phosphonylmethoxy group brings about a marked change in the activity spectrum of (S)-DHPA. Whereas (S)-HPMPA is a

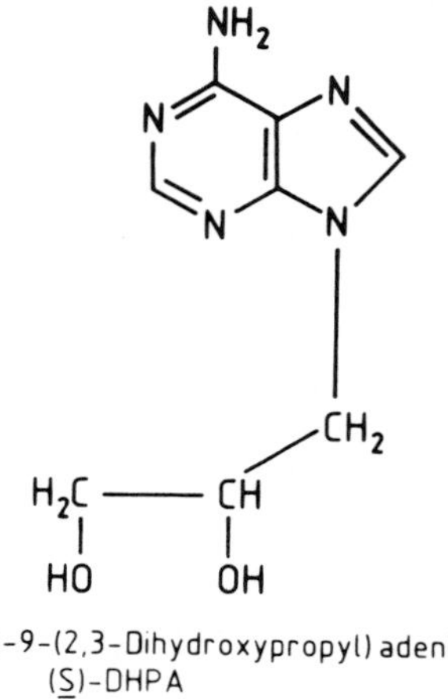

(S)-9-(2,3-Dihydroxypropyl) adenine
(S)-DHPA

FIG. 26. (S)-DHPA.

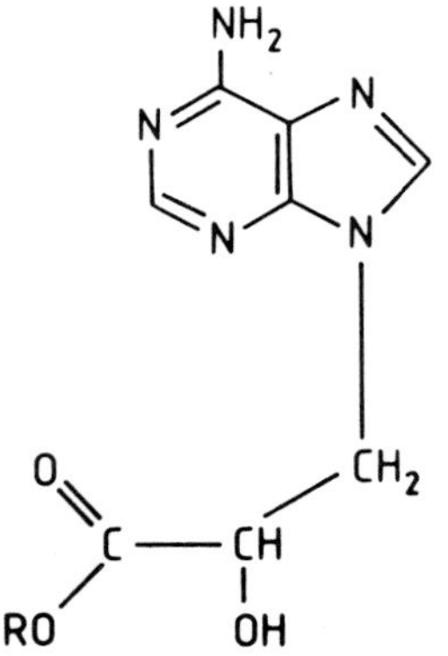

$$NH_2$$

(structure of adenine ring shown)

O
‖
C — CH
/ |
RO   OH
                CH₂

(RS)-3-Adenin-9-yl-2-hydroxypropanoic acid
[(RS)-AHPA] alkyl esters

FIG. 27. (RS)-AHPA.

typically broad-spectrum anti-DNA virus agent, is (S)-DHPA primarily active against the single-stranded (−)RNA viruses [rhabdo (rabies virus, vesicular stomatitis virus, infectious haematopoietic necrosis virus of fish), paramyxo (parainfluenza virus, measles virus)], double-stranded (±)RNA viruses [reo (reovirus, rotavirus, infectious pancreatic necrosis virus of fish)] and, among the DNA viruses, only poxviruses (vaccinia) and iridoviruses (African swine fever virus) (De Clercq *et al.*, 1978, 1984; Kitaoka *et al.*, 1986; De Clercq, 1987f). (S)-DHPA is not active against (+)RNA viruses such as rhino- and enteroviruses (polio, Coxsackie, Echo), and togaviruses (Sindbis, Semliki forest, tick-borne encephalitis). Yet, the plant (+)RNA viruses (i.e. potex-, poty- and tymovirus) appear to be sensitive to the compound (De Fazio *et al.*, 1987). Following (S)-DHPA, other adenosine analogues, i.e. (RS)-AHPA (Fig. 27) (De Clercq and Holý, 1985), C-c³Ado (Fig. 28) (Montgomery *et al.*, 1982; De Clercq and Montgomery, 1983) and *neplanocin A* (Fig. 29) (Borchardt *et al.*, 1984; De Clercq, 1985c) have been described which exhibit an antiviral activity spectrum that is remarkably similar to that of (S)-DHPA. What could all these compounds have in common that makes them active against the same viruses? The most obvious common trait is their inhibitory effect on S-adenosylhomocysteine (SAH) hydrolase. SAH hydrolase is a key enzyme in transmethylation reactions depending on S-adenosylmethionine (SAM) as the methyl donor. SAM-dependent methyltransferases have long since been considered as potential

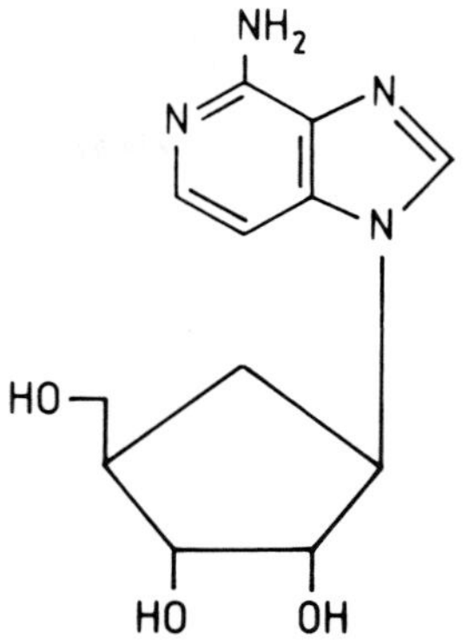

(±)-9-[trans-2, trans-3-Dihydroxy-4-(hydroxymethyl) cyclo-
pentyl]-3-deazaadenine
    Carbocyclic 3-deazaadenosine (C-c³ Ado)

FIG. 28. C-c³Ado.

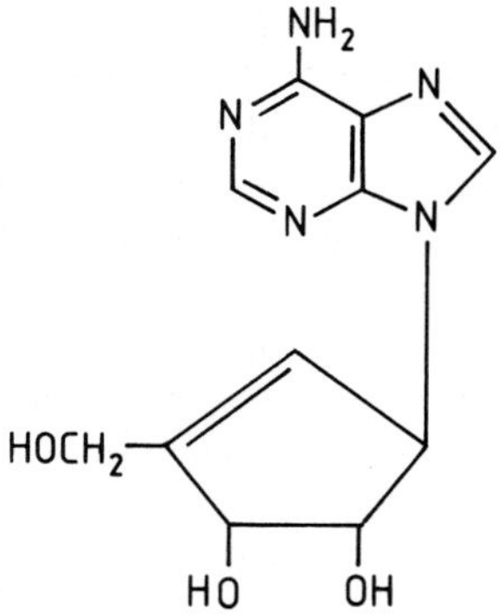

(-)-9- [trans-2, trans-3-Dihydroxy-4-(hydroxymethyl) cyclo-
pent-4-enyl] adenine
    Neplanocin A

FIG. 29. Neplanocin A.

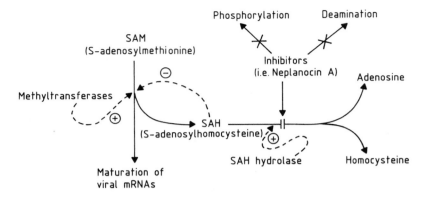

Fig. 30. Mechanism of action of neplanocin A and other SAH hydrolase inhibitors.

targets for chemotherapeutic agents (Borchardt, 1980). Such methyl-transferases are required for the maturation of viral mRNAs, i.e. for 5'-capping, and, as SAH is not only the product but also an inhibitor of the SAM-dependent transmethylation reactions, inhibitors of SAH hydrolase may be expected to interfere with viral mRNA methylation processes through the accumulation of SAH (Fig. 30). In fact, a close correlation ($r = 0.986$) has been found between the antiviral potency of (S)-DHPA, (RS)-AHPA, C-c^{3}Ado and neplanocin A (against vesicular stomatitis virus) and their inhibitory effects (K_i/K_m) on beef liver SAH hydrolase (activity measured in the direction of SAH synthesis) (De Clercq and Cools, 1985). An even closer correlation ($r = 0.993$) was found when the antiviral potency of (S)-DHPA, (RS)-AHPA, C-c^{3}Ado and neplanocin A (against vaccinia virus) was plotted as a function of their inhibitory effect (K_i) on the SAH hydrolase extracted from the same cells (murine L929 cells) as used for the antiviral assays (De Clercq, 1988b; M. Cools and E. De Clercq: unpublished data). These findings point to SAH hydrolase as the target for the antiviral action of (S)-DHPA, (RS)-AHPA, C-c^{3}Ado and neplanocin A (De Clercq, 1988b), and it is likely that the antiviral action of other adenosine analogues, i.e. adenosine dialdehyde, also stems from an inhibitory effect on SAH hydrolase (Keller and Borchardt, 1987).

Of the adenosine analogues which act as inhibitors of SAH hydrolase, *3-deazaneplanocin A* (Fig. 31) would, according to the K_i value that has been reported for this compound (5×10^{-11} M), be the most potent (Glazer *et al.*, 1986a). In contrast with neplanocin A, 3-deazaneplanocin A is only slightly cytotoxic (Glazer *et al.*, 1986b). Its antiviral activity is being examined. For neplanocin A and other adenosine analogues to act preferentially at the SAH hydrolase level they should not be phosphorylated (i.e. by adenosine kinase) or deaminated (i.e. by adenosine deaminase). Phosphorylation

(-)-9- [trans-2, trans-3-Dihydroxy-4-(hydroxymethyl) cyclo-
pent-4-enyl] -3-deazaadenine
3-Deazaneplanocin A

FIG. 31. 3-Deazaneplanocin A.

would make the compounds cytotoxic (i.e. due to inhibition of viral RNA synthesis by the 5'-triphosphates) (Cools *et al.*, 1987), and deamination would make them biologically inert. Both the phosphorylation route and deamination route require an intact 5'-hydroxyl group. In attempts to avoid these routes, and hence to facilitate an interaction with the SAH hydrolase, Keller and Borchardt (1988) synthesized the "decapitated" cyclopentenyl derivatives of neplanocin A and 3-deazaneplanocin A, *DHCA* and *DHCDA* (Fig. 32). The expectations were borne out. DHCA and DHCDA gained in

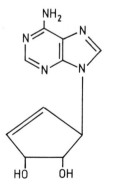

(-)-9-(trans-2, trans-3-Dihydroxy-
cyclopent-4-enyl) adenine
DHCA

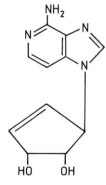

(-)-9-(trans-2, trans-3-Dihydroxy-
cyclopent-4-enyl)-3-deazaadenine
DHCDA

FIG. 32. Neplanocin A derivatives DHCA and DHCDA.

selectivity as both SAH hydrolase inhibitors and antiviral agents, which further strengthens the role of SAH hydrolase in the antiviral activity of this class of compounds.

4.2 RIBAVIRIN, 3-DEAZAGUANINE AND PYRAZOFURIN

Although ribavirin (Fig. 5) is a broad-spectrum antiviral agent active against both DNA and RNA viruses (Sidwell *et al.*, 1972), its major clinical potentials lie in the treatment of RNA virus infections, in particular respiratory syncytial virus (RSV) infections (Hall *et al.*, 1983, 1985) and influenza A or B virus infections (Gilbert *et al.*, 1985), where it can be administered as a small-particle aerosol. Ribavirin is effective in the therapy of Lassa fever when given orally at 15 mg/kg/day for 10 days (McCormick *et al.*, 1986), and other haemorrhagic fever virus infections might also respond favourably to ribavirin. The mechanism of action of ribavirin is multipronged. It inhibits the conversion of IMP to XMP by IMP dehydrogenase, which results in a depletion of the intracellular GTP pools, but, in addition, ribavirin also interferes with the 5'-cap formation of viral mRNAs, preventing both the initiation of transcription and the elongation of viral mRNA. The latter holds particularly for influenza virus (Gilbert and Knight, 1986), and this may explain why the compound has some selectivity towards influenza. Numerous derivatives of ribavirin have been synthesized. Best known are tiazofurin (2-β-D-ribofuranosylthiazole-4-carboxamide) and selenazofurin (2-β-D-ribofuranosylselenazole-4-carboxamide) (Kirsi *et al.*, 1983). The latter is pursued for its effectiveness against influenza virus infections (Sidwell *et al.*, 1986), the former for its potential as an antileukaemic agent (Jayaram *et al.*, 1986).

Two other compounds which display a broad antiviral activity spectrum similar to that of ribavirin are *3-deazaguanine* (Fig. 33) and *pyrazofurin*

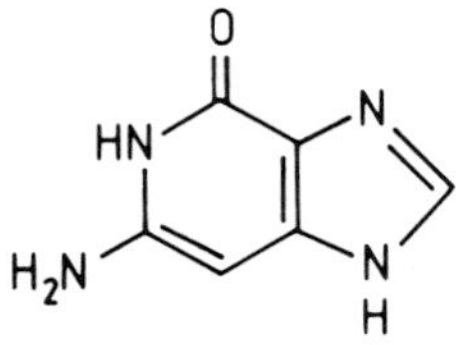

3-Deazaguanine

Fig. 33. 3-Deazaguanine.

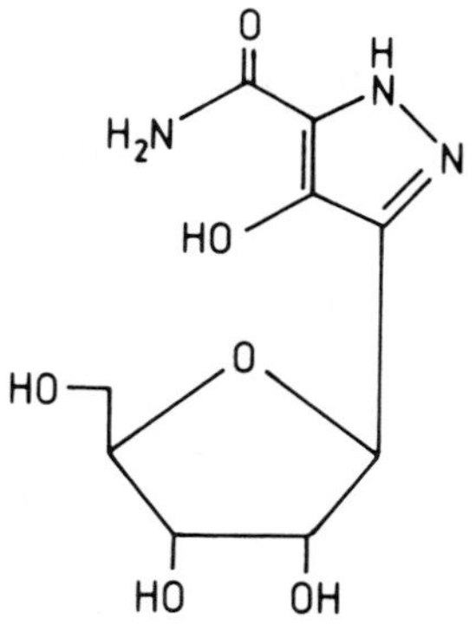

4-Hydroxy-3-β-D-ribofuranosylpyrazole-
5-carboxamide
Pyrazomycin
Pyrazofurin

FIG. 34. Pyrazofurin.

(Fig. 34). 3-Deazaguanine is accredited with activity against several DNA and RNA viruses (Allen et al., 1977; Revankar et al., 1984). Of a series of purine nucleoside analogues examined for their activity against rhinoviruses, 3-deazaguanine proved to be the most selective (De Clercq et al., 1986a). Against RSV 3-deazaguanine is active at a concentration of 1.65 μg/ml, yet not becoming toxic up to concentrations of 400 μg/ml. This makes 3-deazaguanine a more selective anti-RSV agent than ribavirin (Kawana et al., 1987). 3-Deazaguanine has also been examined for its inhibitory activity against a wide variety of influenza A, B and C strains, and here 3-deazaguanine and ribavirin showed a comparable potency and selectivity (Shigeta et al., 1988). Although pyrazofurin has been known for almost two decades, it has received only scant attention as an antiviral agent. Yet, pyrazofurin is inhibitory to a wide range of viruses (i.e. vesicular stomatitis, measles, Sindbis, polio) at a concentration that is approximately 1000-fold lower than the concentration at which ribavirin inhibits these viruses (Descamps and De Clercq, 1978). Moreover, pyrazofurin does not inhibit host cell DNA, RNA or protein synthesis unless it is added to the cells at doses 1000- to 10 000-fold higher than those that are inhibitory to virus replication. These observations have recently been extended to respiratory syncytial virus and influenza virus (types A, B and C), which were inhibited by pyrazofurin at a concentration of 0.07 (RSV) and 0.15 μg/ml (influenza virus) and a selectivity index of approximately 3000 (Kawana et al., 1987;

Shigeta *et al.*, 1988). Although pyrazofurin has a high degree of selectivity *in vitro*, it is markedly toxic for mice (50% lethal dose: approximately 5 mg/kg/day) when given systemically. In patients, pyrazofurin has been pursued primarily as an anticancer agent (Cadman *et al.*, 1978). Limiting factors to the systemic usage of pyrazofurin are mucositis, leukopenia and anaemia. Whether pyrazofurin is also toxic upon topical administration has not been assessed, and, in view of the marked potency and selectivity shown by pyrazofurin against respiratory syncytial virus and influenza (types A, B and C) viruses (Kawana *et al.*, 1987; Shigeta *et al.*, 1988), it may well seem worth envisaging its potential use, as an aerosol, in the topical treatment of respiratory tract virus infections. Certain derivatives of pyrazofurin have been synthesized, some of which might be less toxic than pyrazofurin itself (Petrie *et al.*, 1986). The biochemical target for both the antiviral and cytotoxic action of pyrazofurin has been identified as OMP decarboxylase, a crucial enzyme in the *de novo* biosynthesis of UTP (Ohnuma *et al.*, 1977), although pyrazofurin also interferes with the *de novo* biosynthesis of purine nucleotides, owing to an inhibitory effect on the formyltransferase that converts AICAR (5-aminoimidazole-4-carboxamide-1-β-D-ribofuranosyl-5'-monophosphate) to its formyl-AICAR, the immediate precursor of IMP (Worzalla and Sweeney, 1980).

5 Rhinovirus Infections

Because of their socioeconomic impact, common cold viruses (rhinoviruses) have been considered an attractive goal for antiviral prophylaxis and chemotherapy. The search for effective anti-rhinovirus agents has yielded a wealth of products belonging to widely varying chemical classes such as thiosemicarbazones, isoquinolines, triazinoindoles, guanidines, benzoates, furanyls, benzimidazoles, thiourea, diketones, flavans, flavones, chalcones, nitrobenzenes and isoxazoles (as reviewed by De Clercq *et al.*, 1986a). Typical examples of highly effective inhibitors of rhinovirus replication are 4',6-dichloroflavan (BW683C) (Bauer *et al.*, 1981), 4'-ethoxy-2'-hydroxy-4,6'-dimethoxychalcone (Ro 09-0410) (Ishitsuka *et al.*, 1982), 2-[(1,5,10,10a-tetrahydro-3H-thiazolo-[3,4b]isoquinolin-3-ylidene)amino]-4-thiazole acetic acid (44 081 R.P.) (Zerial *et al.*, 1985) and the isoxazoles 5-[7-[4-(4,5-dihydro-2-oxazolyl)phenoxy]heptyl]-3-methylisoxazole (*WIN 51711*) and 5-[7-[4-(4-methyl-4,5-dihydro-2-oxazolyl)phenoxy]heptyl]-3-methylisoxazole (*WIN 52084*) (Fig. 35) (Diana *et al.*, 1985; Otto *et al.*, 1985; Smith *et al.*, 1986). These compounds are highly discriminative in their anti-rhinovirus activity in that they are much more active against some rhinovirus types than others. Also, the activity spectrum of many of the

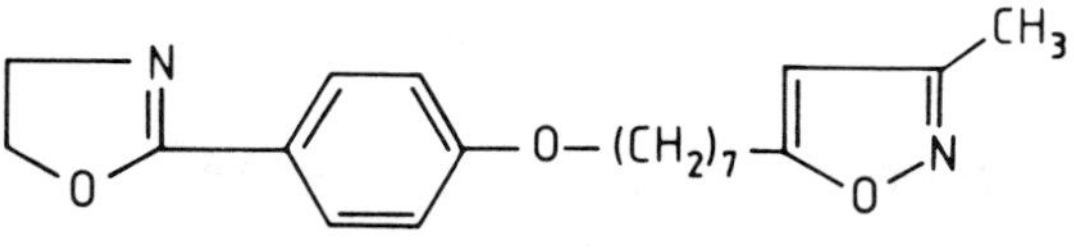

5-[7-[4-(4,5-dihydro-2-oxazolyl) phenoxy] heptyl]-
3-methylisoxazole
WIN   51711

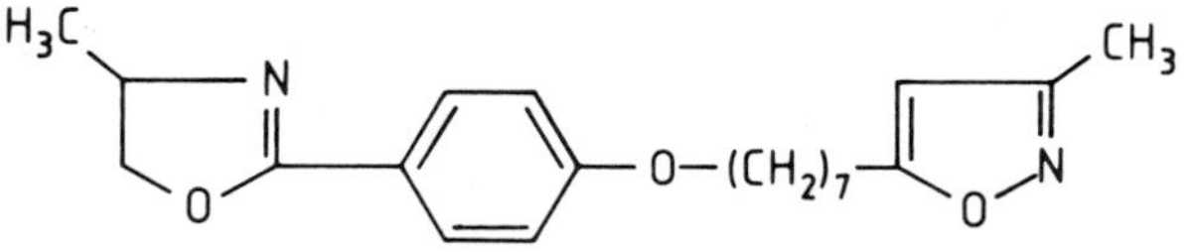

5-[7-[4-(4-methyl-4,5-dihydro-2-oxazolyl)phenoxy]
heptyl]-3-methylisoxazole
WIN   52084

FIG. 35. WIN 51711 and WIN 52084.

compounds, in particular the isoxazoles, extends to other picornaviruses such as polio, Coxsackie and Echo. Despite their disparate chemical structure, BW683C, Ro 09-0410, 44 081 R.P. and WIN 51711 appear to share a common mechanism of action: they specifically bind to the viral capsid, stabilize virus conformation, and thereby inhibit uncoating of the viral RNA (Tisdale and Selway, 1983; Ninomiya *et al.*, 1984; Alarcon *et al.*, 1986; Fox *et al.*, 1986). In fact, such mode of action was first demonstrated for arildone (4-[6-(2-chloro-4-methoxyphenoxy)hexyl]-3,5-heptanedione), the predecessor of WIN 51711, which, in the mean time, has been abandoned as a clinical drug candidate (McSharry *et al.*, 1979). The interaction of WIN 51711 and WIN 52084 with rhinovirus type 14 has been resolved at the atomic level (Smith *et al.*, 1986; Rossmann *et al.*, 1987): as shown in Fig. 36, WIN 52084 binds into a hydrophobic pocket within the viral capsid protein VP1. The oxazolyl moiety of WIN 52084 covers the entrance to the pocket. This entrance corresponds to the pore that is left in the floor of the "canyon" formed by VP1. Virus uncoating may be inhibited by preventing the collapse of the VP1 hydrophobic pocket or by blocking the flow of ions into the virus interior (Smith *et al.*, 1986). Notwithstanding the elegant elucidation of their mechanism of action, it remains to be seen whether WIN 52084, WIN 51711, or for that matter any other anti-rhinovirus agent, would ever be clinically useful. WIN 51711 is effective in reducing paralysis due to poliovirus in mice given the compound p.o. shortly after infection (McKinlay and Steinberg,

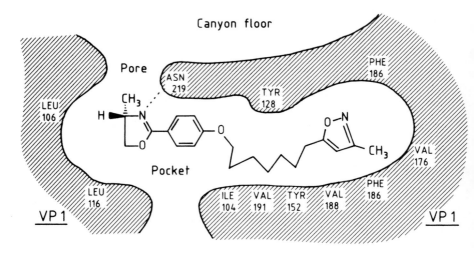

FIG. 36. Mechanism of action of anti-rhinovirus compound WIN 52084.

1986), but this does not necessarily mean that the drug would also be effective against rhinovirus infection (or picornavirus infections in general) in man. The failures obtained with both orally and intranasally administered 4′,6-dichloroflavan (Phillpotts *et al.*, 1983; Al-Nakib *et al.*, 1987) clearly illustrate that the treatment of rhinovirus infections should not be taken light-heartedly. For any drug to be successful in the treatment of rhinovirus infection it has to be delivered such that it sustains adequate concentrations at the site of virus replication, i.e. for rhinoviruses the ciliated nasal epithelial cells.

6 Retrovirus Infections

6.1 NON-NUCLEOSIDE ANALOGUES

Shortly after the discovery of reverse transcriptase (RNA-directed DNA polymerase) as the key enzyme in the replicative cycle of retroviruses (then termed RNA tumour viruses), several compounds were shown to selectively inhibit the replication of retroviruses (Shannon, 1977), and an even greater number of compounds was found to inhibit the retrovirus-associated reverse transcriptase (for a review, see De Clercq, 1986c). By the end of the 1970s both reverse transcriptase inhibitors and retroviruses were agents looking for a disease, and the search for anti-retrovirus compounds became far from fashionable. The advent of AIDS, and the identification of a retrovirus [human immunodeficiency virus (HIV)] as the causative agent of AIDS, has changed all this, and, at present, the efforts to develop an effective chemotherapy of AIDS outweigh the chemotherapeutic attempts for all other virus infections combined. Several interesting compounds have emerged from this burgeoning field, and Table 2 presents the compounds that have received most attention as anti-HIV agents. *Suramin*, a drug that has been used for many decades to treat African trypanosomiasis (sleeping sickness), was the first compound found effective in blocking the infectivity and cytopathogenicity of HIV (Mitsuya *et al.*, 1984). The use of suramin as a candidate anti-HIV agent was prompted by an earlier observation of De Clercq (1979) that suramin inhibits the reverse transcriptase activity of various animal retroviruses. Although it should be recognized that suramin is far from specific as a reverse transcriptase inhibitor and is known to interact with a multitude of proteins and enzymes, it is inhibitory to HIV *in vitro* at concentrations which are non-toxic to the host cells and readily attainable in humans (De Clercq, 1987h). Consequently, suramin has been given to patients with AIDS or ARC (Broder *et al.*, 1985; Collins *et al.*, 1986), where it has proved virustatic without offering much clinical or immunological improvement following a 6-week course. Suramin has also been shown to suppress the propagation of retroviruses in murine models (Ruprecht *et al.*, 1985). As its antiviral action is reversible, long-term administration of suramin may be necessary to achieve any clinical benefit, and, although suramin itself does not seem suitable for such long-term use because of accruing toxicity, some of its less toxic derivatives (Jentsch *et al.*, 1987) may be more useful in this regard. Also, the anionic compounds Evans Blue and aurintricarboxylic acid (an anionic triphenylmethane dye) represent two interesting leads in the development of future anti-HIV agents (Balzarini *et al.*, 1986a,b).

Suramin is not the only compound which was originally described as a reverse transcriptase inhibitor and later found inhibitory to HIV. Other examples are the ammonium 21-tungsto-9-antimoniate *HPA-23* (Chermann *et al.*, 1975; Dormont *et al.*, 1985), *foscarnet* (Sundquist and Öberg, 1979; Sandstrom *et al.*, 1985; Sarin *et al.*, 1985b; Vrang and Öberg, 1986) and the rifamycins (Yang *et al.*, 1972; Anand *et al.*, 1986). HPA-23 is inhibitory to HIV reverse transcriptase (Dormont *et al.*, 1985), but there is no evidence that it inhibits HIV replication at non-toxic concentrations (Balzarini *et al.*, 1986a). Preliminary indications of a beneficial effect of HPA-23 in AIDS patients (Rozenbaum *et al.*, 1985) have so far not been confirmed. The results of the clinical trials that have been initiated with foscarnet in AIDS patients are also awaited. Many of the substances, other than suramin, HPA-23 and PFA, which were described in the 1970s as potent reverse transcriptase inhibitors, i.e. poly(dUz) [poly(2'-azido-2'-deoxyuridic acid)]

TABLE 2

Antiviral drugs which have been found active against HIV

Suramin[a] and suramin derivatives
Evans Blue
Aurintricarboxylic acid (ATA)
Ribavirin (Virazole, 1-β-D-ribofuranosyl-1,2,4-triazole-3-carboxamide)[a]
Foscarnet (Phosphonoformate, PFA)[a]
Interferon (HuIFN-αA)[a]
D-Penicillamine (3-mercapto-D-valine)[a]
HPA-23 (ammonium 21-tungsto-9-antimoniate)[a]
Rifabutin (Ansamycin LM 427)
Amphotericin B methyl ester
Dithiocarb (Diethyldithiocarbamate sodium salt, Imuthiol)[a]
Glycyrrhizin
Heparin and dextran sulfate
Poly(I)·poly(C_{12},U) (Ampligen)[a]
Avarol (a sesquiterpenoid hydroquinone)
AL-721 (lipid mixture composed of glycerides, phosphatidylcholine and
    phosphatidylethanolamine in a 7:2:1 ratio)[a]
Peptide T (octapeptide: Ala-Ser-Thr-Thr-Thr-Asn-Tyr-Thr)[a]
2-Deoxy-D-glucose and other glycosylation inhibitors (i.e. castanospermine)
Oligodeoxynucleotide [i.e., $(dC)_{28}$] phosphorothioates
Azidothymidine (Retrovir, AZT, AzddThd, 3'-azido-2',3'-dideoxythymidine)[a]
2',3'-Dideoxycytidine (ddCyd)[a]
2',3'-Dideoxycytidinene (ddeCyd)
2',3'-Dideoxy-5-fluorocytidine (ddFCyd)
3'-Fluoro-2',3'-dideoxycytidine (FddCyd)
2',3'-Dideoxythymidine (ddThd)
2',3'-Dideoxythymidinene (ddeThd)
3'-Fluoro-2',3'-dideoxythymidine (FddThd)
3'-Fluoro-2',3'-dideoxyuridine (FddUrd)
2',3'-Dideoxyadenosine (ddAdo)
2',3'-Dideoxyinosine (ddIno)
3'-Azido-2',3'-dideoxyadenosine (AzddAdo)
2',3'-Dideoxy-2,6-diaminopurineriboside (ddDAPR)
2',3'-Dideoxyguanosine (ddGuo)
3'-Azido-2',3'-dideoxyguanosine (AzddGuo)
3'-Azido-2',3'-dideoxy-2,6-diaminopurineriboside (AzddDAPR)

[a]Has also been used in patients for the treatment of AIDS or ARC.

(De Clercq et al., 1975), poly(dAz) [poly(2'-azido-2'-deoxyadenylic acid)] (De Clercq et al., 1979a) and poly(fl^2A) [poly(2-fluoroadenylic acid)] (Fukui and De Clercq, 1982) have not yet been examined for their inhibitory effects on HIV replication. The broad-spectrum antiviral agent ribavirin has been investigated for its inhibitory effect on HIV replication, and while it proved inhibitory to the virus in some cell systems (McCormick et al., 1984), in others it did not (Balzarini et al., 1986a; Baba et al., 1987d). Whether ribavirin achieves any benefit in AIDS patients is, at present, a controversial issue. Other known antiviral compounds which gained renewed interest because of their potential use in the treatment of AIDS include: glycyrrhizin, a derivative of glycyrrhizic acid (Pompei et al., 1979; Ito et al., 1987b), interferon (Ho et al., 1985), the mismatched double-stranded RNA poly(I)·poly(C_{12},U) (Mitchell et al., 1987; Carter et al., 1987), the glycosylation inhibitors (i.e. 2-deoxy-D-glucose) (Blough et al., 1986) and the sulphated polysaccharides heparin and dextran sulphate (Ito et al., 1987a; Ueno and Kuno, 1987).

The mismatched double-stranded RNAs and sulphated polysaccharides deserve some further comments. Double-stranded RNA's have long since (Carter and De Clercq, 1974) been accredited with an important role in the recovery from virus infections, due to the induction of interferon and other lymphokines. Mismatching, i.e. introduction of an unpaired base (U) in the poly(C) strand [poly(I)·poly(C_{12},U) (Ampligen)] or the poly(I) strand [poly(I_{10},U)·poly(C) (De Clercq et al., 1979b)], allows the double-stranded RNA to retain its interferon-inducing activity while losing (part of its) toxic potential. Due to the induction of interferon and other lymphokines, mismatched double-stranded RNAs may, on the one hand, control HIV replication, and, on the other hand, stimulate the recovery of T and B cell functions, and this dual effect would, according to Carter et al. (1987), explain the favourable clinical, immunological and virological response of AIDS and ARC patients to treatment with Ampligen.

The antiviral properties of polyanionic substances such as polyacrylic acid (PAA), polymethacrylic acid (PMAA), polyvinyl sulphate, dextran sulphate, heparin have been known for a long time (De Somer et al., 1968a,b). These polyanionic substances interfere with the virus adsorption process. Virus adsorption was considered as a possible target, and polyanionic substances such as dextran sulphate were considered as a chemotherapeutic approach towards the treatment of AIDS (De Clercq, 1986c). This premise has been borne out by the recent discovery of Ito et al. (1987a) and Ueno and Kuno (1987) that dextran sulphate and heparin inhibit HIV replication at concentrations far below the cytotoxicity threshold. In fact, the selectivity indexes demonstrated by dextran sulphate and heparin are among the greatest ever achieved by any anti-HIV agent in vitro.

There are a number of compounds that in the past have been used or pursued for other purposes and that were later evaluated and proved active against the AIDS virus, i.e. the divalent cation-chelating agent D-penicillamine (Chandra and Sarin, 1986), the polyene macrolide antifungal agent amphotericin B methyl ester (Schaffer *et al.*, 1986), the antileukaemic sesquiterpenoid hydroquinone avarol (Müller *et al.*, 1987), the immunomodulator diethyldithiocarbamate (Pompidou *et al.*, 1985), the lipid mixture AL-721 (Sarin *et al.*, 1985a) and the vasoactive intestinal polypeptide homologue "peptide T" (Pert *et al.*, 1986; Ruff *et al.*, 1987). The latter is supposed to block HIV infectivity by preventing the adsorption of the virus to its receptor (CD4). However, it is at present a matter of conjecture whether "peptide T" has any effect on HIV infectivity or adsorption.

6.2 2′,3′-DIDEOXYNUCLEOSIDE ANALOGUES

The 2′,3′-dideoxynucleoside analogues form a class apart among the anti-retrovirus agents. The prototype of this class of compounds, *retrovir* (*azidothymidine*, *AZT*) (Fig. 6), has passed the drug regulatory review process with unusual speed. Azidothymidine was first shown to inhibit Friend murine lymphatic leukaemia helper virus (Ostertag *et al.*, 1974) before Mitsuya *et al.* (1985) demonstrated its selective inhibitory effect on HIV replication. Ruprecht *et al.* (1986) and Tavares *et al.* (1987) established the efficacy of AZT in suppressing or preventing retrovirus infections in mice and cats, respectively; and Yarchoan *et al.* (1986) were the first to demonstrate clinical utility with a short (6-week) course of AZT in AIDS (or ARC) patients. Preliminary evidence of Yarchoan *et al.* (1987) suggests that AZT may also lead to an improvement of the neurological abnormalities which are often associated with HIV infections. From a multi-centred double-blind placebo-controlled trial it has become clear that AZT can decrease mortality and reduce the frequency of opportunistic infections in a selected group of subjects with AIDS or advanced ARC (Fischl *et al.*, 1987). The compound is recommended at a dosage of 3.5 mg/kg/day p.o. every 4 hours (= 21 mg/kg/day p.o.) or, if oral administration is not feasible, at a dosage of 2.5 mg/kg/day i.v. every 4 hours (= 15 mg/kg/day i.v.). Oral bioavailability of the drug is approximately 60%, its plasma half-life is about 60 min, and 50–80% of the drug is eliminated in the urine as its 5′-glucuronidate. Furthermore, AZT readily crosses the blood–brain barrier, which may explain why HIV-associated neurological abnormalities seem to respond favourably to AZT therapy. Yet, the drug has to be administered with caution because severe side effects, particularly bone marrow suppression, may develop in a subset of patients (Richman *et al.*, 1987); the resulting

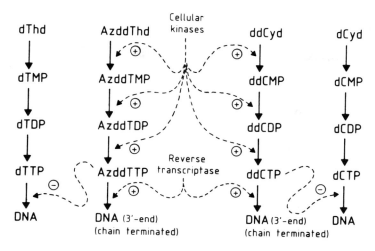

Fig. 37. Mechanism of action of AzddThd and ddCyd against human immunodeficiency virus (HIV).

anaemia and leukopenia may necessitate blood transfusion, reduction of the AZT dosage or even cessation of therapy. Measures to prevent or reverse the toxic effects of AZT should be investigated. The mechanism of action of AZT (Fig. 37) is in line with what could be expected from a 2′,3′-dideoxynucleoside (Waqar et al., 1984). The compound is non-selectively phosphorylated by cellular enzymes to the 5′-monophosphate (AzddTMP), 5′-diphosphate (AzddTDP), and 5′-triphosphate (AzddTTP). The latter then has the dual ability to act as a competitive inhibitor or alternate substrate (both with respect to dTTP) of HIV reverse transcriptase (Furman et al., 1986; Ono et al., 1986; Vrang et al., 1987). The incorporation of AzddTTP into DNA obviously leads to chain termination. AzddTTP inhibits HIV reverse transcriptase 100-fold better than cellular DNA polymerase α, which evidently explains its selective inhibition of HIV replication (Furman et al., 1986).

Various 2′,3′-dideoxynucleoside analogues (Table 2) have recently been described which show an anti-HIV potency and selectivity comparable to that of AZT (De Clercq, 1987e). Foremost among these 2′,3′-dideoxynucleosides are 2′,3′-dideoxycytidine (Fig. 38) (Mitsuya and Broder, 1986), whose mechanism of action is quite similar to that of AzddThd (Fig. 37) (Balzarini and Broder, 1988); 2′,3′-dideoxycytidinene (Fig. 39) (Balzarini et al., 1986c, 1987a; Lin et al., 1987) and the related 2′,3′-didehydro derivative

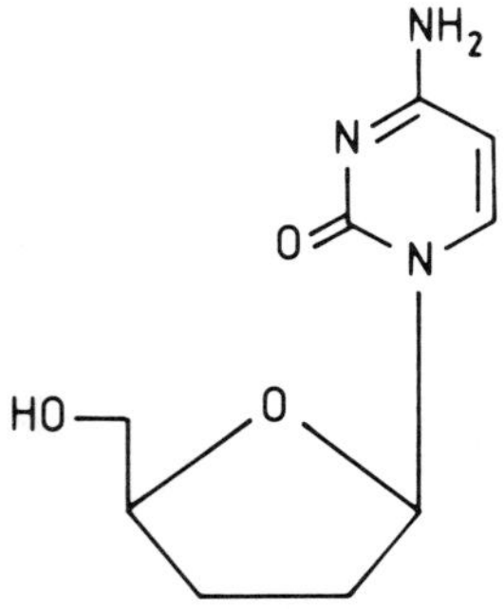

2', 3' - Dideoxycytidine
ddCyd

Fig. 38. ddCyd.

of 2',3'-dideoxythymidine, 2',3'-dideoxythymidinene (Fig. 39) (Baba et al., 1987e); 2',3'-dideoxyadenosine and its deamination product, 2',3'-dideoxyinosine (Fig. 40) (Mitsuya and Broder, 1986); 2',3'-dideoxy-2,6-diaminopurineriboside and its deamination product, 2',3'-dideoxyguanosine (Fig. 41) (Balzarini et al., 1987b,c); and 3'-azido-2',3'-dideoxy-2,6-diaminopurine riboside and its deamination product, 3'-azido-2',3'-dideoxyguanosine (Fig. 42) (Baba et al., 1987c). Among the 2',3'-dideoxycytidine analogues, both the 3'-fluoro- and 5-fluoro-substituted

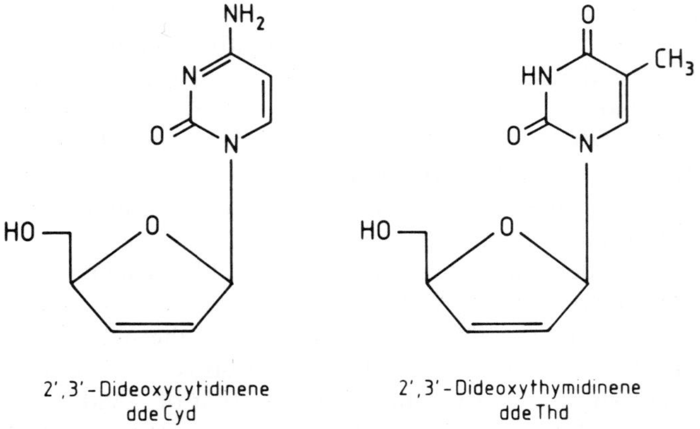

2',3'-Dideoxycytidinene
dde Cyd

2',3'-Dideoxythymidinene
dde Thd

Fig. 39. ddeCyd and ddeThd.

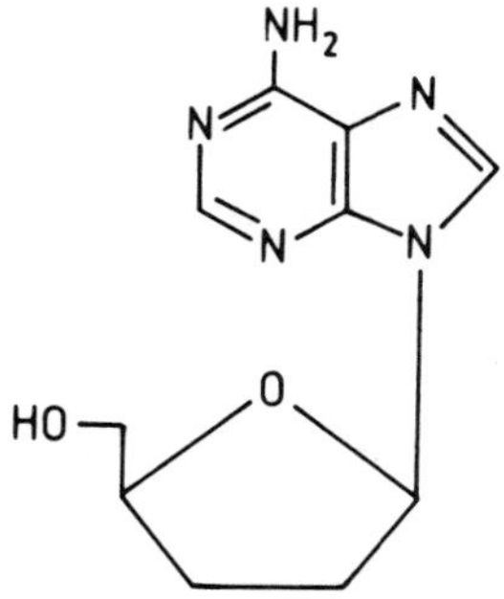

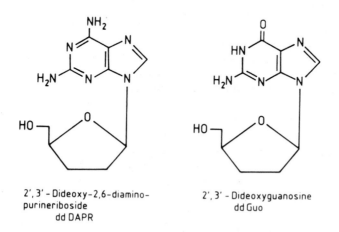

2′,3′ - Dideoxyadenosine
dd Ado

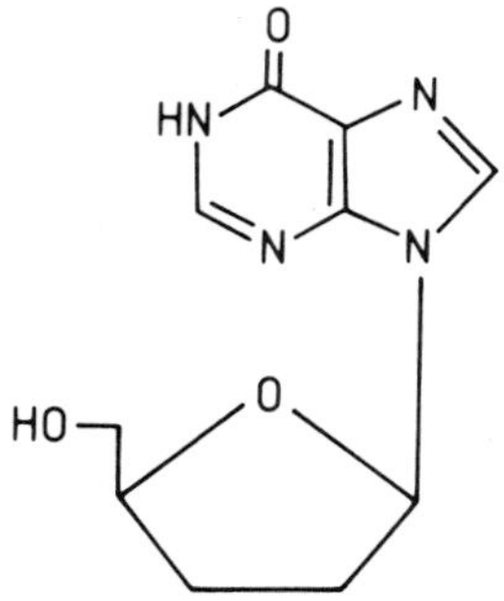

2′,3′ - Dideoxyinosine
dd Ino

FIG. 40. ddAdo and ddIno.

derivatives [termed FddCyd and ddFCyd, respectively (Table 2)] appear to be potent and selective inhibitors of HIV (Herdewijn *et al.*, 1987a; Kim *et al.*, 1987). Of a series of 2′,3′-dideoxyadenosine analogues, the 2′-fluoro ("up")-derivative emerged as the most selective inhibitor of HIV, although it was not quite as potent as 2′,3′-dideoxyadenosine itself (Herdewijn *et al.*, 1987b). The inhibitory effects of the 2′,3′-dideoxynucleoside analogues AZT, 2′,3′-dideoxycytidinene and 2′,3′-dideoxythymidinene on HIV replication have been confirmed in several laboratories (Nakashima *et al.*, 1986;

2′,3′ - Dideoxy-2,6-diamino-
purineriboside
dd DAPR

2′,3′ - Dideoxyguanosine
dd Guo

FIG. 41. ddDAPR and ddGuo.

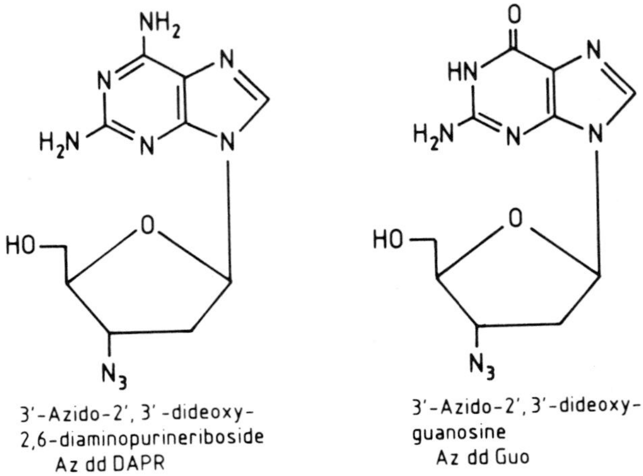

3'-Azido-2',3'-dideoxy-
2,6-diaminopurineriboside
Az dd DAPR

3'-Azido-2',3'-dideoxy-
guanosine
Az dd Guo

FIG. 42. AzddDAPR and AzddGuo.

Hamamoto *et al.*, 1987). Initial biochemical studies have pointed out that 2',3'-dideoxycytidine and 2',3'-dideoxycytidinene are anabolized, albeit less efficiently than the natural substrate (dCyd), to their 5'-triphosphates; ddCyd and ddeCyd are essentially resistant to catabolic enzymes (deaminases, phosphorylases) (Cooney *et al.*, 1986; Balzarini *et al.*, 1987a). 2',3'-Dideoxyadenosine, however, is more prone to enter catabolic pathways, leaving only a minor fraction of the drug available for anabolism to its 5'-triphosphate (Cooney *et al.*, 1987).

Combination chemotherapy is an interesting prospect for the treatment of many virus infections, including retrovirus infections, as such combinations of two or more drugs may result in: (i) enhanced activity, i.e. through positive feedback interactions with kinases involved in the anabolism of the compounds; (ii) diminished toxicity, through reduction in the doses of the individual compounds; and (iii), possibly, decreased risk of emergence of drug-resistant variants (assuming that such virus–drug resistance would arise following single use of the compounds). Various combinations of anti-HIV agents have already been explored and in several instances synergism was noted *in vitro*: retrovir + acyclovir (Mitsuya and Broder, 1987), retrovir + dextran sulphate (Ueno and Kuno, 1987), retrovir + poly(I)·poly(C_{12},U) (Mitchell *et al.*, 1987), foscarnet + human interferon α2A (Hartshorn *et al.*, 1986), retrovir + human interferon α2A (Hartshorn *et al.*, 1987). Ribavirin, which by itself has no anti-HIV activity in our assay systems, was found to potentiate the anti-HIV activity of the purine 2',3'-

dideoxynucleosides ddAdo and ddGuo, while counteracting that of the pyrimidine 2′,3′-dideoxynucleosides AzddThd, ddCyd, ddeCyd and ddeThd (Baba *et al.*, 1987d). Antagonism between AzddThd and ribavirin occurs under varying experimental conditions and can be attributed to the inhibition of AzddThd phosphorylation by ribavirin (Vogt *et al.*, 1987). Thus, drug combinations do not invariably lead to an increased antiviral activity, an important notion that should be taken into account when considering clinical studies with drug combinations.

7 Conclusion

For a long time viral diseases were considered to be intractable by chemotherapeutic means because of the innate alliance between the virus's replicative cycle and the cells' own metabolism. This view has been dramatically changed with the advent of the highly selective anti-herpesvirus and anti-rhinovirus agents. With AIDS added to the array of virus infections in most urgent need of an effective chemotherapy, the development of antivirals has gained an enormous momentum. In the last two to three years, a great number of compounds have been found to be active against the AIDS virus, some of these compounds having been dormant for many years before they were re-discovered as selective anti-HIV agents. At present there are perhaps too many, rather than too few, candidate compounds for the treatment of AIDS, and the prolific number of anti-herpesvirus and anti-rhinovirus agents now available again makes the right choice difficult. For viruses such as papilloma and hepatitis B, however, we still fall short in efficient antiviral drugs, essentially because of the absence of adequate *in vitro* assay systems. For those virus infections where a plethora of candidate drugs are at hand the burden of proof rests with the clinicians who must design the proper clinical trials so as to unequivocally assess the efficacy (and safety) of the compounds and to estimate the efficacy (and safety) of one compound relative to another. Based on a more detailed knowledge of the structure–function relationship of the different classes of compounds, combined with a better insight in their mechanism of action and the viral targets they interact with, the design of antiviral drugs has become more rationally defined. This should bear fruit in the future development of new antiviral compounds. Where the compound appears sufficiently promising from *in vitro* and *in vivo* efficiency studies, it should without further delay be submitted to the necessary pharmacokinetic and toxicological evaluations. This would in turn facilitate the planning of the clinical trials, expedite the handling by the drug-regulatory institutions, and, if the compound passes all these tests, ultimately lead to its success as an antiviral drug.

Acknowledgements

My original investigations are supported by grants from the Belgian F.G.W.O. (Fonds voor Geneeskundig Wetenschappelijk Onderzoek: Projects no. 3.0040.83 and no. 3.0097.87) and the Belgian G.O.A. (Geconcerteerde Onderzoeksacties: Project no. 85/90-79). I gratefully acknowledge the excellent editorial help of Christiane Callebaut in preparing the typescript.

Appendix: List of Abbreviations

ACV	9-(2-hydroxyethoxymethyl)guanine, acyclovir
ACVDP	ACV diphosphate
ACVMP	ACV monophosphate
ACVTP	ACV triphosphate
AHPA	3-adenin-9-yl-2-hydroxypropanoic acid
AICAR	5-aminoimidazole-4-carboxamide-1-β-D-ribofuranosyl-5'-monophosphate
AIDS	acquired immune deficiency syndrome
Ara-A	9-β-D-arabinofuranosyladenine, adenine arabinoside
Ara-Hx	9-β-D-arabinofuranosylhypoxanthine
ARC	AIDS-related complex
ATA	aurintricarboxylic acid
AzddAdo	3'-azido-ddAdo
AzddDAPR	3'-azido-ddDAPR
AzddGuo	3'-azido-ddGuo
AzddTDP	AzddThd diphosphate
AzddThd	see AZT
AzddTMP	AzddThd monophosphate
AzddTTP	AzddThd triphosphate
AZT	3'-azido-2',3'-dideoxythymidine, azidothymidine
BCV	(R)-9-(3,4-dihydroxybutyl)guanine, buciclovir
BCVTP	BCV triphosphate
BHV	bovid herpesvirus
BVaraU	see BVAU
BVaraUTP	BVaraU triphosphate
BVAU	(E)-5-(2-bromovinyl)-1-β-D-arabinofuranosyluracil, bromovinyluracil arabinoside
BVDU	(E)-5-(2-bromovinyl)-2'-deoxyuridine
BVDUDP	BVDU diphosphate
BVDUMP	BVDU monophosphate
BVDUTP	BVDU triphosphate
C-Ara-A	carbocyclic Ara-A
C-BVDU	carbocyclic BVDU
C-c^{3}Ado	carbocyclic 3-deazaadenosine
CEDU	5-(2-chloroethyl)-2'-deoxyuridine

C-IVDU	carbocyclic IVDU
CMV	cytomegalovirus
cNDGMP	9-[(2-hydroxy-1,3,2-dioxaphosphorinan-5-yl)-oxymethyl]guanine P-oxide, 2′-nor-cGMP
dCDP	dCyd diphosphate
dCMP	dCyd monophosphate
dCTP	dCyd triphosphate
dCyd	2′-deoxycytidine
ddAdo	2′,3′-dideoxyadenosine
ddCDP	ddCyd diphosphate
ddCMP	ddCyd monophosphate
ddCTP	ddCyd triphosphate
ddCyd	2′,3′-dideoxycytidine
ddDAPR	2′,3′-dideoxy-2,6-diaminopurineriboside
ddeCyd	2′,3′-dideoxycytidinene
ddeThd	2′,3′-dideoxythymidinene
ddFCyd	5-fluoro-ddCyd
ddGuo	2′,3′-dideoxyguanosine
ddIno	2′,3′-dideoxyinosine
ddThd	2′,3′-dideoxythymidine
dGDP	dGuo diphosphate
dGMP	dGuo monophosphate
dGTP	dGuo triphosphate
dGuo	2′-deoxyguanosine
DHBG	*see* BCV
DHCA	(−)-9-(*trans*-2,*trans*-3-dihydroxycyclopent-4-enyl)-adenine
DHCDA	(−)-9-(*trans*-2,*trans*-3-dihydroxycyclopent-4-enyl)-3-deazaadenine
DHPA	9-(2,3-dihydroxypropyl)adenine
DHPG	*see* 2′NDG
dTDP	dThd diphosphate
dThd	2′-deoxythymidine
dTMP	dThd monophosphate
dTTP	dThd triphosphate
dUrd	2′-deoxyuridine
EBV	Epstein-Barr virus
EDU	5-ethyl-2′-deoxyuridine
EHV	equid herpesvirus
FBVAU	fluorobromovinyl*lara*uracil
FCEAU	fluorochloroethyl*lara*uracil
FddCyd	3′-fluoro-ddCyd
FddThd	3′-fluoro-ddThd
FddUrd	3′-fluoro-2′,3′-dideoxyuridine
FEAU	1-β-D-(2-deoxy-2-fluoroarabinofuranosyl)-5-ethyluracil, fluoroethyl*lara*uracil
FIAC	1-β-D-(2-deoxy-2-fluoroarabinofuranosyl)-5-iodocytosine, fluoroiodo*ara*cytosine
FIAU	1-β-D-(2-deoxy-2-fluoroarabinofuranosyl)-5-iodouracil, fluoroiodo*ara*uracil
FMAU	1-β-D-(2-deoxy-2-fluoroarabinofuranosyl)-5-methyluracil, fluoromethyl*lara*uracil

GMP	guanosine monophosphate
GTP	guanosine triphosphate
HHEMG	*see* 2'NDG
HIV	human immunodeficiency virus
HPMPA	9-(3-hydroxy-2-phosphonylmethoxypropyl)adenine
HPMPC	9-(3-hydroxy-2-phosphonylmethoxypropyl)cytosine
HSV	herpes simplex virus
HVP	herpesvirus platyrrhinae
IDU	5-iodo-2'-deoxyuridine, idoxuridine
IMP	inosine monophosphate
iNDG	9-(2,3-dihydroxy-1-propoxymethyl)guanine
IVDU	(*E*)-5-(2-iodovinyl)-2'-deoxyuridine
2'NDG	2'-nor-2'-deoxyguanosine
OMP	orotidine monophosphate
PAA	polyacrylic acid
PFA	phosphonoformate
PHV	phocid herpesvirus
PMAA	polymethacrylic acid
PMEA	9-(2-phosphonylmethoxyethyl)adenine
RSV	respiratory syncytial virus
SAH	S-adenosylhomocysteine
SAM	S-adenosylmethionine
SHV	suid herpesvirus
SVV	simian varicella virus
TFT	5-trifluoro-2'-deoxythymidine, trifluridine
TK⁻	dThd kinase deficient
VZV	varicella-zoster virus
UTP	uridine triphosphate
XMP	xanthosine monophosphate

References

Alarcon, B., Zerial, A., Dupiol, C., and Carrasco, L. (1986). *Antimicrob. Agents Chemother.* **30**, 31–34.

Alenius, S., Berg, M., Broberg, F., Eklind, K., Lindborg, B., and Öberg, B. (1982). *J. Infect. Dis.* **145**, 569–573.

Allaudeen, H. S., Kozarich, J. W., Bertino, J. R., and De Clercq, E. (1981). *Proc. Natl. Acad. Sci. USA* **78**, 2698–2702.

Allaudeen, H. S., Chen, M. S., Lee, J. J., De Clercq, E., and Prusoff, W. H. (1982a). *J. Biol. Chem.* **257**, 603–606.

Allaudeen, H. S., Descamps, J., Sehgal, R. K., and Fox, J. J. (1982b). *J. Biol. Chem.* **257**, 11 879–11 882.

Allen, L. B., Huffman, J. H., Cook, P. D., Meyer, R. B. Jr., Robins, R. K., and Sidwell, R. W. (1977). *Antimicrob. Agents Chemother.* **12**, 114–119.

Al-Nakib, W., Willman, J., Higgins, P. G., Tyrrell, D. A. J., Shepherd, W. M., and Freestone, D. S. (1987). *Arch. Virol.* **92**, 255–260.

Anand, R., Moore, J., Feorino, P., Curran, J., and Srinivasan, A. (1986). *Lancet* **i**, 97–98.

Ashton, W. T., Karkas, J. D., Field, A. K., and Tolman, R. L. (1982). *Biochem. Biophys. Res. Commun.* **108**, 1716–1721.

Ashton, W. T., Canning, L. F., Reynolds, G. F., Tolman, R. L., Karkas, J. D., Liou, R., Davies, M.-E. M., DeWitt, C. M., Perry, H. C., and Field, A. K. (1985). *J. Med. Chem.* **28**, 926–933.

Ayisi, N. K., De Clercq, E., Wall, R. A., Hughes, H., and Sacks, S. L. (1984). *Antimicrob. Agents Chemother.* **26**, 762–765.

Ayisi, N. K., Wall, R. A., Wanklin, R. J., Machida, H., De Clercq, E., and Sacks, S. L. (1987). *Mol. Pharmacol.* **31**, 422–429.

Baba, M., Konno, K., Shigeta, S., and De Clercq, E. (1987a). *Eur. J. Clin. Microbiol.* **6**, 158–160.

Baba, M., Mori, S., Shigeta, S., and De Clercq, E. (1987b). *Antimicrob. Agents Chemother.* **31**, 337–339.

Baba, M., Pauwels, R., Balzarini, J., Herdewijn, P., and De Clercq, E. (1987c). *Biochem. Biophys. Res. Commun.* **145**, 1080–1086.

Baba, M., Pauwels, R., Balzarini, J., Herdewijn, P., De Clercq, E., and Desmyter, J. (1987d). *Antimicrob. Agents Chemother.* **31**, 1613–1617.

Baba, M., Pauwels, R., Herdewijn, P., De Clercq, E., Desmyter, J., and Vandeputte, M. (1987e). *Biochem. Biophys. Res. Commun.* **142**, 128–134.

Bach, M. C., Bagwell, S. P., Knapp, N. P., Davis, K. M., and Hedstrom, P. S. (1985). *Ann. Intern. Med.* **103**, 381–382.

Balzarini, J., and Broder, S. (1988). *In* "Clinical Use of Antiviral Drugs" (E. De Clercq, ed.) (in press). Klurver Academic Publishers, Norwell, Massachusetts.

Balzarini, J., De Clercq, E., Verbruggen, A., Ayusawa, D., and Seno, T. (1985). *Mol. Pharmacol.* **28**, 581–587.

Balzarini, J., Mitsuya, H., De Clercq, E., and Broder, S. (1986a). *Int. J. Cancer* **37**, 451–457.

Balzarini, J., Mitsuya, H., De Clercq, E., and Broder, S. (1986b). *Biochem. Biophys. Res. Commun.* **136**, 64–71.

Balzarini, J., Pauwels, R., Herdewijn, P., De Clercq, E., Cooney, D. A., Kang, G.-J., Dalal, M., Johns, D. G., and Broder, S. (1986c). *Biochem. Biophys. Res. Commun.* **140**, 735–742.

Balzarini, J., Kang, G.-J., Dalal, M., Herdewijn, P., De Clercq, E., Broder, S., and Johns, D. G. (1987a). *Mol. Pharmacol.* **32**, 162–167.

Balzarini, J., Pauwels, R., Baba, M., Robins, M. J., Zou, R., Herdewijn, P., and De Clercq, E. (1987b). *Biochem. Biophys. Res. Commun.* **145**, 269–276.

Balzarini, J., Robins, M. J., Zou, R., Herdewijn, P., and De Clercq, E. (1987c). *Biochem. Biophys. Res. Commun.* **145**, 277–283.

Bauer, D. J., Selway, J. W. T., Batchelor, J. F., Tisdale, M., Caldwell, J. C., and Young, D. A. B. (1981). *Nature* **292**, 369–373.

Benoit, Y., Laureys, G., Delbeke, M.-J., and De Clercq, E. (1985). *Eur. J. Pediatr.* **143**, 198–202.

Biron, K. K., Stanat, S. C., Sorrell, J. B., Fyfe, J. A., Keller, P. M., Lambe, C. U., and Nelson, D. J. (1985). *Proc. Natl. Acad. Sci. USA* **82**, 2473–2477.

Biron, K. K., Fyfe, J. A., Stanat, S. C., Leslie, L. K., Sorrell, J. B., Lambe, C. U., and Coen, D. M. (1986). *Proc. Natl. Acad. Sci. USA* **83**, 8769–8773.

Blough, H. A., Pauwels, R., De Clercq, E., Cogniaux, J., Sprecher-Goldberger, S., and Thiry, L. (1986). *Biochem. Biophys. Res. Commun.* **141**, 33–38.

Borchardt, R. T. (1980). *J. Med. Chem.* **23**, 347–357.

Borchardt, R. T., Keller, B. T., and Patel-Thombre, U. (1984). *J. Biol. Chem.* **259**, 4353–4358.

Broder, S., Yarchoan, R., Collins, J. M., Lane, H. C., Markham, P. D., Klecker, R. W., Redfield, R. R., Mitsuya, H., Hoth, D. F., Gelmann, E., Groopman, J. E., Resnick, L., Gallo, R. C., Myers, C. E., and Fauci, A. S. (1985). *Lancet* **ii**, 627–630.

Burns, W. H., Saral, R., Santos, G. W., Laskin, O. L., Lietman, P. S., McLaren, C., and Barry, D. W. (1982). *Lancet* **i**, 421–423.

Cadman, E. C., Dix, D. E., and Handschumacher, R. E. (1978). *Cancer Res.* **38**, 682–688.

Carter, W. A., and De Clercq, E. (1974). *Science* **186**, 1172–1178.

Carter, W. A., Strayer, D. R., Brodsky, I., Lewin, M., Pellegrino, M. G., Einck, L., Henriques, H. F., Simon, G. L., Parenti, D. M., Scheib, R. G., Schulof, R. S., Montefiori, D. C., Robinson, W. E., Mitchell, W. M., Volsky, D. J., Paul, D., Paxton, H., Meyer III, W. A., Kariko, K., Reichenbach, N., Suhadolnik, R. J., and Gillespie, D. H. (1987). *Lancet* i, 1286–1292.

Cassiman, J. J., De Clercq, E., and van den Berghe, H. (1983). *Mut. Res.* **117**, 317–327.

Chandra, P., and Sarin, P. S. (1986). *Arzneim.-Forsch./Drug Res.* **36**, 184–186.

Cheng, Y.-C., Grill, S. P., Dutschman, G. E., Nakayama, K., and Bastow, K. F. (1983a). *J. Biol. Chem.* **258**, 12 460–12 464.

Cheng, Y.-C., Huang, E.-S., Lin, J.-C., Mar, E.-C., Pagano, J. S., Dutschman, G. E., and Grill, S. P. (1983b). *Proc. Natl. Acad. Sci. USA* **80**, 2767–2770.

Chermann, J.-C., Sinoussi, F. C., and Jasmin, C. (1975). *Biochem. Biophys. Res. Commun.* **65**, 1229–1236.

Chou, T.-C., Lopez, C., Colacino, J. M., Feinberg, A., Watanabe, K. A., Fox, J. J., and Philips, F. S. (1984). *Mol. Pharmacol.* **26**, 587–593.

Coen, D. M., Aschman, D. P., Gelep, P. T., Retondo, M. J., Weller, S. K., and Schaffer, P. A. (1984). *J. Virol.* **49**, 236–247.

Colacino, J. M., and Lopez, C. (1985). *Antimicrob. Agents Chemother.* **28**, 252–258.

Colla, L., De Clercq, E., Busson, R., and Vanderhaeghe, H. (1983). *J. Med. Chem.* **26**, 602–604.

Collaborative DHPG Treatment Study Group (1986). *New Engl. J. Med.* **314**, 801–805.

Collins, J. M., Klecker, R. W. Jr., Yarchoan, R., Lane, H. C., Fauci, A. S., Redfield, R. R., Broder, S., and Myers, C. E. (1986). *J. Clin. Pharmacol.* **26**, 22–26.

Cookson, R. C., Dudfield, P. J., Newton, R. F., Ravenscroft, P., Scopes, D. I. C., and Cameron, J. M. (1985). *Eur. J. Med. Chem.* **20**, 375–377.

Cools, M., De Clercq, E., and Drach, J. C. (1987). *Nucleosides & Nucleotides* **6**, 423–424.

Cooney, D. A., Dalal, M., Mitsuya, H., McMahon, J. B., Nadkarni, M., Balzarini, J., Broder, S., and Johns, D. G. (1986). *Biochem. Pharmacol.* **35**, 2065–2068.

Cooney, D. A., Ahluwalia, G., Mitsuya, H., Fridland, A., Johnson, M., Hao, Z., Dalal, M., Balzarini, J., Broder, S., and Johns, D. G. (1987). *Biochem. Pharmacol.* **36**, 1765–1768.

Corey, L., and Spear, P. G. (1986). *New Engl. J. Med.* **314**, 749–757.

Crumpacker, C. S., Schnipper, L. E., Marlowe, S. I., Kowalsky, P. N., Hershey, B. J., and Levin, M. J. (1982). *New Engl. J. Med.* **306**, 343–346.

Davies, M.-E. M., Bondi, J. V., Grabowski, L., Schofield, T. L., and Field, A. K. (1987). *Antiviral Res.* **7**, 119–125.

De Clercq, E. (1979). *Cancer Lett.* **8**, 9–22.

De Clercq, E. (1982). *Trends Pharmacol. Sci. (TIPS)* **3**, 492–495.

De Clercq, E. (1985a). In "Scientific Basis of Antimicrobial Chemotherapy" (D. Greenwood and F. O'Grady, eds), pp. 155–184. Cambridge University Press, Cambridge.

De Clercq, E. (1985b). In "Approaches to Antiviral Agents" (M. R. Harnden, ed.), pp. 57–99. Macmillan, London.

De Clercq, E. (1985c). *Antimicrob. Agents Chemother.* **28**, 84–89.

De Clercq, E. (1986a). In "The Antimicrobial Agents Annual/1" (P. K. Peterson and J. Verhoef, eds), pp. 526–535. Elsevier, Amsterdam, New York, Oxford.

De Clercq, E. (1986b). *Verh. K. Acad. Geneeskd. Belg.* **48**, 261–290.

De Clercq, E. (1986c). *J. Med. Chem.* **29**, 1561–1569.

De Clercq, E. (1987b). *ISI Atlas of Science (Pharmacology)* **1**, 20–24.

De Clercq, E. (1987c). In "Trends in Medicinal Chemistry" (E. Mutschler and E. Winterfeldt, eds), pp. 487–501. VCH Verlagsgesellschaft, Weinheim.

De Clercq, E. (1987d). *In* "Proceedings of the CHEMRAWN V Conference on Current and Future Contributions of Chemistry to Health, The New Frontiers" (H. Machleidt, ed.), Vol. 2, pp. 121–143. VCH Verlagsgesellschaft, Weinheim.

De Clercq, E. (1987e). *Trends Pharmacol. Sci. (TIPS)* **8**, 339–345.

De Clercq, E. (1987f). *Biochem. Pharmacol.* **36**, 2567–2575.

De Clercq, E. (1987g). *Annali dell'Istituto Superiore di Sanita* (in press).

De Clercq, E. (1987h). *Antiviral Res.* **7**, 1–10.

De Clercq, E. (1988a). Clinical use of antiviral drugs. *In* "Developments in Medical Virology" (Y. Becker, series ed.) (in press). Klurver Academic Publishers, Norwell, Massachusetts.

De Clercq, E. (1988b). *In* "Antiviral Drug Development: A Multidisciplinary Approach" (E. De Clercq and R. T. Walker, eds) (in press). NATO ASI Series, Series A: Life Sciences. Plenum Press, New York and London.

De Clercq, E., and Bernaerts, R. (1987). *J. Biol. Chem.* (in press).

De Clercq, E., and Cools, M. (1985). *Biochem. Biophys. Res. Commun.* **129**, 306–311.

De Clercq, E., and Holý, A. (1985). *J. Med. Chem.* **28**, 282–287.

De Clercq, E., and Montgomery, J. A. (1983). *Antiviral Res.* **3**, 17–24.

De Clercq, E., and Robins, M. J. (1986). *Antimicrob. Agents Chemother.* **30**, 719–724.

De Clercq, E., and Rosenwirth, B. (1985). *Antimicrob. Agents Chemother.* **28**, 246–251.

De Clercq, E., and Shugar, D. (1975). *Biochem. Pharmacol.* **24**, 1073–1078.

De Clercq, E., and Walker, R. T. (1984). *Pharmac. Ther.* **26**, 1–44.

De Clercq, E., and Walker, R. T. (1986). *In* "Progress in Medicinal Chemistry" (G. P. Ellis and G. B. West, eds), Vol. 23, pp. 187–218. Elsevier Science Publishers, Amsterdam.

De Clercq, E., Billiau, A., Hobbs, J., Torrence, P. F., and Witkop, B. (1975). *Proc. Natl. Acad. Sci. USA* **72**, 284–288.

De Clercq, E., Descamps, J., De Somer, P., and Holý, A. (1978). *Science* **200**, 563–565.

De Clercq, E., Fukui, T., Kakiuchi, N., and Ikehara, M. (1979a). *Cancer Lett.* **7**, 27–37.

De Clercq, E., Huang, G.-F., Bhooshan, B., Ledley, G., and Torrence, P. F. (1979b). *Nucleic Acids Res.* **7**, 2003–2014.

De Clercq, E., Descamps, J., Balzarini, J., Fukui, T., and Allaudeen, H. S. (1983). *Biochem. J.* **211**, 439–445.

De Clercq, E., Bergstrom, D. E., Holý, A., and Montgomery, J. A. (1984). *Antiviral Res.* **4**, 119–133.

De Clercq, E., Balzarini, J., Bernaerts, R., Herdewijn, P., and Verbruggen, A. (1985a). *Biochem. Biophys. Res. Commun.* **126**, 397–403.

De Clercq, E., Bernaerts, R., Balzarini, J., Herdewijn, P., and Verbruggen, A. (1985b). *J. Biol. Chem.* **260**, 10621–10628.

De Clercq, E., Desgranges, C., Herdewijn, P., Sim, I. S., and Walker, R. T. (1985c). *In* "Proceedings of the VIIIth International Symposium on Medicinal Chemistry" (R. Dahlbom and J. L. G. Nilsson, eds), Vol. 1, pp. 198–210. Swedish Pharmaceutical Press, Stockholm.

De Clercq, E., Bernaerts, R., Bergstrom, D. E., Robins, M. J., Montgomery, J. A., and Holý, A. (1986a). *Antimicrob. Agents Chemother.* **29**, 482–487.

De Clercq, E., Holý, A., Rosenberg, I., Sakuma, T., Balzarini, J., and Maudgal, P. C. (1986b). *Nature* **323**, 464–467.

De Clercq, E., Balzarini, J., Madej, D., Hansske, F., and Robins, M. J. (1987a). *J. Med. Chem.* **30**, 481–486.

De Clercq, E., Sakuma, T., Baba, M., Pauwels, R., Balzarini, J., Rosenberg, I., and Holý, A. (1987b). *Antiviral Res.* (in press).

De Fazio, G., Vicente, M., and De Clercq, E. (1987). *Antiviral Res.* **8**, 163–169.

Derse, D., Cheng, Y.-C., Furman, P. A., St. Clair, M. H., and Elion, G. B. (1981). *J. Biol. Chem.* **256**, 11 447–11 451.

Descamps, J., and De Clercq, E. (1978). In "Current Chemotherapy" (W. Siegenthaler and R. Lüthy, eds), pp. 354–357. American Society for Microbiology, Washington D.C.

Descamps, J., and De Clercq, E. (1981). J. Biol. Chem. 256, 5973–5976.

Descamps, J., Sehgal, R. K., De Clercq, E., and Allaudeen, H. S. (1982). J. Virol. 43, 332–336.

Desgranges, C., Razaka, G., Rabaud, M., Bricaud, H., Balzarini, J., and De Clercq, E. (1983). Biochem. Pharmacol. 32, 3583–3590.

Desgranges, C., Razaka, G., Drouillet, F., Bricaud, H., Herdewijn, P., and De Clercq, E. (1984). Nucleic Acids Res. 12, 2081–2090.

Desgranges, C., De Clercq, E., Razaka, G., Drouillet, F., Belloc, I., and Bricaud, H. (1986). Biochem. Pharmacol. 35, 1647–1653.

Diana, G. D., McKinlay, M. A., Brisson, C. J., Zalay, E. S., Miralles, J. V., and Salvador, U. J. (1985). J. Med. Chem. 28, 748–752.

De Somer, P., De Clercq, E., Billiau, A., Schonne, E., and Claesen, M. (1968a). J. Virol. 2, 878–885.

De Somer, P., De Clercq, E., Billiau, A., Schonne, E., and Claesen, M. (1968b). J. Virol. 2, 886–893.

Dolin, R. (1985). Science 227, 1296–1303.

Dormont, D., Spire, B., Barré-Sinoussi, F., Montagnier, L., and Chermann, J. C. (1985). Ann. Inst. Pasteur/Virol. 136E, 75–83.

Duke, A. E., Smee, D. F., Chernow, M., Boehme, R., and Matthews, T. R. (1986). Antiviral Res. 6, 299–308.

Ericson, A.-C., Larsson, A., Aoki, F. Y., Yisak, W.-A., Johansson, N.-G., Öberg, B., and Datema, R. (1985). Antimicrob. Agents Chemother. 27, 753–759.

Ernberg, I., and Andersson, J. (1986). J. Gen. Virol. 67, 2267–2272.

Felsenstein, D., D'Amico, D. J., Hirsch, M. S., Neumeyer, D. A., Cederberg, D. M., de Miranda, P., and Schooley, R. T. (1985). Ann. Intern. Med. 103, 377–380.

Field, A. K., Davies, M. E., DeWitt, C., Perry, H. C., Liou, R., Germershausen, J., Karkas, J. D., Ashton, W. T., Johnston, D. B. R., and Tolman, R. L. (1983). Proc. Natl. Acad. Sci. USA 80, 4139–4143.

Field, A. K., Davies, M. E. M., DeWitt, C. M., Perry, H. C., Schofield, T. L., Karkas, J. D., Germershausen, J., Wagner, A. F., Cantone, C. L., MacCoss, M., and Tolman, R. L. (1986). Antiviral Res. 6, 329–341.

Fischl, M. A., Richman, D. D., Grieco, M. H., Gottlieb, M. S., Volberding, P. A., Laskin, O. L., Leedom, J. M., Groopman, J. E., Mildvan, D., Schooley, R. T., Jackson, G. G., Durack, D. T., Phil, D., King, D., and the AZT Collaborative Working Group (1987). New Engl. J. Med. 317, 185–191.

Fox, M. P., Otto, M. J., and McKinlay, M. A. (1986). Antimicrob. Agents Chemother. 30, 110–116.

Frank, K. B., Chiou, J.-F., and Cheng, Y.-C. (1984). J. Biol. Chem. 259, 1566–1569.

Freitas, V. R., Smee, D. F., Chernow, M., Boehme, R., and Matthews, T. R. (1985). Antimicrob. Agents Chemother. 28, 240–245.

Fukui, T., and De Clercq, E. (1982). Biochem. J. 203, 755–760.

Furman, P. A., St. Clair, M. H., Fyfe, J. A., Rideout, J. L., Keller, P. M., and Elion, G. B. (1979). J. Virol. 32, 72–77.

Furman, P. A., Fyfe, J. A., St. Clair, M. H., Weinhold, K., Rideout, J. L., Freeman, G. A., Nusinoff-Lehrman, S., Bolognesi, D. P., Broder, S., Mitsuya, H., and Barry, D. W. (1986). Proc. Natl. Acad. Sci. USA 83, 8333–8337.

Fyfe, J. A. (1982). Mol. Pharmacol. 21, 432–437.

Fyfe, J. A., Keller, P. M., Furman, P. A., Miller, R. L., and Elion, G. B. (1978). J. Biol. Chem. 253, 8721–8727.

Galasso, G. J. (1988). In "Clinical Use of Antiviral Drugs" (E. De Clercq, ed.) (in press). Klurver Academic Publishers, Norwell, Massachusetts.

Germershausen, J., Bostedor, R., Field, A. K., Perry, H., Liou, R., Bull, H., Tolman, R. L., and Karkas, J. D. (1983). Biochem. Biophys. Res. Commun. 116, 360–367.

Germershausen, J., Bostedor, R., Liou, R., Field, A. K., Wagner, A. F., MacCoss, M., Tolman, R. L., and Karkas, J. D. (1986). Antimicrob. Agents Chemother. 29, 1025–1031.

Gilbert, B. E., and Knight, V. (1986). Antimicrob. Agents Chemother. 30, 201–205.

Gilbert, B. E., Wilson, S. Z., Knight, V., Couch, R. B., Quarles, J. M., Dure, L., Hayes, N., and Willis, G. (1985). Antimicrob. Agents Chemother. 27, 309–313.

Gil-Fernándes, C., and De Clercq, E. (1987). Antiviral Res., 7, 151–160.

Glazer, R. I., Hartman, K. D., Knode, M. C., Richard, M. M., Chiang, P. K., Tseng, C. K. H., and Marquez, V. E. (1986a). Biochem. Biophys. Res. Commun. 135, 688–694.

Glazer, R. I., Knode, M. C., Tseng, C. K. H., Haines, D. R., and Marquez, V. E. (1986b). Biochem. Pharmacol. 35, 4523–4527.

Goodchild, J., Porter, R. A., Raper, R. H., Sim, I. S., Upton, R. M., Viney, J., and Wadsworth, H. J. (1983). J. Med. Chem. 26, 1252–1257.

Griengl, H., Bodenteich, M., Hayden, W., Wanek, E., Streicher, W., Stütz, P., Bachmayer, H., Ghazzouli, I., and Rosenwirth, B. (1985). J. Med. Chem. 28, 1679–1684.

Griengl, H., Wanek, E., Schwartz, W., Streicher, W., Rosenwirth, B., and De Clercq, E. (1987). J. Med. Chem. 30, 1199–1204.

Hall, C. B., McBride, J. T., Walsh, E. E., Bell, D. M., Gala, C. L., Hildreth, S., Ten Eyck, L. G., and Hall, W. J. (1983). New Engl. J. Med. 308, 1443–1447.

Hall, C. B., McBride, J. T., Gala, C. L., Hildreth, S. W., and Schnabel, K. C. (1985). J. Am. Med. Assoc. 254, 3047–3051.

Hamamoto, Y., Nakashima, H., Matsui, T., Matsuda, A., Ueda, T., and Yamamoto, N. (1987). Antimicrob. Agents Chemother. 31, 907–910.

Hartshorn, K. L., Sandstrom, E. G., Neumeyer, D., Paradis, T. J., Chou, T.-C., Schooley, R. T., and Hirsch, M. S. (1986). Antimicrob. Agents Chemother. 30, 189–191.

Hartshorn, K. L., Vogt, M. W., Chou, T.-C., Blumberg, R. S., Byington, R., Schooley, R. T., and Hirsch, M. S. (1987). Antimicrob. Agents Chemother. 31, 168–172.

Herdewijn, P., De Clercq, E., Balzarini, J., and Vanderhaeghe, H. (1985). J. Med. Chem. 28, 550–555.

Herdewijn, P., Balzarini, J., De Clercq, E., Pauwels, R., Baba, M., Broder, S., and Vanderhaeghe, H. (1987a). J. Med. Chem. 30, 1270–1278.

Herdewijn, P., Pauwels, R., Baba, M., Balzarini, J., and De Clercq, E. (1987b). J. Med. Chem. 30, 2131–2137.

Hilleman, M. R. (1987). In "Frontiers in Microbiology: From Antibiotics to AIDS" (E. De Clercq, ed.), pp. 185–196. Martinus Nijhoff Publishers, Dordrecht.

Ho, D. D., Hartshorn, K. L., Rota, T. R., Andrews, C. A., Kaplan, J. C., Schooley, R. T., and Hirsch, M. S. (1985). Lancet i, 602–604.

Ishitsuka, H., Ninomiya, Y. T., Ohsawa, C., Fujiu, M., and Suhara, Y. (1982). Antimicrob. Agents Chemother. 22, 617–621.

Ito, M., Baba, M., Sato, A., Pauwels, R., De Clercq, E., and Shigeta, S. (1987a). Antiviral Res. 7, 361–367.

Ito, M., Nakashima, H., Baba, M., Pauwels, R., De Clercq, E., Shigeta, S., and Yamamoto, N. (1987b). Antiviral Res. 7, 127–137.

Jayaram, H. N., Pillwein, K., Nichols, C. R., Hoffman, R., and Weber, G. (1986). Biochem. Pharmacol. 35, 2029–2032.

Jentsch, K. D., Hunsmann, G., Hartmann, H., and Nickel, P. (1987). J. Gen. Virol. 68, 2183–2192.

Karkas, J. D., Ashton, W. T., Canning, L. F., Liou, R., Germershausen, J., Bostedor, R., Arison, B., Field, A. K., and Tolman, R. L. (1986). *J. Med. Chem.* **29**, 842–848.

Kawana, F., Shigeta, S., Hosoya, M., Suzuki, H. and De Clercq, E. (1987). *Antimicrob. Agents Chemother.* **31**, 1225–1230.

Keller, B. T., and Borchardt, R. T. (1987). *Mol. Pharmacol.* **31**, 485–492.

Keller, B. T., and Borchardt, R. T. (1988). *In* "Antiviral Drug Development: A Multidisciplinary Approach" (E. De Clercq and R. T. Walker, eds) (in press). NATO ASI Series, Series A: Life Sciences. Plenum Press, New York and London.

Kim, C.-H., Marquez, V. E., Broder, S., Mitsuya, H., and Driscoll, J. S. (1987). *J. Med. Chem.* **30**, 862–866.

Kirsi, J. J., North, J. A., McKernan, P. A., Murray, B. K., Canonico, P. G., Huggins, J. W., Srivastava, P. C., and Robins, R. K. (1983). *Antimicrob. Agents Chemother.* **24**, 353–361.

Kit, S., Ichimura, H., and De Clercq, E. (1987a). *Antiviral Res.* **7**, 53–67.

Kit, S., Ichimura, H., and De Clercq, E. (1987b). *Antiviral Res.* **8**, 41–51.

Kitaoka, S., Konno, T., and De Clercq, E. (1986). *Antiviral Res.* **6**, 57–65.

Klintmalm, G., Lönnqvist, B., Öberg, B., Gahrton, G., Lernestedt, J.-O., Lundgren, G., Ringdén, O., Robert, K.-H., Wahren, B., and Groth, C.-G. (1985). *Scand. J. Infect. Dis.* **17**, 157–163.

Krenitsky, T. A., Hall, W. W., de Miranda, P., Beauchamp, L. M., Schaeffer, H. J., and Whiteman, P. D. (1984). *Proc. Natl. Acad. Sci. USA* **81**, 3209–3213.

Larder, B. A., and Darby, G. (1984). *Antiviral Res.* **4**, 1–42.

Larsson, A., Öberg, B., Alenius, S., Hagberg, C.-E., Johansson, N.-G., Lindborg, B., and Stening, G. (1983). *Antimicrob. Agents Chemother.* **23**, 664–670.

Larsson, A., Sundqvist, A., and Parnerud, A.-M. (1986). *Mol. Pharmacol.* **29**, 614–621.

Laskin, O. L., Stahl-Bayliss, C. M., Kalman, C. M., and Rosecan, L. R. (1987). *J. Infect. Dis.* **155**, 323–327.

Lin, J.-C., Smith, M. C., Cheng, Y.-C., and Pagano, J. S. (1983). *Science* **221**, 578–579.

Lin, J.-C., Smith, M. C., and Pagano, J. S. (1984). *J. Virol.* **50**, 50–55.

Lin, J.-C., Smith, M. C., and Pagano, J. S. (1985). *Antimicrob. Agents Chemother.* **27**, 971–973.

Lin, J.-C., De Clercq, E. and Pagano, J. S. (1987). *Antimicrob. Agents Chemother.* **31**, 1431–1433.

Lin, T.-S., Schinazi, R. F., Chen, M. S., Kinney-Thomas, E., and Prusoff, W. H. (1987). *Biochem. Pharmacol.* **36**, 311–316.

Lopez, C., Watanabe, K. A., and Fox, J. J. (1980). *Antimicrob. Agents Chemother.* **17**, 803–806.

Machida, H. (1986). *Antimicrob. Agents Chemother.* **29**, 524–526.

Mancini, W. R., De Clercq, E., and Prusoff, W. H. (1983). *J. Biol. Chem.* **258**, 792–795.

Mansuri, M. M., Ghazzouli, I., Chen, M. S., Howell, H. G., Brodfuehrer, P. R., Benigni, D. A., and Martin, J. C. (1987). *J. Med. Chem.* **30**, 867–871.

Mar, E.-C., Cheng, Y.-C., and Huang, E.-S. (1983). *Antimicrob. Agents Chemother.* **24**, 518–521.

Mar, E.-C., Patel, P. C., Cheng, Y.-C., Fox, J. J., Watanabe, K. A., and Huang, E.-S. (1984). *J. Gen. Virol.* **65**, 47–53.

Marquardt, H., Westendorf, J., De Clercq, E., and Marquardt, H. (1985). *Carcinogenesis* **6**, 1207–1209.

Martin, J. C., Dvorak, C. A., Smee, D. F., Matthews, T. R., and Verheyden, J. P. H. (1983). *J. Med. Chem.* **26**, 759–761.

Maudgal, P. C., and De Clercq, E. (1985). *Arch. Ophthalmol.* **103**, 1393–1397.

Maudgal, P. C., and De Clercq, E. (1988). *In* "Clinical Use of Antiviral Drugs" (E. De Clercq, ed.) (in press). Klurver Academic Publishers, Norwell, Massachusetts.

Maudgal, P. C., De Clercq, E., Descamps, J., and Missotten, L. (1984). *Arch. Ophthalmol.* **102**, 140–142.

Maudgal, P. C., De Clercq, E., and Huyghe, P. (1987). *Invest. Ophthalmol. Vis. Sci.* **28**, 243–248.

McCormick, J. B., Getchell, J. P., Mitchell, S. W., and Hicks, D. R. (1984). *Lancet* **ii**, 1367–1369.

McCormick, J. B., King, I. J., Webb, P. A., Scribner, C. L., Craven, R. B., Johnson, K. M., Elliott, L. H., and Belmont-Williams, R. (1986). *New Engl. J. Med.* **314**, 20–26.

McGuirt, P. V., Shaw, J. E., Elion, G. B., and Furman, P. A. (1984). *Antimicrob. Agents Chemother.* **25**, 507–509.

McKendrick, M. W., McGill, J. I., White, J. E., and Wood, M. J. (1986). *Br. Med. J.* **293**, 1529–1532.

McKinlay, M. A., and Steinberg, B. A. (1986). *Antimicrob. Agents Chemother.* **29**, 30–32.

McLaren, C., Chen, M. S., Barbhaiya, R. H., Buroker, R. A., and Oleson, F. B. (1985a). *In* "Herpes Viruses and Virus Chemotherapy" (R. Kono, ed.), pp. 57–61. Elsevier Science Publishers, Amsterdam.

McLaren, C., Chen, M. S., Ghazzouli, I., Saral, R., and Burns, W. H. (1985b). *Antimicrob. Agents Chemother.* **28**, 740–744.

McSharry, J. J., Caliguiri, L. A., and Eggers, H. J. (1979). *Virology* **97**, 307–315.

Miller, W. H., and Miller, R. L. (1980). *J. Biol. Chem.* **255**, 7204–7207.

Miller, W. H., and Miller, R. L. (1982). *Biochem. Pharmacol.* **31**, 3879–3884.

Mindel, A., Kinghorn, G., Allason-Jones, E., Woolley, P., Barton, I., Faherty, A., Jeavons, M., Williams, P., and Patou, G. (1987). *Lancet* **i**, 1171–1173.

Mitchell, W. M., Montefiori, D. C., Robinson, W. E. Jr., Strayer, D. R., and Carter, W. A. (1987). *Lancet* **i**, 890–892.

Mitsuya, H., and Broder, S. (1986). *Proc. Natl. Acad. Sci. USA* **83**, 1911–1915.

Mitsuya, H., and Broder, S. (1987). *Nature* **325**, 773–778.

Mitsuya, H., Popovic, M., Yarchoan, R., Matsushita, S., Gallo, R. C., and Broder, S. (1984). *Science* **226**, 172–174.

Mitsuya, H., Weinhold, K. J., Furman, P. A., St. Clair, M. H., Nusinoff-Lehrman, S., Gallo, R. C., Bolognesi, D., Barry, D. W., and Broder, S. (1985). *Proc. Natl. Acad. Sci. USA* **82**, 7096–7100.

Montgomery, J. A., Clayton, S. J., Thomas, H. J., Shannon, W. M., Arnett, G., Bodner, A. J., Kim, I.-K., Cantoni, G. L., and Chiang, P. K. (1982). *J. Med. Chem.* **25**, 626–629.

Müller, W. E. G., Sobel, C., Diehl-Seifert, B., Maidhof, A., and Schröder, H. C. (1987). *Biochem. Pharmacol.* **36**, 1489–1494.

Nakashima, H., Matsui, T., Harada, S., Kobayashi, N., Matsuda, A., Ueda, T., and Yamamoto, N. (1986). *Antimicrob. Agents Chemother.* **30**, 933–937.

Ninomiya, Y., Ohsawa, C., Aoyama, M., Umeda, I., Suhara, Y., and Ishitsuka, H. (1984). *Virology* **134**, 269–276.

Öberg, B. (1983). *Pharmac. Ther.* **19**, 387–415.

Öberg, B., Behrnetz, S., Eriksson, B., Jozwiak, H., Larsson, A., Lernestedt, J. O. and Lindsö Åberg, V. (1988), *in* "Clinical Use of Antiviral Drugs" (E. De Clercq, ed.) (in press). Klurver Academic Publishers, Norwell, Massachusetts.

Ohnuma, T., Roboz, J., Shapiro, M. L., and Holland, J. F. (1977). *Cancer Res.* **37**, 2043–2049.

Ono, K., Ogasawara, M., Iwata, Y., Nakane, H., Fujii, T., Sawai, K., and Saneyoshi, M. (1986). *Biochem. Biophys. Res. Commun.* **140**, 498–507.

Osterhaus, A. D. M. E., Groen, J., and De Clercq, E. (1987). *Antiviral Res.* **7**, 221–226.

Ostertag, W., Roesler, G., Krieg, C. J., Kind, J., Cole, T., Crozier, T., Gaedicke, G., Steinheider, G., Kluge, N., and Dube, S. (1974). *Proc. Natl. Acad. Sci. USA* **71**, 4980–4985.

Otto, M. J., Fox, M. P., Fancher, M. J., Kuhrt, M. F., Diana, G. D., and McKinlay, M. A. (1985). *Antimicrob. Agents Chemother.* **27**, 883–886.

Pelling, J. C., Drach, J. C., and Shipman, C. Jr. (1981). *Virology* **109**, 323–335.

Perlman, M. E., Watanabe, K. A., Schinazi, R. F., and Fox, J. J. (1985). *J. Med. Chem.* **28**, 741–748.

Pert, C. B., Hill, J. M., Ruff, M. R., Berman, R. M., Robey, W. G., Arthur, L. O., Ruscetti, F. W., and Farrar, W. L. (1986). *Proc. Natl. Acad. Sci. USA* **83**, 9254–9258.

Petrie III, C. R., Revankar, G. R., Dalley, N. K., George, R. D., McKernan, P. A., Hamill, R. L., and Robins, R. K. (1986). *J. Med. Chem.* **29**, 268–278.

Phillpotts, R. J., Wallace, J., Tyrrell, D. A. J., Freestone, D. S., and Shepherd, W. M. (1983). *Arch. Virol.* **75**, 115–121.

Pompei, R., Flore, O., Marccialis, M. A., Pani, A., and Loddo, B. (1979). *Nature* **281**, 689–690.

Pompidou, A., Zagury, D., Gallo, R. C., Sun, D., Thornton, A., and Sarin, P. S. (1985). *Lancet* ii, 1423.

Prisbe, E. J., Martin, J. C., McGee, D. P. C., Barker, M. F., Smee, D. F., Duke, A. E., Matthews, T. R., and Verheyden, J. P. H. (1986). *J. Med. Chem.* **29**, 671–675.

Revankar, G.R., Gupta, P. K., Adams, A. D., Dalley, N. K., McKernan, P. A., Cook, P. D., Canonico, P. G., and Robins, R. K. (1984). *J. Med. Chem.* **27**, 1389–1396.

Richman, D. D., Fischl, M. A., Grieco, M. H., Gottlieb, M. S., Volberding, P. A., Laskin, O. L., Leedom, J. M., Groopman, J. E., Mildvan, D., Hirsch, M. S., Jackson, G. G., Durack, D. T., Phil, D., Nusinoff-Lehrman, S., and the AZT Collaborative Working Group (1987). *New Engl. J. Med.* **317**, 192–197.

Rosenwirth, B., Griengl, H., Wanek, E., and De Clercq, E. (1985). *Antiviral Res.*, Suppl. 1, 21–28.

Rosenwirth, B., Streicher, W., De Clercq, E., Wanek, E., Schwarz, W., and Griengl, H. (1987). *Antiviral Res.* **7**, 271–287.

Rossmann, M. G., Arnold, E., Griffith, J. P., Kamer, G., Luo, M., Smith, T. J., Vriend, G., Rueckert, R. R., Sherry, B., McKinlay, M. A., Diana, G., and Otto, M. (1987). *Trends Biochem. Sci. (TIBS)* **12**, 313–318.

Rozenbaum, W., Dormont, D., Spire, B., Vilmer, E., Gentilini, M., Griscelli, C., Montagnier, L., Barré-Sinoussi, F., and Chermann, J. C. (1985). *Lancet* i, 450–451.

Ruff, M. R., Martin, B. M., Ginns, E. I., Farrar, W. L., and Pert, C. B. (1987). *FEBS Lett.* **211**, 17–22.

Ruprecht, R. M., Rossoni, L. D., Haseltine, W. A., and Broder, S. (1985). *Proc. Natl. Acad. Sci. USA* **82**, 7733–7737.

Ruprecht, R. M., O'Brien, L. G., Rossoni, L. D., and Nusinoff-Lehrman, S. (1986). *Nature* **323**, 467–469.

Ruth, J. L., and Cheng, Y.-C. (1981). *Mol. Pharmacol.* **20**, 415–422.

Sági, J., Czuppon, A., Kajtár, M., Szabolcs, A., Szemzö, A., and Ötvös, L. (1982). *Nucleic Acids Res.* **10**, 6051–6066.

Sági, J., De Clercq, E., Szemzö, A., Csárnyi, A. H., Kovács, T. and Ötvös, L. (1987). *Biochem. Biophys. Res. Commun.* **147**, 1105–1112.

Sandstrom, E. G., Kaplan, J. C., Byington, R. E., and Hirsch, M. S. (1985). *Lancet* i, 1480–1482.

Sarin, P. S., Gallo, R. C., Scheer, D. I., Crews, F., and Lappa, A. S. (1985a). *New Engl. J. Med.* **313**, 1289–1290.

Sarin, P. S., Taguchi, Y., Sun, D., Thornton, A., Gallo, R. C., and Öberg, B. (1985b). *Biochem. Pharmacol.* **34**, 4075–4079.

Schaffer, C. P., Plescia, O. J., Pontani, D., Sun, D., Thornton, A., Pandey, R. C., and Sarin, P. S. (1986). *Biochem. Pharmacol.* **35**, 4110–4113.

Schinazi, R. F., Peters, J., Sokol, M. K., and Nahmias, A. J. (1983). *Antimicrob. Agents Chemother.* **24**, 95–103.

Schinazi, R. F., Scott, R. T., Peters, J., Rice, V., and Nahmias, A. J. (1985). *Antimicrob. Agents Chemother.* **28**, 552–560.

Schinazi, R. F., del Bene, V., Scott, R. T., and Dudley-Thorpe, J.-B. (1986). *J. Antimicrob. Chemother.* **18**, Suppl. B, 127–134.

Schwartz, J., Ostrander, M., Butkiewicz, N. B., Lieberman, M., Lin, C., Lim, J., and Miller, G. H. (1987). *Antimicrob. Agents Chemother.* **31**, 21–26.

Selby, P., Powles, R. L., Blake, S., Stolle, K., Mbidde, E. K., McElwain, T. J., Hickmott, E., Whiteman, P. D., and Fiddian, A. P. (1984). *Lancet* **ii**, 1428–1430.

Shannon, W. M. (1977). *Ann. N.Y. Acad. Sci.* **284**, 472–507.

Shannon, W. M., Westbrook, L., Arnett, G., Daluge, S., Lee, H., and Vince, R. (1983). *Antimicrob. Agents Chemother.* **24**, 538–543.

Shaw, M., King, M., Best, J. M., Banatvala, J. E., Gibson, J. R., and Klaber, M. R. (1985). *Br. Med. J.* **291**, 7–9.

Shealy, Y. F., O'Dell, C. A., Shannon, W. M., and Arnett, G. (1983). *J. Med. Chem.* **26**, 156–161.

Shealy, Y. F., O'Dell, C. A., Arnett, G., and Shannon, W. M. (1986). *J. Med. Chem.* **29**, 79–84.

Shepp, D. H., Dandliker, P. S., de Miranda, P., Burnette, T. C., Cederberg, D. M., Kirk, L. E., and Meyers, J. D. (1985). *Ann. Intern. Med.* **103**, 368–373.

Shepp, D. H., Dandliker, P. S., and Meyers, J. D. (1986). *New Engl. J. Med.* **314**, 208–212.

Sherker, A. H., Hirota, K., Omata, M., and Okuda, K. (1986). *Gastroenterology* **91**, 818–824.

Shigeta, S., Yokota, T., Iwabuchi, T., Baba, M., Konno, K., Ogata, M., and De Clercq, E. (1983). *J. Infect. Dis.* **147**, 576–584.

Shigeta, S., Konno, K., Yokota, T., Nakamura, K., and De Clercq, E. (1988). *Antimicrob. Agents Chemother.* Submitted.

Shiota, H., Naito, T., and Mimura, Y. (1987). *Current Eye Res.* **6**, 241–245.

Sibrack, C. D., Gutman, L. T., Wilfert, C. M., McLaren, C., St. Clair, M. H., Keller, P. M., and Barry, D. W. (1982). *J. Infect. Dis.* **146**, 673–682.

Sidwell, R. W., Huffman, J. H., Khare, G. P., Allen, L. B., Witkowski, J. T., and Robins, R. K. (1972). *Science* **177**, 705–706.

Sidwell, R. W., Huffman, J. H., Call, E. W., Alaghamandan, H., Cook, P. D., and Robins, R. K. (1986). *Antiviral Res.* **6**, 343–353.

Sköldenberg, B., Forsgren, M., Alestig, K., Bergström, T., Burman, L., Dahlqvist, E., Forkman, A., Frydén, A., Lövgren, K., Norlin, K., Norrby, R., Olding-Stenkvist, E., Stiernstedt, G., Uhnoo, I., and de Vahl, K. (1984). *Lancet* **ii**, 707–711.

Smee, D. F., Martin, J. C., Verheyden, J. P. H., and Matthews, T. R. (1983). *Antimicrob. Agents Chemother.* **23**, 676–682.

Smee, D. F., Boehme, R., Chernow, M., Binko, B. P., and Matthews, T. R. (1985). *Biochem. Pharmacol.* **34**, 1049–1056.

Smith, K. O., Galloway, K. S., Kennell, W. L., Ogilvie, K. K., and Radatus, B. K. (1982). *Antimicrob. Agents Chemother.* **22**, 55–61.

Smith, R. A. (1980). *In* "Ribavirin: A Broad Spectrum of Antiviral Agent", pp. 99–119. Academic Press, New York.

Smith, T. J., Kremer, M. J., Luo, M., Vriend, G., Arnold, E., Kamer, G., Rossmann, M. G., McKinlay, M. A., Diana, G. D., and Otto, M. J. (1986). *Science* **233**, 1286–1293.

Soike, K. F., Gibson, S., and Gerone, P. J. (1981). *Antiviral Res.* **1**, 325–337.

Soike, K. F., Baskin, G., Cantrell, C., and Gerone, P. (1984). *Antiviral Res.* **4**, 245–257.

Soike, K. F., Cantrell, C., and Gerone, P. J. (1986). *Antimicrob. Agents Chemother.* **29**, 20–25.

Spruance, S. L., Crumpacker, C. S., Haines, H., Bader, C., Mehr, K., MacCalman, J.,

Schnipper, L. E., Klauber, M. R., Overall, J. C. Jr., and the Collaborative Study Group (1979). *New Engl. J. Med.* **300**, 1180–1184.

Spruance, S. L., Freeman, D. J., and Sheth, N. V. (1985). *Antimicrob. Agents Chemother.* **28**, 103–106.

Spruance, S. L., Freeman, D. J., and Sheth, N. V. (1986). *Antimicrob. Agents Chemother.* **30**, 196–198.

St. Clair, M. H., Furman, P. A., Lubbers, C. M., and Elion, G. B. (1980). *Antimicrob. Agents Chemother.* **18**, 741–745.

St. Clair, M. H., Miller, W. H., Miller, R. L., Lambe, C. U., and Furman, P. A. (1984). *Antimicrob. Agents Chemother.* **25**, 191–194.

Stenberg, K., Larsson, A., and Datema, R. (1986). *J. Biol. Chem.* **261**, 2134–2139.

Straus, S. E., Takiff, H. E., Seidlin, M., Bachrach, S., Lininger, L., DiGiovanna, J. J., Western, K. A., Smith, H. A., Nusinoff Lehrman, S., Creagh-Kirk, T., and Alling, D. W. (1984). *New Engl. J. Med.* **310**, 1545–1550.

Su, T.-L., Watanabe, K. A., Schinazi, R. F., and Fox, J. J. (1986). *J. Med. Chem.* **29**, 151–154.

Sundquist, B., and Öberg, B. (1979). *J. Gen. Virol.* **45**, 273–281.

Tavares, L., Ronecker, C., Johnston, K., Nusinoff Lehrman, S., and de Noronha, F. (1987). *Cancer Res.* **47**, 3190–3194.

Tisdale, M., and Selway, J. W. T. (1983). *J. Gen. Virol.* **64**, 795–803.

Tocci, M. J., Livelli, T. J., Perry, H. C., Crumpacker, C. S., and Field, A. K. (1984). *Antimicrob. Agents Chemother.* **25**, 247–252.

Tolman, R. L., Field, A. K., Karkas, J. D., Wagner, A. F., Germershausen, J., Crumpacker, C., and Scolnick, E. M. (1985). *Biochem. Biophys. Res. Commun.* **128**, 1329–1335.

Tricot, G., De Clercq, E., Boogaerts, M. A., and Verwilghen, R. L. (1986). *J. Med. Virol.* **18**, 11–20.

Ueno, R., and Kuno, S. (1987). *Lancet* **i**, 1379.

Vilde, J. L., Bricaire, F., Huchon, A., and Brun-Vezinet, F. (1983). *J. Med. Virol.* **12**, 149–153.

Vince, R., and Daluge, S. (1977). *J. Med. Chem.* **20**, 612–613.

Vince, R., Daluge, S., Lee, H., Shannon, W. M., Arnett, G., Schater, T. W., Nagabhushan, T. L., Reichert, P., and Tsai, H. (1983). *Science* **221**, 1405–1406.

Vinckier, F., Boogaerts, M., Declerck, D., and De Clercq, E. (1987). *J. Oral Maxillofacial Surgery* **45**, 723–728.

Vogt, M. W., Hartshorn, K. L., Furman, P. A., Chou, T.-C., Fyfe, J. A., Coleman, L. A., Crumpacker, C., Schooley, R. T., and Hirsch, M. S. (1987). *Science* **235**, 1376–1379.

Votruba, I., Bernaerts, R., Sakuma, T., De Clercq, E., Merta, A., Rosenberg, I., and Holý, A. (1987). *Mol. Pharmacol.* **32**, 524–529.

Vrang, L., and Öberg, B. (1986). *Antimicrob. Agents Chemother.* **29**, 867–872.

Vrang, L., Bazin, H., Remaud, G., Chattopadhyaya, J., and Öberg, B. (1987). *Antiviral Res.* **7**, 139–149.

Wade, J. C., McLaren, C., and Meyers, J. D. (1983). *J. Infect. Dis.* **148**, 1077–1082.

Wahren, B., Larsson, A., Rudén, U., Sundqvist, A. and Sølver, E. (1987). *Antimicrob. Agents Chemother.* **31**, 317–320.

Wallin, J., Lernestedt, J.-O., Ogenstad, S., and Lycke, E. (1985). *Scand. J. Infect. Dis.* **17**, 165–172.

Waqar, M. A., Evans, M. J., Manly, K. F., Hughes, R. G., and Huberman, J. A. (1984). *J. Cell. Physiol.* **121**, 402–408.

Watanabe, K. A., Reichman, U., Hirota, K., Lopez, C., and Fox, J. J. (1979). *J. Med. Chem.* **22**, 21–24.

Watanabe, K. A., Su, T.-L., Klein, R. S., Chu, C. K., Matsuda, A., Chun, M. W., Lopez, C., and Fox, J. J. (1983). *J. Med. Chem.* **26**, 152–156.

Watanabe, K. A., Su, T.-S., Reichman, U., Greenberg, N., Lopez, C., and Fox, J. J. (1984). *J. Med. Chem.* **27**, 91–94.

Whiteman, P. D., Bye, A., Fowle, A. S. E., Jeal, S., Land, G., and Posner, J. (1984). *Eur. J. Clin. Pharmacol.* **27**, 471–475.

Whitley, R. J., Ch'ien, L. T., Dolin, R., Galasso, G. J., Alford, C. A. Jr., and the Collaborative Study Group (1976). *New Engl. J. Med.* **294**, 1193–1199.

Whitley, R. J., Soong, S.-J., Dolin, R., Galasso, G. J., Ch'ien, L. T., Alford, C. A., and the Collaborative Study Group (1977). *New Engl. J. Med.* **297**, 289–294.

Whitley, R. J., Soong, S.-J., Hirsch, M. S., Karchmer, A. W., Dolin, R., Galasso, G., Dunnick, J. K., Alford, C. A., and the NIAID Collaborative Antiviral Study Group (1981). *New Engl. J. Med.* **304**, 313–318.

Whitley, R. J., Soong, S.-J., Dolin, R., Betts, R., Linnemann, C. Jr., Alford, C. A., and the NIAID Collaborative Antiviral Study Group (1982). *New Engl. J. Med.* **307**, 971–975.

Whitley, R. J., Alford, C. A., Hirsch, M. S., Schooley, R. T., Luby, J. P., Aoki, F. Y., Hanley, D., Nahmias, A. J., Soong, S.-J., and the NIAID Collaborative Antiviral Study Group (1986). *New Engl. J. Med.* **314**, 144–149.

Wildiers, J., and De Clercq, E. (1984). *Eur. J. Cancer Clin. Oncol.* **20**, 471–476.

Worzalla, J. F., and Sweeney, M. J. (1980). *Cancer Res.* **40**, 1482–1485.

Yang, S. S., Herrera, F. M., Smith, R. G., Reitz, M. S., Lancini, G., Ting, R. C., and Gallo, R. C. (1972). *J. Natl. Cancer Inst.* **49**, 7–25.

Yarchoan, R., Klecker, R. W., Weinhold, K. J., Markham, P. D., Lyerly, H. K., Durack, D. T., Gelmann, E., Nusinoff Lehrman, S., Blum, R. M., Barry, D. W., Shearer, G. M., Fischl, M. A., Mitsuya, H., Gallo, R. C., Collins, J. M., Bolognesi, D. P., Myers, C. E., and Broder, S. (1986). *Lancet* **i**, 575–580.

Yarchoan, R., Berg, G., Brouwers, P., Fischl, M. A., Spitzer, A. R., Wichman, A., Grafman, J., Thomas, R. V., Safai, B., Brunetti, A., Perno, C. F., Schmidt, P. J., Larson, S. M., Myers, C. E., and Broder, S. (1987). *Lancet* **i**, 132–135.

Young, C. W., Schneider, R., Leyland-Jones, B., Armstrong, D., Tan, C. T. C., Lopez, C., Watanabe, K. A., Fox, J. J., and Philips, F. S. (1983). *Cancer Res.* **43**, 5006–5009.

Zerial, A., Werner, G. H., Phillpotts, R. J., Willmann, J. S., Higgins, P. G., and Tyrrell, D. A. J. (1985). *Antimicrob. Agents Chemother.* **27**, 846–850.

Recent Developments in the Field of Cephem Antibiotics

WALTER DÜRCKHEIMER, FRIEDHELM ADAM, GERD FISCHER
and REINER KIRRSTETTER

Pharma-Synthese, Hoechst AG, Frankfurt/Main 80, FRG

Dedicated to Professor Dr. Wilhelm Bartmann on the occasion of his 60th birthday

ADVANCES IN DRUG RESEARCH, VOL. 17
ISBN 0-12-013317-2

The following abbreviations are used in this article: Ac, acetyl; 7-ACA, 7-aminocephalosporanic acid; 7-ADCA, 7-aminodeacetoxycephalosporanic acid; 6-APA, 6-aminopenicillanic acid; AUC, area under the curve; BH, benzhydryl; Boc, *tert*-butoxycarbonyl; Bu, butyl; Bz, benzyl; CNS, central nervous system; CSF, cerebrospinal fluid; DAC, deacetylcephalosporin C_1 DBU, 1,8-diazabicyclo[5.4.0]undec-7-ene; DCC, dicyclohexylcarbodiimide; DMF, dimethylformamide; DMSO, dimethylsulphoxide; Et, ethyl; h, hour, hours; HPLC, high pressure liquid chromatography; i.m., intramuscular; i.v., intravenous; LDA, lithium di-isopropylamide; LLD-ACV, (L-α-aminoadipoyl)-L-cysteinyl-D-valine; MBC, minimal bactericidal concentration; MCPBA, m-chloroperbenzoic acid; Me, methyl; MIC, minimal inhibitory concentration; MRS, methicillin-resistant Staphylococci; Ms, methanesulphonyl; Nu, nucleophile; PBP, penicillin-binding protein; Ph, phenyl; Phth, phthalimido; PNB, *p*-nitrobenzyl; r.t., room temperature; SAR, structure–activity relationships; s.c., subcutaneous; t, tertiary; TCE, trichloroethyl; TEA, triethylamine; Tet, 1-methyltetrazol-5-yl; TFA, trifluoroacetic acid; THF, tetrahydrofuran; TMSCl, trimethylsilyl chloride; Ts, toluenesulphonyl; UR, urinary recovery.

1 Introduction

The number of natural and synthetic antibiotics is increasing year by year. This tendency will continue. More than 6000 natural antibiotics have been discovered so far (Omura, 1986) and the number of semisynthetic variations is in the order of tens of thousands. A few classes dominate the market: β-lactams, tetracyclines, aminoglycosides and macrolides. The β-lactam family of antibiotics played a dominant role from their introduction in the 1940s and had a tremendous impact on public health and chemotherapeutic research due to their high selectivity, great safety, low toxicity and unique

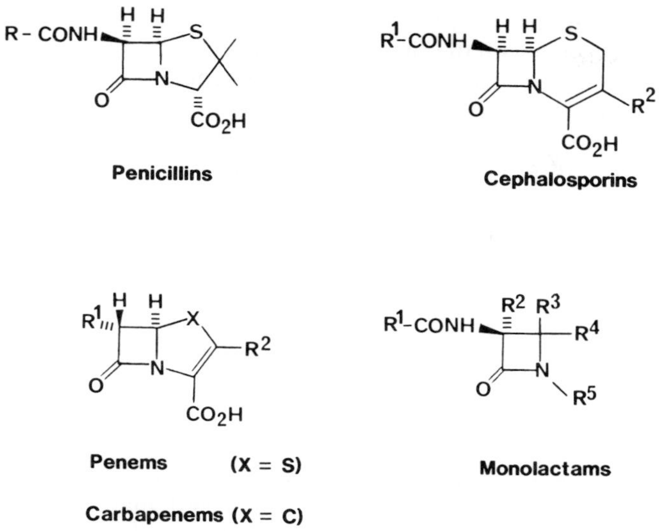

R-CONH— S / CO₂H

Penicillins

R¹-CONH— S / R² CO₂H

Cephalosporins

R¹— X / R² CO₂H

Penems (X = S)

Carbapenems (X = C)

R¹-CONH— R² R³ / R⁴ / R⁵

Monolactams

FIG. 1. Basic structures of important categories of β-lactam antibiotics.

versatility. Currently β-lactams account for about 60% of the total antibiotic market. The β-lactam family is divided into five main groups according to their basic ring structures: penicillins, cephalosporins, penems, carbapenems and monolactams (Fig. 1). Semisynthetic cephalosporins, often more simply marked as cephems, gained outstanding clinical importance during the last decade and are worldwide the dominating and fastest growing group among β-lactams. Pharmaceutical research has made considerable efforts in developing derivatives which improved antibacterial activity and extended the spectrum in such a way that pathogens which are resistant to the older antibiotics of different structural types are inhibited by the new cephalosporins. Moreover, the pharmacokinetic properties and the β-lactamase stability were improved; adverse reactions were reduced as well. Three generations of cephalosporins are already on the market and many more derivatives are in extended evaluation or are about to be released.

This review attempts to summarize the biosynthesis, chemistry, biological activity and mode of action of cephem antibiotics and related structures, focusing on derivatives that have recently gained significance in clinical practice or are now being clinically tested. Structures made by semi- or total synthesis that might point the route for further developments or have been of interest in connection with SAR investigations are also presented. Due to the limitless amount of literature the chapter is mainly based on a selection of recent publications. There are already a number of detailed monographs and reviews, dealing with the chemistry, antibacterial activity, biosynthesis, microbiology and mechanism of action of cephem antibiotics. Many references in this chapter give detailed lists of review articles and newer original research papers that the reader can use as a guide for more detailed studies. Yearly updates of the current literature available up to 1986 (Dunn, 1986) are given in the Annual Reports in Medicinal Chemistry. Very recently, a special issue on several topics of cephalosporins has been published (Drugs, 1987).

2 General Aspects and Characteristics

2.1 NOMENCLATURE

The parent structure of cephalosporins consists of a bicyclic β-lactam-Δ^3-dihydrothiazine ring system designated in a semisystematic nomenclature as 3-cephem. The corresponding ring system without a double bond is called cepham. Figure 2 gives the nomenclature and numbering of the skeleton. Names that are followed by a star apply to the compounds with the indicated double bond in the six-membered ring. Most cephalosporins are acyl-derivatives of 7-amino-3-acetoxymethyl-3-cephem-4-carboxylic acid which is also called 7-aminocephalosporanic acid (7-ACA). 7-ACA is the most important starting material for semisynthetic cephalosporins and prepared by chemical cleavage of cephalosporin C.

When the cephem ring is substituted with a 7-methoxy group, the resultant 7-methoxycephalosporin is called a cephamycin because natural β-lactams of this structural type were first named this way. Correspondingly natural 7-formylamidocephalosporins are called chitinovorins. 1-Oxacephems and 1-carbacephems have been coined to define the ring system in which an oxygen or a —CH_2— unit replaces the sulphur of a cephem ring. Other nuclear analogues are designated similarly. A systematic nomenclature for cephalosporins is necessary to define a compound more precisely, especially for chemical and patent purposes. The systematic names for the 3-cephems and 1-oxa and 1-carba analogues are also given in Fig. 2. They are generally avoided because of their complexity.

2.2 CLASSIFICATION

Several attempts have been made to subdivide the cephalosporins into various generations based upon stability to β-lactamases, potency, anti-

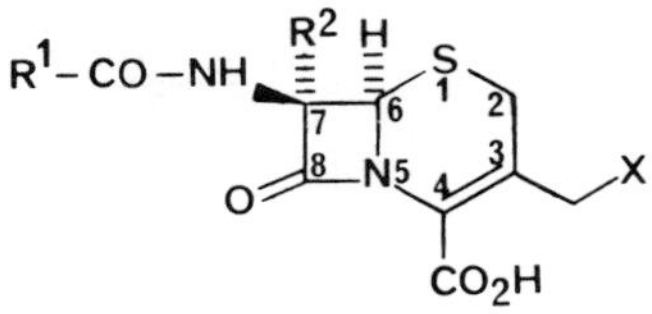

Cephalosporins: R^2 = H (1945)

Cephamycins: R^2 = OCH$_3$ (1971)

Chitinovorins: R^2 = NHCHO (1984)

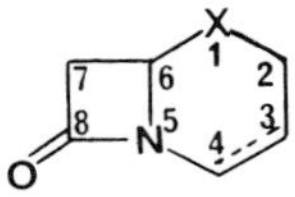

X = S   Cepham,   3-Cephem*

X = O   1-Oxacepham, 1-Oxacephem*

X = CH$_2$ 1-Carbacepham , 1-Carba-3-cephem*

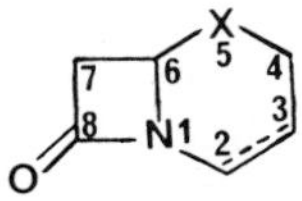

X = S   5-Thia-1-azabicyclo [4.2.0] octan-8-one
           5-Thia-1-azabicyclo [4.2.0] oct-2-en-8-one*

X = O   5-Oxa-1-azabicyclo [4.2.0] octan-8-one
          5-Oxa-1-azabicyclo [4.2.0] oct-2-en-8-one*

X = CH$_2$ 1-Azabicyclo [4.2.0] oct-2-en-8-one
          1-Azabicyclo [4.2.0] oct-2-en-8-one*

FIG. 2. Nomenclature and numbering of β-lactam skeletons. Names that are followed by an asterisk refer to the compounds with the indicated double bond in the six-membered ring.

bacterial spectrum and pharmacological properties. No classification whatsoever has been generally accepted. A comparison of different classifications
which are relatively arbitrary, and sometimes made more on a commercial
than a scientific basis, has been published by Kühn and Zimmermann
(1986). For practical reasons a simple subdivision into oral agents and
parenteral agents is justified. A more detailed classification in terms of
generations has proved to be suitable. First generation parenteral cephalosporins, e.g. cephalothin or cefazolin, possess reasonable activity against
Gram-positive bacteria, but a relatively narrow spectrum against Gram-
negative species due to their lability to β-lactamases. All older oral cephalosporins, e.g. cephalexin and related glycylcephalosporins, belong to the first
generation.

Second generation cephalosporins, e.g. cefamandole and cefuroxime,
generally possess enhanced activity against *Haemophilus influenzae* and a
number of Enterobacteriaceae due to their better β-lactamase stability, but
this has often compromised their potency against Gram-positive bacteria.
The cephamycins (7-methoxycephalosporins), e.g. cefoxitin and cefotetan,
resemble second generation cephalosporins but possess, due to their excellent β-lactamase stability, a pronounced activity against *Bacteroides fragilis*.

Third generation cephalosporins, e.g. cefotaxime (**207**), ceftazidime (**266**)
and cefoperazone (**244**), have several important advantages over both the
first and second generation cephalosporins and many previous penicillins.
They exhibit a broader spectrum of activity, especially against Enterobacteriaceae, *Pseudomonas aeruginosa* and *Acinetobacter* spp. They exhibit
increased resistance to most plasmid- and chromosomally-mediated β-
lactamases. Third generation cephalosporins are inferior to first generation
agents in respect to Gram-positive bacteria and, like all other cephalosporins, are inactive against methicillin-resistant Staphylococci.

Cefpirome (HR-810) (**220**) and cefepime (BMY-28 142) (**221**) have been
recently classified as fourth generation cephalosporins because of their
surpassing activity against Enterobacteriaceae and enhanced activity against
Ps. aeruginosa (Amsterdam *et al.*, 1985).

2.3 STRUCTURE AND BIOLOGICAL ACTIVITY

The antibiotic activity of cephalosporins not only depends on the high
reactivity of the β-lactam ring, but is also strongly influenced by the nature
of the peripheral substituents and their spatial relationships. They potentiate
antimicrobial properties by providing additional affinity for the bacterial
targets, by imparting β-lactamase stability, by altering the permeability and
by changing the pharmacokinetics.

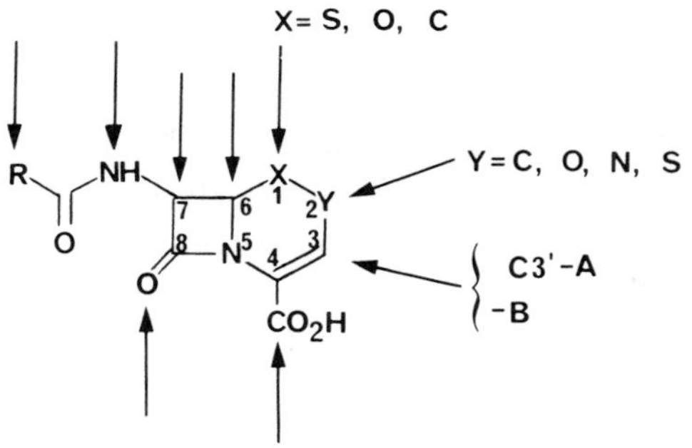

FIG. 3. Structural variations of the cephem skeleton. The numbered arrows indicate the positions of modification.

Major chemical variations around and within the cephalosporin nucleus are portrayed in Fig. 3. Exceptional importance for antibacterial activity is attributed to the 7β-acylamino side chain, the nature and spatial orientation of the substituents being contributory factors. Aromatically and hetero-aromatically substituted acetic acid residues with polar substituents, e.g. hydroxy, carboxy, sulpho, ureido and oxyimino, proved to be particularly advantageous. Secondly, the substituents at C-3 (B in Fig. 3) or C-3' (A in Fig. 3) are extensively variable and affect antibacterial activity, metabolic stability, pharmacokinetics and adverse effects. C-2 has been substituted with the possibility of α- or β-isomers. Substitution at C-7 strongly influenced β-lactamase stability and binding to PBPs. The carboxylic function at C-4 has been the site of transformations to esters, prodrug esters, aldehyde-, alcohol-, tetrazolyl- and acyl derivatives or homologous and vinylogous carboxylic derivatives.

Many studies on nuclear analogues have been carried out with the hope of discovering more potent antibacterial agents and furthering knowledge about structure–activity relationships (SAR). Modification of the nuclear skeleton will alter the molecular geometry and the reactivity of the β-lactam ring and consequently the affinity to the target enzymes. The most interesting modifications concern the sulphur at atom 1, which can be replaced by oxygen or a —CH$_2$— unit or be moved to the C-2 position. These and other variations are discussed in the section on nuclear analogues (Section 4.2).

Structure-activity relationship studies in different series of cephalosporins have been made and are entirely empirical. They are mostly centred around *in vitro* parameters such as, for example, the minimal inhibitory concentration (MIC), the minimal bactericidal concentration (MBC), and the relative β-lactamase stability. A direct comparison of MIC-values from one laboratory to the other is inadvisable, because *in vitro* test results vary from study to study and are strongly influenced by the test methodology, the size of the inoculum and the number and sensitivity of organisms. A single parameter is almost useless for a critical evaluation. Furthermore, laboratory test results may not correlate with clinical results which may be better or worse than would be expected on the basis of *in vitro* tests. The main reasons for this lie in important differences of cephalosporins in clinicopharmacological parameters and in their complex, not fully understood interactions with the causative microorganisms and the infected host. *In vitro* comparisons for many cephalosporin derivatives have been reviewed, e.g. in monographs edited by Perlman (1977), Salton and Shockman (1981), Morin and Gorman (1982), Neu (1982d), Brown and Roberts (1985), Sykes *et al.* (1985), Thornsberry (1985) and Peterson and Verhoef (1986).

The *in vitro* activity of a number of representative oral and parenteral cephalosporins and nuclear analogues are listed in Table 1. This table includes examples of all generations which are either in clinical use or have been developed to a stage sufficient for a microbiological and pharmacokinetic evaluation. The often used classification of the *in vitro* activity against Gram-positive or Gram-negative bacteria and β-lactamase stability is only a rough synoptic guide, as many bacterial species show wide variations in their MICs. Some species said to be resistant may include sensitive strains. More detailed microbiological data for individual drugs will be given later, but a full description of antibacterial spectra of cephalosporins is far beyond the scope of this review because a bewildering number of papers on microbiological data has been published.

With the introduction of second and third generation cephalosporins there has been progress in respect to higher activity against Gram-negative bacteria and broader spectrum together with high β-lactamase stability. An opposite trend has been a decrease of activity against *Staphylococcus aureus* compared to first generation cephalosporins. A typical example is ceftazidime (**266**), which is the best cephalosporin against *Ps. aeruginosa*, but is 10- to 100-fold less active than cephalothin and cephaloridine against Staphylococci and Streptococci (Knothe and Dette, 1981; Phillips *et al.*, 1981). Only in the series of quaternary ammonio cephalosporins, some betain-like derivatives, e.g. cefpirome (**220**), have MICs against *Staph. aureus* comparable to cephalothin. Methicillin-resistant Staphylococci (MRS) and *Streptococcus faecalis* are not sufficiently susceptible to cephalosporins. A similar situation exists toward anaerobic bacteria, especially β-lactamase-forming Gram-negative anaerobes including the *B. fragilis* group. This is a major distinguishing factor between the rather labile aminothiazole cephalosporins and the highly stable 7-methoxycephalosporins (cephamycins) and 7-methoxy-1-oxacephems (Sykes *et al.*, 1985).

TABLE 1

Comparative *in vitro* antibacterial activities of representative oral and parenteral cephalosporins (modified from Kühn and Zimmermann, 1986). The asterisk indicates that the *in vitro* activity of the parent compound cefteram is given

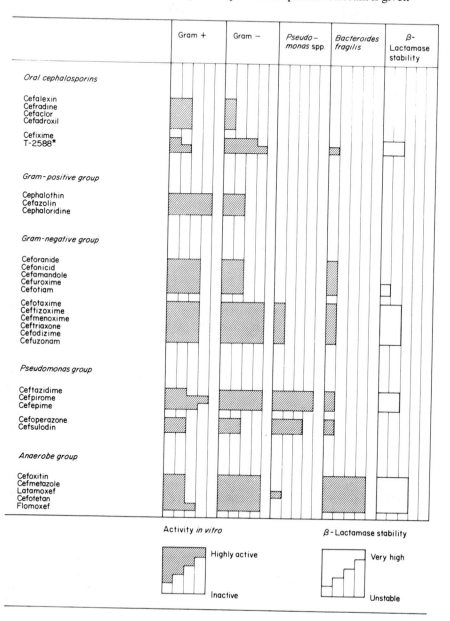

Most compounds with favourable broad spectrum activity are not orally absorbed. Factors affecting enteral absorption are not well understood. Major improvements have been achieved by preparation of prodrugs of parenteral cephalosporins with increased lipophilicity, adjusted acid stability and rapid cleavage by enzymes in the intestinal lumen and blood. Structural parameters which determine such properties are discussed in Section 5.2 on oral cephalosporins.

2.4 PHARMACOLOGICAL AND CLINICAL ASPECTS

The clinical pharmacology of cephalosporins has been recently reviewed (Neu, 1982b; Adam *et al.*, 1982; Klastersky, 1983; Barriere and Flaherty, 1984; Sykes *et al.*, 1985; Sanders and Sanders Jr., 1986a; Walther and Meyer, 1987). Many details for individual drugs are given in later sections. Beside the antibacterial potency and spectrum of a cephalosporin, its pharmacokinetic profile in human is of great importance. It is valuable to tailor dosage schedules, to optimize therapeutic effects and to minimize side effects and drug interactions. Antibacterial concentrations must be achieved and maintained at the various sites of infections. A variety of animal models of infection are used to determine pharmacokinetic parameters. They are good indicators, but not a substitute for extensive clinical trials. A number of reasonably well-defined pharmacokinetic parameters are often used by clinicians as a guide to differentiate cephalosporins: concentration of antibiotic in serum and body fluids (e.g. cerebrospinal fluid, interstitial fluid, peritoneal fluid, bile and in sputum), tissues (e.g. lung, bone, muscles, pericardium and fat) and in urine after oral or parenteral administration, besides volume of distribution, area under the curve (AUC), protein binding, serum elimination half-life, clearance (total/renal) and effect of probenicid.

Pharmacokinetic parameters vary from person to person and from study to study and should be interpreted with care. A summary of clinical pharmacokinetics of the third generation cephalosporins has been published (Balant *et al.*, 1985). Distribution properties of i.v. cephalosporins in man have also been reviewed and compared (Ganzinger, 1987). Table 2 gives some characteristic human pharmacokinetic data of a number of cephalosporins. Values from three different sources (referred to as A, B and C) are mentioned to indicate the degree of deviations in different studies. Binding of cephalosporins to serum protein is a reversible interaction and is considered as a concentration-dependent reversible equilibrium in serum and in body fluids. It may become a slow release depot mechanism in case of high binding and decreases the rate of elimination. The influence of protein

TABLE 2

Characteristic human pharmacokinetic parameters of representative oral and parenteral cephalosporins. Values from three different sources are mentioned to indicate the degree of deviations in different studies (Ref. A: Walther and Meyer, 1987; Ref. B: Bergan, 1984; Ref. C: Wise, 1982)

Drug	Proteinbinding (%)			Serum half-life (h)			Urinary recovery (%)			
	Ref. A	Ref. B	Ref. C	Ref. A	Ref. B	Ref. C	Ref. A 6 h	Ref. A 24 h	Ref. B	Ref. C
Oral cephalosporins										
Cefalexin	10–35	10	18–20	0.6–1.2	0.75	0.9	70–90	>90	95	88
Cefradine	5–30	5	10–20	0.5–1.5	0.75	0.9	70–90	86–100	90	86
Cefadroxil	17–20	20	18–20	1.2–1.7	1.6	1.6	70	<85	90	88
Cefaclor	25	25	25	0.6–0.9	0.75	0.6	50–70	<90	60	54
Gram-positive group										
Cephalothin[a]	50–75	65	72	0.3–1.0	0.7	0.6	40–60	70–90	70	50
Cefazolin	60–90	80	80	1.1–3.0	1.5	1.8	60–80	>90	85	90
Cephaloridine	10–30	20	20	0.8–1.8	1.4	1.3	60	90	60	80
Gram-negative group										
Cefamandole	50–75	75	70	0.5–2.0	0.8	0.8	70–80	90–100	80	75
Cefuroxime	25–40	30	35	1.0–2.0	1.2	1.4	90	100	95	80
Cefotiam	40	40	40	0.75–2.0	0.75	0.75	50–60	69–72	70	70
Cefotaxime[a]	30–50	35	40	0.7–1.8	1.2	0.9	33–60	60–70	80	50
Ceftizoxime	31	30	30	1.2–1.8	1.3	1.4	80–85	—	85	90
Cefmenoxime	43–75	60	52	0.6–1.2	1.4	0.9	—	>80	60	70
Ceftriaxone[b]	50–96	95	95	5.0–11.3	8.5	8.5	35–45	55–60	65	65
Cefodizime	81[d]	—	—	2.5–3.1[c]	3.0[d]	3.8[e]	—	—	80[c]	—

Continued

TABLE 2

Continued

Drug	Proteinbinding (%)			Serum half-life (h)			Urinary recovery (%)			
	Ref. A	Ref. B	Ref. C	Ref. A	Ref. B	Ref. C	Ref. A		Ref. B	Ref. C
							6 h	24 h		
Pseudomonas group										
Ceftazidime	17–26	20	17	1.5–2.8	2.0	1.8	—	75–92	80	88
Cefpirome	—	—	—	1.9–2.1	—	—		87		
Cefoperazone[b]	70–94	90	90	1.6–2.6	2.0	1.7	33	35	30	25
Cefsulodin	25–35	30	34	1.4–1.7	1.5	1.5	65	70	70	90
Anaerobe group										
Cefoxitin	20–35	55	75	0.6–2.0	0.7	0.7	90	>90	80	90
Cefmetazole	—	85	—	0.7–1.4	1.0	—	66	>90	75	—
Cefotetan	—	90	87	2.0–4.0	3.5	3.0	65	83	70	80
Latamoxef	—	—	40	2.0	2.5	2.5	84	—	50	88

[a] Deacetylation *in vivo*.
[b] High biliary excretion.
[c] Dagrosa *et al.* (1987).
[d] Schäfer-Korting *et al.* (1986).
[e] Humbert *et al.* (1985).

binding on the pharmacokinetics, e.g. distribution, metabolism and elimination, is discussed by Dette (1986) and by Limbert and Seibert (1986). There is no direct correlation between protein binding and serum half-life. Only those cephalosporins with higher protein binding rates (>80%) tend to give longer half-lives and lower renal clearance rates. The serum half-life for many cephalosporins ranges from 1–2 hours. It reaches the highest value for ceftriaxone (5–11 h). A prolonged duration of effective antibacterial concentrations allows a less frequent and more convenient dosing regimen, easier use in outpatient therapy and financial benefits.

The difficulties of predicting the pharmacokinetic data from the rate of protein binding alone arise from the different routes of elimination. The main route of elimination of most cephalosporins in normal subjects is via renal excretion. Biliary excretion is significant for a few agents such as cefoperazone (244) or ceftriaxone (210). In subjects with renal or hepatic impairment the pharmacokinetic parameters can be substantially affected and dose modifications may thus be required. Excretion of cephalosporins can be governed by glomerular filtration or by tubular secretion.

Knowledge of the degree of metabolism of a cephalosporin is essential for its proper clinical use. Metabolism may influence the potency, spectrum of antibacterial activity, toxicity, pharmacokinetic properties and may interfere in bioassay determinations. Partial inactivation of cephalosporins results from spontaneous hydrolysis of the β-lactam ring in an aqueous medium or by enzymatic degradation, especially in cases where a labile 3-acetoxymethyl substituent is present, e.g. in cephalothin or cefotaxime (207). Most 3'-substituents are liberated to a small extent and may cause adverse reactions, e.g. in the case of cephalosporins possessing a 3'-1-methyltetrazol-5-ylthio moiety. A 100% recovery of the administered dose is not reached, even in cases where no metabolism has been observed.

Improvement of the pharmacokinetic profile of cephalosporins aim towards the following aspects: improved oral absorption, reduced protein binding, prolonged half-life, low degree of metabolism, high penetration to extravascular body sites and high excretion of active drugs into urine, bile and sputum.

The antibacterial spectra of cephalosporins, their favourable pharmacokinetic properties and their safety profile allow their application in many clinical situations, especially in the initial treatment of serious life-threatening infections. The clinical efficacy and safety of new agents is evaluated in the course of controlled clinical studies. Due to the high potency and broad spectrum of the newer agents, an effective treatment can be expected for many typical human infections, e.g.:

- lower respiratory tract infections;
- skin and skin structure infections;
- urinary infections;
- gynaecologic and obstetric infections;
- sexually transmitted diseases;
- bone and joint infections;
- abdominal infections;
- central nervous system infections;
- bacteraemia;
- post-operative infections (prophylactic use).

Clinical studies are difficult to evaluate because there are no nationally or internationally recognized and standardized criteria for the rate of success. The often used evaluations, i.e. the percentage of clinical cure, clinical improvement and failure, is a rough guide, but many other parameters should be considered. First of all, safety and tolerance have to be assessed in depth during all clinical phases, and also in a subsequent postmarketing surveillance. Cephalosporins are in general safe and well-tolerated anti-biotics. Most clinical adverse effects are transient, mild or moderate in nature; severe or fatal reactions are very rare. Typical reported side effects are similar in type and frequency for different β-lactam groups and can be classified as follows:

- local reactions;
- hypersensitivity reactions;
- CNS reactions;
- gastrointestinal reactions;
- bacterial or fungal superinfections;
- alcohol intolerance;
- laboratory abnormalities (haematological, hepatic, renal and urinary).

The value of cephalosporins is not only expressed by their property as single agents, but also in combination with other anti-infectives. There are microbiological and clinical reasons for a combined therapy. The synergistic combination of cephalosporins with aminoglycosides has been in common use for many years and is based on an improved bactericidal effect, extension of antibacterial spectrum and prevention of resistance. Clinical reasons for a synergistic or additive combination therapy are of varying importance and there may be reduction of dose, improved pharmaco-kinetics, and shorter duration of therapy. The literature on the clinical aspects of cephalosporins is vast. For specific details the reader is referred to standard textbooks and references cited in later sections.

2.5 SYNTHETIC ROUTES

The methods available for the synthesis of cephalosporins and many of their nuclear analogues have been given in monographs (Morin and Gorman, 1982; Brown and Roberts, 1985) and review articles (Dürckheimer *et al.*, 1985 and references cited therein). Reviews on the synthesis and biological properties of the most interesting group of aminothiazole cephalosporins have been given by Newall (1985) and Dürckheimer *et al.* (1982).

On account of the high sensitivity of the cephalosporin nucleus to acids and bases, all synthetic procedures require selectively activating reagents, protecting groups that can be split off gently, and mild reaction temperatures. The most common route for a semisynthetic cephalosporin starting from 7-ACA can be described as follows:

- displacement of the 3'-acetoxy residue in 7-ACA by nucleophiles;
- synthesis of the 7-side chain acid and, if necessary, protection of functional groups;
- coupling of the side chain acid to the 7-aminocephem nucleus optionally followed by deprotection of functional groups;
- preparation of stable, non-toxic salts of sufficient solubility at a physiological pH value.

The nucleophilic displacement of the 3'-acetoxy group can also be performed on cephems already bearing the appropriate 7-acyl side chain. Some cephem structures, as well as nuclear analogues, are not accessible from 7-ACA. In such cases more synthetic steps are necessary. Examples are given in later sections. Methods for activating side chain acid and protecting functional groups have been already reviewed (Dürckheimer *et al.*, 1985).

3 Naturally Occurring Cephalosporins

3.1 CEPHALOSPORIN C

Cephalosporin C (Ceph. C), the first natural cephalosporin, is produced along with penicillin N by *Cephalosporium acremonium*. This was cultivated by Brotzu from seawater near a sewage outlet on the coast of Sardinia in 1945. The degree of antibacterial activity was moderate. The property which attracted most attention was the high degree of resistance to staphylococcal penicillinase. The spur to further research came from Florey and Abraham. Abraham and Newton purified Ceph. C and elucidated its structure

(Abraham and Newton, 1961a,b). The final structural proof by X-ray analysis from Crowfoot-Hodgkin and Malen (1961). The biosynthetic pathway of Ceph. C and the origin of its precursors (D-α-aminoadipic acid, L-cysteine, L-valine, acidic acid) was elucidated by ^{14}C-labelling (Trown and Sharp, 1963; Demain, 1963). Woodward *et al.* (1966) reported the first total synthesis of Ceph. C.

Because the antibacterial activity of Ceph. C is low, attempts were made to improve it by replacing the 7-β-acyl side chain using the experience gained from the study of penicillin chemistry. Great efforts were devoted to the cleavage of Ceph. C by chemical or enzymatic methods to 7-ACA, an ideal starting material for semisynthetic modifications. The first chemical process for the conversion of Ceph. C to 7-ACA was found by a research group at Lilly (Morin *et al.*, 1962a) using nitrosyl chloride in formic acid. The most important technical route to 7-ACA consists of the silylation of Ceph. C with trimethylchlorosilane, conversion to a 7-imidochloride intermediate with phosphorous pentachloride, and subsequent solvolysis (Fechtig, 1968). An interesting ring expansion from penicillin sulphoxide esters to the skeleton of cephalosporins was discovered by Morin *et al.* (1962b) and by Kukolja *et al.* (1976).

The enzymatic cleavage of Ceph. C to 7-ACA by several microorganisms has also been claimed (Huang, 1963). However, no acylase has yet been reported to be capable of removing in one step the D-α-aminoadipoyl chain in Ceph. C or cephamycines in reasonable yields. Discovery of such an enzyme would greatly facilitate the production of semisynthetic cephalosporins. However, in 1972, deamination of Ceph. C to a keto derivative was achieved using D-amino acid oxidase from yeast and pig kidney (Mazzeo and Romeo, 1972), to produce 7-ACA with a glutaryl side chain. An analogous enzymatic degradation of Ceph. C by a D-aminoacid oxidase system from *Trigonopsis variabilis* has been published (Szwajcer and Mosbach, 1985). Keto adipic-7-ACA is spontaneously transformed to glutaryl-7-ACA and simultaneously hydrogen peroxide is formed. Reports have appeared of an acylase that will hydrolyse the side chain of glutaryl-7-ACA to 7-ACA (Shibuya *et al.*, 1981; Szwajcer and Mosbach, 1985 and references cited therein).

The molecular cloning and structure of a gene for cephalosporanic acid acylase from a *Pseudomonas* strain, as well as the purification and characterization of cloned isopenicillin N synthetase, have been reported (Matsuda and Ichikomaton, 1985; Baldwin *et al.*, 1987).

3.2 7α-SUBSTITUTED CEPHALOSPORINS

After the discovery of cephalosporins, an intensive screening of micro-organisms producing new types of β-lactam antibiotics was launched. More than 20 years elapsed before the next major, naturally occurring variation of a β-lactam structure, the cephamycins, were observed (Gordon and Sykes, 1982b; Southgate and Elson, 1985). These cephalosporins all possess a 7α-methoxy substituent and an α-amino-adipic acid side chain, but vary in the substitution pattern at C-3. Table 3 lists some of the cephamycins discovered. Their antibacterial activity is too weak for clinical application, but they are interesting starting materials for semisynthetic variations due to their intrinsically high resistance to hydrolysis by β-lactamases compared to the analogues without the 7α-methoxy group. In particular, cephamycin C (2) is a valuable starting material for cefoxitin (104), the first 7α-methoxycephalosporin introduced into the clinic.

Cephabacins M_1–M_6 (11a–f) (Table 4) are naturally occurring cephem antibiotics which were isolated from the culture filtrate of the bacterial strain *Xanthomonas lactamgena* Yk-431 (Nozaki *et al.*, 1985; Tsubotani *et al.*, 1985). These weakly active antibiotics have a 7α-methoxy-3'-deacetyl-cephalosporin C skeleton linked with oligopeptides at C-3'. Related to the cephabacin M series are the cephabacins F_1–F_9 and H_1–H_6 (12a–p) (Table 5) and the chitinovorins (13a–e) (Table 6), discovered by research groups at Takeda (Ono *et al.*, 1984; Tsubotani *et al.*, 1984) and Shionogi (Shoji *et al.*, 1984). They possess as a new structural feature a 7α-formylamido substituent. Squibb (Singh *et al.*, 1984) isolated further derivatives, SQ-28 516 (13d) and SQ-28 517 (13e) (Table 6). 7α-Formylamidocephems also show weak antimicrobial activity. The affinity for penicillin-binding proteins (PBPs) has been studied for cephabacins F_1 (12a), H_1 (12k) and M_1 (11a) (Nozaki *et al.*, 1984, 1985). For cephabacin M_1 (11a) the primary targets are PBP 1 in *Escherichia coli* and PBP 4 in *Bacteroides subtilis*. Cephabacins F_1 (12a) and H_1 (12k) show the same binding pattern. Comparison with deacetylcephalosporin C and 7α-formyldeacetylcephalosporin C led to the conclusion that the oligopeptide side chain increases the affinity for PBPs, whereas the formylamido substituent does not significantly affect binding to them.

In the 7α-methoxy series a few compounds have been introduced into the market or are presently under clinical evaluation (Section 5.1). The 7α-methoxy and 7α-formylamido groups can be introduced into cephalosporins by several high yielding selective methods (Section 4.1.6.1).

TABLE 3

Naturally occurring 7α-methoxycephalosporins

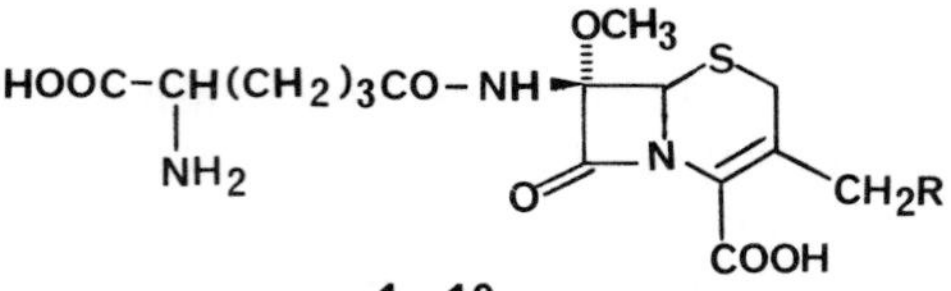

1 – 10

No	COMPOUND	R
1	7-METHOXYCEPHALOSPORIN C (A 16884 A)	$-OCOCH_3$
2	A 16886 B CEPHAMYCIN C	$-OCONH_2$
3	CEPHAMYCIN A	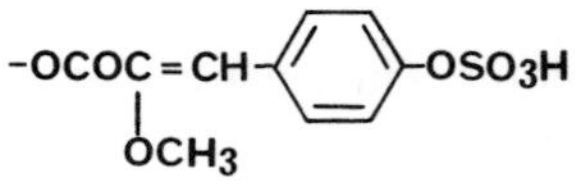
4	CEPHAMYCIN B	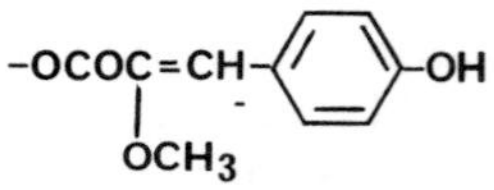
5	C 2801 X	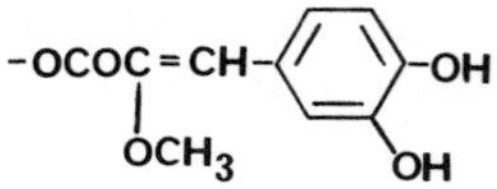
6	OGANOMYCIN A	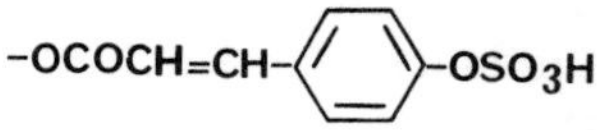
7	OGANOMYCIN G	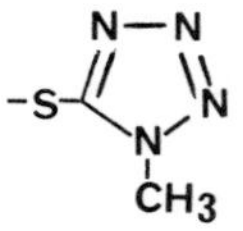
8	OGANOMYCIN F	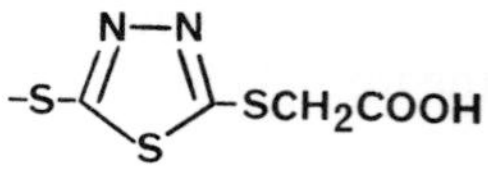
9	OGANOMYCIN H	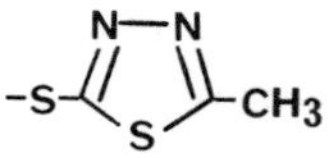
10	OGANOMYCIN I	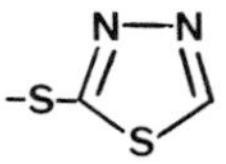

TABLE 4

Structures of cephabacins M_1–M_6 **11a–f**

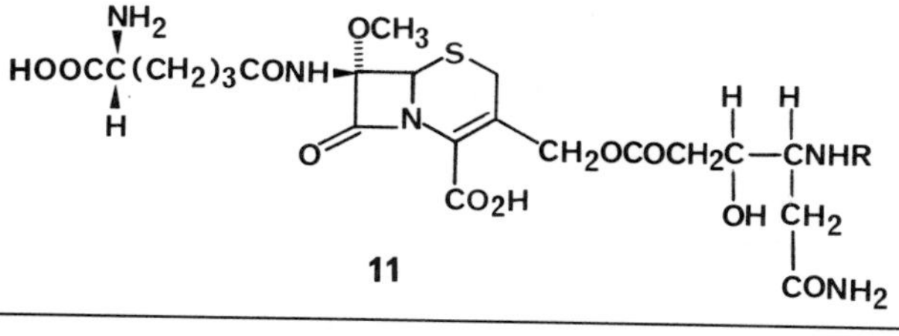

$$\text{HOOCC(CH}_2)_3\text{CONH} \quad \overset{NH_2}{\underset{H}{|}}$$

Structure **11**: cephem core with OCH_3 substituent, CO_2H, and side chain $CH_2OCOCH_2C-CNHR$ with OH, CH_2, $CONH_2$ groups.

11

No.	Cephabacin		R			
a	M_1	L-Val	L-Orn			
b	M_2	L-Val	L-Orn	L-Ser		
c	M_3	L-Val	L-Orn	L-Ser	L-Ala	
d	M_4	L-Val	L-Orn	L-Ser	L-Orn	
e	M_5	L-Val	L-Orn	L-Val	L-Orn	L-Ser
f	M_6	L-Val	L-Orn	L-Val	L-Orn	L-Ser	L-Ala

TABLE 5

Structures of cephabacins F_1–F_9 **12a–i** and cephabacins H_1–H_6 **12k–p**

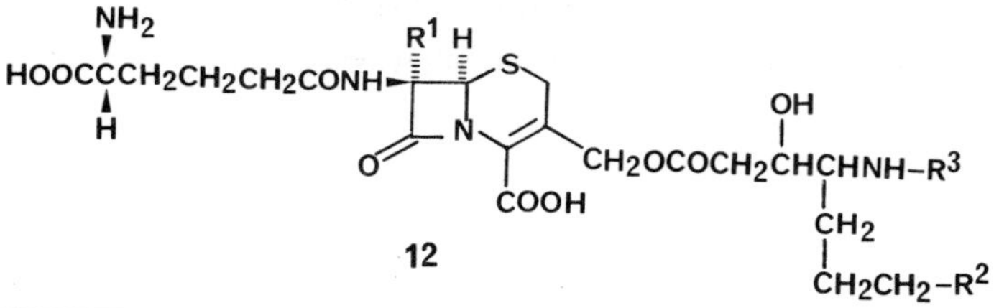

$$\text{HOOCCCH}_2\text{CH}_2\text{CH}_2\text{CONH} \quad \overset{NH_2}{\underset{H}{|}}$$

Structure **12**: cephem core with R^1 substituent, $COOH$, and side chain $CH_2OCOCH_2CHCHNH-R^3$ with OH, CH_2, $CH_2CH_2-R^2$ groups.

12

No.	Cephabacin	R_1	R_2	R_3
a	F_1	—NHC(=O)H	—NHC(=NH)NH$_2$	-L-Ala
b	F_2	—NHC(=O)H	—NHC(=NH)NH$_2$	-L-Ala-L-Ala
c	F_3	—NHC(=O)H	—NHC(=NH)NH$_2$	-L-Ala-L-Ala-L-Ala
d	F_4	—NHC(=O)H	—NHC(=NH)NH$_2$	-L-Ser
e	F_5	—NHC(=O)H	—NHC(=NH)NH$_2$	-L-Ser-L-Ser
f	F_6	—NHC(=O)H	—NHC(=NH)NH$_2$	-L-Ser-L-Ser-L-Ala
g	F_7	—NHC(=O)H	—CH$_2$NH$_2$	-L-Ser
h	F_8	—NHC(=O)H	—CH$_2$NH$_2$	-L-Ser-L-Ser
i	F_9	—NHC(=O)H	—CH$_2$NH$_2$	-L-Ser-L-Ser-L-Ala
k	H_1	—H	—NHC(=NH)NH$_2$	-L-Ala
l	H_2	—H	—NHC(=NH)NH$_2$	-L-Ala-L-Ala
m	H_3	—H	—NHC(=NH)NH$_2$	-L-Ala-L-Ala-L-Ala
n	H_4	—H	—NHC(=NH)NH$_2$	-L-Ser
o	H_5	—H	—NHC(=NH)NH$_2$	-L-Ser-L-Ser
p	H_6	—H	—NHC(=NH)NH$_2$	-L-Ser-L-Ser-L-Ala

TABLE 6

Structures of chitinovorins A–C **13a–c** and SQ-28 156 **13d** and SQ-28 517 **13e**

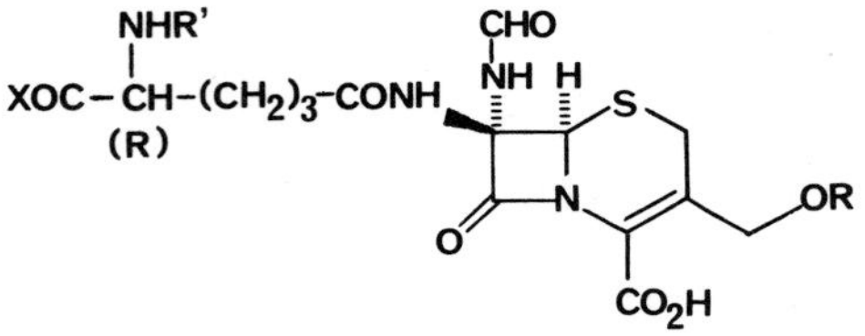

13

No	Compound	R	R'	X
a	Chitinovorin C	H	H	OH
b	Chitinovorin A	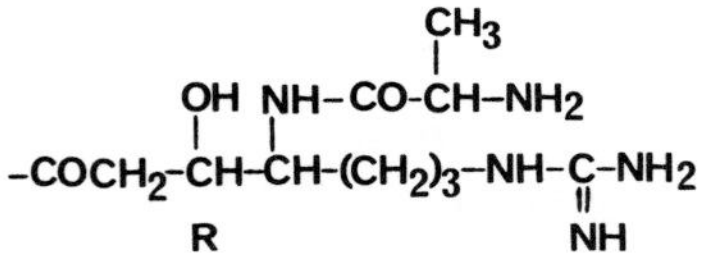 $-COCH_2-CH-CH-(CH_2)_3-NH-C-NH_2$ with OH, NH–CO–CH(CH_3)–NH_2, R, and $=NH$ substituents	H	OH
c	Chitinovorin B	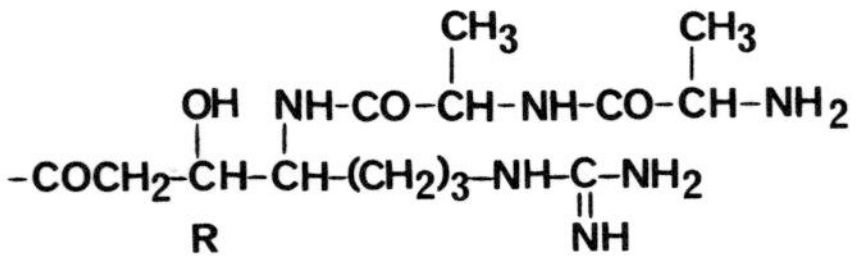 $-COCH_2-CH-CH-(CH_2)_3-NH-C-NH_2$ with OH, NH–CO–CH(CH_3)–NH–CO–CH(CH_3)–NH_2, R, and $=NH$ substituents	H	OH
d	SQ 28 156	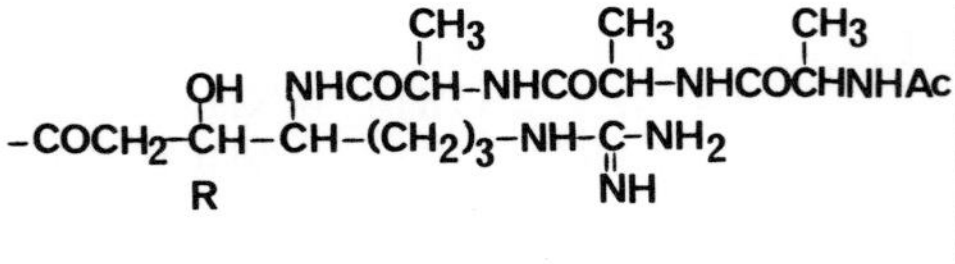 $-COCH_2-CH-CH-(CH_2)_3-NH-C-NH_2$ with OH, NHCOCH(CH_3)–NHCOCH(CH_3)–NHCOCHNHAc(CH_3), R, and $=NH$ substituents	Ac	OH
e	SQ 28 517	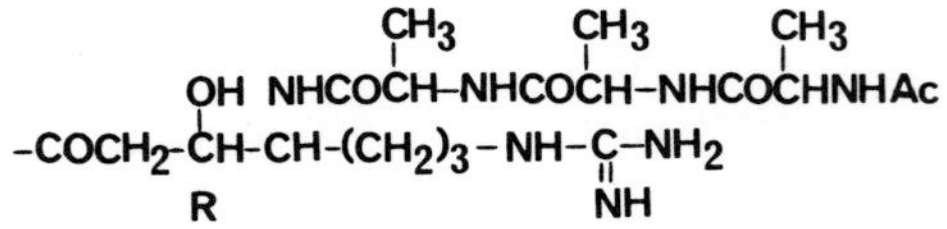 $-COCH_2-CH-CH-(CH_2)_3-NH-C-NH_2$ with OH, NHCOCH(CH_3)–NHCOCH(CH_3)–NHCOCHNHAc(CH_3), R, and $=NH$ substituents	Ac	NH_2

3.3 BIOSYNTHESIS

Our knowledge of the biosynthesis of cephalosporins has grown gradually and has developed parallel to the work on the biosynthesis of penicillins. In recent years biochemists have made significant contributions by the purification of the enzymes involved and by establishing suitable cell-free systems, which allow mechanistic aspects to be studied. Newer results have been summarized in a series of papers (Baldwin, 1984, 1985; Baldwin *et al.*, 1986a–f; Abraham, 1986; Demain and Brana, 1986; Martin *et al.*, 1986; Demain and Wolfe, 1987). The biosynthetic pathways to penicillins and cephalosporins are outlined in Scheme 1.

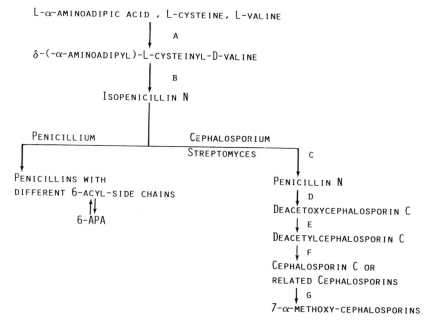

SCHEME 1. Biosynthetic pathways to penicillins and cephalosporins, modified after Abraham (1986).

It has been unequivocally established that the natural penicillins and cephalosporins derive from the same three L-amino acids, which condense to form the so-called Arnstein-tripeptide (L-α-aminoadipoyl)-L-cysteinyl-D-valine (LLD-ACV). L-Valine is isomerized to D-valine during tripeptide formation. LLD-ACV undergoes an oxidative cyclization catalysed by isopenicillin N synthetase. This enzyme from *Acremonium crysogenum* and

Penicillium descrysogenum has been characterized and purified. The tripeptide LLL-ACV is not a substrate for this enzyme. By the use of ^{13}C- and ^1H-NMR techniques and ^{14}C- and ^3H-isotopically labelled precursors, the substrate specificity and the stereochemistry of ring closures have been determined. One molecule of oxygen is required to convert one molecule of ACV to isopenicillin N. Oxygen is not incorporated, but reduced to water, and the configuration at the valine β-site is retained. Baldwin (1985) postulated for the Fe^{2+}-ion-dependent isopenicillin N-synthetase a free radical mechanism involving iron-oxo intermediates. In cephalosporin- and cephamycin-producing microorganisms isopenicillin N is converted to penicillin N by isopenicillin N isomerase. This labile epimerase converts the L-aminoadipic moiety to the D-isomer and does not require Fe^{2+} or other metal ions. The ring expansion of penicillin N to deacetoxycephalosporin C is achieved by the deacetoxycephalosporin C synthetase, also called ring-expanding enzyme or expandase. It shows high specificity for the acyl side chain attached to the penicillin nucleus, expands the thiazolidine ring of penicillin N, but does not accept the isomeric isopenicillin N, penicillin C or 6-APA. The expandase of *Streptococcus clavuligerus* (mol. wt about 30 000) strongly requires Fe^{2+} ions, α-ketoglutarate and ascorbate as cofactors. Deacetoxycephalosporin C is hydroxylated to deacetylcephalosporin C (DAC) by an α-ketoglutarate-requiring intermolecular dioxygenase using molecular oxygen. Acetylation of DAC to cephalosporin C is the terminal reaction in cephalosporin-producing fungi. The enzyme is called deacetyl-cephalosporin C acetyltransferase.

Further enzymatic reactions are involved in the introduction of the 7α-methoxy group and the attachment of different C-3′ groups during the biosynthesis of cephamycins in actinomyces. Several side chains may be attached to the C-3′ hydroxymethyl group of DAC, e.g. a carbamoyl residue in cephamycin C (2), an acetyl group in 7α-methoxycephalosporin C (1) and aromatic acyl groups in cephamycins A (3), B (4) and C-2801X (5). The methoxy group at C-7 of cephamycins is derived from molecular oxygen and methionine and is incorporated by an enzyme system containing a dioxygenase and methyltransferase.

In view of the great importance of cephalosporins, the application of isolated isopenicillin N synthetase and deacetoxycephalosporin C synthetase for the enzymatic synthesis of modified cephalosporins has been extensively tested. All changes made in the L-cysteinyl residue of LLD-ACV destroy the ability of the peptide to compete with the natural substrate. Tripeptides with C-terminal D-α-aminobutyric acid, D-isoleucine and D-alloisoleucine produced penicillin in which the normal terminal dimethyl group was replaced by hydrogen or an ethyl group (Baldwin *et al.*, 1981; Abraham, 1986 and references cited therein). These penicillins are transformed to the corre-

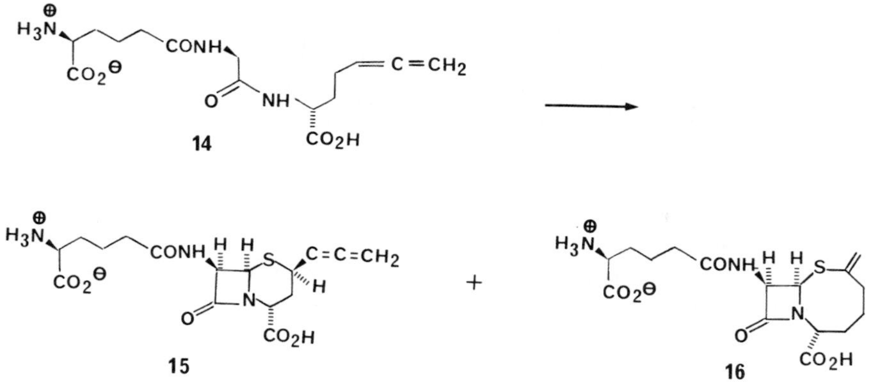

SCHEME 2. Enzymatic cyclization of a synthetic tripeptide to β-lactams.

sponding cephalosporins in the presence of epimerase and deacetoxy-cephalosporin C synthetase from *Strep. clavuligerus*. A synthetic tripeptide 14 with an appropriate C-terminal residue could be enzymatically converted to cepham (15) and the bicyclic β-lactam (16) (Scheme 2) (Baldwin *et al.*, 1986e).

A better understanding of the biosynthetic steps will probably allow the synthesis of new cephalosporins as starting materials for semisynthesis. Work on the cloning of genes that encode the enzymes involved is in progress, and success will open new possibilities in this field.

4 Chemical Variations and Biological Activity

4.1 SEMISYNTHETIC VARIATIONS AT THE CEPHEM NUCLEUS

4.1.1 1-Position

As stated in several reports (Dürckheimer *et al.*, 1981), oxidation of the ring sulphur in cephalosporins to a sulphoxide or sulphone usually diminishes or destroys the antibacterial activity. De Koning *et al.* (1977) compared the (R)- and (S)-sulphoxides of several cephalosporins, including those of cephalothin and cefalexin (23), with their parent compounds, and found *in vitro* activity for (R)-sulphoxides. In contrast to these observations, the (S)-sulphoxide of cefotaxime is more active than its (R)-sulphoxide and is characterized by higher β-lactamase stability and good penetration of the outer membrane of Gram-negative bacteria, but is inactive against

Staphylococci. Even the corresponding sulphone retained a portion of the antibacterial properties. CM-40 874 (271a) is a newer (S)-sulphoxide with high resistance to cephalosporinases (Drugs of the Future, 1985b).

Sulphoxides of cephalosporins are easily prepared by oxidation with peracids (Dürckheimer et al., 1981; Micetich et al., 1984). Cooper et al. (1969, 1970) found a preferential or exclusive formation of (S)-sulphoxides when a 7-acylamido side chain is present in the cephalosporin molecule. A hydrogen bond between the 7β-amido hydrogen and the oxidant seems to exert a directing influence and favors the attack of the oxidants from the β-side. Lack of an amide hydrogen bridge, for example in a Schiff's base, leads to a dominant attack from the α-side and formation of (R)-sulphoxides.

The oxidation of cephalosporins to sulphones needs more drastic conditions and an excess of peracid. The acidity of the hydrogen atoms at C-2 in sulphoxides and sulphones leads to a rapid deuterium exchange at this position and a slower deuterium exchange at C-7 accompanied by epimerization in the presence of a base (Sassiver and Shepherd, 1969). Cephalosporin sulphones containing a 7α-substituent are potent inhibitors of human leukocyte elastase (Doherty et al., 1986). The degradative activity of this enzyme seems to be implicated in the development of pulmonary emphysema and the pathogenesis of respiratory disease states.

4.1.2 2-Position

Modifications at C-2 in cephalosporins were reviewed by Jung et al. (1980). Starting from a 2-exomethylenecephem sulphoxide of type 17a (obtained from cephalosporin sulphoxide esters under Mannich reaction conditions) and also from 2-diazocephem sulphoxide of type 17b (obtained from cephem sulphoxide by diazotransfer) a number of 2,2-disubstituted cephalosporins have been prepared. Table 7 gives examples of C-2 modified cephalosporins. Most of the resulting compounds are biologically inactive, and only 2-alkyl and 2-alkylidene derivatives 17c and 17e are reported to exhibit antibacterial activity. In the ceftizoxime series it could be demonstrated that the configuration at C-2 for 2-methyl derivatives plays an important role for antibacterial activity. The 2α-methylceftizoxime FR-13374 of type 17c, once selected by Fujisawa but not further developed, shows considerably more antibacterial activity than the corresponding 2β-methyl diastereomer 17d. Its activity is comparable to that of ceftizoxime (209) (Takaya et al., 1982). A stereoselective synthesis of 2α- and 2β-methyl-3-cephems (17c and 17d) with different 3- and 7-substitution patterns was performed. In some cases, a good overall antibacterial activity was observed (Mizokami et al., 1983).

A convenient preparation of C-2 substituted cephalosporins is achieved by displacement of the 2-acetoxy or 2-methoxy group with nucleophiles,

TABLE 7

Modification at C-2 in cephalosporins **17** (R^1, R^2, R^3 = different substitution; R^4 = alkyl, cycloalkyl, aryl or acetyl; R^5 = Cl, Br)

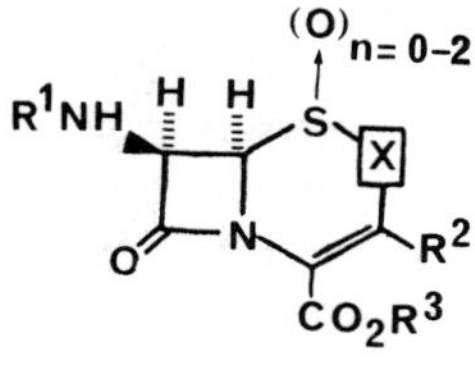

17

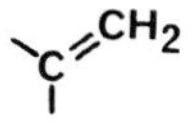

a 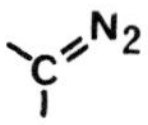   b 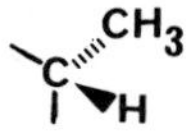   c 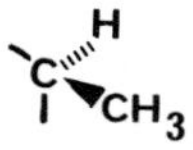   d

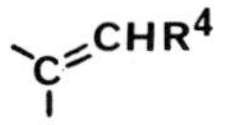

e 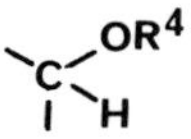   f 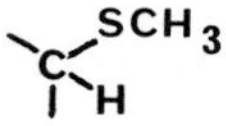   g 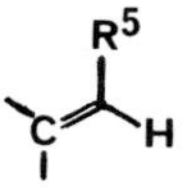   h

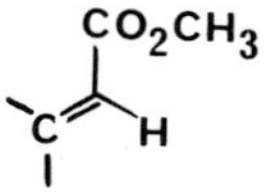

i 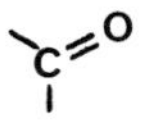   k 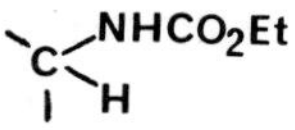   l 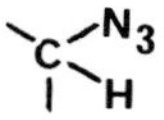   m

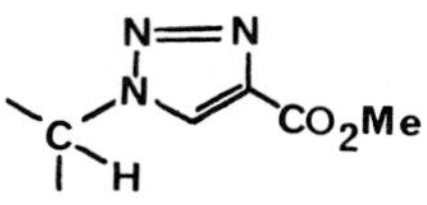

n 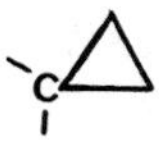   o 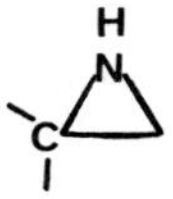   p 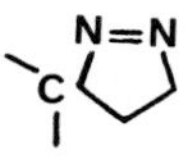   q e.g. furan, 2-methylfuran, 2-methylthiophene, N-methylpyrrole, alkyl and heteroaryl thiols and allylic alcohol (Torii et al., 1983c). Only (S)-sulphoxides and sulphones react under Mannich reaction conditions to form 2-exomethylene derivatives **17a**, whereas the corresponding (R)-sulphoxides remain unchanged (Jaszberenyi et al., 1982).

2-Alkoxycephalosporins **17f** have been produced by several methods (Jung et al., 1980). Recently, a new simple method of producing stereospecific 2α-alkoxylation was reported using cerium(IV)ammonium nitrate in an alcoholic medium (Humber and Roberts, 1985; Fletton et al., 1985). Compound **17g** has also been prepared (Jung et al., 1980). Regiospecific 2-methylthiolation of cephalosporin sulphoxides was accomplished by addition of methylthio mesylate ($CH_3SO_2SCH_3$) to a previously formed C-2 carbanion (Applegate et al., 1979). The synthesis of 4- and 7-methylthio-substituted cephems was also described in the same publication.

2-Vinylchloro- and 2-vinylbromocephems **17h** were obtained from 2-exomethylenecephem sulphoxides **17a** by reaction with dimethyl immonium halide in a Pummerer type rearrangement (Spry, 1980a). Reactions of 2-vinylhalocephem sulphoxides of type **17h** with primary and secondary amines, thiols, tetramethylguanidinium formate, Grignard reagents and lithium dimethylcuprate have been reported (Spry, 1980b). Treatment of cephalosporin sulphoxide esters with lithium di-isopropylamide and methyl bromoacetate yields 2-(methoxycarbonyl)methylene cephalosporins (**17i**), which display antibacterial activity against Gram-positive bacteria (Kim et al., 1984).

The synthesis of 2-oxocephalosporins of type **17k** have been achieved by several routes:

(a) by a brief treatment of 2-exomethylene cephalosporins **17a** with ozone at low temperature (Kim et al., 1979);
(b) by a rearrangement of 2-diazocephem sulphoxides **17b** under rhodium acetate catalysis (Ebbinghaus et al., 1979);
(c) from penicillins including an intramolecular Wittig condensation as a key step (Ernest, 1979, 1980); and
(d) from penicillin V via 4-mercaptoazetidinones as intermediates (Hagiwara et al., 1981).

In general, 2-oxocephem esters **17k** are quite labile under basic conditions and fairly stable in acidic media. The free acids possess only a limited half-life in a neutral buffer. Antibacterial activity of these compounds has been reported to be low, probably due to their instability under test conditions (Hagiwara et al., 1981). The 2-oxo analogue of cephalothin is much less active than cephalothin itself (Kim et al., 1979).

Reaction of 2-cephems with ethoxycarbonyl nitrene yielded a cephem possessing an aziridine annelated via C-2 and C-3 and as a byproduct

2-ethoxycarbonylamino-3-cephem **17l** (Hoshide and Ogawa, 1982). Reaction of 2-cephems with iodo azide afforded 2-azido-3-cephems **17m** and 2-azido-2-cephems (Hoshide *et al.*, 1982a). Thermolysis of a 2-azido-3-cephem **17m** led to ring enlargement and a β-lactam with a seven-membered ring, whereas refluxing of a 2-azido-2-cephem in benzene gave a penam derivative. Condensation of **17m** with acetylenes gave 2-triazolyl-3-cephems **17n**. 2-Azido-2-cephems reacted with triphenylphosphine and carbon disulphide to form 2-isothiocyanato-2-cephems, which can be further derivatized. Antibacterial activities of all tested compounds were lower than that of cefalexin (**23**) (Hoshide *et al.*, 1982b).

The photochemical rearrangement of 2-diazocephem sulphoxides **17b** produced 1-oxo-carbapenems (Rosati *et al.*, 1982). Electrolytic chlorination of a thiazolo-azetidinone yielded 2,3′-dithio-substituted cephalosporins (Torii *et al.*, 1983a). 2-Spirocephems **17o–q** have been prepared from 2-exomethylenecephem sulphoxides **17a** (Jung *et al.*, 1980).

4.1.3 3-Position

4.1.3.1 Introduction. The following sections (4.1.3.2–4.1.3.6) will give an overview of newer synthetic methods for the preparation of 3-substituted cephems, including 3-vinylcephems, and will also describe their basic biological properties. 3-Modified cephalosporins which are on the market or under extended evaluation are discussed in Sections 5.1 and 5.2. The 3-substituted cephem derivatives, prepared by partial synthesis from penicillins, have been accessible since about 1970, after several methods for the preparation of 3-exomethylencephams had been developed. The chemistry of 3-modified cephems and their properties have already been reviewed in detail (Sammes, 1980; Kukolja and Chauvette, 1982). The 3-position of cephems has not been derivatized to the same extent as the 3′-position (Section 4.1.4). Nevertheless, variations have led to cephalosporins with interesting bacteriological and pharmacological properties, which have been also exploited clinically.

The 3-substituent has a marked electronic influence on the β-lactam carbonyl system. Electronegative substituents at C-3 facilitate β-lactam cleavage initiated by addition of nucleophiles to the amide carbonyl group. Relevant physicochemical parameters of the cephem molecule, for instance the pK_a value of the 4-carboxylic group, can be influenced by the 3-substituent. The antimicrobial properties and pharmacokinetic parameters are changed as well. Small 3-substituents like methyl in cefalexin (**23**), methoxy in cefroxadine (**279**), or chlorine in cefaclor (**275**), promote the enteral absorption of glycyl cephalosporins. The 3-substituent also modulates the enteral absorption in carboxymethyl cephalosporins.

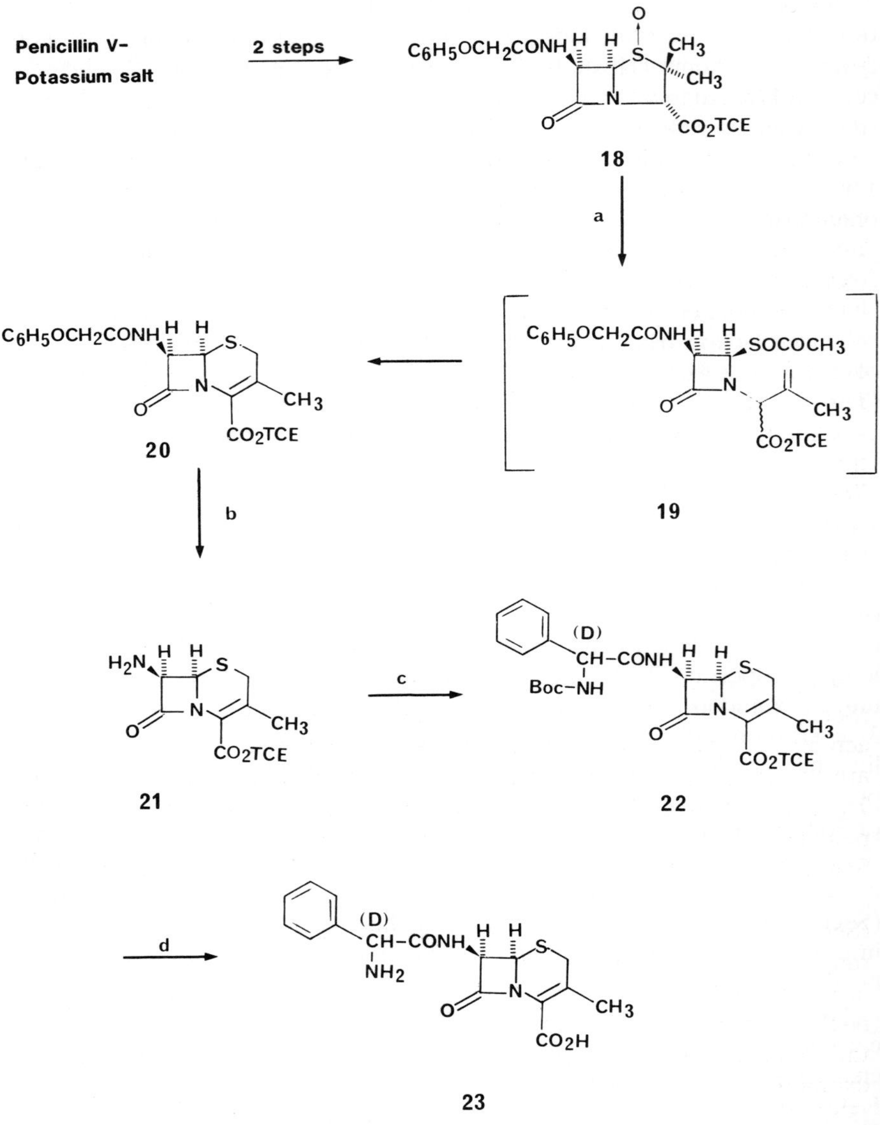

SCHEME 3. Synthesis of cefalexin (**23**). (a) (Ac)₂O, DMF, 130°C; (b) side chain cleavage sequence (1) PCl₅, pyridine, benzene; (2) CH₃OH; (3) H₂O; (c) acylation with (D)-N-Boc-phenylglycine, ClCO₂CH₃, triethylamine; (d) deprotection (1) Zn, HOAc, DMF, 0°C; (2) pTsOH, CH₃CN (3) H₂O, triethylamine, pH 4.8 (isolation). TCE = trichloroethyl.

4.1.3.2 Derivatives of 7-Aminodeacetoxycephalosporanic Acid (7-ADCA). The 3-methylcephalosporin nucleus (deacetoxycephalosporins) is part of several important cephalosporin antibiotics. The 3-methylcephem compounds are readily available from two sources: firstly, from 7-ACA derivatives by removal of the 3'-acetoxy group, e.g. by hydrogenation in the presence of a palladium catalyst; secondly, from penicillin sulphoxide esters by Lewis acid-catalysed penicillin–cephalosporin rearrangement, as exemplified in the synthesis of cefalexin (**23**) (Scheme 3). Penicillin V 1-S-oxide trichloroethyl ester (**18**), readily prepared from penicillin V, is treated with acetic anhydride in DMF to yield a ring-opened sulphenic acid intermediate (**19**) that recyclizes to the biprotected 7-ADCA derivative (**20**) (*Morin–Jackson* rearrangement). Synthesis is completed via the deacylation of the 7-amido function, reacylation with Boc-protected phenylglycine, and removal of the protecting groups.

The chemistry of penicillin–cephalosporin rearrangements has been thoroughly reviewed elsewhere (Cooper and Spry, 1972; Murphy and Webber, 1972a,b; Sammes, 1976, 1980; Cooper and Koppel, 1982). Recent work in this field has been published by Torii *et al.* (1986) (see also references cited therein).

4.1.3.3 3-Exomethylenecephams. Unlike the isomeric 3-methylcephems (Section 4.1.3.2), 3-exomethylene-2-cephams are devoid of antimicrobial activity. They are important precursors for 3-modified cephalosporins and are mostly prepared by ring expansion of penicillin derivatives or from 7-ACA derivatives. The synthetic routes to 3-exomethylenecephams from penicillins have been reviewed (Cooper and Spry, 1972; Kukolja, 1976; Sammes, 1976, 1980; Kukolja and Chauvette, 1982). Upon ozonolysis, 3-exomethylenecephams are further transformed to 3-hydroxycephems (Section 4.1.3.4) as versatile synthetic intermediates. The *Kukolja* rearrangement starting from penicillin V 1-oxide *p*-nitrobenzyl ester (**24**) is used in a technical process as outlined in Scheme 4. Compound **24** reacts with N-chlorosuccinimide to a ring-opened product **25**, similar to that formed in the synthesis of cefalexin **23** (Scheme 3). Product **25** cyclizes to the exomethylene sulphoxide **26** in an ene-type reaction catalysed by $SnCl_4$ (Kukolja *et al.*, 1976; Chou, 1977). Starting from 7-ACA derivatives of general structure **27**, 3-exomethylenecephams of type **28** are accessible by reductive elimination using metals or metal salts as catalysts (Table 8, I–IV). Of special interest is the application of electrochemical methods for this transformation (Table 8, V).

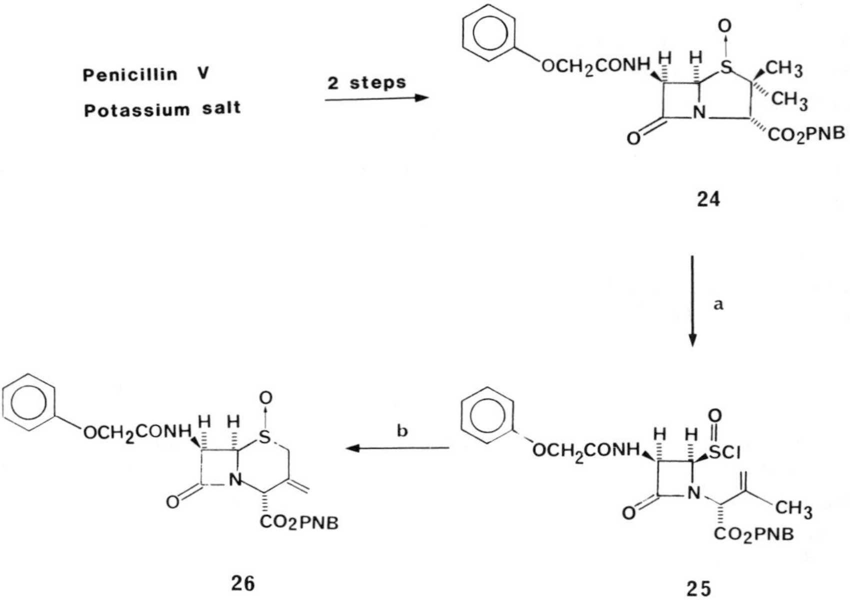

SCHEME 4. Synthesis of 3-exomethylenecephams **26** from penicillin V (a) N-chlorosuccinimide; (b) SnCl$_4$.

4.1.3.4 3-Hydroxycephems and Derivatives.

3-Hydroxycephems **34** which exhibit only poor antimicrobial activity are important key intermediates for the synthesis of a variety of 3-substituted cephalosporins. Table 9 shows a selection of 3-substituted cephems from the literature or recent patent applications. For earlier reviews see Kukolja and Chauvette (1982) and Sammes (1980). Scartazzini and Bickel (1977) focused on the 3-substituent and its influence on the enteral absorption of cephalosporins. Cephalosporins with relevant antibacterial and clinical properties emerged from the series of 3-H (**29a**), 3-CH$_3$ (**29b**), 3-OCH$_3$ (**29m**), 3-SR (of types **29n–o**) and 3-Cl-cephems (**29q**). Other modifications did not receive so much attention due to reduced antimicrobial activities or low chemical stability.

In general, the synthesis of 3-hydroxycephems **31** and **34** and their derivatives **32** and **35** (Scheme 5) starts from 3-methylenecephams **33** (Section 4.1.3.3) and their S-oxides **30**, which are ozonolysed. The S-oxides are reduced prior to or after ozonolysis. The subsequent introduction of the 3-substituent completes the sequence. In some cases the sulphoxide reduction is performed after the introduction of the 3-substituent in order to avoid

TABLE 8

Preparation methods for 3-exo-methylenecephams **28** from 7-ACA-derivatives **27**. References: (I) Fujisawa Pharmaceutical Co. Ltd. (1982, 1983); (II) McShane and Dunigan (1986); (III) McShane (1985); (IV) Nishimura (1986); (V) Torii *et al.* (1983, 1986). PG = protecting group

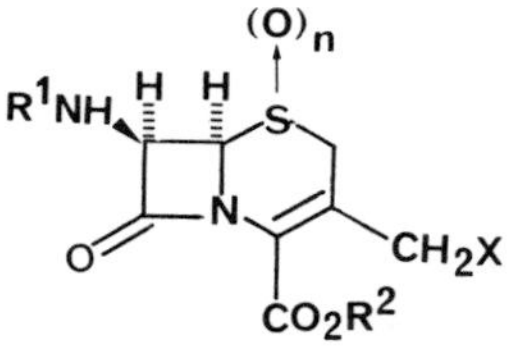

		Starting material			
	R^1	R^2	X	n	Reagents
I	H	H	OAc	0	$CaCl_2$, $TiCl_3$, HCl, H_2O pH 7–8
II	Acyl	BH	OAc	1	Zn, DMF-H_2O, 0–5°C
III	H	H	SHet	0	Zn, NH_4Cl, DMF $(CH_3)_3SiCH_2CONH_2$
IV					Mg, $(NH_4)_2SO_4$, H_3PO_4, H_2O pH 8–9, 3–7°C
V	Acyl	PG	Cl SHet	0	THF-$LiClO_4$, Pb-cathode or CH_3CN, EtOH, $LiClO_4$, NH_4ClO_4, Pb-cathode

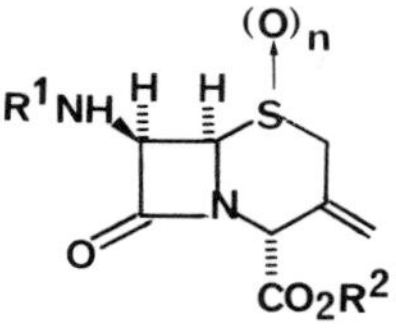

Δ^3–Δ^2 isomerization during the substitution. Alternatively, 3-hydroxy-cephems **37** are obtained by cyclization of seco-penicillins **36** without 3-methylenecephams as intermediates (Hamashima *et al.*, 1976) (Scheme 6). Seco-penicillins **36** are obtained via ring-opening of penicillins, e.g. in the *Morin* reaction or related processes (for reviews see Cooper and Spry, 1972; Sammes, 1980; Cooper and Koppel, 1982; Kukolja and Chauvette, 1982).

Representative methods for the preparation of 3-substituted cephems starting from cephems **32** or **35** or cephem 1-oxides of type **38** are given in Table 10. 3-Hydroxycephems **34** with protected 7-amino and 4-carboxyl groups are more susceptible to nucleophilic substitution at C-3 when they are transformed to their 3-chloro, 3-tosylate, 3-mesylate or —OP(O) $(OC_6H_5)_2$

TABLE 9

Examples of 3-substituted cephems **29**. Only the modified part of the basic structure **29** is shown. Cephems of type **29a**, **29b**, **29e**, **29h**, **29i**, **29l**, **29m**, **29n–o** and **29q** are discussed throughout the text. Additional references: Boswell and Brittelli (1975) (**29c**); Kawano et al. (1980); Watanabe et al. (1980) (**29d**); Sugawara et al. (1979b) (**29f**); Takao et al. (1980) (**29k**); Kukolja and Chauvette (1982) (for **29g** and **29p**)

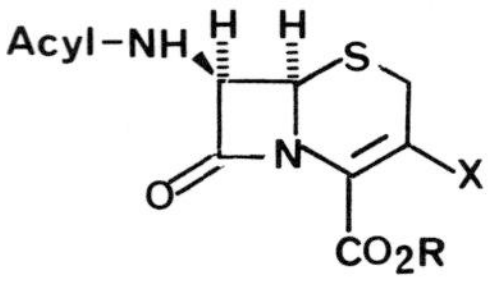

29

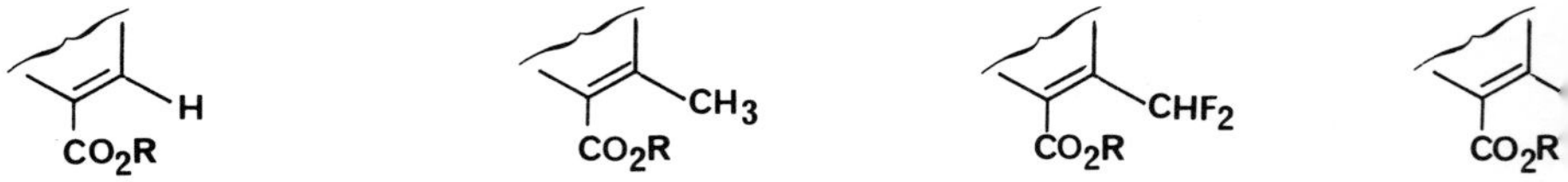

a   b   c   d

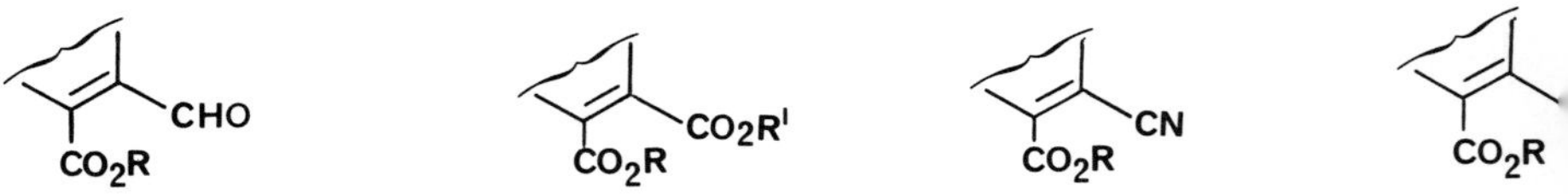

e   f   g   h

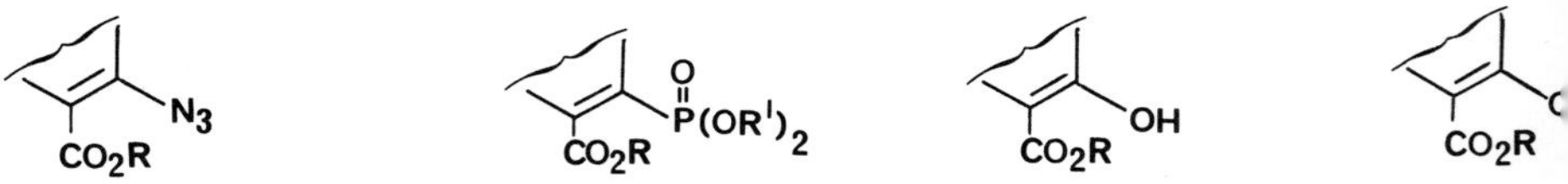

i   k   l   m

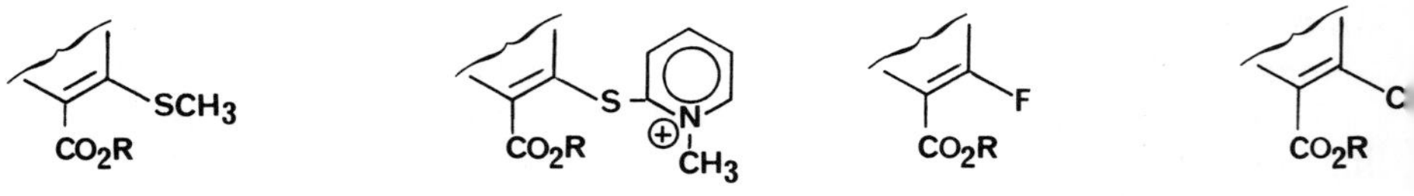

n   o   p   q

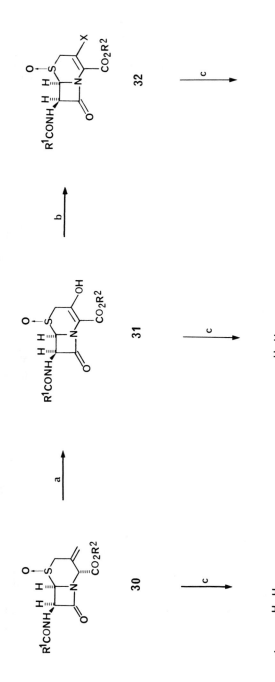

SCHEME 5. Synthetic routes to 3-hydroxycephems **34** and cephems **35** with varying 3-substituents. (a) Ozonolysis; (b) introduction of 3-substituent (X); (c) sulphoxide reduction (PBr$_3$, PCl$_3$ or CH$_3$COCl). (R^{1}CO, R^2 = protecting groups.)

derivatives, because these substituents are better leaving groups and more easily displaced by nucleophiles than the hydroxy group. 3-Thiocephems are readily prepared by this route (Table 10, IX). Alternatively, 3-mercaptocephems are alkylated (Table 10, XI). Compared to their 3-alkoxy-

TABLE 10

Preparation methods for 3-substituted cephems **32** and **35**. BH = benzhydryl, TCE = trichloroethyl, PNB = *para*-nitrobenzyl

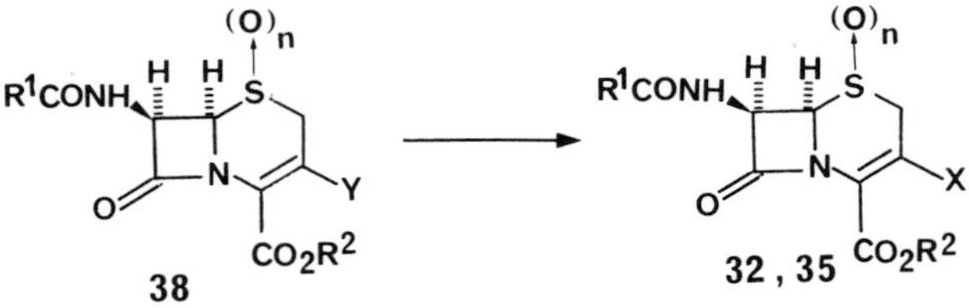

Starting material					Product
R^1	R^2	n	Y	Reagents (yield)	X
I $C_6H_5CH_2$	BH	0	Cl	Zn, HOAc	
II $C_6H_5CH_2$	TCE	0	OTs	Zn, HOAc (78%)	H
III $C_6H_5CH_2$	BH	0	OH	(1) $NaBH_4$; (2) Ac_2O; (3) TEA	
IV $C_6H_5OCH_2$	CH_3	0	Cl	Me_2CuLi, THF, $-50°C$ (50%)	CH_3
V $C_6H_5CH_2$	BH	0	OH	NH_4Cl, pyridine, EtOH	NH_2
VI ⟨thienyl⟩CH_2	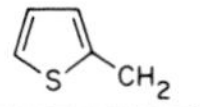 PNB	0	OTs	NaN_3, DMF (80–90%)	N_3
VII $C_6H_5CH(NH_2)$	BH	0	OH	CH_2N_2	OCH_3
VIII $C_6H_5OCH_2$	PNB	0	OH	$MeO_2C—N{=}N—CO_2Me$, PPh_3, ROH (60–90%)	OR
IX 7-NH_2	BH	0	OMS	$AgSCH{=}CH—R'$	
X $C_6H_5CH_2$	BH	1	OTs	$HSCH_2CO_2CH_3$	SR
XI $C_6H_5OCH_2$	PNB	0	OH	(1) NaHS; (2) $BrCH_2CH{=}CH_2$	
XII ⟨thienyl⟩CH_2	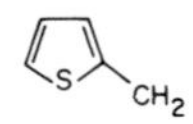 PNB	0	OH	$SOCl_2$	Cl

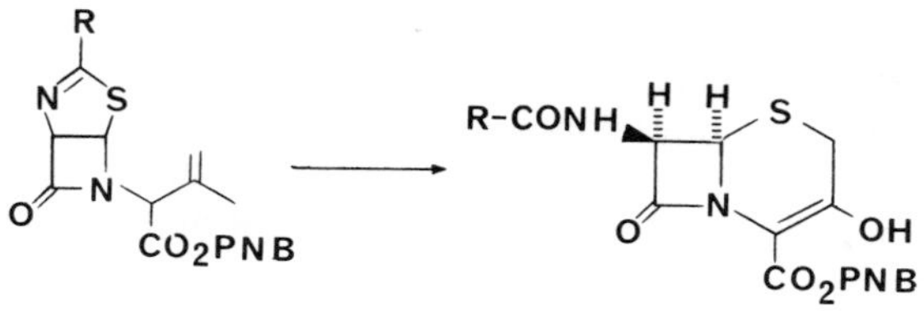

SCHEME 6. A synthetic route to 3-hydroxycephems 37 via an azetidinone derivative.

analogues, 3-thiocephems exhibit a somewhat higher antibacterial activity *in vitro*. Several 3-thiocephems **39** carrying aminothiazolyl side chains possess a broad spectrum of antibacterial activity (Takaya *et al.*, 1985d; Takatani *et al.*, 1986). Moreover, 3-thiocephems of type **39** carrying aminothiazolyl or glycyl side chains are claimed to be enterally absorbed in animals (Ishimaru, 1983, 1984; Csendes, 1985; Y. Watanabe *et al.*, 1987a,b,c). CGP-33098 A (**290**) (Section 5.2) is one example of this type undergoing extended evaluation.

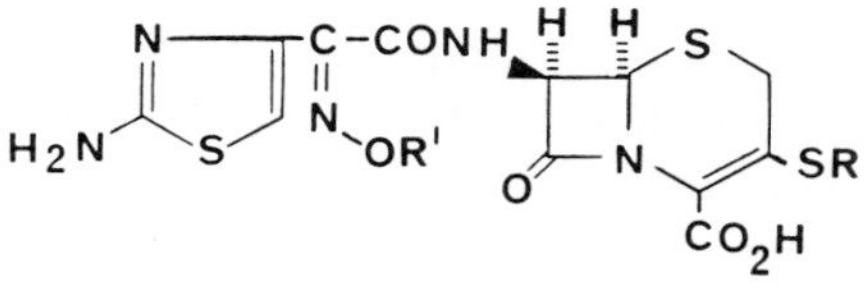

39

Several research groups have reported the synthesis and biological activities of 3-alkoxycephems **29m** [R' = CH$_3$, C$_2$H$_5$, *n*—C$_4$H$_9$ or CH(C$_6$H$_5$)$_2$] (Scartazzini and Bickel, 1977, 1983). 3-Hydroxycephems of type **34** are mostly O-alkylated with dimethylsulphate, alkylhalides, *Meerwein*'s reagent, triazenes or diazoalkanes (Table 10, VII). In contrast, *Williamson*'s ether synthesis leads preferentially to C-4-alkylated cephems instead of O-alkylated products. 3-Methoxycephems like cefroxadine (**279**) bearing a 7-glycylamido side chain exhibit favourable enteral absorption and good antimicrobial activity (Section 5.2). 3-Methoxycephems **40** with aminothiazolyl side chains do not surpass other convenient 3'-substituted cephalosporins with respect to antimicrobial activity.

A new synthetic approach to 3-alkoxycephems **29m** consists of a redox-condensation of **38** (R^1 = C$_6$H$_5$CH(NH$_2$)—, R^2 = benzhydryl, n = 0, Y = OH) with alcohols (ROH) using *Mitsunobu* reaction conditions (Table 10,

VIII) (Spry, 1986; Spry and Bhala, 1986a). Triphenylphosphine and an azodicarboxylic ester serve as redox reagents. The yield and nature of byproducts (C-4-alkyl- and hydrazine derivatives) strongly depend on the nature of the reducing agent. Using dimethyl diazodicarboxylate and methanol, cephem **40** and the corresponding C-4-methylated product are

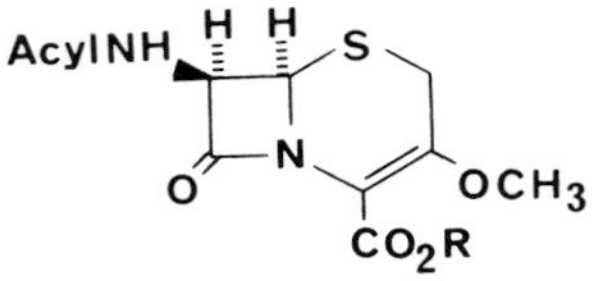

40

obtained in 60% and 10% yields, respectively. 3-Hydroxycephems **34** can be treated with ammonium chloride to yield 3-aminocephems (Table 10, V) (Scartazzini *et al.*, 1975). Another approach to 3-N-derivatives consists of a displacement of the 3-hydroxy group by an azide group (Table 10, VI). 3-Azidocephems of type **35** (X = N_3) are reduced with thiophenol or hydrogen on palladium/charcoal to **35** (X = NH_2). Acylation of 3-aminocephems (**41b**) gives rise to 3-N-acylderivatives **35** (X = NHAcyl), which exhibit only moderate antimicrobial activity when a 7-phenylglycylamido side chain is attached to the cephem nucleus.

    3-Azidocephem **41a** reacts with *Grignard* reagents to a triazine derivative which decomposes on chromatography to 3-aminocephem **41b**. This compound is also obtained upon hydrogenation, whereas the azido group is inert to Zn–HCl reduction conditions (Spry and Bhala, 1984). Moreover, 3-azidocephems **41a** react with electron-rich dipolarophiles to amidines,

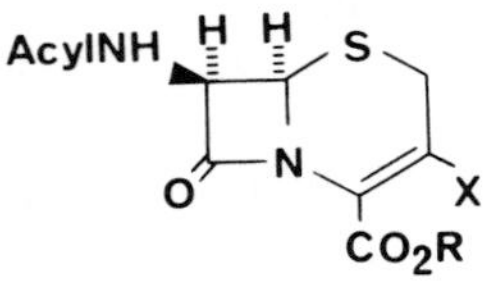

41

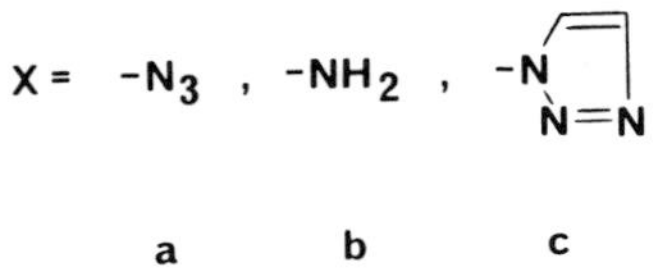

imidates, imino lactones, and aziridines; triazoles **41c** and tetrazolyl cephems are not formed (Spry and Bhala, 1984; Spry, 1985). The major products from the thermolysis and photolysis of 3-azidocephems (**41a**) in methanol are ring-expanded 1,4,6-thiadiazepine azetidinones (Spry et al., 1984).

Cefaclor (**275**) (Section 5.2) was the first semisynthetic oral cephem antibiotic on the market with a non-classical substitution pattern at C-3. 3-Chlorocephems with non-glycyl side chains have recently been described as orally active antibiotics (Section 5.2). The chloro atom at C-3 is introduced by reaction of **34** with chlorinating agents. Phosphorus trichloride (Chauvette and Pennington, 1975; Chauvette and Chauvette, 1981) and thionyl chloride are convenient to use (Table 10, XII). In an elegant approach, **42** reacts with $(C_6H_5O)_3PCl_2$ (prepared from $(C_6H_5O)_3P$ and PCl_3) to **43** (Hatfield et al., 1980a). Deacylation of the 7-amido group via an imino chloride, reduction of the sulphoxide and displacement of the hydroxyl group by chlorine occur in a single step (Scheme 7).

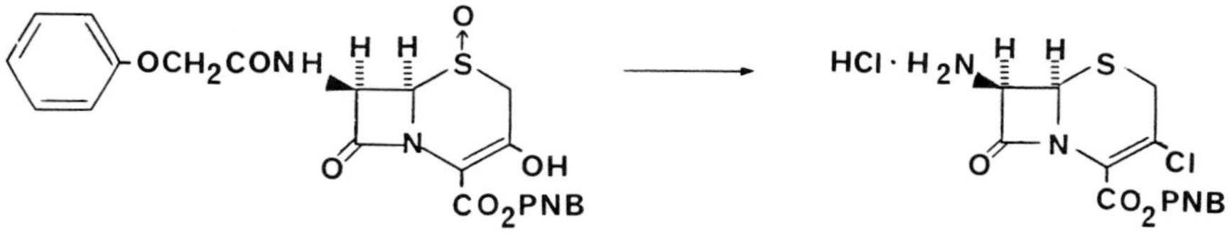

SCHEME 7. Preparation of 3-chlorocephem nucleus **43** from 3-hydroxycephems **42**.

Broad spectrum cephalosporins ceftizoxime (**209**) (Section 5.1), 7432-S (**289**), and FK-089 (**288**) (Section 5.2) are the most prominent members of the series of 3-H-cephems **29a**. They are readily prepared by partial synthesis. 3-Formylcephems of type **29e**, important synthetic intermediates for both 3-H- and 3-vinylcephems, are readily accessible by oxidation of 3-hydroxymethylcephalosporins (DMSO/acetic anhydride or Collins reagent) (Sugawara et al., 1980a). **29e** is decarbonylated to 3-H-cephems **29a** in good yields using a rhodium catalyst, e.g. RhCl(Ph$_3$P)$_3$ (Peter and Bickel, 1974). Another approach to 3-H-cephalosporins **29a** is by reduction of 3-hydroxy-, 3-chloro- or 3-tosyloxycephems (Table 10, I–II) (Takaya et al., 1978). In a three-step sequence, 3-hydroxycephem **38** ($R^1 = C_6H_5CH_2$—, $R^2 = BH$, $n = O$, $Y = OH$) is reduced to the corresponding 3-hydroxycepham with sodium borohydride and then acetylated. Subsequent elimination of acetic acid gives 3-unsubstituted cephems **35** ($X = H$) (Table 10, III).

4.1.3.5 3-Vinylcephems. 3-Vinylcephems **50** have been intensively studied in recent years following the finding that derivatives such as cefixime (**53**) (Section 5.2) exhibit not only remarkable antimicrobial properties, but also are enterally absorbed. Semisynthetic approaches to 3-vinylcephems starting from 7-ACA derivatives have been known for some time. Early observations that 3-vinylcephems **50** with electron-attracting substituents (—CO_2H, —$CO_2C_2H_5$ or —C≡N) attached to the vinyl group, revealed a favourable effect on MIC values against Gram-negative bacteria compared with their 3-acetoxymethyl analogues, encouraged the synthesis of new vinyl derivatives. Table 11 shows a selection from the recent literature and patent applications. Several structural variations have been already discussed by earlier reviews (Webber and Ott, 1977; Sammes, 1980; Kukolja and Chauvette, 1982).

Synthetic routes to 3-vinylcephems starting from 7-ACA or cephalosporin C, respectively, are outlined in Scheme 8. Initial saponification of the 3′-acetoxy group of cephalosporin C **45** (R′CO = protected aminoadipoyl residue) followed by 7-amido side chain cleavage yields 7-aminodeacetyl-cephalosporanic acid, which can be further transformed to protected 3-hydroxymethylcephems **46** (R^1CO, R^2 = protecting groups). Various protecting groups for the 7-amino and the 4-carboxylic group are used at this stage. Even the protected aminoadipoyl residue (R^1CO—) can be carried throughout the synthesis. The transformation of 3-hydroxymethylcephems **46** to 3-vinylcephems **50** proceeds via two complementary approaches using a *Wittig* olefination as the crucial step. Thus, oxidation of **46** to the 3-formylcephem **48** and subsequent reaction with phosphonium ylides gives rise to protected 3-vinylcephems **50** with varying substitution pattern (R^3, R^4), depending on the phosphonium ylide used. On the other hand, halogen–hydroxyl exchange to 3-chloro- or bromomethylcephems **47a** or **47b** is achieved using phosphorus tri- or pentahalogenides, whereas the more reactive 3-iodomethylcephems **47c** are obtained by subsequent halogen exchange. Conversion of 3-halomethylcephems to ylids **49** proceeds via a phosphonium salt **47d**. *Wittig* reaction of **49** with appropriate aldehydes also gives access to protected 3-vinylcephems **50**. Aldehydes other than formaldehyde and unsymmetrically substituted ylides ($R^3 \neq R^4$) yield isomeric (E,Z)-mixtures that can be separated by chromatography. The ratio of these isomers can be controlled by appropriate reaction conditions. The choice of either approach to 3-vinylcephems **50** depends on the accessibility of the aldehydes (R^3R^4C=O) or phosphonium ylides (R^3R^4C=PPh$_3$), as well as on the (E,Z)-ratio desired. Protected 3-vinylcephems **50** are further derivatized by removal of the protecting groups and reacylation at the 7-amino group by standard procedures.

Several 3-vinylcephem **50** analogues are prepared by the routes outlined in Scheme 8. For instance, the synthesis of cefixime (**53**) (Section 5.2) has

TABLE 11

Examples of 3-vinylcephems **44**. Only the modified part of the basic structure **44** is shown. Cephems of type **44a–f** and **44i–p** are discussed throughout the text. Additional references: see Kukolja and Chauvette (1982) (**44g–h**)

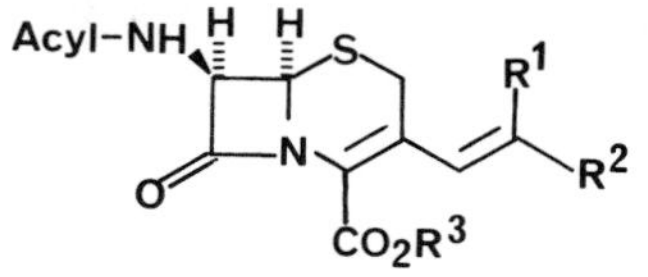

44

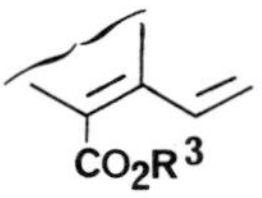

a

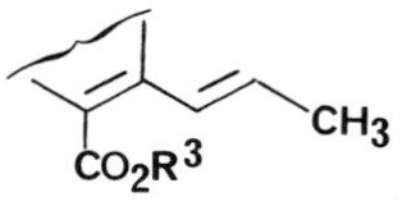

b

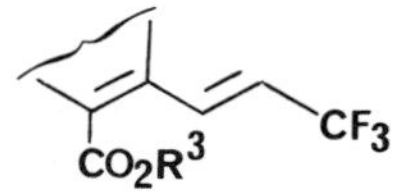

c

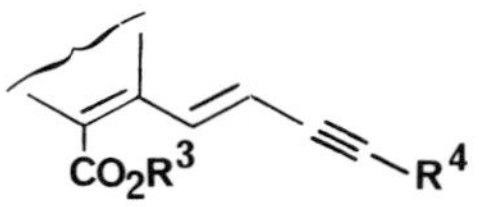

d

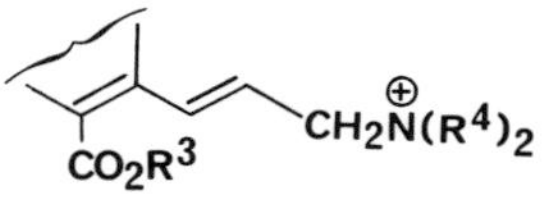

e

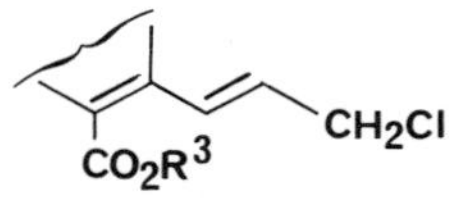

f

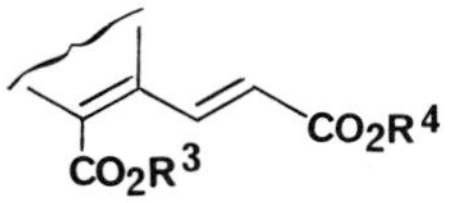

g

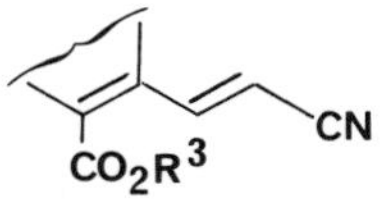

h

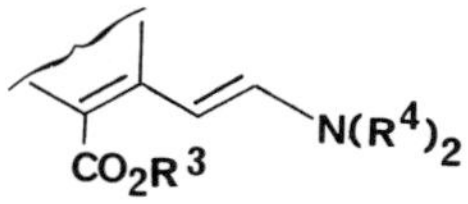

i

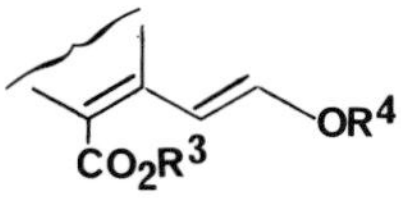

k

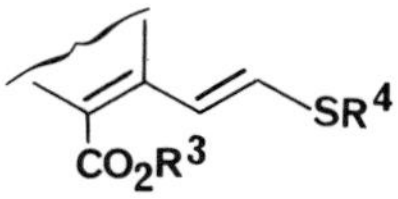

l

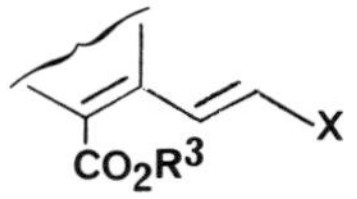

X = F, Cl, Br

m

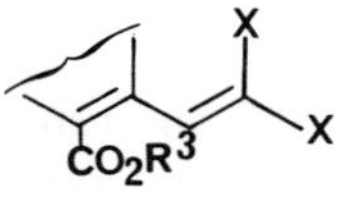

X = F, Cl, Br

n

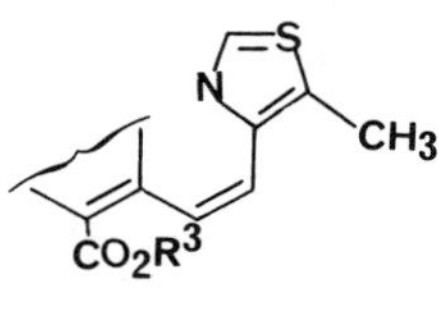

o

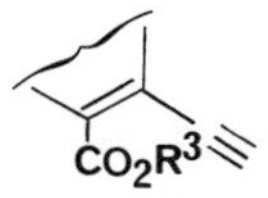

p

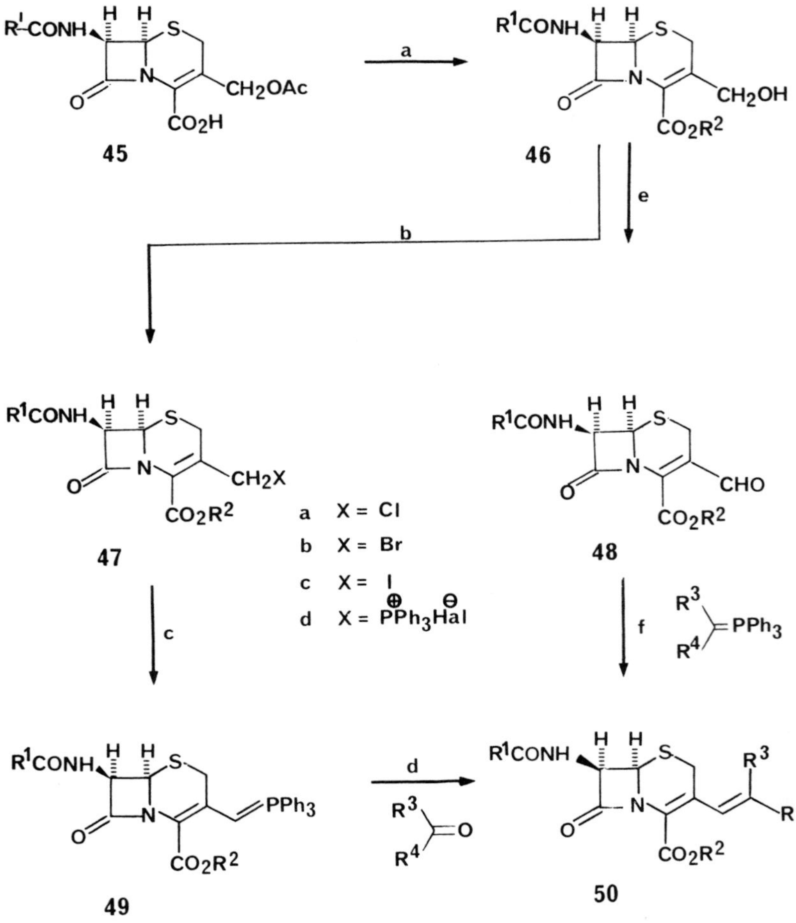

SCHEME 8. General synthetic routes to 3-vinylcephems. (R^1CO = acyl residue or protecting group). (a) Saponification of **45** ($R'CO$ = prot. aminoadipoyl); deacylation of the 7-amido group; reacylation at 7-NH$_2$ and protection of 4-CO$_2$H-group; (b) hydroxyl–halogen exchange: 3'-OH → 3'-Cl (PCl$_3$), 3'-OH → 3'-I (NaI, acetone); formation of phosphonium salt: 3'-Cl, 3'-Br or 3'-I → 3'-PPh$_3$X$^-$ (PPh$_3$); (c) aqueous base (from **47d** only); (d) *Wittig*-reaction; (e) DMSO, (CH$_3$CO)$_2$O or *Collins*-reagent; (f) *Wittig*-reaction.

been worked out on alternative routes (Yamanaka *et al.*, 1985b and references cited therein). The final synthetic steps are outlined in Scheme 9. BMY-28 100 (**280**) (Section 5.2) is synthesized starting from 3-chloromethyl-cephem **47a** (R^1 = N-Boc-*p*-hydroxyphenylglycine, R^2 = benzhydryl) via

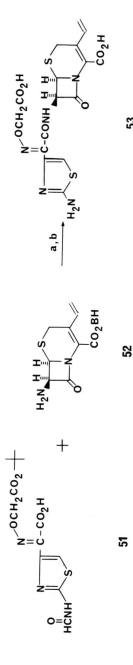

SCHEME 9. Synthesis of cefixime (53). (a) Acylation with the acid chloride of 51; (b) cleavage of protecting groups. (BH = benzhydryl.)

the corresponding 3-iodomethylcephem **47c**, (R^1 = N-Boc-p-hydroxy-phenylglycine, R^2 = benzhydryl) and phosphonium salt **47c** (2c, R^1 = N-Boc-p-hydroxyphenylglycine, R^2 = benzhydryl, X = PPh$_3$I) (Naito *et al.*, 1985, 1987). Treatment with aqueous base gives the phosphonium ylide **49** (R^1 = N-Boc-p-hydroxyphenylglycine, R^2 = benzhydryl), which upon *Wittig* reaction with acetaldehyde in the presence of lithium bromide yields an (E,Z)-mixture of 3-(1-propen-1-yl)-3-cephems **50** [R^3 = CH$_3$, R^4 = H and R^3 = H, R^4 = CH$_3$, respectively; R^1 and R^2 defined as above (E : Z = 1 : 5)], which are separated by preparative HPLC after removal of protecting groups. Overall, 40% of the (Z)-isomer **50** (R^1 = p-hydroxyphenylglycine, R^2 = H, R^3 = CH$_3$, R^4 = H) and 2% of the corresponding (E)-isomer are isolated. Other examples include (E)-3-(3,3,3-trifluoropropenyl)-3-cephem of type **50** (R^1 = C$_6$H$_5$CH$_2$—, R^2 = benzhydryl, R^3 = H, R^4 = CF$_3$) (Yamamoto *et al.*, 1986) and 3-(3-chlor-1-propenyl)-3-cephem of type **50** (R^1, R^2 = protecting groups, R^3 = H, R^4 = —CH$_2$Cl), a versatile synthetic intermediate. It is transformed to the corresponding iodo derivatives of type **50** (R^3 = H, R^4 = —CH$_2$I) and reacts with tertiary amines to 3-(3-ammonium-1-propenyl)cephems of type **44e** (Oka *et al.*, 1985). Some derivatives **54** of this series inhibit penicillin-resistant Staphylococci and *Pseudomonas* strains.

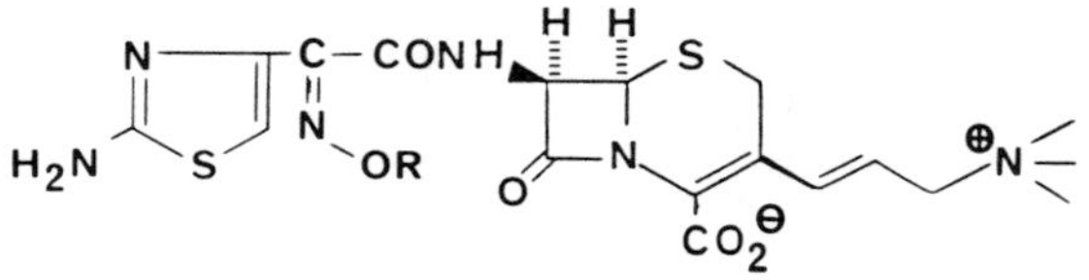

54

R = alkyl ; $\overset{\oplus}{-N}\overset{\diagup}{\diagdown}$ = cyclic or acyclic ammonio group

3-Vinylcephems of type **44o** with heterocyclic substituents attached to the vinyl group are prepared by *Wittig* reaction of 3-formylcephem **48** and, for example, 3-pyridylmethyltriphenylphosphoniumylide. Inversely, nicotin-aldehyde and ylide **49** yield the same product (Takaya *et al.*, 1985c). The reaction product of **49** (R^1 = C$_6$H$_5$OCH$_2$—, R^2 = benzhydryl) and 4-methyl-1,3-thiazol-5-aldehyde is a key intermediate for the synthesis of the orally active cephalosporin ME-1207 (**294**) (Section 5.2) (Atsumi *et al.*, 1986). 3-(2,2-Dihalovinyl)cephems of type **44n** have been described by Kawabata *et al.* (1986b). Dichloro- and dibromovinylderivatives **50** (R^3 = R^4 = Cl or R^3 = R^4 = Br) are obtained by reaction of a 3-formyl-2-cephem and dihalocarbenes, prepared *in situ* from tetrachloromethane or tetra-bromomethane in the presence of triphenylphosphin and zinc dust. The less stable difluoro compound **50** ($R^3 = R^4 = F$) is synthesized from di-bromodifluoromethane using hexamethylphosphorus triamide instead of triphenylphosphine. Dihalovinyl cephems **55a–c** display high antimicrobial activity against both Gram-negative and Gram-positive bacteria, surpassing the activity of cefixime (**53**) towards Staphylococci. They are only poorly absorbed by the oral route. 3-(2,2-Dibromovinyl)cephems of type **44n** (X = Br) are further transformed to (E)-3-bromovinylcephems **50** ($R^1 = H, R^2 = $ H or protecting group, $R^3 = H, R^4 = Br$) or 3-ethynylcephems of type **44p** (Kawabata *et al.*, 1986c). (E)-3-Chlorovinylcephems of type **44m** are obtained by hydroxyl–chloro exchange of enolized aldehydes **58** using phosphorus trichloride. (E)-3-Chlorovinylcephem **55f** surpasses cefixime (**53**) in the degree of enteral absorption (Takaya *et al.*, 1984). 3-Ethynyl-cephem **55e** exhibits good antistaphylococcal activity and moderate enteral absorption (Kawabata *et al.*, 1986c).

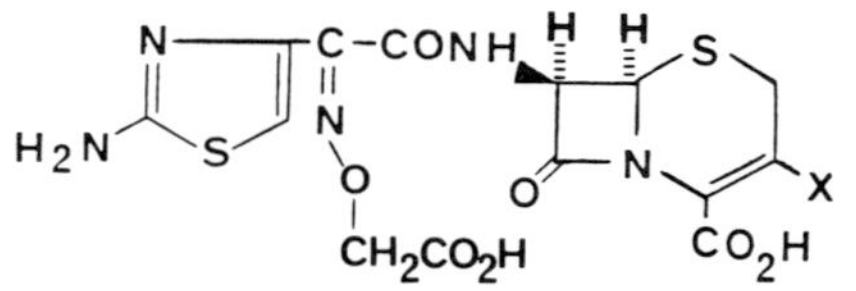

55

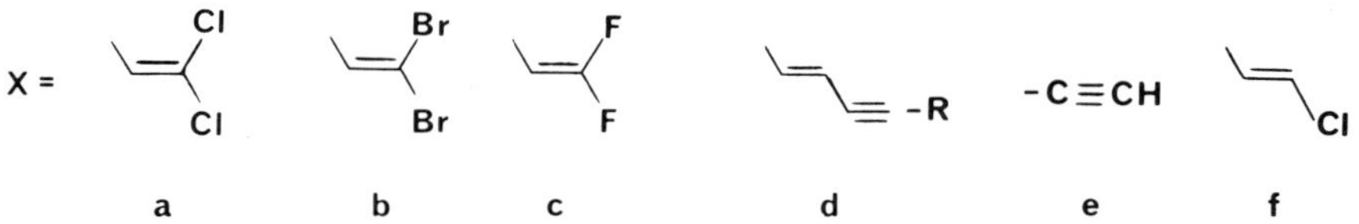

3-Alkyl-1-en-3-ynyl-substituted cephems **55d** (R = H, alkyl) were patented by Glaxo (Bell *et al.*, 1985). Some derivatives bearing the car-boxymethyl side chain of cefixime (**53**) exhibit broad spectrum activity. Compounds with an (E)-substituted 3-vinyl group are enterally absorbed and exhibit prolonged serum half-lives in animals.

An elegant approach to a variety of 3-vinylcephems uses the reaction of deacetoxycephalosporins with orthoamides (Scheme 10). 3-Dial-kylaminovinylcephalosporins **57** are formed in a high-yielding reaction under mild conditions from **56** and tert-butoxy-bis(dimethyl-amino) methane. The enamine **57** is a versatile key intermediate and can be further

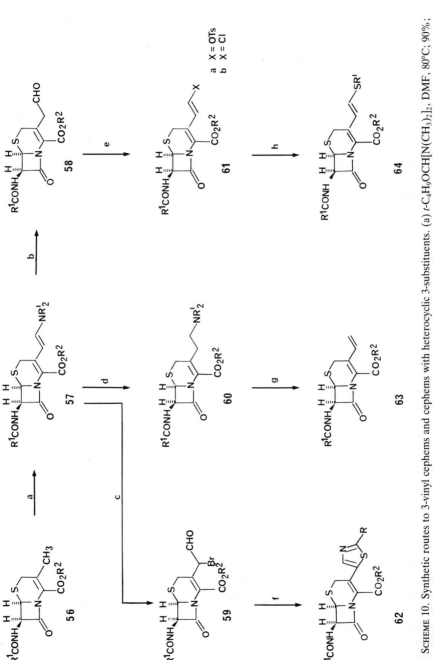

SCHEME 10. Synthetic routes to 3-vinyl cephems and cephems with heterocyclic 3-substituents. (a) t-$C_4H_9OCH[N(CH_3)_2]_2$, DMF, 80°C; 90%; (b) HCl/EtOAc; (c) Br_2, H_2O; (d) TFA, NaBH$_3$CN; (e) (Pho)$_3$PCl$_2$; MCPBA; PCl$_3$ (for **61b**); pTsCl, Et$_3$N (for **61a**); (f) RCSNH$_2$, PCl$_3$; (g) MCPBA, PCl$_3$; (h) HSR', base; acylation, removal of protecting groups are achieved by standard methods. (R^1 = Boc, R^2 = benzhydryl.)

modified as outlined in Scheme 10 (Peyronel *et al.*, 1985). Hydrolysis of **57** under acidic conditions yields 3′-formylcephems **58** which react either with tosyl chloride and triethylamine to the (E)-enol tosylate **61a** or with $(C_6H_5O)_3PCl_2$ to the chlorovinylcephem **61b**. Both products are subsequently transformed to 3-thiovinyl derivatives **64** in analogy with procedures developed for 3-thio derivatives (Section 4.1.3.3). For instance, reaction of the (E)-enol tosylate **61a** with thiols in the presence of base yields 3-thiovinyl derivatives as exemplified by the synthesis of ceftiolene **(213)** (*Drugs of the Future*, 1984d).

Alternatively, reductive elimination leads from **61b** to 3-ethynylcephems of type **44p**. Reduction of the enamine double bond of **57** yields 3-(2-dialkylamino)ethylcephem **60** which is transformed to unsubstituted 3-vinyl derivatives of type **63** by N,S-bisoxidation and subsequent *Cope* elimination of dimethylhydroxyl amine. Bromination of **57** is a route to 3-(1-bromo-2-ethanal) **59**, which reacts with thioamides in a cyclization reaction to 3-(2-substituted-1,3-thiazol-5-yl)cephems **62**.

Cephems with 1,2,4-thiadiazol-2-yl substituents attached to C-3 have been shown to display good antimicrobial activities (Hashimoto *et al.*, 1978; Sugawara *et al.*, 1979a, 1980b). 3-Pyrazolyl-, 3-isoxazolyl-, 3-allenyl-, 3-propenyl- and 3-acylpyrazoles have been synthesized from 3-(1-hydroxy-propenyl)cephem (Spry and Bhala, 1985). Cyclic dithioketals of 3-formyl-cephems **29e** have also been prepared (Nagano *et al.*, 1986a,b).

4.1.3.6 Miscellaneous Synthetic Transformations. Alkylation of cephems bearing —Cl, —SC_6H_5, —OCH_3, —$N(C_2H_4)_2O$, —OSO_2CH_3 or —$OP(O)(OC_6H_5)_2$ substituents at C-3 has been achieved using cuprate reagents (Spry and Bhala, 1985): addition of lithium dimethylcuprate or lithium di-*n*-butylcuprate to 3-chlorocephem yielded a 7-ADCA derivative and a 3-*n*-butylcephem in moderate yield, whereas addition of lithium diallylcuprate produced a 3-allyl-3-cephem. Addition of lithium di-*n*-butyl-cuprate to a 3-vinyl-3-cephem **44a** yielded predominantly the corresponding 1,6-addition product.

4.1.4 3′-Position

4.1.4.1 Synthetic Aspects. Chemical variations in the 3′-position of cephalosporins have been intensively studied (for reviews see Gorman and Ryan, 1972b; Murphy and Webber, 1972; Hatfield *et al.*, 1980b; Dürckheimer *et al.*, 1985 and references cited therein). Displacement of the 3′-acetoxy group by S- and N-nucleophiles is usually achieved in aqueous solution (pH about 6) between 40 and 90°C. Similarly, the 3′-acetylacetoxy group (Tsushima et al., 1979; Ochiai et al., 1981b) and the 3'-carbamoyloxy group (Gordon and Sykes, 1982: pp. 315–318) can be replaced. Hydrolysis of the β-lactam ring and the acetoxy group are observed as side reactions. Kinetic data, salt and solvent effects of the 3'-displacement support an S_N1-type reaction. Formation of a resonance-stabilized allylic cation seems to be the rate-determining step. By protection of the amino group as a *Schiff* base, 3'-substitution of 7-aminocephalosporanic acid (7-ACA) with heterocyclic thiols can be improved with regard to yield and purity (Palomo-Coll et al., 1985). Pyridine bases react more easily in the presence of a high molar excess of potassium iodide or potassium thiocyanate (Spencer et al., 1967). The catalytic role of these salts has not yet been fully clarified. Oxygen nucleophiles do not react under these conditions.

A 3'-displacement in aprotic solvents, e.g. acetonitrile or 1,2-dichloroethane, is accomplished by addition of acids or Lewis acids. A series of boron trifluoride catalysed nucleophilic reactions with 7-ACA to 3'-substituted cephalosporins of type **65** are summarized in Scheme 11. Preparation of 3-CH$_2$-S-R cephems **65a,b** (R = alkyl, aryl and heterocycles) are described by Saikawa et al. (1985). By this method 3-CH$_2$-C **65c,d** and 3-CH$_2$-N **65e–h** cephalosporins can also be synthesized (Sadaki et al., 1986a,b). An example of 3'-displacement by an O-nucleophile to **65i** is given by Prager and Sturm (1986). In spite of the acidic reaction medium, the formation of 7-ACA lactone is not observed.

3-Halomethylcephalosporins are highly useful starting materials for 3'-displacement reactions. They are prepared by a number of routes. For instance, 3-bromomethyl-3-cephem derivatives **67** (X = Br) can be prepared (Scheme 12):

- by treatment of 3-exomethylenecepham **66** with DBU and bromine (Koppel et al., 1977);
- by allylic bromination of 3-methyl-3-cephem esters **68** (R^3 = H) with N-bromosuccinimide (Murphy and Webber, 1972);
- or from 3-hydroxymethyl-3-cephems **68** (R^3 = OH) (Section 4.1.3.5).

The synthesis of 3-methoxymethyl-3-cephems by methanolysis of 3-bromomethyl-2-cephems followed by isomerization to the Δ^3-isomers via 1-sulphoxides is well known (Webber et al., 1971). 3-(2- and 4-Pyridon-1-yl-methyl)-3-cephems (Edwards and Erickson, 1979) and 3-CH$_2$-O-Het-3-cephem esters (Kishi et al., 1979) have been similarly prepared. Reaction of 3-bromomethyl-3-cephems with aqueous dimethylformamide leads to 3-formyloxymethyl-3-cephems (Balsamo et al., 1981). Aliphatic or heterocyclic S-nucleophiles condense to 3-thiomethyl-3-cephem esters (Miskolczi et al., 1981; Cowley et al., 1983a). Lithium dimethyl and diphenylcuprate react with 3-bromomethyl-3-cephems to 3-ethyl and 3-benzyl deriva-

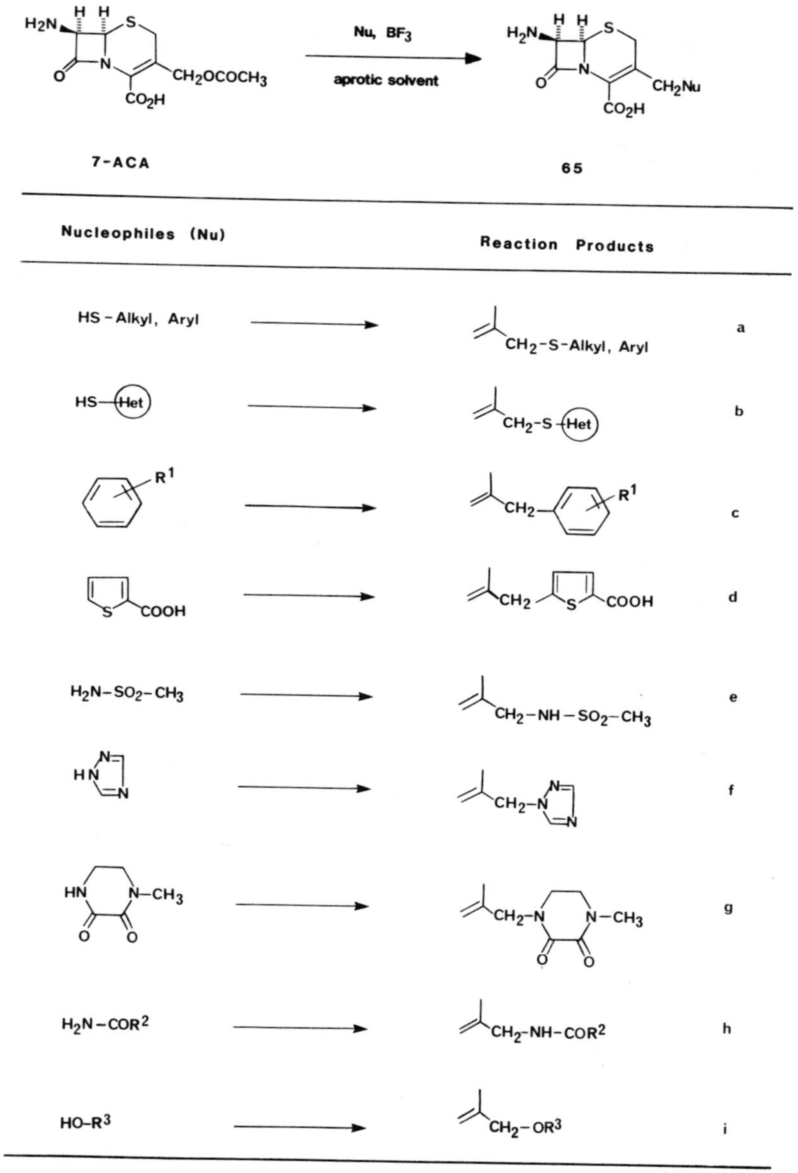

SCHEME 11. 3'-Displacement reactions catalysed by boron trifluoride BF_3. (R^1 = H, OH; R^2 = alkyl, aryl; R^3 = lower alkyl.)

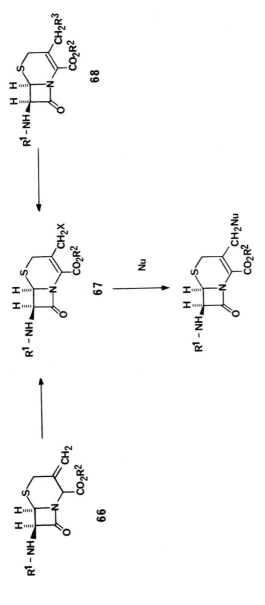

SCHEME 12. Synthesis and reaction of 3-halomethyl cephalosporins **67** with various nucleophiles (Nu), e.g. S-nucleophiles (HS-alkyl, HS-aryl, HS-heterocycles); N-nucleophiles (HNR$_2$, cyclic amines, pyridines); O-nucleophiles (HO-alkyl, HO-heterocycles, carboxylic acids); C-nucleophiles (lithium dialkyl cuprates, phenols). (R^1 = H, protecting group, acyl; R^2 = H, protecting group; R^3 = H, OH, OAc; X = Cl, Br, I.)

tives (Cowley *et al.*, 1983b). Phenols yield C-alkylated products (Animati *et al.*, 1983). Reaction of 3-bromomethyl-3-cephems and the more reactive isomeric 2-cephems with several salts of carboxylic acids yields 3-CH$_2$O-acyl derivatives without isomerization of the double bond (Botta *et al.*, 1985).

A decisive progress in the semisynthesis of 3'-modified cephalosporins has been achieved by preparing 3-iodomethyl cephalosporins **67** (X = I) from appropriate 3-acetoxymethyl derivatives **68** (R^3 = OAc) using iodo-trimethylsilane as reagent (Bonjouklian, 1981; Bonjouklian and Phillips, 1981). The 3-iodomethyl intermediates react either *in situ* or after isolation with S-, N-, or O-nucleophiles. The reaction pathway to such 3'-substituted cephalosporins does not necessarily proceed via a reactive 3-iodomethyl-3-cephem. In the reaction of cefotaxime with pyridine derivatives and iodotrimethylsilane, there is no indication for the existence of a 3-iodomethyl intermediate (Kirrstetter *et al.*, 1984). Other applications are given in several papers. Typical examples are the displacement reactions with S-nucleophiles (Bonjouklian and Phillips, 1981; Wheeler *et al.*, 1986a), with substituted and bicyclic pyridines (Lunn and Shadle, 1982; Lunn and Vasileff, 1983; Smith, 1983; Katner, 1985), with quinolines and isoquinolines (Lunn, 1983; Lunn and Shadle, 1983; Lattrell *et al.*, 1984), with substituted thiazoles (Morin and Leonard, 1986), with isothiazoles (Skotnicki and Strike, 1986), and with O-nucleophiles (Mobashery *et al.*, 1986; Mobashery and Johnston, 1986b).

More recently, the synthesis of 3-iodomethyl-3-cephems by phase-transfer catalysis and their direct conversion to 3'-substituted cephems has been described (Farina, 1986). The introduction of a 3'-carbamoyloxy group which improves the metabolic stability is achieved by reacting 3-hydroxy-methyl-3-cephems with isocyanates (Humber *et al.*, 1981; Wilson, 1984). Using dichlorophosphoryl isocyanate (Cl$_2$P(O)NCO) 3'-phosphonocar-bamoyl-3-cephems can be obtained similarly (Humber *et al.*, 1981).

4.1.4.2 Influence of 3'-Substituents on Stability and Reactivity of the β-Lactam Ring. Substituents at the 3'-position strongly influence the chemical reactivity of the β-lactam ring (Boyd, 1984). Quantitative correlations between the rate of hydrolysis of the β-lactam ring and spectroscopic data (^{13}C-NMR and IR) of 3-substituted cephalosporins have been found (Boyd, 1983; Nishikawa and Tori, 1984; Coene *et al.*, 1984). A relationship has been confirmed between β-lactam ring-opening rates and either the ^{13}C-chemical shift differences of C-3 and C-4, or the β-lactam C=O frequency in the IR spectra, as expressing the electronic effects of the substituents at the 3'-position. The nucleophilic attack on the β-lactam carbonyl carbon seems to be largely simultaneous with the departure of the 3'-leaving group, but the mechanism is still controversially discussed (Page, 1984; Boyd, 1985).

There is good evidence in some cases that elimination of a good leaving group at the 3'-position does not need to be in concert with the cleavage of the β-lactam ring (Faraci and Pratt, 1984; Page and Proctor, 1984). Grabowski et al. (1985) were able to characterize an intermediate which arises from the opening of the β-lactam ring before the 3'-group is expelled. Ester cleavage of the 3'-acetoxy group in cefotaxime (207) in strong alkaline media (pH > 12) is much faster than β-lactam ring opening (Dürckheimer and Seliger, 1982). The hydrolysis of the 3'-acetoxy group in cephalothin was studied using isotopically labelled $H_2^{18}O$ and [2-^{13}C]acetate anion and proceeds by two ways: an acyl-oxygen bond cleavage and a reversible alkyl-oxygen bond cleavage (Indelicato et al., 1985).

In recent papers on the degradation of 7α-methoxy-1-oxacephems with various 3'-substituents, it was pointed out that the chemical reactivity of the β-lactam ring is dependent on the electron-withdrawing character of the 3'-substituents (Narisada et al., 1987; Nishikawa et al., 1987 and references cited therein).

4.1.4.3 3-Thiomethyl Derivatives. The 1-methyltetrazol-5-yl-thio group has been introduced into the 3'-position of many semisynthetic cephalosporins (70a in Table 12). It considerably improves the antibacterial activity, especially against Gram-negative bacteria and is found as a characteristic structural element in many parenteral cephalosporins either on the market or under extended evaluation, e.g. cefamandole, cefbuperazone (106), cefmenoxime (208), cefmetazole, cefminox (107), cefoperazone (244), cefotetan (105), cefpiramide (245), latamoxef (273), CPW-86 363, KIT-180 (246), L-640 876 (255), NY-1675, UG-FA-132 (108) and VX-VD2 (Section 5).

Some adverse reactions of cephalosporins seem to be connected with this 3'-substituent, which is cleaved off in small amounts as 1-methyltetrazol-5-thiol. Two types of coagulopathy have been observed. The first involves hypoprothrombinaemia and can be prevented by administration of vitamin K. The second is associated with prolonged bleeding time and impairment of platelet function; it is not influenced by vitamin K (Sattler et al., 1986, and references therein). Disulfiram-like reactions with increased blood concentrations of acetaldehyde following alcohol consumption have also occurred (Sanders and Sanders, 1986b). In the rat, the latter effect is more pronounced with cefamandole, cefbuperazone (106), cefmetazol and latamoxef (273) than with cefmenoxime (208), cefminox (107), and cefotetan (105), and can be triggered by administering 1-methyltetrazol-5-thiol alone (Kamei et al., 1986). Testicular toxicity of 3'-(1-methyltetrazol-5-yl-thio)cephalosporins in juvenile rats has also been reported (Comereski et al., 1987). The

3'-tetrazol-5-yl-thio moiety in cephalosporins has been manifoldly substituted at the 1-nitrogen by acidic or basic groups, as outlined in Table 12.

The N-substituted tetrazole rings of structures **70b–e** (Table 12) are found at the 3'-position of ceforanide (type **70b**), cefonicide (type **70c**), cefotiam (type **70d**), E-0702 (type **70b**), SKF-80 303 (type **70c**) and SKF-88 070 (type **70d**). Many other five-membered N- and N,S-heterocyclic moieties, mostly containing more than one heteroatom, have been linked via a 3'-thioether bridge, e.g. 1,2,3-triazol-4-yl in **70f** [in cefatrizine (**277**) and ICI-156 488 (**250**)], 1,2,3-thiadiazol-5-yl in **70g** [in cefuzonam (**216**) and CGP-31 523 A (**272**)], 1,3,4-thiadiazol-2-yl in **70h** (in ceftezole), 5-methyl-1,3,4-thiadiazol-2-yl in **70h** [in cefazolin, cefazedone and KY-087 (**249**)], 3-hydroxy-4-carboxy-isothiazol-5-yl in **70i** [in YM-13 115 (**264**)] and 5-carboxymethyl-4-methylthiazol-2-yl in **70k** [in cefodizime (**211**)]. Structure–activity relationships in the cefodizime (**211**) series were recently described (Blumbach *et al.*, 1987). Thus, esterification of the mercaptothiazol-carboxy group in cefodizime (**211**) improved in some cases (allyl and propargyl ester) MIC values against Gram-positive strains. In the Gram-negative range, the esters are slightly less active compared to **211**. Concerning pharmacokinetic data in mouse and dog, only the chlorobenzyl ester has comparably balanced properties.

The 6-hydroxy-2-methyl-5-oxo-1,2,4-triazin-3-ylthio moiety in **70l** confers to ceftriaxone (**210**) outstanding pharmacokinetic properties (Section 5.1). N-Substituted 4-pyridinium rings of structure **70m–o** are found in CM-40 874 (**271a**), CM-40 876 (**271b**), ME-1220 (**263a**), and ME-1228 (**263c**). Some interesting bicyclic heterocycles are also listed in Table 12, e.g. pyrazolo[2,3-a]-pyrimidine in **70p** [in M-14 638 (**262a**), M-14 643 (**262b**) and M-14 659 (**262e**)], tetrazolo[1,5-b]pyridazine in **70q** [in FCE-20 485 (**217**), FCE-20 635, K-13 102 (**258**) and K-13 176 (**257**)] and N-substituted 2,3-cyclopentenopyridines in **70r** [in ME-1221 (**263b**) and MT-382 (**225**)]. Synthesis and structure–activity relationships of cephalosporins bearing a thiotetrazolo[1,5-b]pyridazine at the 3'-position as in **70q** have been intensively investigated (Nannini *et al.*, 1981b; Alpegiani *et al.*, 1983). In this series, FCE-20 485 (**217**) was selected for further studies because of its long serum half-life and good *in vivo* activity. The most interesting compounds are described in Section 5.1.

4.1.4.4 3-Oxymethyl Derivatives. Besides 3'-acetoxy- and 3'-carbamoyloxycephalosporins, only a few 3-oxymethyl derivatives are known. 3-Alkoxymethylcephalosporins of the first generation have been investigated (Sassiver and Lewis, 1977). An interesting compound with a 2-aminothiazole moiety in the 7-acyl side chain is the orally active prodrug

TABLE 12

3-Thiomethylcephalosporins **70** with different 7-side chains

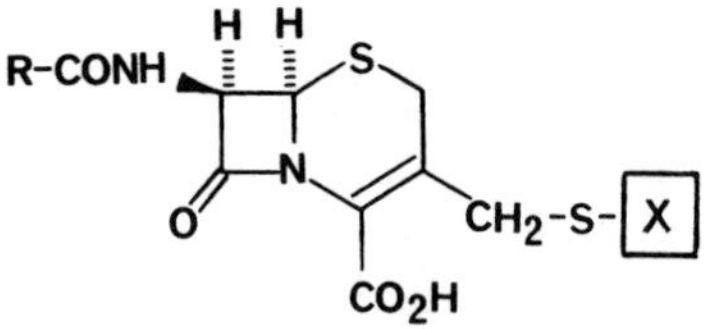

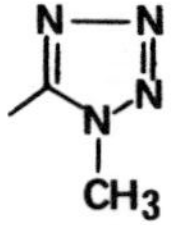

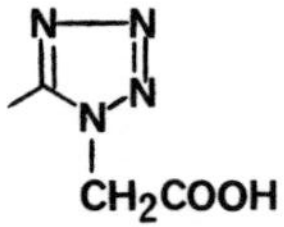

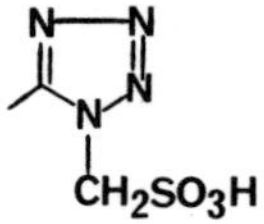

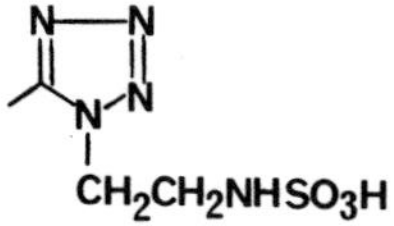

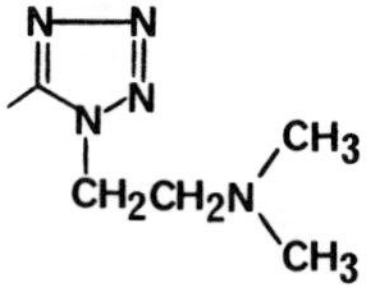

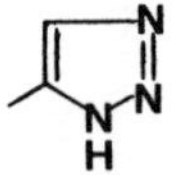

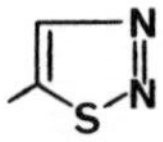

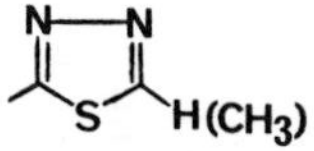

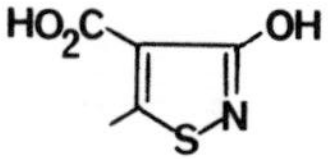

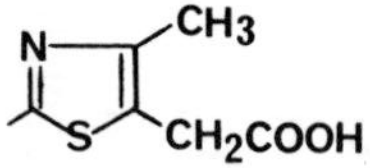

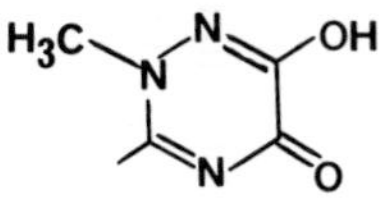

CH_2 COOH

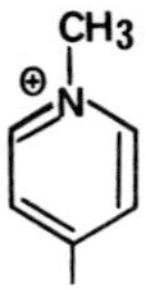

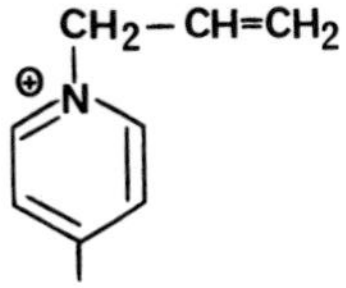

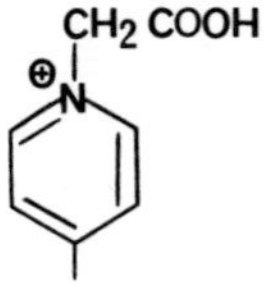

o

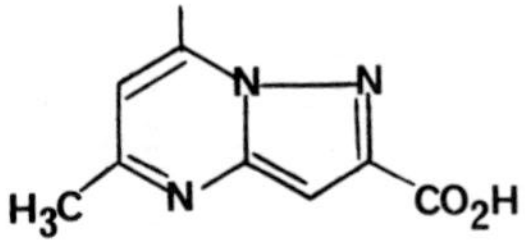

CH_2—CH=CH_2

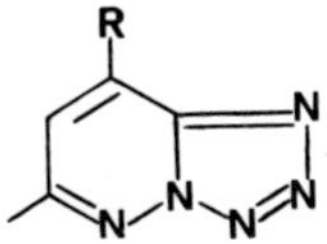

n

CH_3

m

OH

l

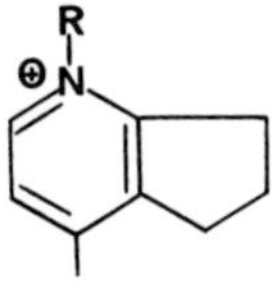

R = CH_3, CH_2COOH

r

R = H, CH_3, COOH, NH_2

q

CO_2H

p

cephalosporin cefpodoxime (CS-807) (**295**) (Section 5.2). 1-Methyl-3-pyridinio-oxymethyl analogues have been reported to have good antibiotic activity (Terachi *et al.*, 1985).

4.1.4.5 3-Ammonio and 3-Aminomethyl Derivatives. Displacement of the acetoxy group by nitrogen nucleophiles has also become attractive. Abraham and Newton (1958) found the first 3′-displacement reaction with pyridine, when cephalosporin C was stored overnight in a pyridine-acetate buffer. Further investigation led to the development of cephaloridine and cefsulodine (**254**) (Section 5.1). 3-Azidomethyl-, 3-aminomethyl- and 3-acylamidomethylcephems were also described (Murphy and Webber, 1972). In the aminothiazole cephalosporin series, the introduction of a pyridinium group resulted in very broad and high antibacterial activity. Ceftazidime (**266**) (Section 5.1) was the first representative of this group.

Another very promising compound is cefpirome (**220**) (Section 5.1), which was selected out of a large series of 3′-pyridinio compounds (Lattrell *et al.*, 1982, 1983a). SAR studies revealed the best overall activity with annelated saturated and unsaturated rings, or cyclopropyl and alkoxy residues at the pyridine moiety (Schwab *et al.*, 1983). General routes for the preparation of 3′-pyridiniocephalosporins **72** are outlined in Scheme 13. 3′-Pyridiniocephalosporins **72** and also other 3-ammoniomethylcephalosporins can be synthesized:

- by displacement of the 3′-acetoxy group in cefotaxime (**207; 71**, R = CH₃) or its analogues **71** with appropriately substituted pyridines or nitrogen-containing heterocycles in aqueous solution or formamide in the presence of alkali iodides or alkali thiocyanates at 50–80°C (route a);
- or from cefotaxime (**207; 71**, R = CH₃) or its analogues **71** and the corresponding nitrogen compounds after addition of iodotrimethylsilane in an organic solvent, such as methylene chloride or chloroform (route b);
- or via the 3-iodomethylcephalosporin derivative which is prepared from cefotaxime (**207; 71**, R = CH₃) or its analogues **71** by silylation with N-methyltrimethylsilyl trifluoroacetamide or bistrimethylsilyl trifluoroacetamide and subsequent treatment with iodotrimethylsilane in an organic solvent. The iodides are converted *in situ* to the desired cephalosporins **72** after addition of the nitrogen base in a suitable aprotic solvent (route c);
- or by condensation of 2-(2-amino-4-thiazolyl)-2-alkoxyimino acetic acid and the corresponding derivatives of 7-aminocephalosporanic acid **73** which are prepared from 7-ACA and pyridines (route d).

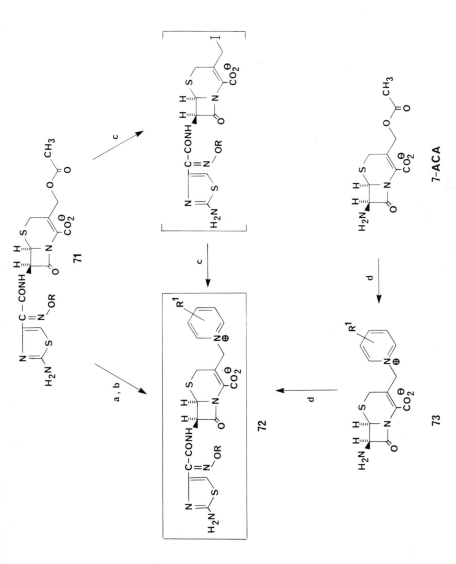

SCHEME 13. Synthesis of 3′-pyridiniocephalosporins **72** on different routes, described in the text.

TABLE 13

3-Ammonio- and 3-aminomethylcephalosporins **74** with different 7-side chains. (In compound **74m–t** the carboxylate group has to be replaced by a carboxylic acid moiety)

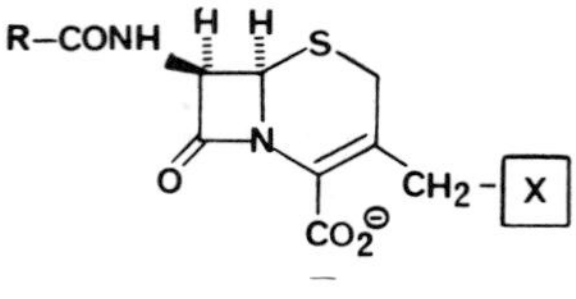

74

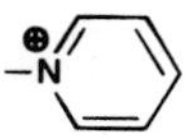

a

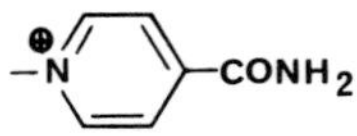

b

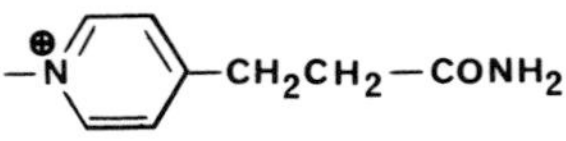

c

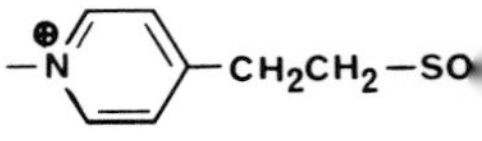

d

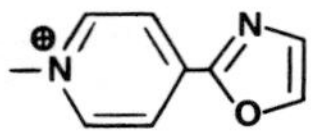

e

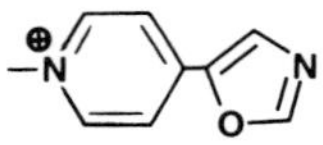

f

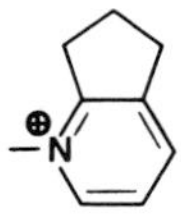

g

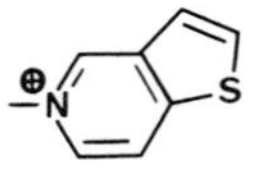

h

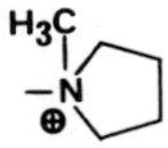

i

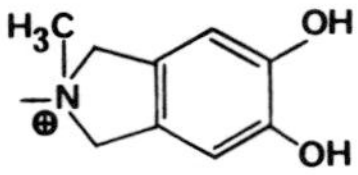

k

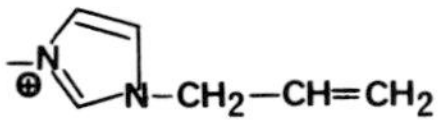

l

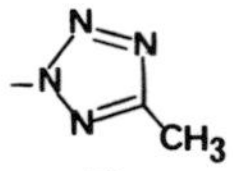

m

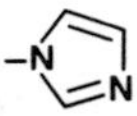

n

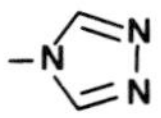

o

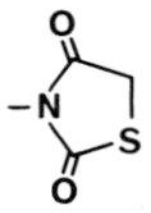

p

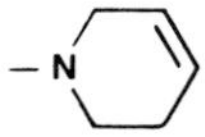

q

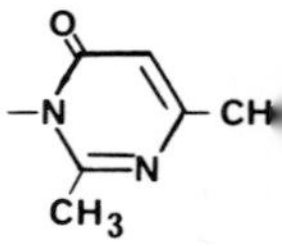

r

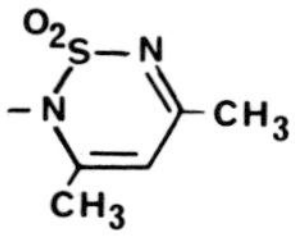

s

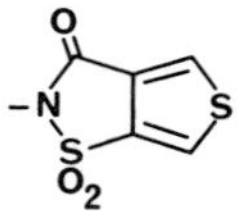

t

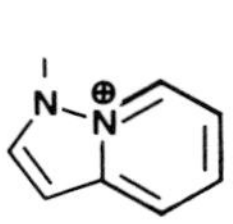

u

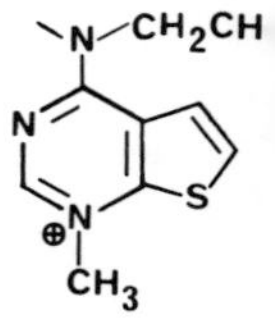

v

Optimum oxyimino substituents were methyl, ethyl and the less accessible difluoromethyl and carbamoylmethyl residues. In comparison, cephalosporins with an acidic function in the oxyimino group showed decreased activity against *Staph. aureus*. The introduction of 3'-aliphatic or cycloaliphatic ammonio groups led to highly active compounds, e.g. cefepime (BMY-28 142) (**221**) (Section 5.1), which in its antibiotic potency is comparable to cefpirome (**220**) (Naito *et al.*, 1986a). Many other 3-ammonio- and 3-aminomethylcephalosporins have also been prepared (Table 13). Cephaloridine and ceftazidime (**266**) are of type **74a**, cefsulodin (**254**) **74b**, cefpirome (**220**) **74g**, and cefepime (**221**) **74i**. The following 3-ammoniomethyl-3-cephems were selected for extended evaluation: DN-9550 (**270**), FR-17 126 (**240**) and GR-32 620 (type **74a**), CGP-22 495 (**238**) (type **74b**), SG-164 (**267**) (type **74c**), cefpimizole (**248**) (type **74d**), DQ-2522 (**222**) (type **74e**), DQ-2556 (**223**) (type **74f**), L-165 433 (**224**) (type **74h**), BO-1232 (**269a**) (type **74k**) and OCS-575 (**268**) (type **74l**). The synthesis of OCS-575 (**268**) is described by Matsumura *et al.* (1987). Recently, SAR studies of 3'-pyridiniocephalosporins with 5-membered heterocycles at the pyridinium group have been reported. In this series DQ-2522 (**222**) and DQ-2556 (**223**) exhibit the best antibacterial activity (Ejima *et al.*, 1987).

In the group of 3-aminomethylcephalosporins, cefteram (**215**) (type **74m**) displays good overall activity (Sadaki *et al.*, 1986b). Its pivaloyloxymethyl ester T-2588 (**293**) has been selected for further studies (Section 5.2). Moreover, characteristic examples of this type claimed in patents are also given in Table 13, e.g. cephems with imidazol-1-yl and substituted imidazol-1-yl of type **74n** (Lattrell *et al.*, 1987), with N-bonded triazolyl **74o** (Sadaki *et al.*, 1982), with 2,4-dioxothiazolidin-3-yl **74p** (Horii *et al.*, 1979), with 1,2,5,6-tetrahydro-1-pyridyl **74q** (Fujisawa Pharmaceutical Co., Ltd, 1985), with 1,6-dihydro-2,4-dimethyl-6-oxo-1-pyrimidinyl **74r** (Toyama Chemical Co., Ltd, 1985a), with 3,5-dimethyl-1,1-dioxo-1,2,6-thiadiazin-2-yl **74s** (Toyama Chemical Co., Ltd, 1985b), with 3-oxothieno[3,4-d]isothiazol-2(3H)-yl **74t** and related compounds (Skotnicki and Strike, 1986), with pyrazolo[1,5-a]pyrimidinium-1-yl **74u** (Miyake *et al.*, 1985), and with N-ethyl-N-(1-methylthieno[2,3-d]pyrimidinium-4-yl)amino **74v** and related compounds (Bradbury *et al.*, 1985). ICI-194 008 is a new injectable cephalosporin of this type **74v** which is now under further evaluation (Hennessey *et al.*, 1987b).

4.1.4.6 3'-Carbon Derivatives. 3'-Carbon cephalosporins have already been reviewed by Murphy and Webber (1972). Newer 3-CH_2-C cephems were reported by Cowley *et al.* (1983b), Animati *et al.* (1983) and Sadaki *et al.* (1986a) (see Section 4.1.4.1). Typical examples are given in Table 14. All compounds show only diminished antibacterial activity.

TABLE 14

3'-Carbon cephalosporins **75** with different 7-side chains

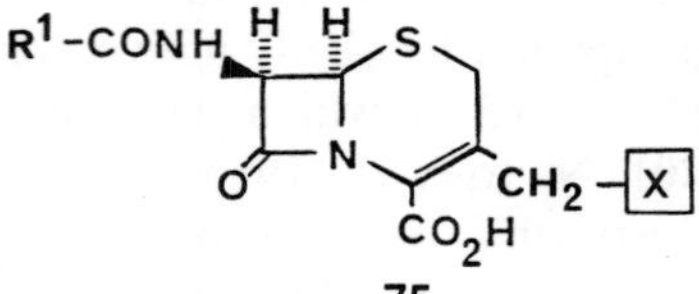

R^1-CONH ... CH$_2$—[X]
CO$_2$H
75

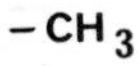

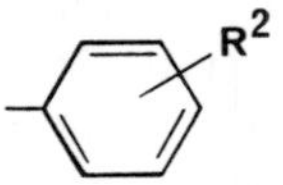

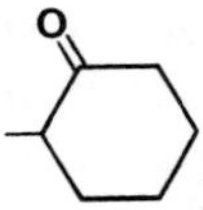

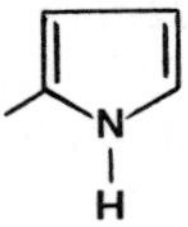

−CH$_3$	R^2		N−H
a	b	c	d
N	CO$_2$H	S CO$_2$H	
e	f	g	

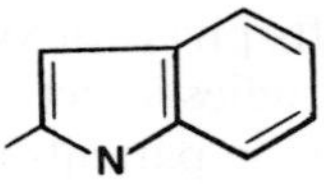

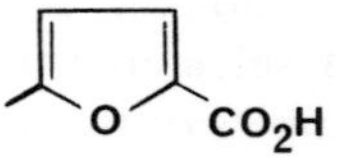

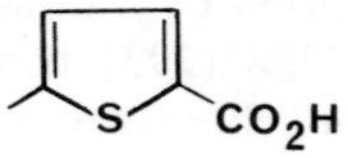

4.1.5 4-Position

4.1.5.1 Various 4-Substituents. With few exceptions, only limited success was achieved in the past by varying the free carboxylic acid function in β-lactams. Examples of the main structural variations that have been made were summarized by Murphy and Webber (1972) and Sammes (1980). Lactones **76a** and lactames **76c** retain some activity against Gram-positive bacteria, whereas thiolactones **76b** do not. Cephems with a 5-tetrazolyl residue at C-4, e.g. **76d**, are synthesized from cephems via a 1,3-dipolar cycloaddition reaction from the 4-nitrile or 4-imine group prepared from the 4-carboxylic acid with sodium azide. They have been found to exhibit significant biological activity against Gram-positive strains (English *et al.*, 1976; Cama and Christensen, 1978; Presslitz, 1978). Cephalosporins

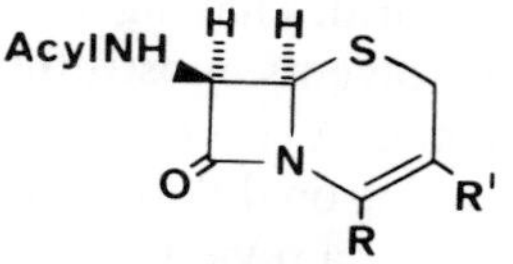

76

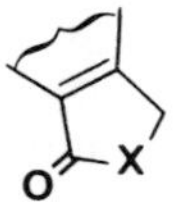

X = O , S , NH

R =

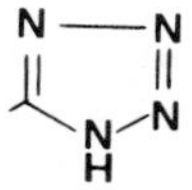

a   b   c   d

with other 4-substituents, e.g. —COCH$_3$, —CHO, —CH=N—OR, —CH$_2$CO$_2$H, or heteroatom substituents, such as —P(O)(OH)$_2$, —SO$_3$H and —SO$_2$NH$_2$, showed no significant antibacterial activities, in some cases in contrast to the penicillin series (see Sammes, 1980, and references cited therein).

4.1.5.2 Ester Derivatives. Cephem esters are important intermediates because many synthetic manipulations of the cephem nucleus require carboxy-protected derivatives. Due to the high sensitivity of the cephem nucleus, only ester-protecting groups which are selectively formed and cleaved under mild conditions have gained importance. The choice of the protecting group depends on the intended chemical transformation and the required reaction conditions. Tertiary butyl-, benzhydryl-, *p*-nitrobenzyl-, *p*-methoxybenzyl-, allyl- and silyl esters are the groups most frequently used [see Greene (1981) for a general review]. Phenoxyethyl has been recently reported as a cephem-protecting group (Alpegiani *et al.*, 1984).

In recent years, the main efforts have focused on the elaboration of oral cephalosporin prodrugs with metabolically cleavable esters (Section 5.2). These prodrugs are mostly acyloxymethyl-, acyloxyethyl- or alkoxycarbonyloxyethyl esters. Besides, prodrug residues of different types, e.g. allyl ester, (5-methyl-2-oxo-1,3-dioxolen-4-yl)methylester, or prodrugs with more complex structures, e.g. *p*-alanyloxybenzoylmethyl ester (Kakeya *et al.*, 1984), have been prepared in several series of physiologically active cephalosporins.

Cephalosporin alkylesters are obtained by reacting either a cephem carboxylic acid with a diazoalkane or an alkali metal or ammonium cephem carboxylates with reactive halides in a S$_N$2-reaction. Iodides and bromides are most frequently used, chlorides having a lower reactivity. The reaction is conducted in inert aprotic solvents, mostly dimethylformamide. Mixtures of Δ^3- and biologically inactive Δ^2-isomeric products are often formed in varying ratios, largely depending on the size of the cephem 3-substituent [see Murphy and Webber (1972) for a review]. It was suggested that isomerization results from the ability of a cephem carboxylate to abstract a proton from the 2-methylene of the 3-cephem ester formed during the reaction (Bentley et al., 1976). Reprotonation occurs at C-2 or C-4, generating the 2- and 3-cephem esters. They cannot be easily separated by conventional chromatographic methods. Isomeric mixtures are mostly not amenable to fractional crystallization. It is therefore advantageous to employ mild reaction conditions which minimize the formation of Δ^2-isomers (low reaction temperature, small excess of base, short reaction time). A pure Δ^3-isomer can be obtained from a Δ^3/Δ^{2-} mixture in a two-step reaction sequence: both the Δ^2- and Δ^3-esters are converted to the corresponding Δ^3-sulphoxide, which is subsequently reduced (Kaiser et al., 1970).

The need for acetyl chloride or a phosphorus trihalide in the sulphoxide reduction step restricts the applicability to esters with functionalities unaffected by these reagents. Several approaches for the preparation of pure Δ^3-esters have been reported (Mobashery and Johnston, 1986a and references cited therein). The esterification by diazoalkanes avoids Δ^3/Δ^{2-} isomerization, but the preparation of the specific diazoalkane is tedious. Other procedures, e.g. reacting cephem acids with alcohols under Mitsunobu reaction conditions, or using DCC as condensing agent, have also been applied in the synthesis of cephem esters [review: Murphy and Webber (1972)]. In the case of esters of the hemiacetal type, this approach has little scope due to the instability of most of the corresponding alcohols.

4.1.6 7α-Position

Cephamycins are a class of naturally occurring cephalosporins formed by different streptomyces species and discovered in screening programmes by Lilly (Nagarajan et al., 1971) and Merck (Stapley et al., 1972). They contain as a typical structural feature a 7α-methoxy substituent which confers on these compounds and their derivatives an excellent β-lactamase stability. All cephamycins isolated and characterized up until 1982 are described in an excellent review (Gordon and Sykes, 1982). The purpose of this section is to give a brief survey of the methodology needed for chemical introduction of a 7α-methoxy group or other substituents such as alkyl, N-formylamido or thioalkyl, at the 7α-position of cephalosporins.

4.1.6.1 7α-Methoxylation of Cephalosporins. Cama *et al.* (1972) developed the first procedure for introducing a 7α-methoxy group in cephalosporins utilizing benzhydryl 7-diazocephalosporanate **79** as a key intermediate. It is obtained by diphenyldiazomethane esterification of 7-ACA *p*-toluene sulfonate **77** and subsequent diazotation (Scheme 14). Reaction with bromoazide gives a mixture of diastereomeric 7-bromo-7-azidoesters **80** which, by reaction with silver tetrafluoroborate in methanol, afford the desired stereoisomer **81**. The observed stereoselectivity is rationalized as proceeding via addition of methanol to a 7-carbenium ion from the less hindered exo-face. Reduction of **81** followed by acylation with thienylacetyl chloride and deprotection give the 7α-methoxycephalothin **82**.

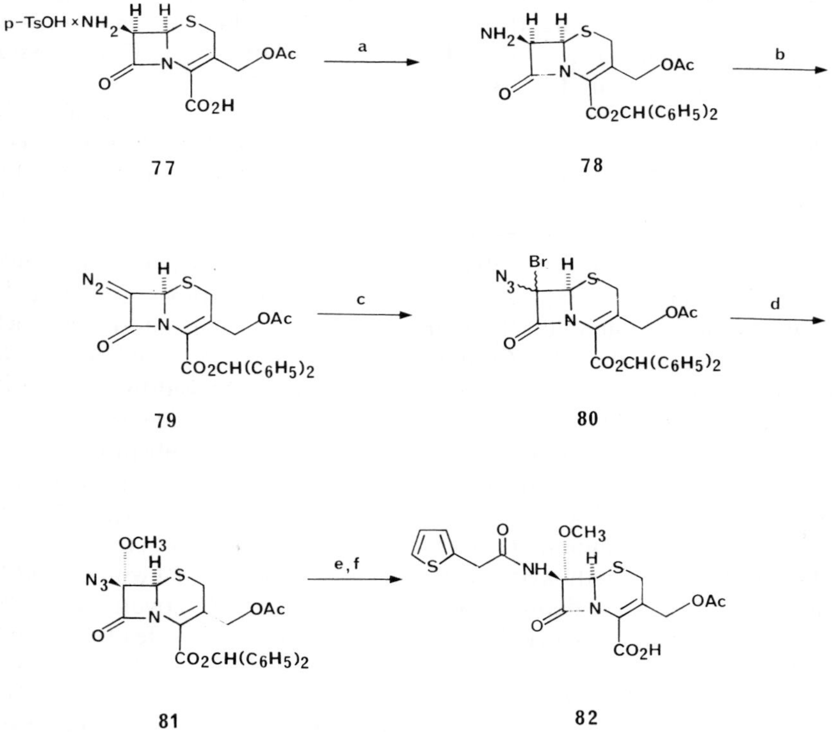

SCHEME 14. Introduction of a 7α-methoxy group via a bromine azide **80**. (a) $(C_6H_5)_2CHN_2$; (b) HNO_2, 0°C, CH_2Cl_2/H_2O; (c) BrN_3 in the presence of excess Et_3N-N_3, -15°C; (d) MeOH/$AgBF_4$, r.t.; (e) PtO_2/H_2, dioxane, followed by acylation with 2-thienylacetyl chloride, pyridine, 0°C; (f) CF_3CO_2H/anisole, 0°C.

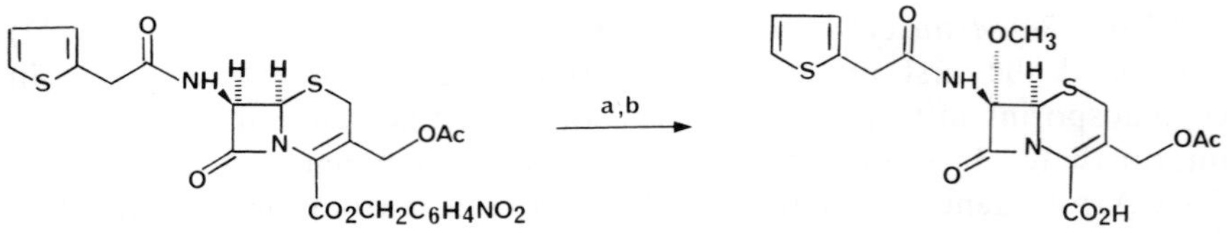

83   82

SCHEME 15. Introduction of a 7α-methoxy group via an acylimine. (a) 3.5 eq. LiOCH$_3$, −80°C, THF, *t*-BuOCl, followed by quenching with CH$_3$CO$_2$H; chromatography, 73%; (b) 5% Pd/C-H$_2$, MeOH/THF.

Koppel and Koehler (1973) developed a method to introduce the 7α-methoxy substituent directly, using *t*-butylhypochlorite and lithium methoxide (Scheme 15). The acylated cephalosporin **83** is treated with lithium methoxide in THF at −78°C, followed by reaction with *t*-butylhypochlorite. After quenching with methanol, **82** is obtained in good yield and with high stereoselectivity. Instead of lithium methoxide, Firestone and Christensen (1973) recommended phenyllithium as a base. Isomerization of the Δ^3-double bond is not observed. Later it was realized that the same procedure can be applied without protection of the carboxyl group (Feyen and Schröck, 1981). Sugimura *et al.* (1976) reported that α-chloroiminochloride **85**, synthesized from **84**, undergoes at −78°C a lithium methoxide initiated 1,4-elimination to **86**, which via intermediate **87** affords the iminoether **88**. Conversion to amide **89** was affected with trimethylchlorosilane in the presence of quinoline followed by hydrolysis (Scheme 16). Another elegant method introduced by Yanagisawa *et al.* (1975) exploits a quinoid imine intermediate to achieve 7α-substitution. The reaction sequence is shown in Scheme 17. Condensation of **78** and **90** to the *Schiff*'s base **91** and subsequent oxidation with freshly prepared lead dioxide produces the labile quinoid **92**. Its treatment with methanol stereospecifically affords the 7α-methoxyimine **93**, which is cleaved into **94** with *Girard* T reagent. Acylation and deprotection of **94** give **95** in a 70% overall yield. A modified procedure uses nickel peroxide instead of lead dioxide (Tsuji *et al.*, 1984).

Nakabayashi *et al.* (1982) reported a "one-pot" procedure which comprises a 1,4-elimination process to form an acylimine without use of *t*-butyl hypochlorite. The procedure is shown in Scheme 18. The imino chloride **96** is treated with silver triflate and pyridine-N-oxide to give **97**. This reacts with triethylamine and methanol via acylimine **98** to **99** in 70% yield.

Groups at Squibb (Gordon *et al.*, 1977, 1980) and Sankyo (Kobayashi *et al.*, 1979) independently developed a procedure using relatively stable

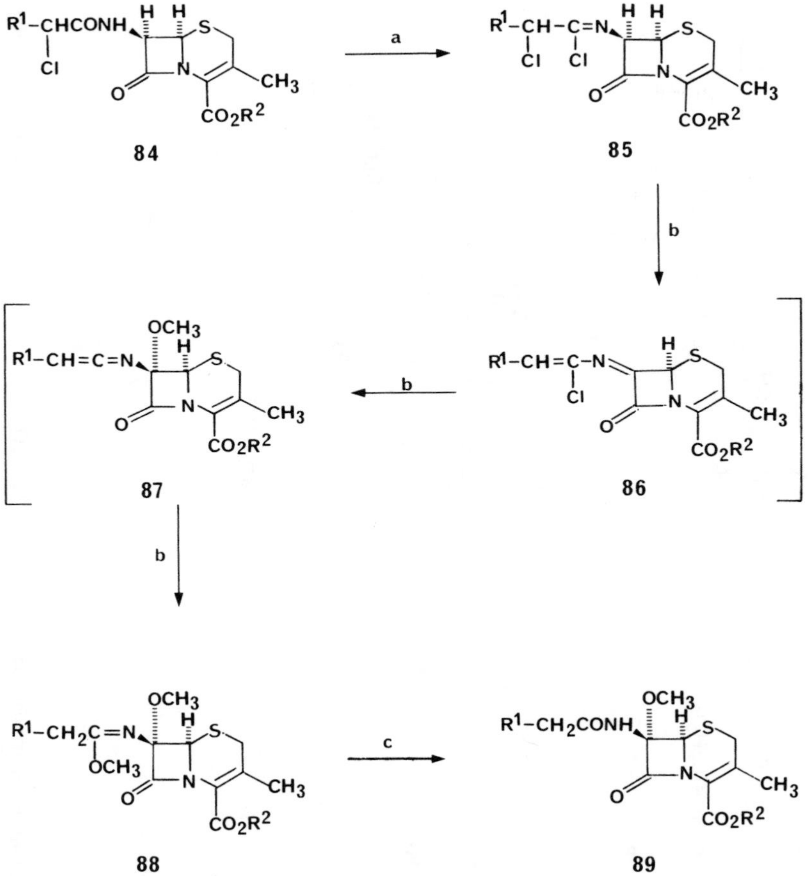

SCHEME 16. Introduction of a 7α-methoxy group via an imidoylchloride **86**. $R^1 = C_6H_5$, $R^2 = CH(C_6H_5)_2$. (a) PCl_5; (b) excess $LiOCH_3/MeOH$, THF, then CH_3CO_2H, 60%, chromatography; (c) excess trimethylsilylchloride, 1 eq. quinoline, $CHCl_3$, r.t.

sulphenimines. They are conveniently obtained by oxidation of sulphenamides with manganese dioxide or by reacting 7-ACA esters with excess of methylsulphenyl chloride (Scheme 19). Reaction of benzhydryl ester **100** with three equivalents of methylsulphenyl chloride in the presence of propylene oxide as an acid scavenger affords the sulphenimine **101** in high yield. When **101** is reacted with triphenylphosphine, mercuric acetate and methanol in CH_2Cl_2, the corresponding 7α-methoxy-derivative **102** is obtained stereospecifically. Acylation and deprotection afford **103**.

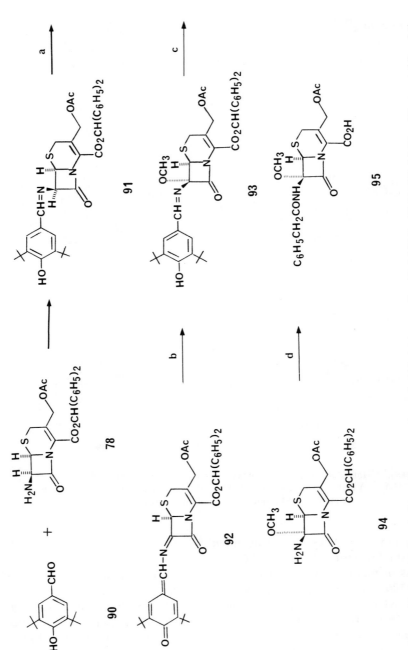

SCHEME 17. Introduction of a 7α-methoxy group via a quinoid imine intermediate **92**. (a) PbO₂; (b) MeOH; (c) *Girard* T reagent; (d) acylation, then deprotection.

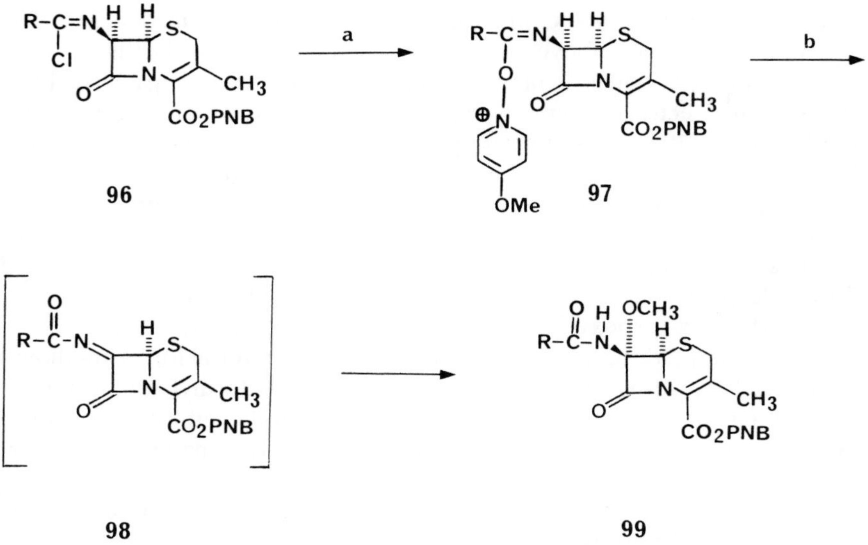

SCHEME 18. Introduction of a 7α-methoxy group via a 1-pyridinium-oxyimino intermediate. (a) Silver triflate, 4-methoxypyridine N-oxide, CH_2Cl_2, −30°C, 2 h; (b) MeOH, triethylamine, −40°C. (R = $C_6H_5OCH_2$.)

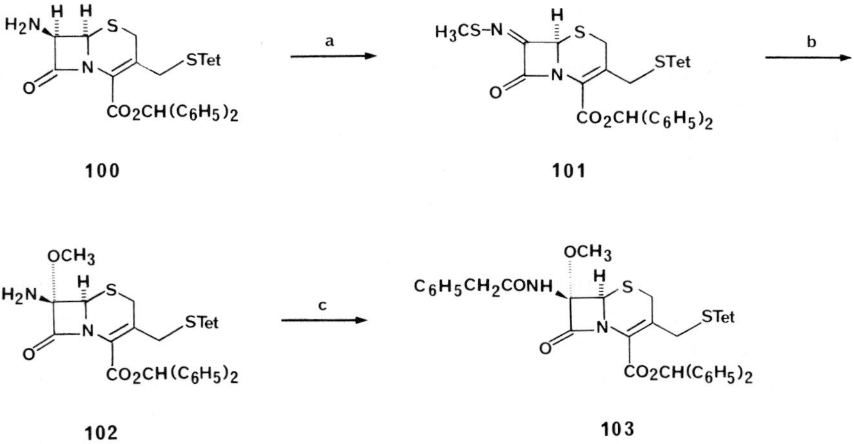

SCHEME 19. Introduction of 7α-methoxy substituent via sulfenimine 101. (a) 3 eq. methyl-sulphenyl chloride, excess propylene oxide; (b) triphenylphosphine, mercuric acetate, methanol in CH_2Cl_2; (c) acylation and deprotection. (Tet = 1-methyltetrazol-5-yl.)

4.1.6.2 7α-Substituted Cephalosporins with Various Substituents. The methods discussed above are also useful for introducing diverse 7α-substituents besides a methoxyl group. Thioalkyl groups have been introduced directly or indirectly via acylimine or carbanionic intermediates (Böhme *et al.*, 1971). In a typical procedure, a *Schiff*'s base is deprotonated by a strong base such as potassium tert-butoxide at low temperature, and the generated anion is quenched with an electrophile such as methylsulphenyl chloride to give 7α-methylthiocephalosporins. By a similar process various 7α-substituted cephalosporins have been prepared, e.g. 7α-methyl- and 7α-ethylcephalothin, 7α-hydroxy-, 7α-hydroxymethyl-, 7α-formyl-, 7α-acetyl- or 7α-carboxy-3-cephems (Gordon and Sykes, 1982).

The 7α-methylthiocephem is a versatile starting material for 7α-methoxy-cephems. It can also be used for the preparation of 7α-formylamidocephems by treating with mercuric acetate and ammonia, followed by formylation. Acetic formic anhydride and N,N-bis (trimethylsilyl)formamide have been used as formylating agents (Milner, 1984; Guest *et al.*, 1987). 7α-Hydroxy-cephems have been prepared by direct hydroxylation (Schröck and Kinast, 1983). Various 7α-ethoxy-, thioalkyl-, cyano-, azido- or phosphonocephems have also been prepared (Gordon and Sykes, 1982).

The 7α-methoxy group in cephalosporins is associated with a high degree of resistance towards β-lactamases, but impairs the bacteriostatic activity for many organisms by altering the affinity to the PBPs. It was shown that the binding to PBPs in *Escherichia coli* is changed when cefotaxime (**207**) is 7α-methoxylated. The ID_{50}-values for PBP 1a and PBP 1b, and particularly for PBP 3, are reduced, whereas the proteins PBP 5 and 6 bind more intensively (Seeger *et al.*, 1983).

Table 15 lists semisynthetic 7α-methoxy cephalosporins that are important antibiotics on the market or have been extensively evaluated. Cefoxitin (**104**) was the first cephamycin to have great success in clinical practice. It is especially useful in the case of mixed infection with β-lactamase-forming anaerobes. Cefotetan (**105**), which possesses a 1-methyltetrazol-5-yl-thiomethyl substituent and a tautomerizing 7β-acyl side chain, is less active against Gram-positive bacteria, but is more active against Gram-negative strains than cefoxitin (**104**) and has a longer half-life. Cefbuperazone (**106**) is excreted in bile and, thus, is suitable for treating infections of the bile duct. Cefminox (**107**) has advantages similar to those of cefotetan (**105**) and cefbuperazone (**106**). UG-FA-132 (**108**) is in its antibacterial activity similar to those compounds described above, but also has some anti-*Pseudomonas* activity (Wetzel *et al.*, 1985). Latamoxef (**273**) was the first 1-oxacephem introduced into the market. In the meantime, two other 1-oxacephem derivatives have come under extended clinical evaluation. More biological data of these compounds will be discussed in Section 5.1.

TABLE 15

Cephamycin derivatives on the market or under evaluation

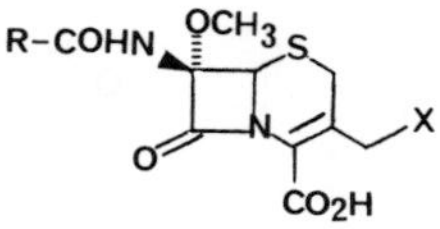

No.	Compound	R	X
104	Cefoxitin	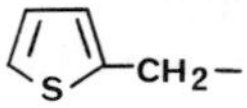	$-OCONH_2$
105	Cefotetan	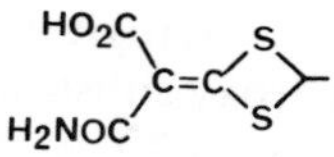	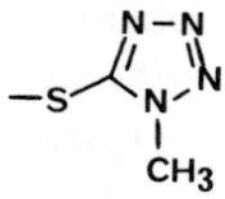
106	Cefbuperazone	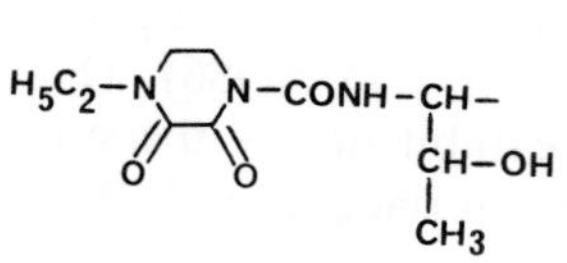	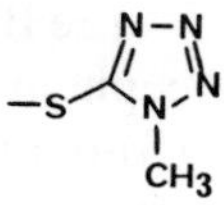
107	Cefminox		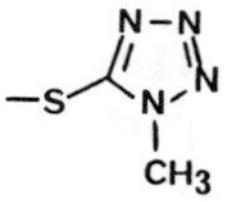
108	UG-FA 132	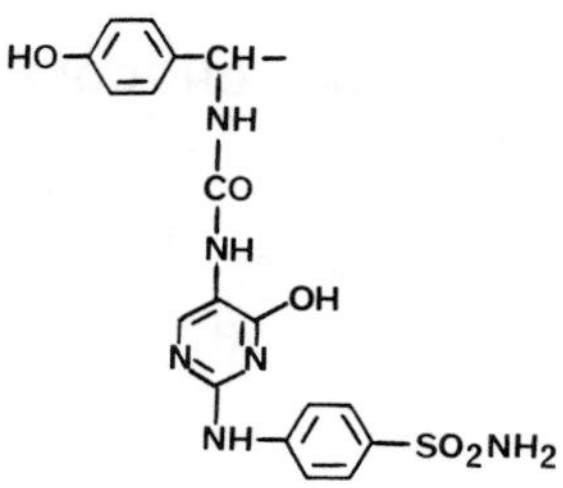	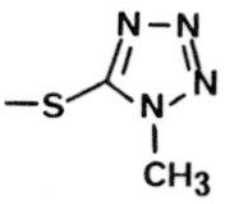

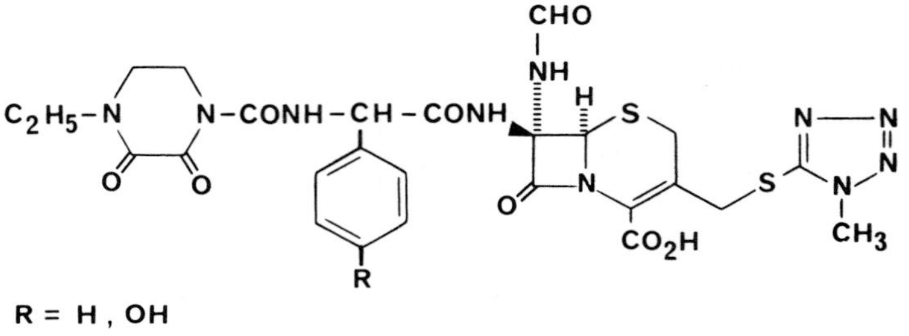

R = H , OH

109

7α-Formylamidocephalosporins of type **109** have been synthesized and tested by the Beecham group (Basker *et al.*, 1986; Branch *et al.*, 1987). The formylamido substituent improves the potency against Gram-negative bacteria, including *Pseudomonas aeruginosa*. Further improvements are observed by introduction of a 1-methyltetrazol-5-ylthiomethyl substituent into the 3-position and a 4-hydroxy substituent into the phenyl ring. In the cefpirome series, introduction of a 7α-methoxy or 7α-formylamido group causes a dramatic drop in biological activity (Dürckheimer and Schrinner, 1985).

The Beecham group also investigated the sulphoxides of 7α-formylamidocephem **109** (Branch *et al.*, 1986). The (R)-sulphoxides are superior to the (S)-oxides and exhibit nearly the same activity as the parent compound against Enterobacteriaceae and *Pseudomonas* strains. With a mercaptoheterocycle at 3'-position, activity against *Staphylococcus aureus* is significantly reduced compared to the parent compound. The oxacephalosporins **110a** and **110b** show similar antibacterial activity to their cephem counterparts (Branch *et al.*, 1986).

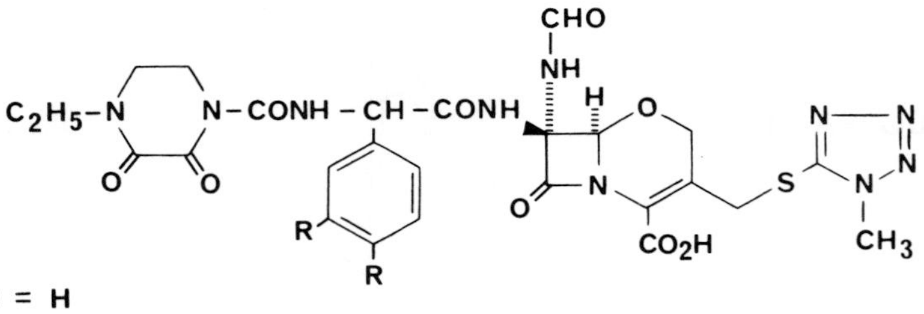

a   R = H

b   R = OAc

110

4.1.7 8-Position

Thiolactam analogues of cephalosporins have been prepared in low yield by treatment of cephem esters with boron sulphide. The free acids display substantially reduced antibacterial activity *in vitro* (Wojtkowski *et al.*, 1975). As yet no further paper concerning C-8 modification has been published.

4.2 NUCLEAR ANALOGUES

Nuclear analogues constitute a fascinating aspect of the chemistry of cephalosporins, and great efforts have been devoted to their synthesis (Holden *et al.*, 1979; Sammes, 1980). It was expected that a structural change of the cephem skeleton might lead to unpredicted superior activity. Introduction of unnatural elements in the skeleton alters the molecular geometry and thus the reactivity of the β-lactam ring, which is due to the strained four-membered ring and an electronic activation by conjugation of the nitrogen lone pair electron with the C-3 double bond in competition with the β-lactam amide resonance (Sweet, 1972; Boyd, 1982). Replacement of sulphur by carbon or small heteroatoms intensifies the pyramidal character of the β-lactam nitrogen, and consequently the reactivity of the β-lactam bond. Furthermore, such structural changes strongly influence the partition parameters of the whole molecule and consequently the protein binding and pharmacokinetic properties.

The synthesis of nuclear analogues is complicated and requires many synthetic steps. Some nuclear analogues are accessible by degradation of penicillin and resynthesis starting from monocyclic building blocks. Many attractive new structures have been made by total synthesis. To construct the nuclear skeleton, some reaction sequences have proven particularly useful, for example: [2 + 2]-cycloaddition between a *Schiff*'s base and a ketene (addition of sulphonyl isocyanate to an olefine) to synthesize the monocyclic azetidinone derivative. Completion of the bicyclic system has been achieved in many appropriate cases by an intramolecular *Wittig* reaction. The examples **111–126** of Table 16 represent cephem, carba-, phospha-, aza-, and oxacephem analogues, including some tricyclic systems. In the following sections examples of each group will be discussed in more detail.

TABLE 16

Different structures of nuclear analogues

111

112

113

114

115

116

117

118

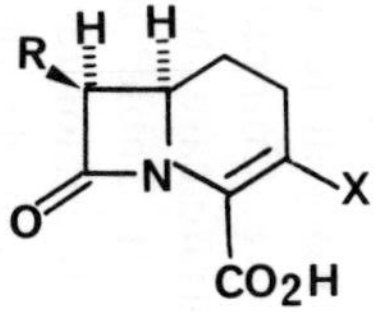

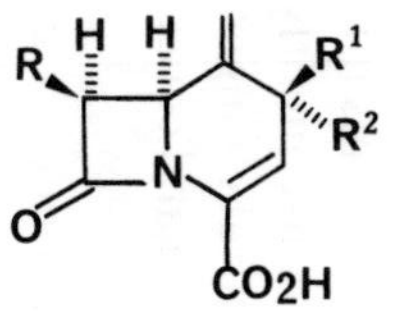

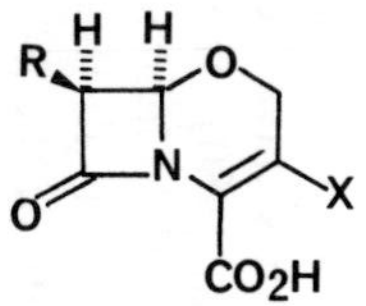

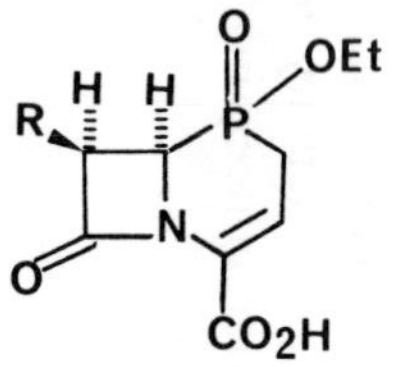

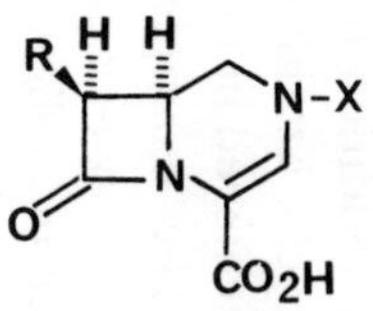

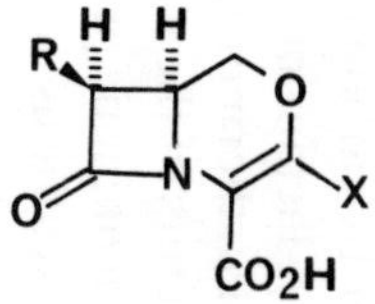

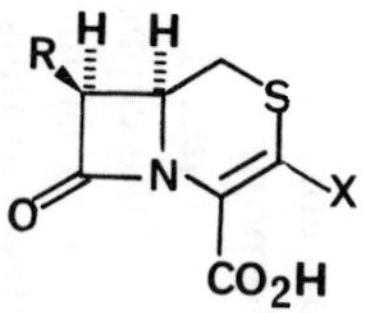

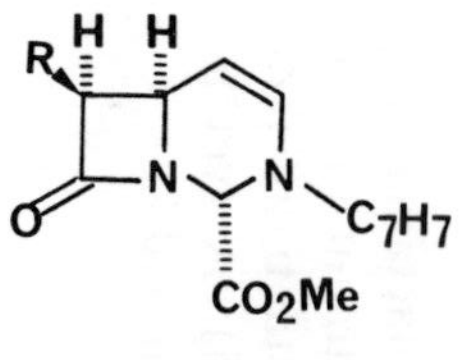

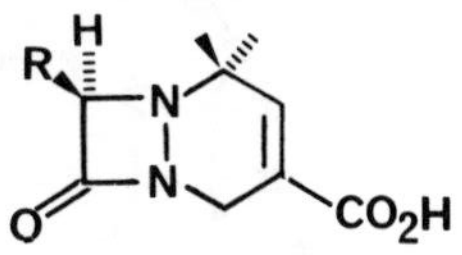

122

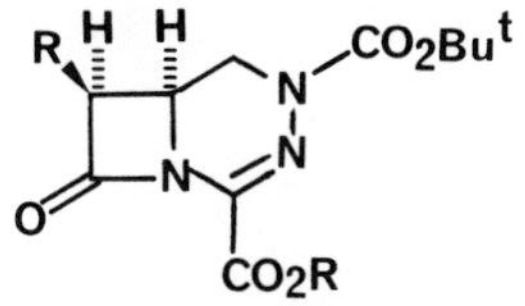

121

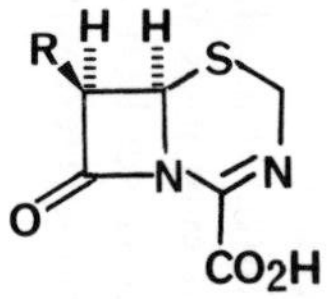

120

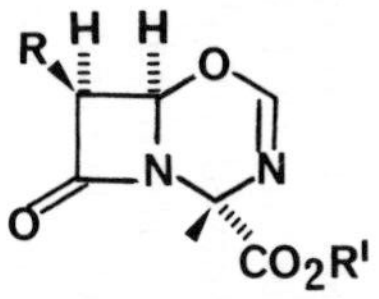

119

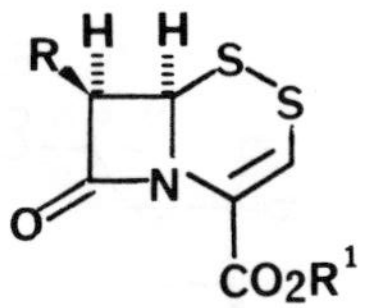

126

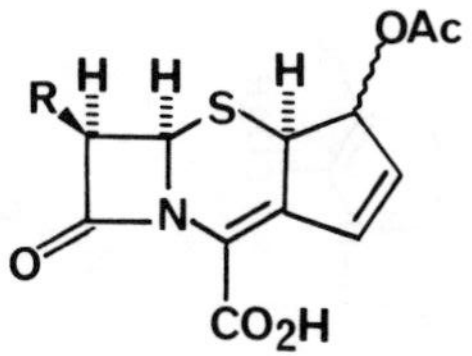

125

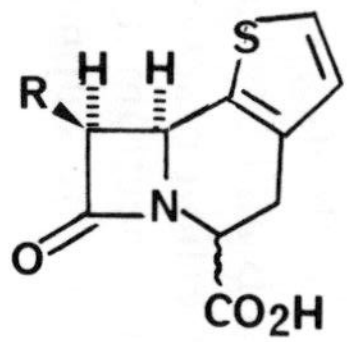

124

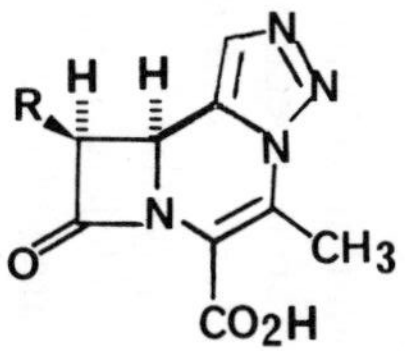

123

4.2.1 1-Oxacephems

1-Oxacephems are the most thoroughly investigated group of nuclear analogues (Nagata *et al.*, 1981; Narisada *et al.*, 1981). Chemists at Merck first synthesized racemic 1-oxacephalothin (Cama and Christensen, 1974) and demonstrated that its antibacterial spectrum was similar to that of cephalothin. A four- to eight-fold increase in activity was observed with the optically active 1-oxacephalothin, synthesized from penicillin (Narisada *et al.*, 1979). Racemic 1-oxacefamandole was twice as active as cefamandole (Christensen *et al.*, 1977). Encouraged by these findings, a research group from Shionogi investigated the effect of various side chains at the positions 3 and 7 on the biological activity of 1-oxa-3-cephem-4-carboxylic acid (Yoshida, 1980).

Scheme 20 shows stereoselective synthetic strategies used to build up the dihydro-oxazin ring. Route A, with its intramolecular acetalization, is claimed to be superior to routes B and C which feature an intramolecular *Wittig* reaction or a carbene insertion reaction. A technical synthesis for latamoxef (**273**), the first broad spectrum 1-oxacephem, is described in Scheme 21. Starting from 6-APA, the sulphoxide **127** is epimerized with

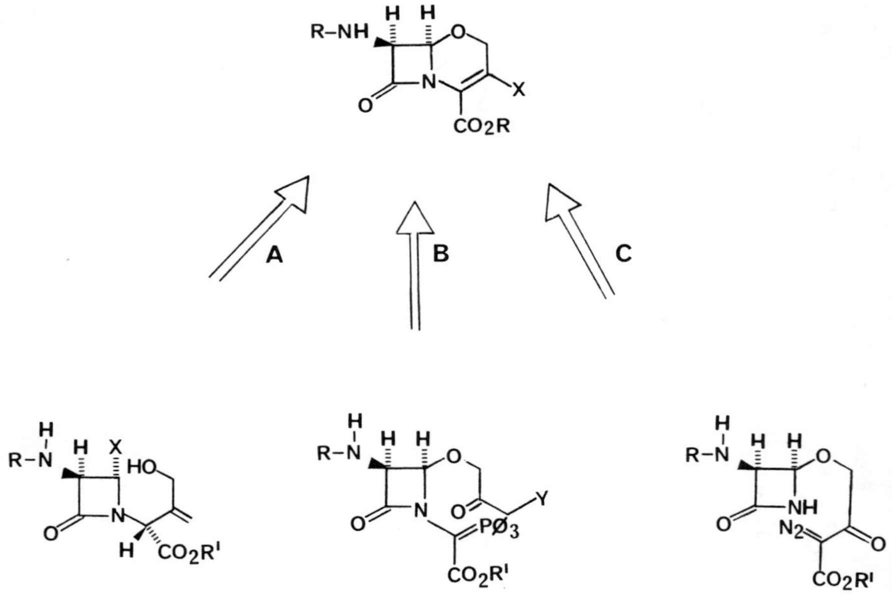

SCHEME 20. Synthetic strategies to 1-oxa-3-cephems.

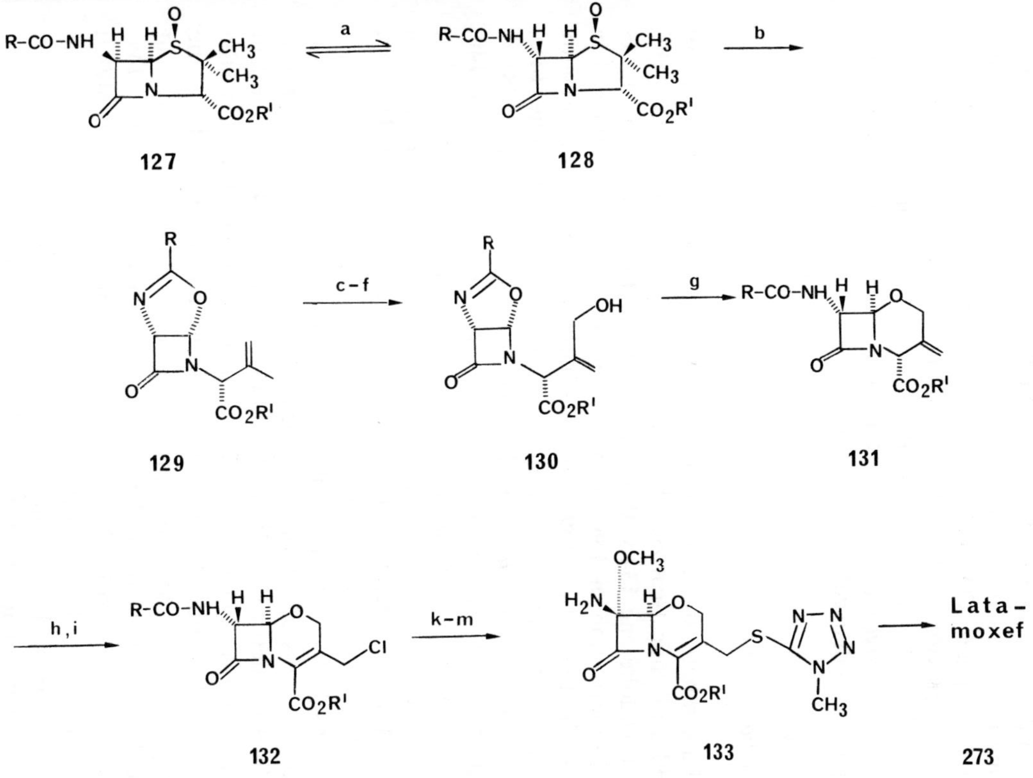

SCHEME 21. Synthesis of latamoxef (273). R = Ph, R¹ = CHPh₂. (a) Base; (b) 80°C, PPh₃; (c) Cl₂; (d) NaHCO₃; (e) NaI; (f) dimethylsulphoxide H₂O/Cu₂O; (g) BF₃ × Et₂O; (h) Cl₂, light; (i) piperidine; (j) ClOtBu, LiOCH₃; (k) sodium 1-methyltetrazole-5-thiolate; (l) PCl₅, pyridine; (m) MeOH.

base at C-6 to give **128**. Opening of the thiazolidine ring by heating with triphenylphosphine results in **129**, which is transformed into the allylic alcohol **130**. Lewis acid-catalysed cyclization proceeds stereospecifically to **131**. Light-induced addition of chlorine and HCl-elimination yield **132**, which is methoxylated and converted into **133** by well known reaction sequences. Latamoxef (**273**) is obtained by reacylation and deprotection.

A novel 2-methyloxacephalosporin without a 7α-methoxy group was recently presented by Shibahara *et al.* (1987b). Compound OCP-9-176, selected from extensive studies on SAR, is more active against Staphylococci and *Ps. aeruginosa* than ceftazidime (**266**).

4.2.2 1-Carbacephems

Following a synthetic strategy developed at Merck, Uyeo and Ona (1980) synthesized a racemic 1-carbacephem as outlined in Scheme 22. A cyclo-addition of azidoketene **134** with the chiral imine **135**, followed by base-catalysed isomerization of **136**, yields **137**, which is then transformed in several steps via **138** and ylid **139** to the 1-carbacephem **140**. Cleavage of the side chain, reacylation and deprotection lead to 1-carbacefmenoxime (**141**), whose antibacterial activity *in vitro* is less than that of cefmenoxime (**208**). A versatile starting material for various 3-substituted 1-carbacephems is **140**. The optically active 1-carba analogue of ceftizoxime (**143**) was obtained by enzymatic deacylation of (6R,7S)-phenylacetyl-1-carbacephem **142a** out of a mixture of **142a** and **142b** (Scheme 23) (Hashimoto *et al.*, 1984). The pure enantiomer **143** is twice as active as its racemate.

An enantioselective synthesis of a 1-carbacephem (Scheme 24) was performed by Evans and Sjogren (1985). The chiral azetidinone **146** is prepared by asymmetric [2 + 2]-cycloaddition from **144** to **145**. Subsequent hydrogenation affords **147**. On reduction with lithium in liquid ammonia the auxiliary oxazolidone ring and the N-protecting group are removed, and the anisole ring is reduced after Boc-protection to give **148** in an excellent overall yield. Ozonolysis and reductive work-up give the β-keto-ester **149**, which is transformed into **150** by a diazo transfer and a titanium-catalysed transesterification. A rhodium-catalysed carbene insertion reaction gives **151**, which can be further transformed into **152**. This high yielding short synthesis allows flexibility in several steps and makes a range of analogous structures readily available.

Vanderhaeghe *et al.* (1986) synthesized 1-exomethylene-3-cephems of type **112** (Table 16). The corresponding cefalexin (**23**) analogues displayed significantly less antibiotic activity. The synthesis of derivatives unsubstituted at C-2 was unsuccessful.

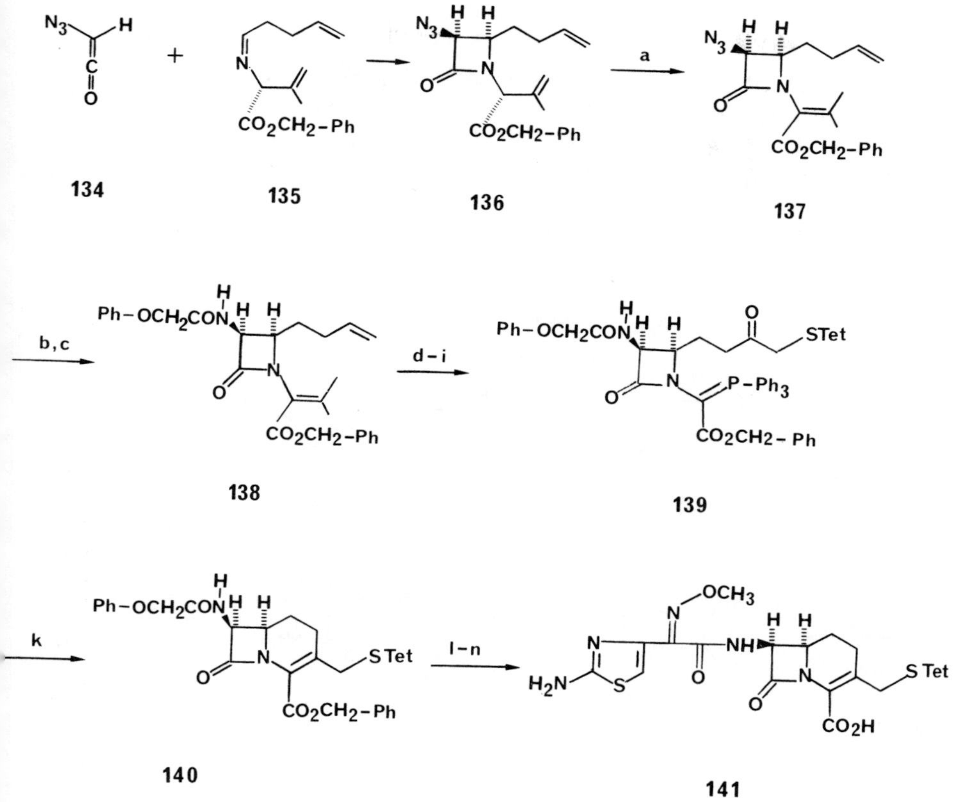

SCHEME 22. Synthesis of 1-carbacephem **141**. (a) NEt₃; (b) Zn, AcOH; (c) reacylation; (d) MCPBA; (e) n-BuLi, then 1-methyltetrazole-5-thiol; (f) CrO₃; (g) O₃, Zn/AcOH; (h) SOCl₂; (i) PPh₃; (k) 10 h in refluxing dioxane, then chromatography, 60%; (l) PCl₅/MeOH; (m) acylation; (n) deprotection. (Tet = 1-methyltetrazol-5-yl.)

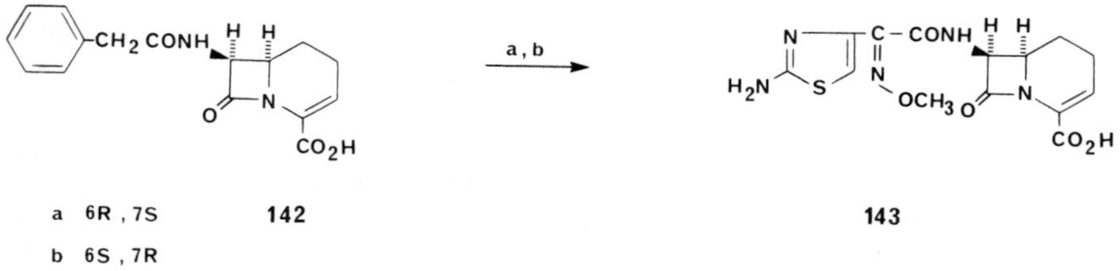

SCHEME 23. Enzymatic synthesis of the 1-carba analogue of ceftizoxime. (a) Incubation with *Kluyvera citrophila KY 7844*; (b) reacylation.

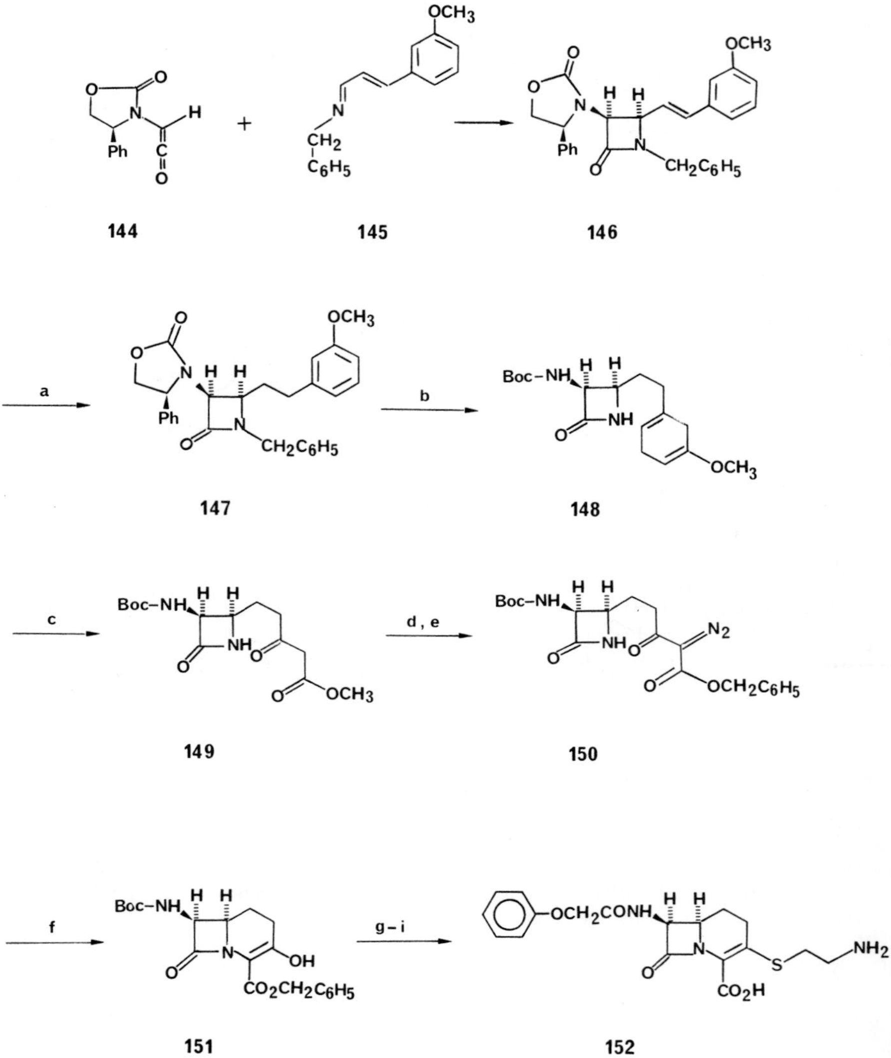

144 145 146 147 148 149 150 151 152

SCHEME 24. Enantioselective synthesis of 1-carbacephem **152**. (a) 10% Pd-C, 1 atm., CH_2Cl_2; (b) Li, NH_3-butanol, 5:1, −78°C, then quenching with NH_4OAc; treatment with *t*-butyl pyrocarbonate, overall yield 74% from **146**; (c) O_3, Me_2S; (d) tosylazide, *Hünig*'s base; (e) 1 eq. titanium tetrabenzyloxide in benzyl alcohol, 36°C, 42 h; (f) 1% Rh_2OAc_4 in refluxing chloroform; (g) 1 eq. trifluoromethanesulphonic anhydride, *Hüning*'s base; (h) CF_3CO_2H/anisole, then acylation, followed by treatment with the *p*-nitrobenzyl carbamate of cysteamine; (i) $AlCl_3$/anisole, then hydrogenolysis.

4.2.3 Hetero-1-carbacephems

Hetero-1-carbacephems synthesized by several groups displayed anti-bacterial activity when appropriately substituted. Scheme 25 presents a versatile route to 1-carba-2-oxacephems **156** and **157** (Doyle *et al.*, 1980). The key reaction is a base-induced intramolecular cyclization of **155**, which is prepared from **153** via **154**. In an analogous manner 1-substituted 1-carba-2-oxacephems can be obtained. Very recently, a new synthesis of 1-carba-2-oxacephems has been described. The key step is the reaction of an azetidinone with an α-diazo-β-keto-ester under rhodium acetate catalysis, followed by a cyclization of the resulting enol (Hrytsak and Durst, 1987). Compound **155** is also useful for the preparation of 3'-substituted derivatives, as well as for the synthesis of 1-carba-2-thia-3-cephems (Scheme 26). Intermediate **155** is mesylated and affords in a base-catalysed elimination allene **158**, which is trapped by bromine and yields **159**. Reaction of **159** with 1-methyltetrazol-5-thiol and triethylamine gives **160**. Reaction of **161**, prepared from **155**, with hydrogen sulphide and triethylamine, affords **162** which is further transformed into **163**. The above mentioned authors have also prepared 1-carba-2-azacephems, which have proved to be more active than their 2-thia- and 2-azacephem analogues. Increased biological activity against non β-lactamase-producing Gram-positive organisms has improved in the 2-oxa series by increasing the hydrophilic character at position 3.

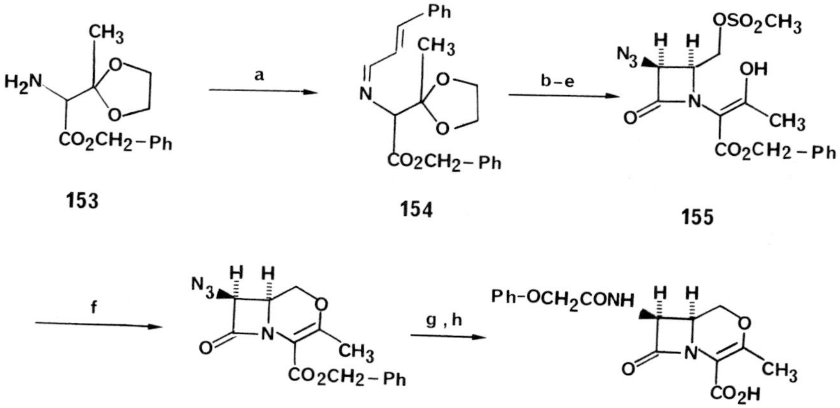

SCHEME 25. Synthesis of 2-oxacephem **157**. (a) Cinnamic aldehyde; (b) azidoacetyl chloride, NEt$_3$; (c) O$_3$; NaBH$_4$; (d) methanesulphonyl chloride; (e) hydrolysis; (f) base; (g) reduction with H$_2$S; (h) acylation, then ester cleavage.

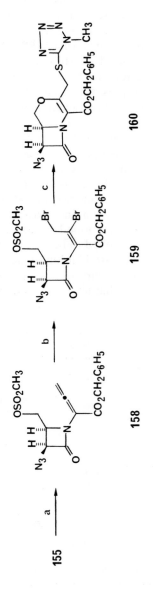

SCHEME 26. Synthesis of 1-carba-2-thiocephem **163**. (a) Methane sulphonyl chloride, excess NEt₃; (b) Br₂; (c) 1-methyltetrazole-5-thiol, NEt₃; (d) H₂S/NEt₃; (e) acylation, then ester cleavage.

Mercaptoheterocycles at the 3'-position further enhance the antibacterial activity. The 1-carba-2-oxacepham analogue of cephalothin shows the same blood level as cephalothin in mice.

A stereocontrolled synthesis of optically active 2-oxa- and 2-thia-3-cephem analogues from L-aspartic acid was described by Hatanaka *et al.* (1987), the key step being the stereoselective introduction of an azide group into **165**, obtained from **164** by reduction, leading to the corresponding azido lactone **166** (Scheme 27). The latter was converted via **167** into the chiral azetidinone **168**. Starting from **168**, nuclear analogue **169** can be obtained

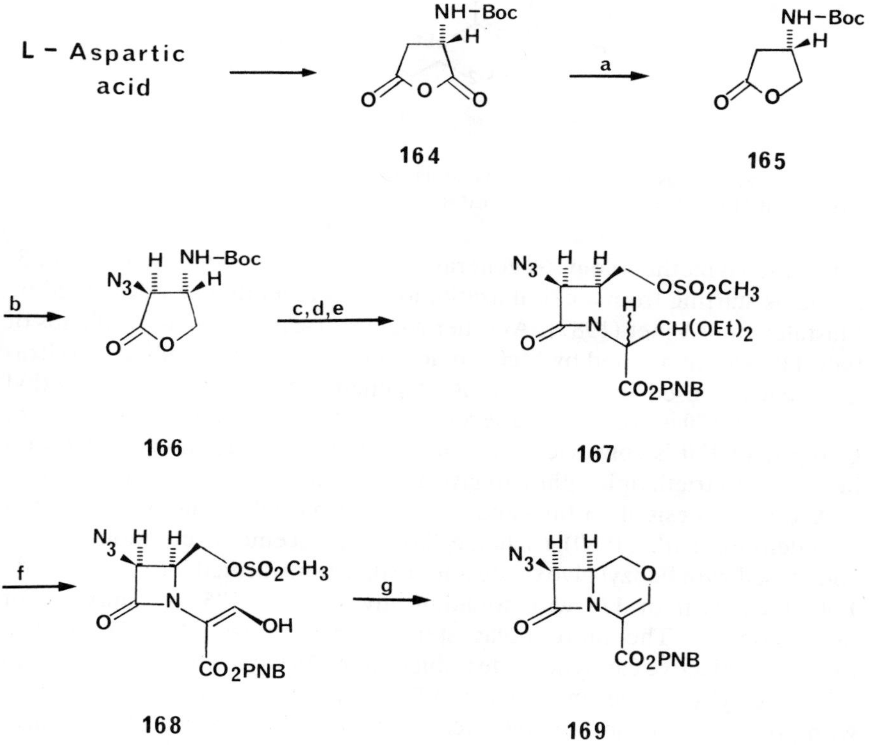

SCHEME 27. Synthesis of an optically active 1-carba-2-oxacephem **169**. (a) 1 eq. NaBH$_4$, −20 to 0°C, followed by benzene, reflux, 3 h; (b) LDA (2.1 eq.), −78 to 20°C, then tosyl azide (1.2 eq.), THF, −78°C, 1 h, followed by TMSCl, −78 to 0°C; (c) CF$_3$CO$_2$H, then MeOH/H$_2$O, Amberlite; (d) (EtO)$_2$CHCHO, *p*-nitrobenzyl isocyanide/MeOH, r.t., 10 h; (e) MsCl, NEt$_3$, then N$_2$O$_4$, CHCl$_3$, AcONa, 0°C, followed by CCl$_4$ reflux; (f) CF$_3$CO$_2$H; (g) NEt$_3$, CH$_2$Cl$_2$, reflux.

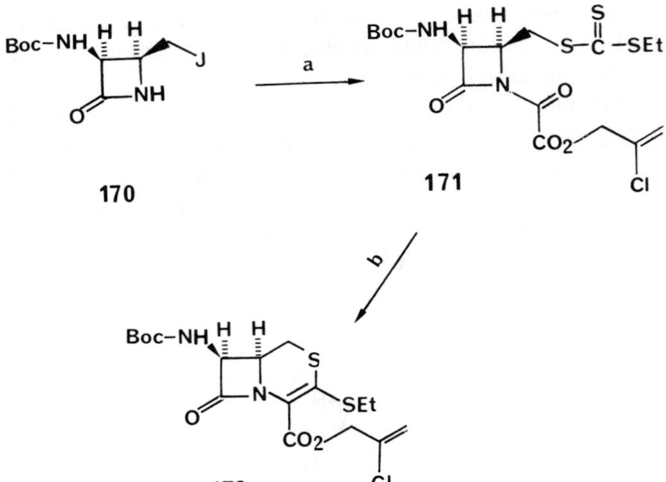

SCHEME 28. Synthesis of a 1-carba-2-thia 3-cephem **172**. (a) NaSCS$_2$Et/DMF; CH$_2$=CClCH$_2$OCOCOCl/iPr$_2$NEt; (b) (EtO)$_3$P, refluxing benzene, 8 h.

using known methodology. A general enantioselective synthesis of 2-oxa-3-cephems starting from a chiral azetidinone has recently been described by Mastalerz and Vinet (1987). Another route to 1-carba-2-thia-3-cephems of type **117** was elaborated by McCombie *et al.* (1986), who applied a cyclization reaction used in the synthesis of penems (Scheme 28). Iodomethyl azetidinone **170** is prepared via several steps by ketene-imine cycloaddition. Compound **170** is converted into the intermediate **171**, which cyclizes on heating with triethylphosphite to give **172** and can be further derivatized.

A total synthesis of a 3-thia- and a 3-aza-1-carbacephem has been reported by Gleason *et al.* (1980) (Scheme 29). The racemic azetidinone **173** is condensed with benzyl glyoxalate and further transformed into the chloride **174**. Treatment of **174** with toluidine gives amine **175** as a mixture of diastereomers. The more polar stereoisomer cyclized to **176** by acid catalysis. Selective catalytic azide reduction of **176** gave, after acylation with thienylacetyl chloride, methylester **177**. By a similar approach **174** reacts with potassium thioacetate and cyclizes to the 3-thiocephem **178**. A 3-aza-

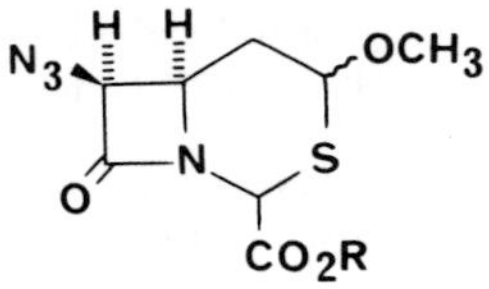

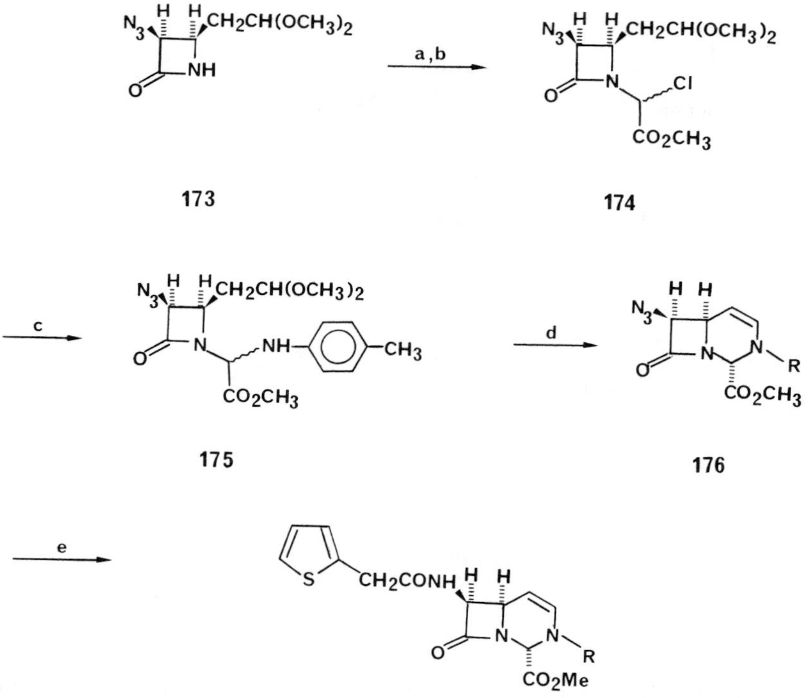

SCHEME 29. Synthesis of a 1-carba-3-aza-cephem **177**. (a) Benzylglyoxylate; SOCl₂, pyridine; (c) toluidine, then chromatography; (d) pTsOH 70%; (e) PtO₂/H₂, 0.5 h, r.t., followed by acylation.

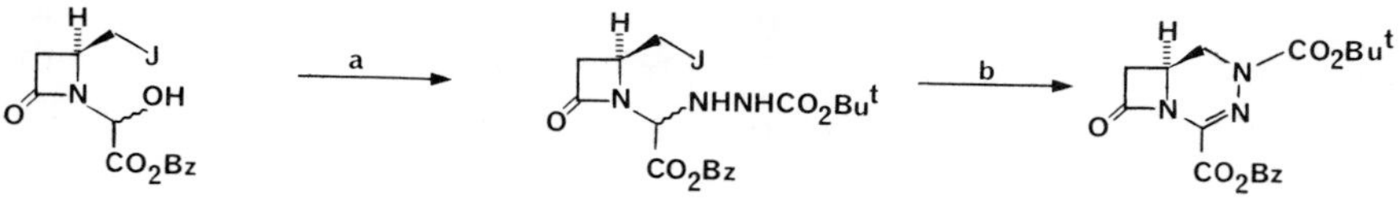

SCHEME 30. Synthesis of a 2,3-diaza-cephem **182**. (a) SOCl₂, 2,6-lutidine, −20°C; then reaction with *tert.* butyl carbazate; (b) Ag₂O in acetonitrile.

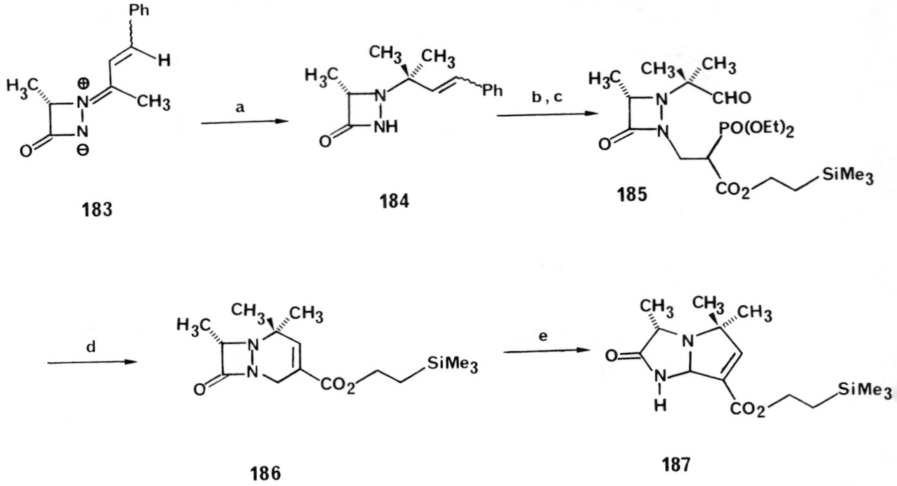

SCHEME 31. Synthesis of a fused 1,2-diazetidinone derivative. (a) MeMgBr, 0°C; (b) 2-trimethylsilylethyl-2-diethoxy-phosphinyl-2-propenoate, **188**, r.t., 18 h, 93%; (c) O₃, Me₂S, −78°C → RT, 2 h, 54%; (d) DBU; (e) 1.5 eq. LDA, −78°C, 26%.

derivative **179** has been prepared by an intramolecular 1,3-cycloaddition (Nagakura, 1981), as also used by the Beecham group (Pearson and Branch, 1982a,b, 1983). Stoodley *et al.* (1984) reported the new 2,3-diaza-analogue **182** obtained from **180** via **181** by cyclization with silver(I) oxide in acetonitrile (Scheme 30). 1,2-Diazetidinone **183** is the starting material for a novel class of highly strained, bridgehead aza-analogues, first described by Taylor and Davies (1986) (Scheme 31). Reaction of the inner salt **183** with methylmagnesium bromide affords **184**, which is then transformed into the

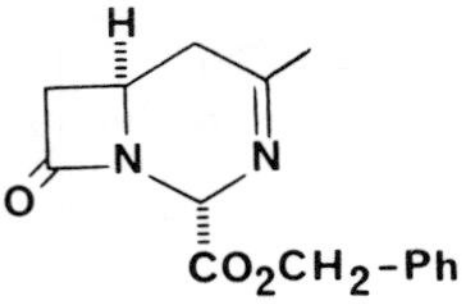

179

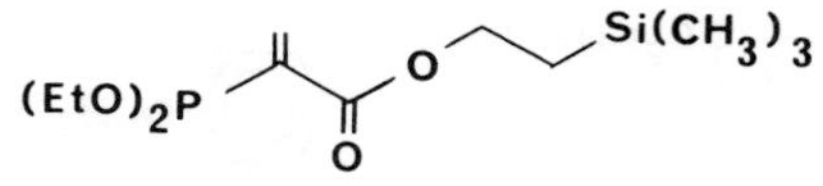

$(EtO)_2P$ ⋯ O ⋯ $Si(CH_3)_3$

188

aldehyde **185** by a *Michael* reaction of **184** with **188**, followed by ozonolysis and reductive work-up. Treatment of crude **185** with DBU affords the cyclized product **186** (*Horner–Emmons* reaction). Treatment of **186** with LDA at low temperature gave the rearranged product **187**.

4.2.4 Cephems with Heteroatoms

As intermediates in penem synthesis Ross *et al.* (1982) prepared 2-thia-3-cephems. Other 2-thiacephalosporins with polar substituents at C-3 have been described by Teutsch *et al.* (1987). Furthermore, 1,2-dithia-cephems of structure **191** have been synthesized starting from the sulphoxide **189** in several steps via the disulphide **190** (Scheme 32) (Perrone *et al.*, 1984b). The

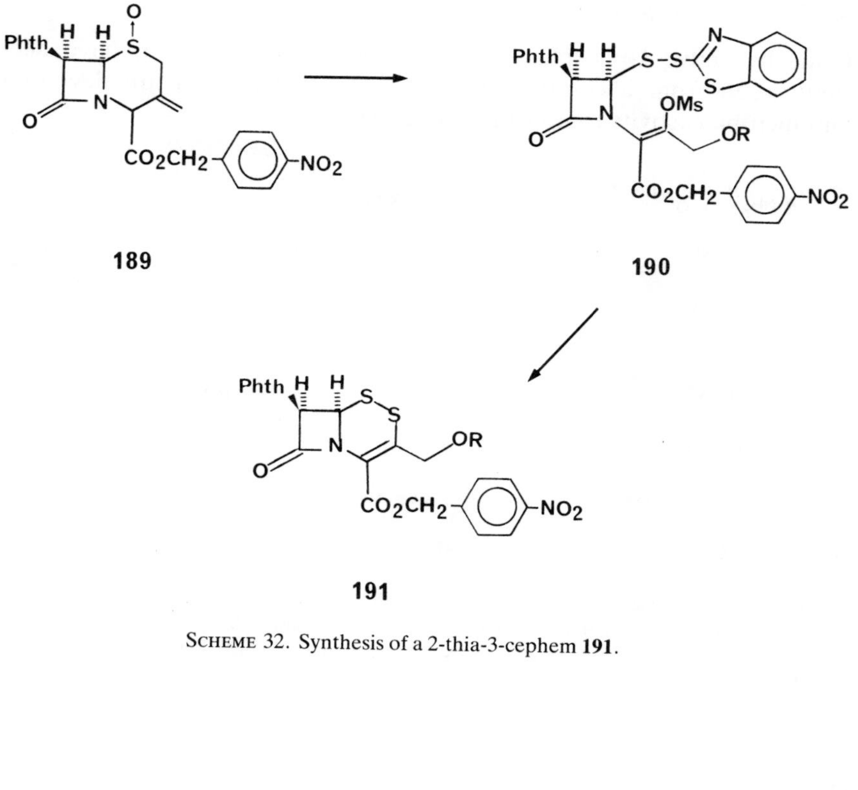

189

190

191

SCHEME 32. Synthesis of a 2-thia-3-cephem **191**.

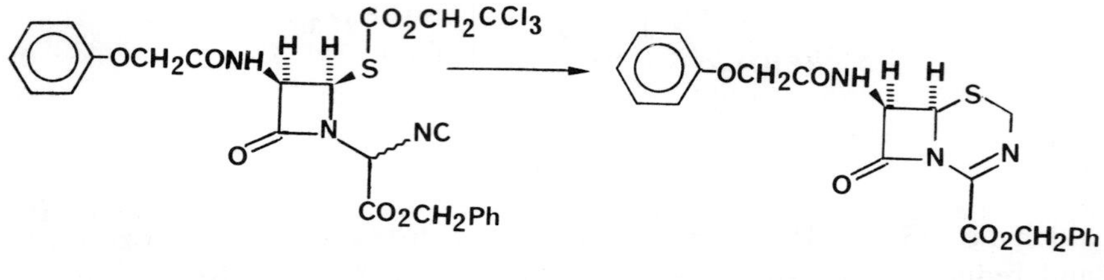

192   **193**

SCHEME 33. Synthesis of a 3-aza-3-cephem **193**.

corresponding seleno compound can be obtained using an analogous sequence (Perrone *et al.*, 1986). Both nuclear analogues yield the penem skeleton when treated with triphenylphosphine.

A 3-aza-3-cephem analogue of structure **193** has been obtained by an intramolecular cyclization of isonitrile **192** (Aratani and Hashimoto, 1980). This compound is very unstable and could not be cleaved into the free acid (Scheme 33).

4.2.5 Various Structures

Optically active 1-phosphacephems of type **114** (Table 16) have been synthesized from a chiral azetidinone intermediate and are devoid of antimicrobial activity (Satoh and Tsuji, 1984).

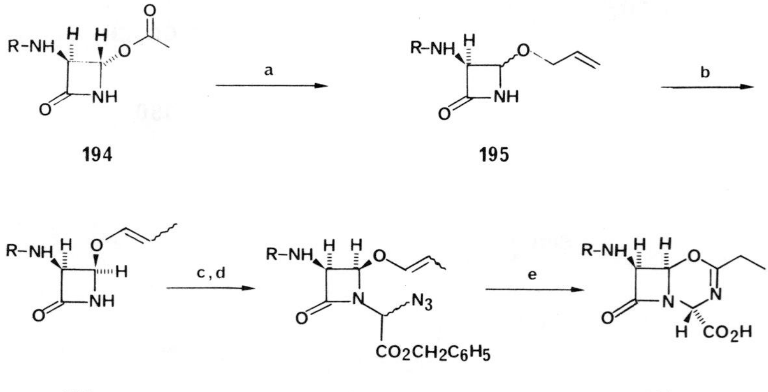

194   **195**

196   **197**   **198**

SCHEME 34. Synthesis of 1-oxa-3-azacephem **198**. (a) Allylic alcohol, ZnOAc, 80°C, 1:1 diastereomeric mixture; (b) *cis*-isomer: 10% Pd-C, dioxane, *Z/E* mixture = 2:1, 89%; (c) benzylglyoxalate; (d) SOCl$_2$, then NaN$_3$; (e) refluxing toluene, then ester cleavage with 10% Pd/C.

1-Oxa-3-azacephem **198** has been prepared by intramolecular cyclo-addition of vinylether **197** (Scheme 34) (Pearson and Branch, 1986). The introduction of the desired vinyl ether functionality was achieved in two steps. The azetidinone **194**, when warmed with allylic alcohol under Lewis acid catalysis, afforded a 1:1 diastereomeric mixture of **195**. The *cis*-isomer was isomerized to **196**, which was then transformed into **197**. Compound **198** was obtained by refluxing in toluene followed by deprotection. It is devoid of antibiotic activity.

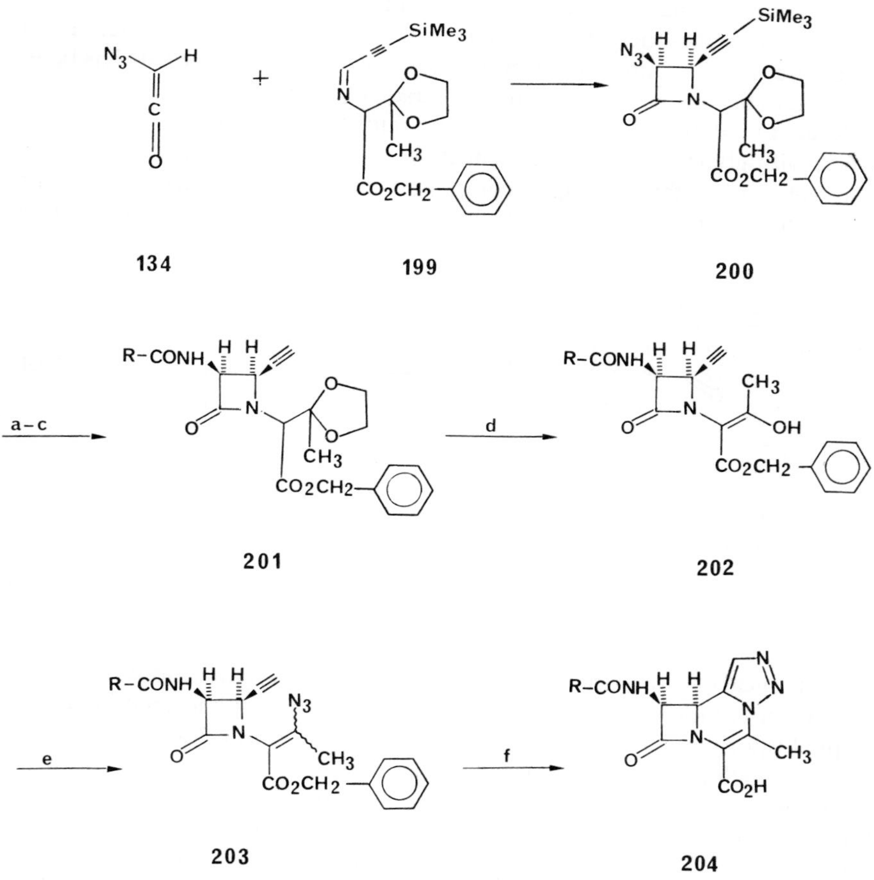

SCHEME 35. Synthesis of a tricyclic triazolo-cephem **204**. (a) Tetrabutylammoniumfluoride, THF; (b) H₂S; (c) phenoxyacetyl chloride, NEt₃; (d) CF₃CO₂H; (e) MsCl, NEt₃, then NaN₃ in DMF; (f) benzene, 15 min, reflux, 49%; then hydrogenation with 10% Pd/C.

4.2.6 Tricyclic Cephem Analogues

The layout of synthesis of three types of tricyclic cephem analogues shall illustrate the principal routes to this type of compounds. The intramolecular 1,3-cycloaddition reaction is useful for the construction of tricyclic cephems. The synthesis of **204** is illustrated in Scheme 35. Cycloaddition of *Schiff*'s base **199** and azidoketene **134** affords a mixture of diastereomeric *trans-β*-lactams and two diastereomeric, separable *cis-β*-lactams **200**. Removal of the trimethylsilyl group from **200**, followed by reduction and acylation, provides the ethynyl derivative **201**, which is hydrolysed to give **202**. Conversion of **202** into the mesylate and nucleophilic substitution with sodium azide gives the vinyl azide **203**, which smoothly cyclizes on heating to give, after deprotection, the tricyclic cephem **204**. Compound **204** has been claimed to be antibacterially active (Pearson *et al.*, 1982b).

Reaction of the 3'-triphenylphosphonium ylide **205** (Hatanaka *et al.*, 1985) with glyoxal gives, after protection of the free hydroxyl with ketene and selective ester cleavage, compound **206**. It shows activity against Gram-positive organisms, but no significant activity against Gram-negative strains.

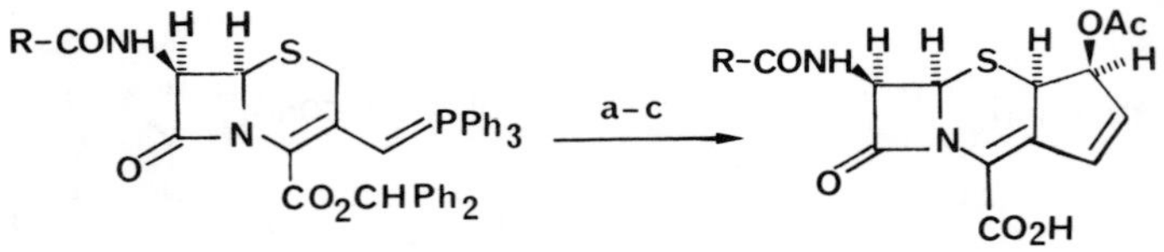

205   **206**

Scheme 36. Synthesis of a tricyclic nuclear analogue **206**. (a) Glyoxal/CH_2Cl_2, r.t., 50%; (b) ketene/pTsOH; (c) CF_3CO_2H.

4.3 VARIATIONS AT THE 7-ACYL SIDE CHAIN

The chemical nature of the 7β-acylamido side chain of cephalosporins and its spatial orientation are of great importance for antibacterial activity. Cephalosporins of different generations possess typical 7-acylamido side chains, which determine the antibacterial profile by creating characteristic affinities to the PBPs and by influencing the permeation properties across the outer membrane of bacteria and β-lactamase stability. Structure–activity relationships in the series of first and second generation cephalosporins have already been described in several reports (Gorman and Ryan, 1972a; Quintiliani *et al.*, 1982; Dürckheimer *et al.*, 1985 and references cited therein). The recent third generation cephalosporins will be considered in more detail in Sections 5.1 and 5.2.

4.3.1 Aminothiazole Cephalosporins and Analogues

The first example was cefotaxime (**207**) (Table 17), discovered in 1975 by Heymes (Bucourt *et al.*, 1977) in a joint venture programme carried out by Hoechst and Roussel-Uclaf. With cefotaxime (**207**), a decisive improvement in the intensity of antibacterial action and spectrum of activity was achieved. Whereas its activity against Gram-positive bacteria is comparable to that of older antibiotics, many Gram-negative bacteria including *Pseudomonas* spp. experience 10- to 100-fold higher inhibitions (see detailed description in Section 5.1). Cefotaxime (**207**) is routinely used in the management of many life-threatening infections, including nosocomial infections. Its outstanding antibiotic properties are due to a favourable interaction of the 7β-(2-aminothiazol-4-yl-acetyl) side chain and the (Z)-methoxyimino group.

All chemically modifiable positions in the cefotaxime molecule have been manifoldly varied, and extensive SAR studies have been carried out. The arrows in the cefotaxime formula (Fig. 4) indicate the positions of modifications. The chemistry and SAR studies in the aminothiazole cephalosporins up to 1982 have been summarized (Dürckheimer *et al.*, 1982). The following sections mainly discuss more recent papers.

4.3.1.1 Successors of Cefotaxime (207) with Identical 7-Side Chain. Out of thousands of derivatives, a number of successors of cefotaxime (**207**) having an identical 7-side chain but with additional modifications at 3- or 3'-position have been chosen. Some are already on the market, others undergoing clinical trials. Biological parameters, like the antibacterial spectrum, protein binding, serum elimination time, or metabolic degradation, can be altered by 3- and 3'-modifications. Table 17 gives the formulae of antibiotics of the

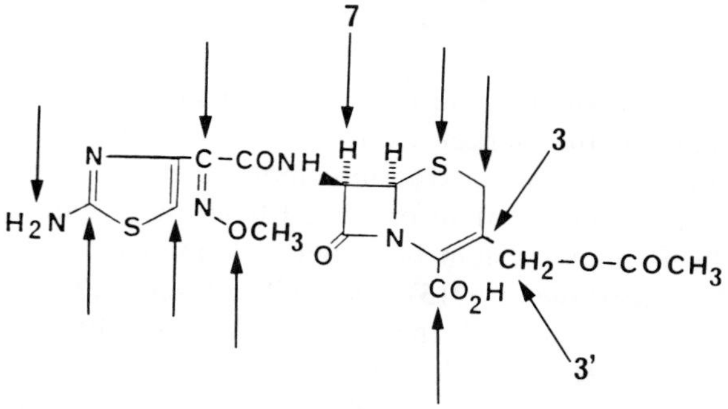

FIG. 4. Structural variations of the cefotaxime molecule. Arrows indicate the positions of modification.

TABLE 17

Aminothiazole cephalosporins of cefotaxime type with neutral 3′-substituents. Prodrug compounds are given in parentheses

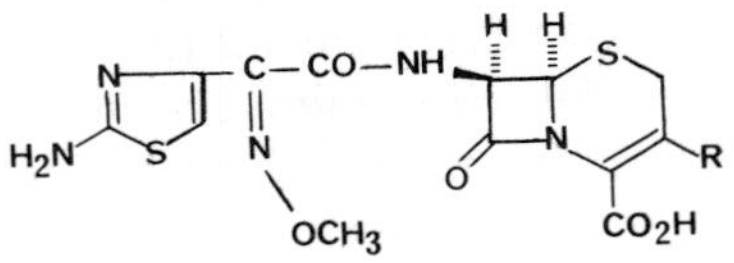

No.	Compound	R	No.	Compound	R
207	Cefotaxime	$-CH_2-O-COCH_3$	214	Cefetamet (RO15-8075)	$-CH_3$
208	Cefmenoxime	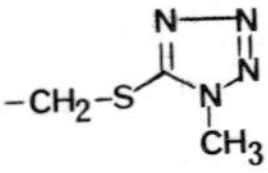 $-CH_2-S-$ (1-methyltetrazol-5-yl)	215	Cefteram (T 2588)	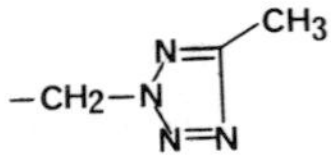 $-CH_2-$ (tetrazolyl-CH$_3$)
209	Ceftizoxime	$-H$	216	Cefuzonam (Baccefuzonam)	$-CH_2-S-$ (thiadiazolyl)
210	Ceftriaxone	$-CH_2-S-$ (triazinone-CH$_3$,OH)	217	FCE 20 485	$-CH_2-S-$ (triazolopyridazine-COOH)
211	Cefodizime	$-CH_2-S-$ (thiazole-CH$_3$,CH$_2$CO$_2$H)	218	ME 1206 (ME 1207)	$- CH=CH-$ (thiazolyl-H$_3$C)
212	Ceftiofur	$-CH_2-S-CO-$ (furyl)	219	R-3763 (CS 807)	$-CH_2-O-CH_3$
213	Ceftiolene	$-CH=CH-S-$ (triazinone-OH, N-CH$_2$CHO)			

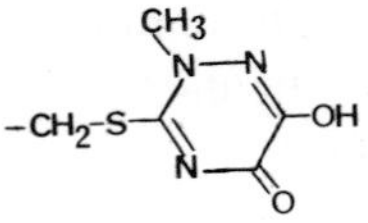

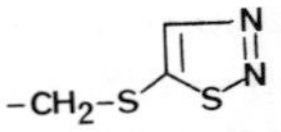

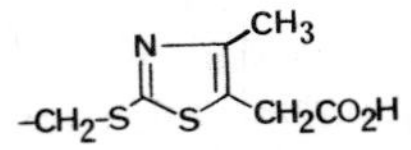

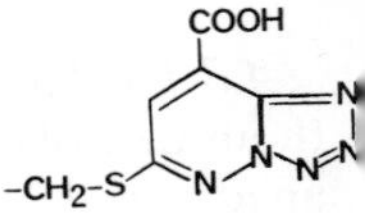

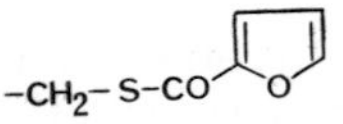

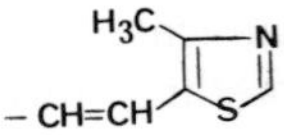

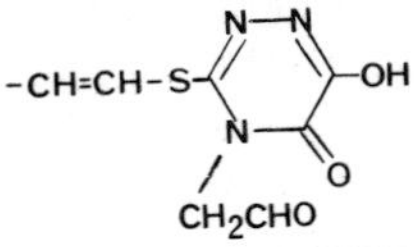

cefotaxime type. Cefmenoxime (**208**), ceftizoxime (**209**) and ceftriaxone (**210**) are already on the market. Ceftriaxone (**210**) is characterized by high protein binding and a prolonged serum elimination time. Cefodizime (**211**) has higher *in vivo* activity than predicted from its *in vitro* data. Positive effects on the immune system have been claimed from animal studies. Ceftiofur (**212**), ceftiolene (**213**) and FCE-20 485 (**217**) have also been intensively tested, but do not bring decisive progress. Other cephalosporins (**214**, **215**, **216**, **218**, **219** in Table 17) are of interest because they are parent compounds of enterally absorbed cephalosporins (see Section 5.2).

Quaternary 3′-ammonio cephalosporins of the aminothiazole type are listed in Table 18. The characteristic feature of this group is the improved

TABLE 18

Aminothiazole cephalosporins of cefotaxime type with polar 3'-substituents

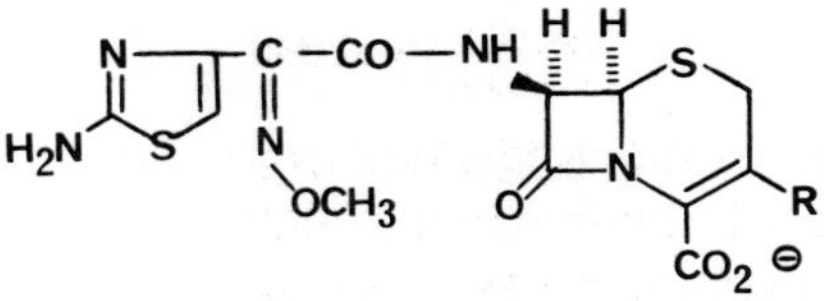

No.	Compound	R
220	Cefpirome	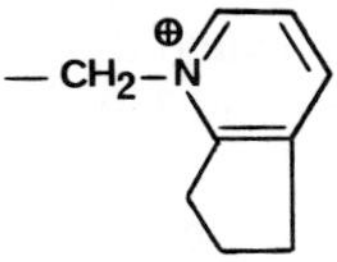
221	Cefepime (BMY 28 142)	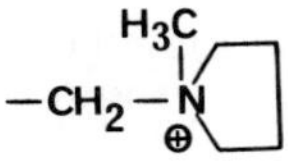
222	DQ 2522	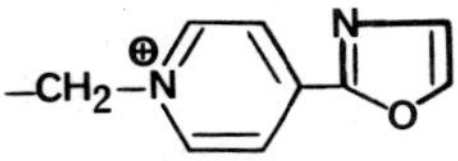
223	DQ 2556	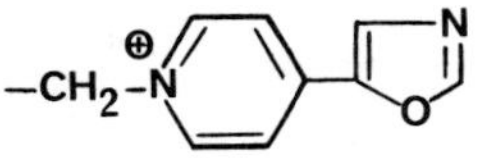
224	L 165 433	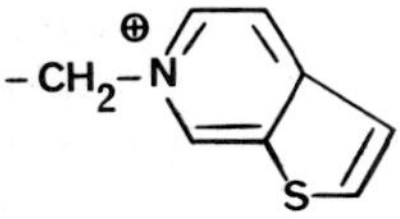
225	MT-382	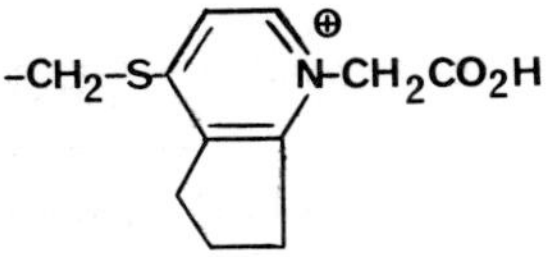
226	MT-383	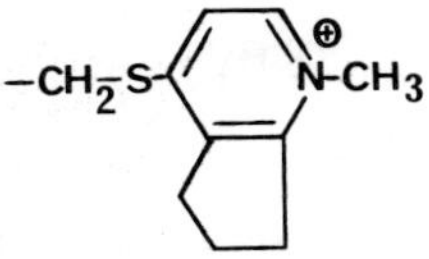

activity against Staphylococci and especially *Pseudomonas* spp. The first representatives of this class are cefpirome (**220**) and cefepime (BMY-28 142) (**221**). For further details of these compounds, see Section 5.1. For SAR studies of 3′-ammonio cephalosporins with cefotaxime side chain, see Section 4.1.4.5.

4.3.1.2 Aminothiazole Side Chain and its Modification.

4.3.1.2 Aminothiazole Side Chain and its Modification. The importance of the aminothiazole side chain for outstanding antibacterial properties is well established. Preparation of this moiety is outlined in Scheme 37. The synthesis starts from acetoacetate **227** which is treated with sodium nitrite and acetic acid. The resulting (Z)-oxime group is methylated by dimethylsulphate. By this procedure, the (Z)-configuration of the oxime group is retained. Bromination at the γ-position and ring closure with thiourea in aqueous medium yield the corresponding ethyl ester, which is saponified to form the desired acid **230**. Other methods for the synthesis of this side chain have been described. For a summary, see Newall (1985).

The presence of the 2-amino group in the thiazole ring is important for broad antibacterial activity and β-lactamase stability. Its shifting to the 4- or 5-position in the ring (Looker and Paternoster, 1985) or its acylation (Dürckheimer *et al.*, 1982) impair antibiotic potency. Desamino derivatives have been synthesized by Hoechst (Bormann *et al.*, 1979), Fujisawa (Takao *et al.*, 1985) and Sumitomo (Yamada *et al.*, 1985). Fujisawa selected the

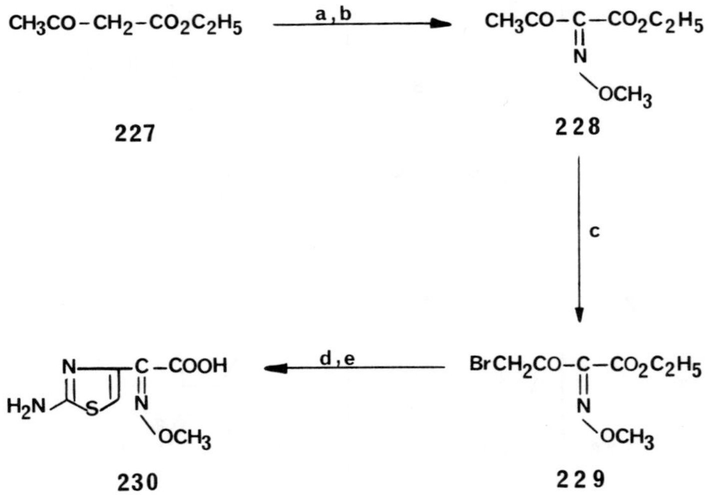

SCHEME 37. Synthesis of 2-(2-aminothiazol-4-yl)-2-methoxyimino acetic acid (**230**). (a) $NaNO_2/H^+$; (b) $(CH_3)_2SO_4$/base; (c) Br_2; (d) H_2NCSNH_2; (e) $NaOH/H_2O$.

desamino compound FK-089 (**288**) for clinical studies because of its good enteral absorption (Section 5.2). A chlorine or bromine substituent at the 5-position of the thiazole ring in the cefotaxime (**207**) (Dürckheimer *et al.*, 1982) and cefpirome (**220**) series (Blumbach *et al.*, 1983) slightly decreases antibiotic activity. SAR studies in the ceftizoxime (**207**) series with a fluorine, chlorine or bromine substituent at the corresponding 5-position demonstrated that the antibacterial activity against Gram-negative bacteria decreases in the order of 5-F ∼ 5-H-[ceftizoxime (**209**)] > 5-Cl- > 5-Br-derivatives (Hamashima and Nagata, 1980). Oxidation of the thiazole ring nitrogen leads to a tautomeric N-oxide derivative displaying moderate activity against Gram-negative bacteria (Perrone *et al.*, 1984a,b).

4.3.1.3 Replacement of the Aminothiazole Ring by Other Heterocycles. The replacement of 2-aminothiazole moiety in the 7-acyl side chain of cephalosporins by related five-membered heteroaromatics has been extensively studied. Examples are given in Table 19. Antibiotic activity comparable to that of cefotaxime (**207**) was found only in the 5-amino-1,2,4-thiadiazole series (Csendes *et al.*, 1983a,b; Goto *et al.*, 1984d). The synthesis is more difficult than that of the aminothiazole ring; one useful synthetic pathway is shown in Scheme 38. The amidino ester **232** is cyclized by a modification of *Goerdeler*'s general procedure (Goerdeler, 1954), formylated and reacted with formaldehyde dimethyldithioacetal S-oxide to **234**. Heating in a mixture of sodium periodate and acetic acid yields **235**. Hydrolysis of **235**, reaction with methoxyamine, and deformylation give the acid **237**.

There are several patent applications on 1,2,4-thiadiazole cephalosporins bearing 3'-ammonio substituents (Teraji *et al.*, 1981, 1982, 1983, 1984; Müller and Csendes, 1982; Dürckheimer *et al.*, 1984; Oka *et al.*, 1985; Takaya *et al.*, 1985b). Compounds CGP-22 495 (**238a**) and CGP-24 042 (**238b**) (Table 20) are examples which display high activity against both Gram-positive and Gram-negative bacteria, including *Ps. aeruginosa* (Csendes *et al.*, 1985). Another selected compound is FR-17 126 (**239**) (Sakane *et al.*, 1984, 1985) with an antibacterial spectrum similar to that of ceftazidime (**266**). In 1987, a novel cephalosporin of this type was presented by N. Watanabe *et al.* (1987a): E-1040 (**240**) with a (4-carbamoyl-1-quinuclidinio)methyl group at C-3 displays high antipseudomonal activity [4–8 fold more active than ceftazidime (**266**)]. It is also extremely potent against *Enterobacter cloacae* and *C. freundii*. Against Gram-positive strains and anaerobes, E-1040 (**240**) is as active as ceftazidime (**266**). When administered intravenously to health volunteers, E-1040 (**240**) is well tolerated (Nakashima *et al.*, 1987). The mean urinary recoveries within 24 h are 74–92%, serum half-lives are about 1.7–1.9 h.

TABLE 19

Replacement of the aminothiazole ring by other 5-ring heterocycles in cephalosporins **231** with different 3-substituents R

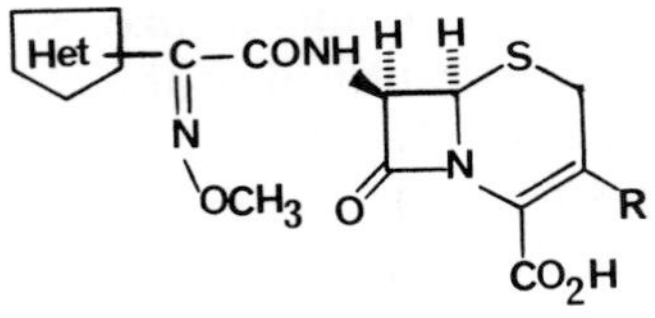

231

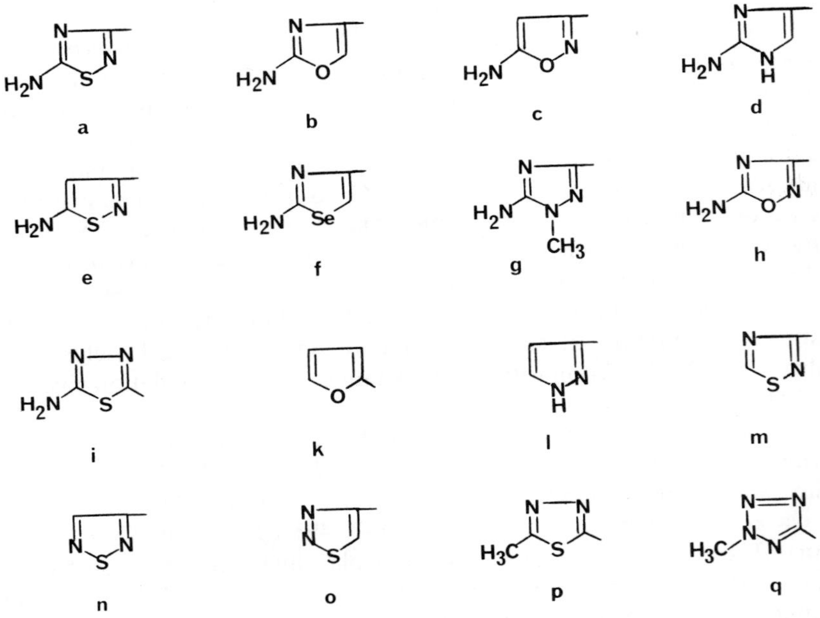

The MIC values of 2-amino-1,3-oxadiazole derivatives **231b** (Table 19) against *Staph. aureus* are comparable to that of cefotaxime (**207**), whereas those against Gram-negative bacteria are impaired (Csendes *et al.*, 1983a; Scartazzini, 1983; Naito *et al.*, 1986b; Wheeler *et al.*, 1986a; Sadaki *et al.*, 1986c). Cephalosporins having other five-membered heterocyclic substituents in the 7-acyl side chain are less active *in vitro*, e.g. 5-amino-isoxazol-3-yl **231c** (Lunn and Wheeler, 1983), 2-aminoimidazol-4-yl **231d** (Newall and Tonge, 1982), 5-amino-isothiazol-3-yl **231e** (Csendes *et al.*, 1983a; Müller, 1981), 2-amino-1,3-selenazol-4-yl **231f** (Reiner and Weiss, 1982),

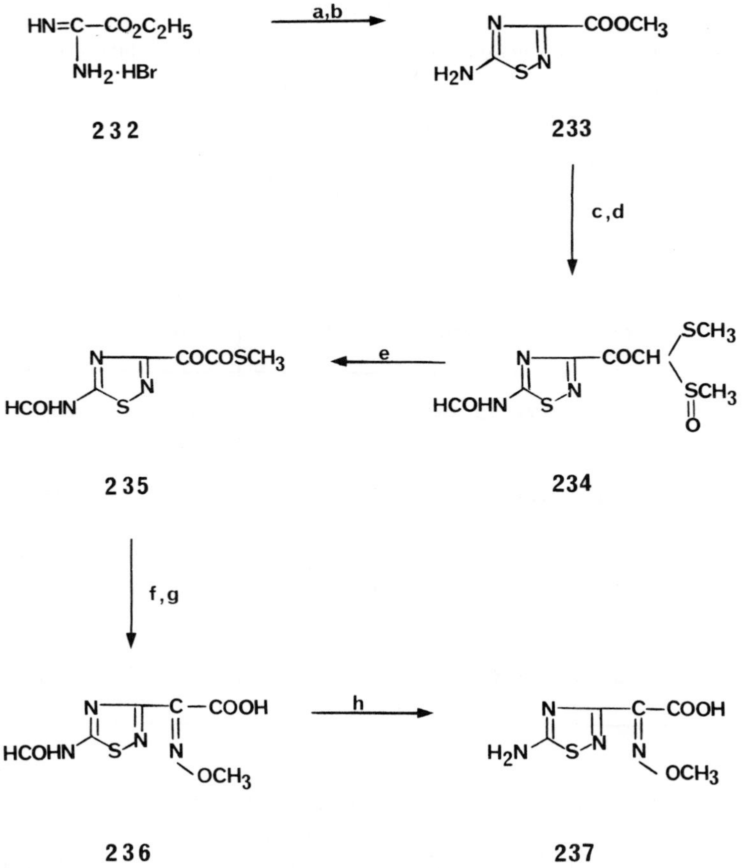

SCHEME 38. Synthesis of 2-(5-amino-1,2,4-thiadiazol-3-yl)-2-methoxyimino acetic acid (237). (a) Br_2; (b) $KSCN/CH_3OH$; (c) $HCOOH/Ac_2O$; (d) $NaH/CH_3SCH_2SOCH_3$; (e) $NaIO_4/AcOH$; (f) OH^-; (g) NH_2OCH_3; (h) OH^-.

3-amino-1,2,4-triazol-5-yl **231g** (Csendes *et al.*, 1983a), 5-amino-1,2,4-oxadiazol-3-yl **231h** (Wheeler *et al.*, 1986a), and 2-amino-1,3,4-thiadiazol-5-yl **232i** (Csendes *et al.*, 1983a; Sakagami *et al.*, 1983). All structures are given in Table 19. As a rule, unsubstituted or methyl substituted heterocyclic moieties in the 7-acyl side chain like 1-H-pyrazol-3-yl **231l** (Lattrell *et al.*, 1985), 1,2,4-thiadiazol-3-yl **231m**, 1,2,5-thiadiazol-3-yl **231n** (Takaya *et al.*, 1983), 1,2,3-thiadiazol-4-yl **231o**, 2-methyl-1,3,4-thiadiazol-5-yl **231p** and 2-methyl-tetrazol-5-yl **231q** (Nakano, 1981), are less interesting. Only 1-H-pyrazol-3-yl-cephem CPW-86 363 of type **231l** seems to be of clinical interest

TABLE 20

Selected cephalosporins in development with a 5-amino-1,2,4-thiadiazole moiety

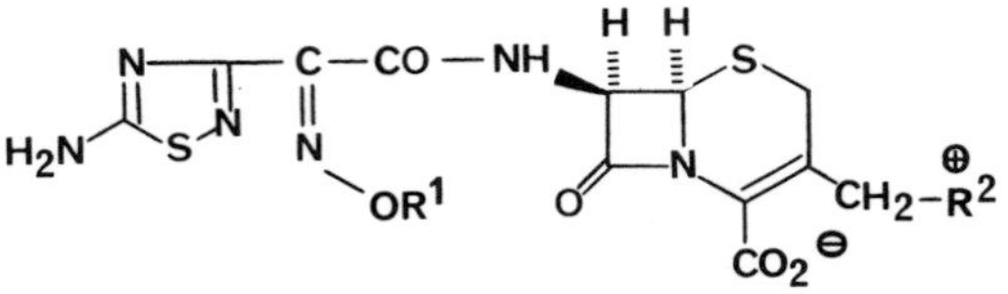

No.	Compound	R^1	R^2
238 a	CGP 22 495	–CH$_3$	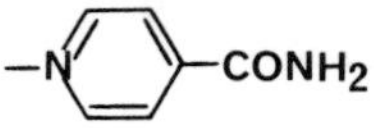
238 b	CGP 24 042	–CH$_3$	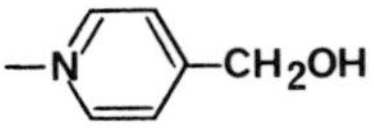
239	FR 17 126	–CH$_2$–CO$_2$H	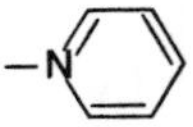
240	E 1040	–CH$_3$	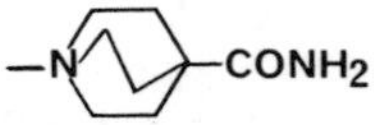

due to its synergistic interactions with host defence mechanisms (Lam *et al.*, 1984; see Section 5.1). Cefuroxime (**298**) formally belonging to this group (of type **231k**) is a clinically established second generation cephalosporin.

Great efforts have been made to replace the thiazole ring in cephalosporins by six-membered heteroaromatics. Typical examples are listed in Table 21. Structure–activity relationships in the cefmenoxime (**208**) series demonstrated that the 2-aminopyridin-6-yl derivative **241a** shows higher activity than the isomers **241b–d** against many tested organisms (Goto *et al.*, 1984b). Replacement of the pyridine ring by 4-aminopyrimidin-2-yl **241e** increased activity, especially against Gram-negative bacteria, while this activity is reduced for 2-aminopyrimidin-6-yl **241f** (Goto *et al.*, 1984c) and 2-amino-3-methyl-1,3,5-triazin-6-yl **241g** derivatives (Lattrell *et al.*, 1985).

4.3.1.4 Modification of the (Z)-Methoxyimino Group. A Z-configurated oxime residue in the α-position of the 7-[2-aminothiazolyl]-acetamido side chain is essential for high antibacterial activity and β-lactamase stability. All

TABLE 21

Replacement of the aminothiazole ring by 6-ring heterocycles in cephalosporins **241** with different 3-substituents R

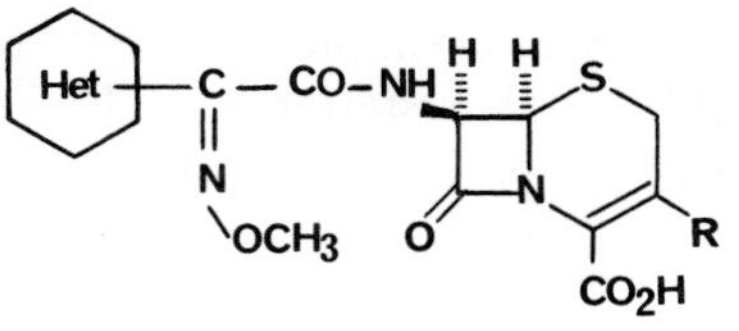

241

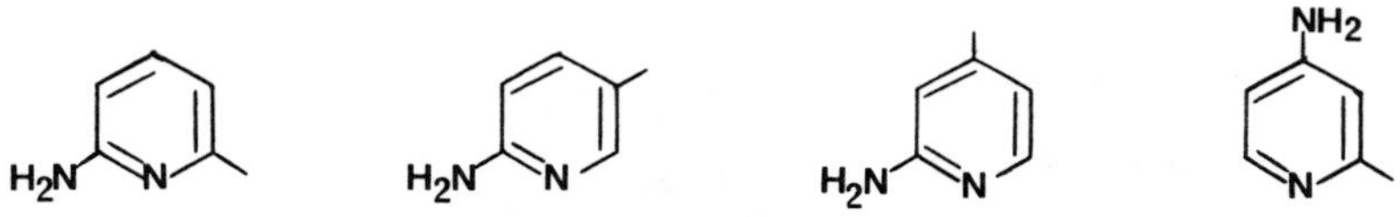

a   b   c   d

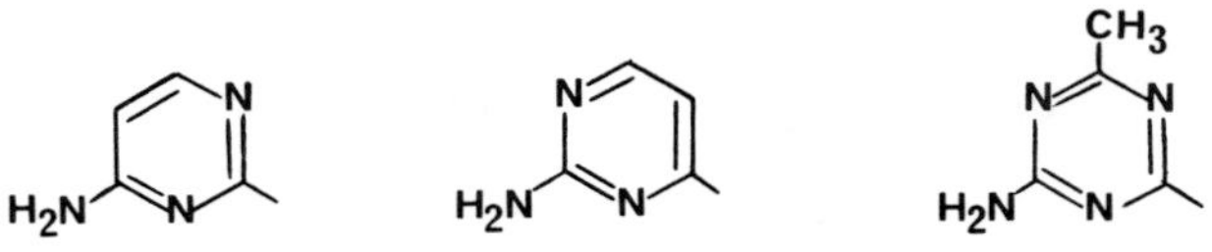

e   f   g

cephalosporins possessing an (E)-configuration of the oxime have low potency (Nakano, 1981; Ochiai *et al.*, 1981b; Dürckheimer *et al.*, 1982; Dunn, 1982). A selective synthesis and structural evidence for the isomeric (E)- and (Z)-2-(2-aminothiazol-4-yl)-2-methoxyiminoacetic acids and their derivatives have been given (Ochiai *et al.*, 1981a). A (Z/E)-isomerization caused by ultraviolet light has been described for cefuroxime (**298**) (Iorio and Nicoletti, 1986). Methylation studies on hydroxyimino compounds of cefotaxime (**207**), cefmenoxime (**208**) or their precursors showed that in most cases the isomeric nitrone compounds are the major products. Nevertheless, by this procedure preparation of labelled cefmenoxime (**208**) has been successful (Ochiai *et al.*, 1981c).

A compound without an oxime group, for example cefotiam (**265**), possesses diminished β-lactamase stability. The effect of substitution in the oxime residue has been studied extensively in several series, e.g. cefotaxime (**207**) (Bucourt *et al.*, 1978, 1981; Dürckheimer *et al.*, 1982; Skotnicki and Steinbaugh, 1986), ceftizoxime (**209**) (Nakano, 1981; Takaya *et al.*, 1981b; Dunn, 1982; Takasugi *et al.*, 1983b; Yamanaka *et al.*, 1985a), cefmenoxime (**208**) (Ochiai *et al.*, 1981b; Arimoto *et al.*, 1986b) and cefpirome (**220**) (Lattrell *et al.*, 1982, 1983b; Kirrstetter *et al.*, 1983). Of the many variations (more than 100), only the most interesting derivatives are shown in Table 22.

TABLE 22

Modification of the Z-methoxyimino group by other residues R^1 in cephalosporins **242** with different 3-substituents R^2

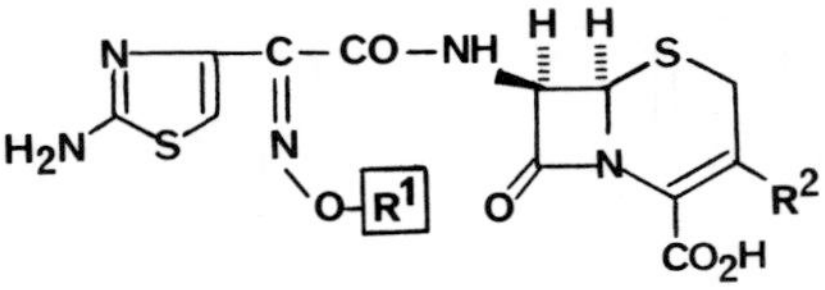

2 4 2

$-CH_2-CH_3$	$-CH_2-CH=CH_2$	$-CHF_2$	$-CH_2F$
a	b	c	d

$-CH_2CO_2H$	$-C(CH_3)_2CO_2H$	$-CH-COOH$
e	f	g

$-CH_2-CH_2NH_2$	$-CH_2-CONR_2$	$-CH_2-CO-N\diagdown NH$
h	i	k

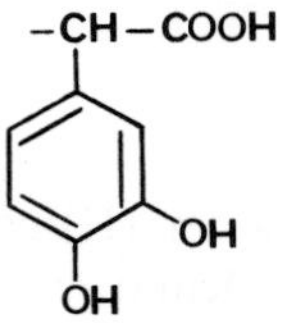

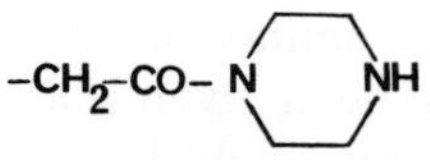

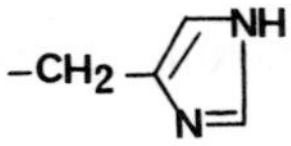

l	m	n	o

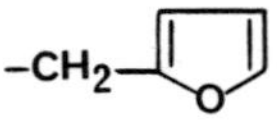

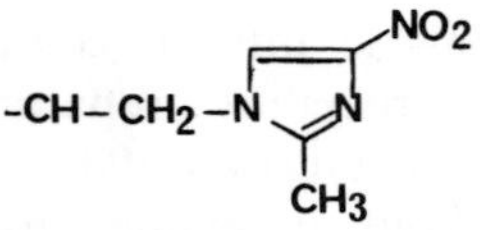

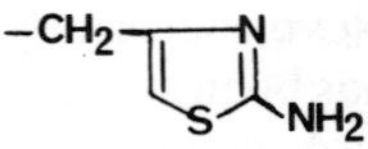

Cephems carrying a methoxy-, ethoxy- (**242a**) [e.g. in BO-1232 (**269a**) and ME-1220 (**263a**)], an allyloxy- (**242b**) [e.g. in OCS-575 (**268**)] or a difluoromethoxyimino group (**242c**) in the (Z)-configuration generally display a balanced antibacterial spectrum over a wide range of Gram-positive and Gram-negative bacteria. Increasing lengths of alkyl- or alkenyl substituents only favour the activity against Gram-positive bacteria at the expense of Gram-negative strains. An unsubstituted (Z)-oxime group has a similar effect. Substitution with alkynyl-, cycloalkyl-, cycloalkylmethyl- or halogenated alkyl groups in the oxime moiety results in lower potencies, with the exception of the difluoromethyl group (**242c**) (Vignau and Heymes, 1981; Fleischmann *et al.*, 1985). *In vitro* data for the recently published fluoromethoxyimino cephems **242d** are not yet available (Bell *et al.*, 1986).

Introduction of acidic groups, e.g. a carboxymethyl or 2-carboxy-2-propyl substituent (**242e** or **242f**), increases the activity against *Pseudomonas* strains at the expense of activity against *Staph. aureus*. Ceftazidime (**266**) is the first interesting representative of a parenteral aminothiazole cephalosporin with an acidic 7β-acyl side chain. Other parenteral compounds selected for further evaluation are BO-1236 (**269b**), CM-40 874 (**271a**), CM-40 876 (**271b**), CPW-86 363, FR-17 126 (**240**), ME-1221 (**263b**) and YM-13 115 (**264**). For more details, see Section 5.1. In a recent paper, synthesis and *in vitro* activity of YM-13 115 (**264**) and some related compounds with an acidic function in the oxyimino group were reported (Nagano *et al.*, 1987). Some carboxymethylcephalosporins of type **242e** are members of a new class of oral antibiotics. Examples of this type are cefixime (**51**), FK-089 (**288**) and CGP-33 098A (**290**) (see Section 5.2).

Introduction of a basic group into the oxime moiety, e.g. **242h–k**, causes a significant decrease in the activity against *Staph. aureus* (Dunn, 1982), but in case of basic-substituted carbamoylmethoxyimino derivatives **242i** a well balanced activity against several strains is observed (Arimoto *et al.*, 1986a). The best compound in this series is claimed to be **242k**.

Substitution of the oxime group with heterocyclic moieties (**242l–o**) also leads to very active compounds, e.g. DN-9550 (**270**), M-14 638 (**262a**) and NY-1675 (Section 5.1). Introduction of the 2-amino-4-thiazolyl residue into the oxime moiety reduces activity (Shibanuma *et al.*, 1984, 1985).

4.3.1.5 Replacement of the Methoxyimino Group by other Functionalities. Replacement of the oxime group by other moieties such as methylene (**243a**), hydroxylmethyl (**243b**), ethyl (**243c**), *i*-propyl (**243d**), carbonyl (**243e**), aminomethyl (**243f**) (Ochiai *et al.*, 1980a,b; Dürckheimer *et al.*, 1982; Takasugi *et al.*, 1983a; Mitsuhashi and Ochiai, 1985), sulphomethyl (**243g**) (Minami *et al.*, 1983) and ureidomethyl (**243h**) (Polacek and Starke, 1980) have already been reviewed. Examples of this type are given in Table

TABLE 23

Replacement of the methoxyimino group by other functionalities X in cephalosporins **243** with different 3-substituents R^2

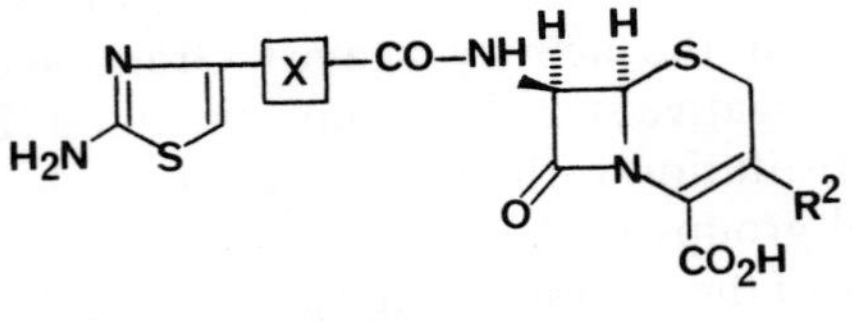

243

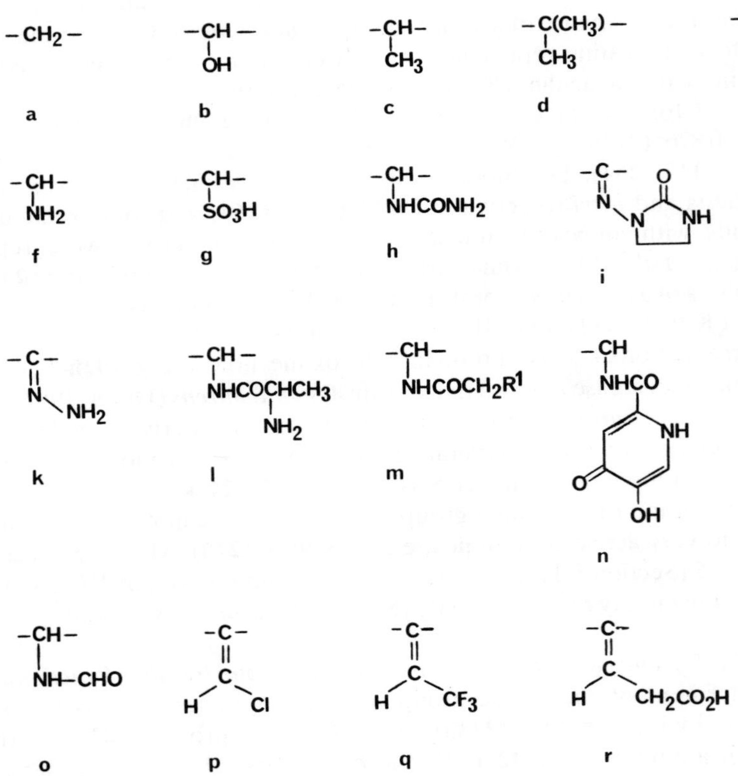

$-CH_2-$	$-CH-$ OH	$-CH-$ CH_3	$-C(CH_3)-$ CH_3	$-C-$ $\parallel$ O
a	**b**	**c**	**d**	**e**

$-CH-$ NH_2	$-CH-$ SO_3H	$-CH-$ $NHCONH_2$	
f	**g**	**h**	**i**

k	**l**	**m**	**n**

$-CH-$ $NH-CHO$			
o	**p**	**q**	**r**

23. Hydrazono analogues like **243i** and **243k** have also been prepared and tested (König and Metzger, 1981). MIC values of (E)-isomers of α-hydrazonobenzylcephalosporins revealed lower activity than cefuroxime (**298**) (Monguzzi *et al.*, 1985). In a series of 2-(2-aminothiazol-4-yl)-2-hydrazonacetamidocephalosporins, the most active compound **243k** bearing a 1-methyltetrazol-5-yl thio group at C-3′, exhibits good antibacterial activity against both Gram-positive and Gram-negative bacteria (Brandt *et al.*, 1987).

Cephalosporins of type **243l** and **243m** having a dipeptide-like 7-side chain display a balanced antibacterial spectrum (Furukawa *et al.*, 1986). 3-Cephems of type **243m** with strongly basic amidino or guanidino residues (R^1 = —C(NH$_2$)=NH or —NH—C(NH$_2$)=NH$_2$) have been prepared. They displayed high antibacterial activity similar to that of cefotaxime (**207**), but lower stability to β-lactamases (Arimoto *et al.*, 1986a). Reduction of the methoxyimino group of cefotaxime (**207**) resulted in an aminothiazolylglycyl derivative as a mixture of two diastereomers **243f**, which was acylated by 5-hydroxy-4-pyridone-2-carboxylic acid to give **243n** (Mochida *et al.*, 1987). Variation of the 3′-position was performed and led to compound KT-4788 having a methylpyridinium-4-thio group. Its antibacterial activity is claimed to be better than that of cefoperazone (**244**).

Recently, some cephalosporins of types **243o–q** with promising antibacterial properties have been reported, namely CGP-31 523 A (**272**) (of type **243o**) and SG-164 (**267**) (of type **243p**), which display overall activity comparable to that of third generation cephalosporins. Analogues of SG 164 (**267**), which contain fluorine instead of chlorine in the 7-side chain, have also been synthesized (Nishide *et al.*, 1987). 7432-S (**289**) (of type **243r**), with activity against Gram-negative bacteria, is an oral cephalosporin (Hamashima, 1985). Synthetic routes to this compound have been described by Yoshioko (1987). For more details see Sections 5.1 and 5.2. Bayer AG (Kinast *et al.*, 1984; Angerbauer *et al.*, 1985a,b) and Meiji Seika Kaisha, Ltd. (Sakagami *et al.*, 1986) have also claimed cephalosporins of this structure and related compounds. Synthesis and SAR studies of ammoniocephalosporins with acrylic side chains (type **243p**, alkyl instead of chlorine) have been recently published (Angerbauer *et al.*, 1987).

4.3.2 Glycylcephalosporins

Glycylcephalosporins are important antibiotics due to their high enteral absorption. Cefalexin (**23**) was the first compound and is still the most commonly used oral cephalosporin. It has been shown that the (D)-

phenylglycine side chain is a more potent antibacterial agent than the (L)-isomer. To improve the biological activity of cefalexin (23) the substitution pattern in the aromatic ring and the substitution at C-3 have been examined in great detail (Webber and Ott, 1977). Only very few structures which are either phenyl substituted or related ring analogues have similar activity, but differ to some extent in the pharmacokinetic profile. As substituents at C-3, small groups are preferred, like methyl, chlorine, and methoxy.

Whereas most of the side chains for glycylcephalosporins are readily available, the side chain of LY 164 846 (281) has to be prepared in several steps from benzothiophene (Kukolja et al., 1985a). Formulae of old and new glycylcephalosporins are given later in Table 31 and discussed in more detail in Section 5.2.

4.3.3 N-Acylated Phenylglycine Cephalosporins

Glycylcephalosporins described in the previous Section (4.3.2) belong to the group of oral cephalosporins with low β-lactamase stability. Acylation of the glycyl-amino group has led to compounds with enhanced stability against β-lactamases and extended antibacterial spectrum to cover a great number of bacterial genera, including Pseudomonas spp. However, these drugs are no longer enterally absorbed. Table 24 summarizes individual compounds. Cefoperazone (244) is a parenteral ureidocephalosporin structurally related to the penicillin piperacillin with a broad antibacterial spectrum including Pseudomonas spp., but diminished activity against TEM β-lactamases forming Escherichia coli (Drugs of the Future, 1981c). Out of a great number of described acyl derivatives cefpiramide (245) (Drugs of the Future, 1986d), KIT-180 (246) (Takada et al., 1983), E-0702 (247) (Drugs of the Future, 1983a) and cefpimizole (AC-1370) (248) (Drugs of the Future, 1987d) have been selected for further development. Cefpimizole (248) augments phagocytosis by macrophages and neutrophils (Ohnishi, 1984). For E-0702 (247) a new mode of transport into the bacterial cell was observed (N. Watanabe et al., 1987b). It coordinates to iron ions via the vicinal phenolic hydroxy group and penetrates the outer membrane via the ton B-dependent transport system for iron.

New ureidocephalosporins and ureidocephamycins containing a catechol moiety in the 7-side chain were recently reported by Ohi et al. (1987). Some of these compounds show remarkable activity against Ps. aeruginosa spp.

TABLE 24

N-Acylated phenylglycine cephalosporins

No	Compound	X	R^1	R^2
244	Cefoperazone	HO		
245	Cefpiramide	HO		
246	KIT-180	HO		
247	E-0702	HO		
248	Cefpimizole	H		

4.3.4 Miscellaneous Cephalosporin Derivatives

Although aminothiazole and N-acylated phenylglycine cephalosporins dominate the newly introduced antibiotics, several other interesting structural types which are mentioned in the literature will be described (Table 25). KY-087 (**249**) bears the mandelic acid side chain of cefamandole. Prodrugs of **249** have been prepared in order to improve enteral absorption (Section 5.2). ICI-156 488 (**250**) is remarkable, because of its non-acyl 7-side chain (Bruneau, 1984). CGP-17 520 (**251**) is a parenteral broad spectrum cephalosporin similar to cefuroxime (**298**). In systemic infections in mice it exhibited better activity than cefuroxime (**298**) and cefoxitin (**104**) against various strains (Kadurugamuwa *et al.*, 1985). SKF-80 303 (**252**) (Brocalli *et al.*, 1983) and ISF-3453 (**253**) (*Drugs of the Future*, 1980) are cephalosporins with a hydroxyimino function. The antimicrobial activity and β-lactamase stability are comparable to those of cefuroxime (**298**). Cefsulodin (**254**) is a marketed narrow spectrum cephalosporin with excellent MIC values against *Pseudomonas* spp. and is discussed in Section 5.1. Compound L-640 876 (**255**), a structurally novel pyridiniocephem, possesses good activity against many Gram-negative and Gram-positive bacteria, with the exception of *Pseudomonas* spp., *Serratia marcescens* and *Streptococcus faecalis* (Koupal *et al.*, 1987). In mouse protection studies **255** was as potent as cefoxitin (**104**) against *Bacteroides* sp.

Compound L-652 813 (**256**) (Pelak *et al.*, 1987), another member of this type, is also a potent antibiotic with high activity against both *Staph. aureus* and Gram-negative bacteria. It is not active against *Ps. aeruginosa* and *Strep. faecalis*, but shows activity against anaerobic bacteria, such as *Bacteroides* spp. The prolonged pharmacokinetics of **256** in mice and in rhesus monkeys resembles that of ceftriaxone (**210**). The therapeutic efficacy in experimental bacteraemias in mice is lower than that of ceftriaxone (**210**).

Table 26 lists parenteral cephalosporins with a S-substituted mercaptoacetamido side chain at C-7. K-13 176 (**257**) is comparable to cefazolin against Staphylococci and more active against Streptococci and Gram-negative species (Nannini, 1981a). The antimicrobial spectrum of K-13 102 (**258**) is similar to that of **257** (Nannini, 1981b). MT-116 (**259**) is a derivative of cefminox with increased activity against Gram-positive bacteria (Inouye *et al.*, 1984).

Fluorine-containing 7-acyl side chains are part of broad spectrum 1-oxa cephalosporins flomoxef (6315-S) (**260**) and 2355-S (**261**) (Table 27), imparting excellent antistaphylococcal activity including clinical isolates of methicillin-resistant Staphylococci (see Section 5.1).

TABLE 25

Miscellaneous cephalosporin derivatives with different side chains

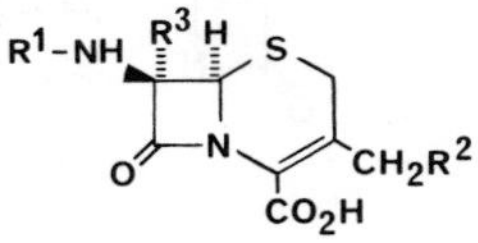

No	Compound	R^1	R^2
249	KY 087	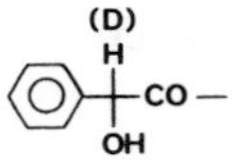	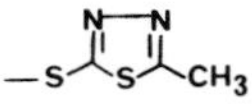
250	ICI 156 488	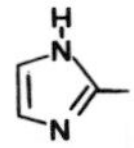	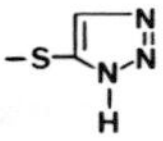
251	CGP 17 520	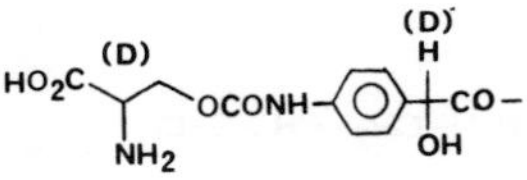	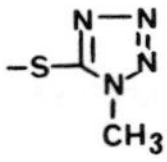
252	SKF 80 303	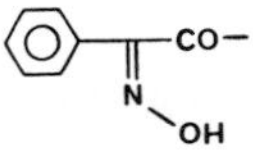	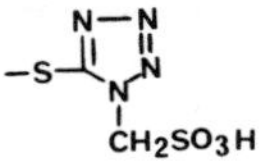
253	ISF 3453	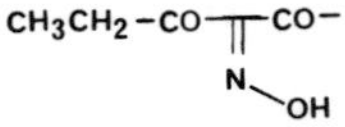	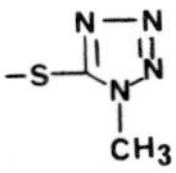
254	Cefsulodin	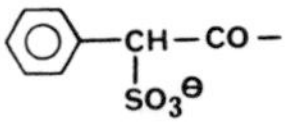	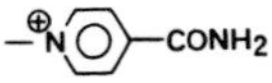
255	L 640 876	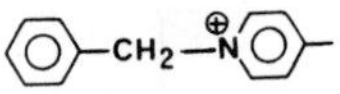	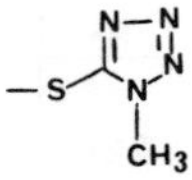
256	L 652 813	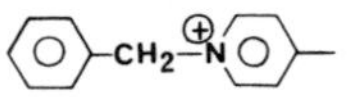	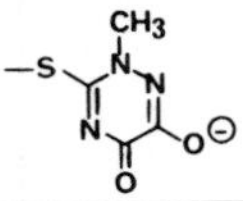

TABLE 26

Cephalosporin derivatives with a S-substituted mercaptoacetamido side chain at C-7

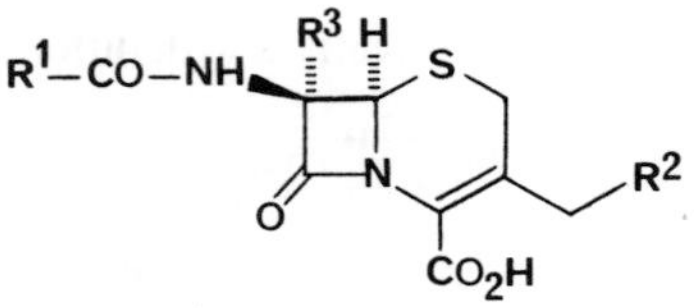

No.	Compound	R^1	R^2	R^3
257	K 13 176	$HO_2C-CH=CH-S-CH_2-$	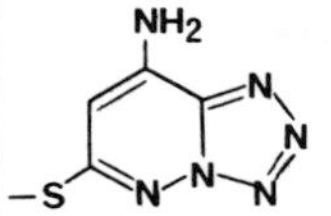	H
258	K 13 102	$HO_2C-CH=CH-S-CH_2-$	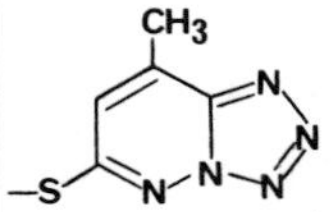	H
259	MT 116	$H_2N-CH_2-CH_2-S-CH_2-$	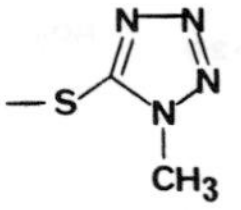	OCH_3

TABLE 27

1-Oxacephems under extended evaluation

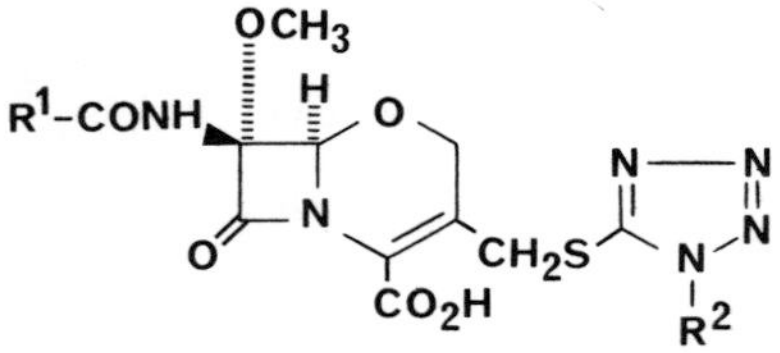

No.	Compound	R^1	R^2
260	Flomoxef (6315-S)	$F_2CH-S-CH_2-$	$-CH_2CH_2OH$
261	2355-S	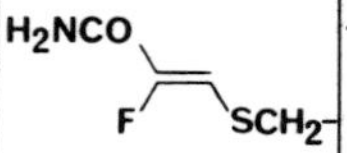	$-CH_2CH_2OH$

5 Compounds on the Market and under Development

5.1 PARENTERAL CEPHALOSPORINS

5.1.1 Introduction

A brief characterization of parenteral cephalosporins which have been launched in recent years or which are currently under development is given. *In vitro* and *in vivo* antimicrobial activities, β-lactamase stability, and pharmacokinetic parameters (e.g. serum half-life, peak serum concentration, main route of excretion, metabolism) are considered. Only preliminary results are available for compounds which are currently in an early state of development. A vast amount of original literature is dealing with cephalosporins [e.g. at least 2500 documents are available concerning cefotaxime (**207**)]. Whenever possible, review articles are cited to give access to further references. Compounds discussed are mostly representatives of the third generation cephalosporins, distinguished from older first and second generation predecessors by a very high stability to β-lactamases with a much broader spectrum of activity and a greater potency against Gram-negative organisms. Newer second generation derivatives are included for completeness, whereas the characteristics of first and older second generation cephalosporins have already been reviewed (Quintiliani *et al.*, 1982; Smith and Lefrock, 1982). Newer reviews summarizing *in vitro* and *in vivo* properties of cephalosporins have been published by Brogard *et al.* (1978), Bonetti (1981), Kuhlmann (1981), Brogard and Comte (1982), Neu (1982a,b), Webber and Wheeler (1982), Wise (1982), Garzone *et al.* (1983). Price and McGregor (1984), Barriere and Flaherty (1984), Bergan (1984), Knothe (1984), Neu (1984c, 1985), Weinstein (1984), Newman (1985), O'Callaghan and Harper (1985), Kühn and Zimmermann (1986), and Rolinson (1986); other comprehensive reviews on several aspects are given in *Fortschritte der Antimikrobiellen, Antineoplastischen Chemotherapie* (1982) and by Mitsuhashi (1981).

Analytical investigations on cephalosporins have been compiled by Van Krimpen *et al.* (1987). This review presents physicochemical properties of cephalosporins, their degradation routes and methods for analysis of these substances in biological and other matrices. Another survey on analytical methods for cephalosporins in biological fluids is given by Toothaker *et al.* (1987).

Clinical experiences for many cephalosporins have been summarized (Simon and Stille, 1985; Neu, 1984a,d). The important aspect of combination therapy with aminoglycosides and other antibiotics has also been reviewed (Klastersky *et al.*, 1986).

Different classification systems for cephalosporins have been proposed (see Section 2.2). Although the classification is not based on structural features, third generation cephalosporins mainly derive from aminothiazole cephalosporins, substituted by neutral or polar groups attached to C-3. Other important representatives belong to N-acylated phenylglycyl cephalosporins, cephamycins or to nuclear analogues of cephalosporins.

Synthesis and SAR studies are discussed in preceding sections. Both the antimicrobial spectrum and the potency of cephalosporins are mainly determined by the affinity of the cephalosporins to cell wall synthesizing enzymes (penicillin binding proteins), the penetration across the cell envelope and their stability against degrading enzymes. For a discussion of the mode of action see Section 6.1. Although cefotaxime (**207**) and other third generation cephalosporins have proved to be effective in clinical practice, further improvement with respect to activity against Staphylococci, *Pseudomonas* spp. and anaerobes is still a major task. The extent of activity against these bacteria has become a key determinant in evaluating new cephalosporins. Table 1 sketches the antibacterial activity and β-lactamase stability for different groups of Gram-positive and Gram-negative bacteria, *Pseudomonas* spp. and *Bacteroides fragilis*. Table 2 summarizes often used pharmacokinetic parameters of cephalosporins (Sections 2.3 and 2.4).

5.1.2 Aminothiazole Cephalosporins

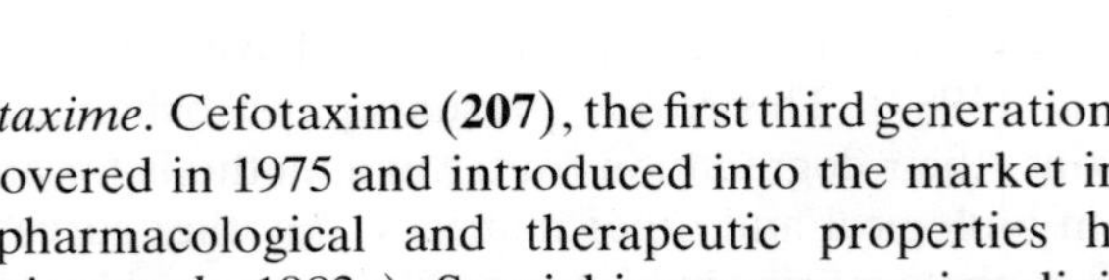

207

5.1.2.1 *Cefotaxime.* Cefotaxime (**207**), the first third generation cephalosporin, was discovered in 1975 and introduced into the market in 1980. Its antibacterial, pharmacological and therapeutic properties have been reviewed (Carmine *et al.*, 1983a). Special issues summarize clinical results (*J. Antimicrob. Chemother.*, 1980, 1984; *Chemotherapy (Tokyo)* 1980a; *Infection*, 1985). Cefotaxime (**207**) exhibits a broad antibacterial spectrum including clinically important Gram-positive and Gram-negative bacteria. MIC values against selected groups of bacteria for cefotaxime (**207**) and other new cephalosporins are listed in Table 28.

TABLE 28

Comparative *in vitro* antibacterial activities of third generation cephalosporins (Seibert *et al.*, 1983a,b)

Bacteria	MIC$_{50}$ (μg/ml)						
	Cefpirome 220	Cefoperazone 244	Cefotaxime 207	Ceftazidime 266	Ceftriaxone 210	Latamoxef 247
Staph. spp. (N = 110)	0.260	1.200	1.300	6.500	2.400	5.700
Staph. spp. (Methicillin-resistant; N = 49)	5.600	18.200	28.800	44.100	61.600	40.000
Strep. spp. (Serogroup A, B, C; N = 49)	0.002	0.034	0.002	0.050	0.002	1.300
Enterococci (N = 73)	1.900	13.100	1.600	106.200	8.800	103.100
E. coli (N = 193)	0.005	0.028	0.004	0.018	0.007	0.022
Citrobacter (N = 54)	0.013	0.200	0.094	0.190	0.094	0.058
Serratia spp. (N = 107)	0.025	0.810	0.093	0.049	0.047	0.130
Salmonella spp. (N = 47)	0.007	0.110	0.029	0.094	0.012	0.032
Enterobacter spp. (N = 95)	0.024	0.240	0.140	0.240	0.180	0.980
Ps. aeruginosa (N = 259)	1.600	4.600	11.400	0.870	10.400	12.500

Against Enterobacteriaceae, the MICs of cefotaxime (**207**) are in many cases more than 100 times better than those of older cephalosporins and broad spectrum penicillins. Furthermore, the drug exhibits a therapeutic activity against *Pseudomonas aeruginosa* (Leone *et al.*, 1982; Okubadejo and Bax, 1982). Cefotaxime (**207**) is highly stable to β-lactamases of both Gram-positive and Gram-negative bacteria. Several reviews on clinical and pharmacokinetic properties of cefotaxime (**207**) and other third generation analogues have been published by Neu (1982a), Noble and Barza (1985) and Balant *et al.* (1985). Cefotaxime (**207**) is mainly excreted by the kidneys and has a serum half-life of about one hour. Probenicid increases its plasma level and half-life, indicating that it is excreted by tubular secretion as well as glomular filtration. About 50–60% of cefotaxime (**207**) is recovered unchanged in the urine after i.v. administration (Geddes *et al.*, 1980; LeFrock *et al.*, 1982). It is partially metabolized in man, the main metabolite being deacetylcefotaxime (about 20%). Other metabolites (e.g. lactone and lactone derivatives with an open β-lactam ring) are formed in smaller amounts (Geddes *et al.*, 1980). Deacetylcefotaxime shows synergistic or additive antibacterial effects with cefotaxime (**207**) (Jones and Wilson, 1982; Limbert *et al.*, 1982).

Cefotaxime (**207**) has a serum protein binding of about 30–50% and penetrates readily body tissues and fluids. Only in patients with severe renal failure is the half-life significantly extended. CSF levels in case of meningeal inflammation are about 10% of the serum concentration, sufficient for the treatment of meningitis. The half-life of deacetylcefotaxime is longer than that of the parent antibiotic (Neu, 1982a).

Ceftizoxime (**209**), cefmenoxime (**208**), and ceftriaxone (**210**), which are already on the market, are potent successors of cefotaxime (**207**). They are discussed in the following sections.

5.1.2.2 Ceftizoxime. Ceftizoxime (FK-749) (**209**) was introduced in 1982 as a so-called "metabolically stable cefotaxime analogue". Summaries of its pharmacological and clinical evaluation have been published (*Chemotherapy (Tokyo)*, 1980b; *J. Antimicrob. Agents Chemother.*, 1982b). Richards and Heel (1985) reviewed the antibacterial activity, pharmacokinetic properties and therapeutic use of ceftizoxime (**209**), which is highly

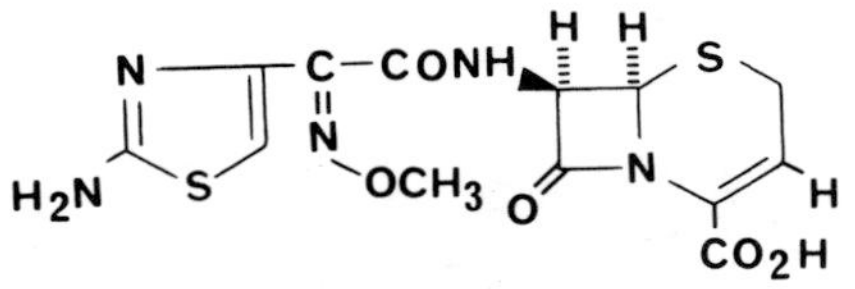

209

active against Enterobacteriaceae, including β-lactamase-producing strains, but has limited activity against *Ps. aeruginosa*. Similarly, its low *in vitro* activity against *B. fragilis* and Enterococci may restrict its usage in infections caused by these pathogens. Ceftizoxime (**209**) is highly β-lactamase resistant. The serum half-life of about 1.9 h is longer than that of cefotaxime (**207**). About 80% of unmetabolized ceftizoxime (**209**) is recovered in urine (Neu, 1984b; Furlanut *et al.*, 1983). Its CSF concentration is slightly higher than that of cefotaxime (**207**). CSF levels of ceftizoxime (**209**) were determined by Ruf (1982). Biliary levels of up to 70 mg/l have been reported (Cunha *et al.*, 1982), exceeding the MIC values of most biliary pathogens.

5.1.2.3 Cefmenoxime. Cefmenoxime (SCE 1365) (**208**) reached the market in 1983. A special issue [*Chemotherapy (Tokyo)*, 1981a] summarizes the clinical evaluation of cefmenoxime (**208**). A review of its antibacterial

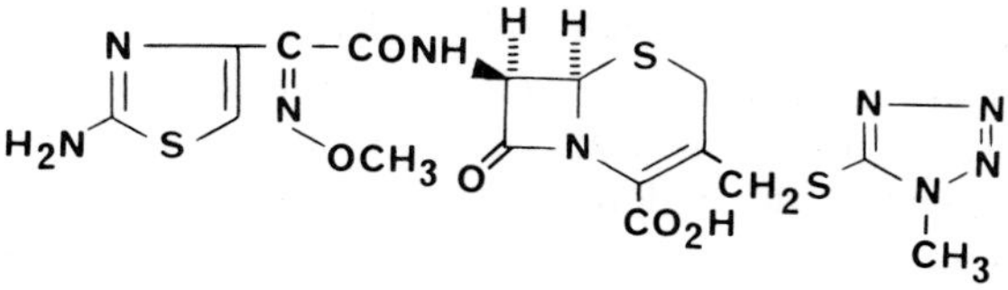

208

activity, pharmacokinetic properties and therapeutic use has been recently published (Campoli-Richards and Todd, 1987). Like cefamandole, cefoperazone (**244**) and latamoxef (**273**), it possesses at C-3' a 1-methyltetrazolylthio substituent. The antimicrobial potency of cefmenoxime (**208**) has been compared to that of cefotaxime (**207**) and second generation cephalosporins (Stamm *et al.*, 1981). It is active against Streptococci, except *Streptococcus faecalis*. Against Staphylococci cefmenoxime (**208**) is slightly less active than cefotaxime (**207**), but more active than latamoxef (**273**). Its activity against *Escherichia coli*, *Klebsiella* spp., *P. mirabilis*, *Salmonella* spp. and *Shigella* spp. is similar to that of cefotaxime (**207**), ceftizoxime (**209**), or latamoxef (**273**). After i.v. or i.m. administration, cefmenoxime (**208**) is rapidly absorbed with nearly complete bioavailability and an elimination half-life of 1.5 h (Fourtillan *et al.*, 1984). More than 70% of the drug is excreted renally.

5.1.2.4 Ceftriaxone. The antibacterial, pharmacological and therapeutic properties of ceftriaxone (RO-139 904) (**210**) (*Drugs of the Future*, 1981b), which has been on the market since 1982, have been reviewed [Richards *et al.*, 1984; special issues: *Chemotherapy (Tokyo)*, 1984c; *Chemotherapy*

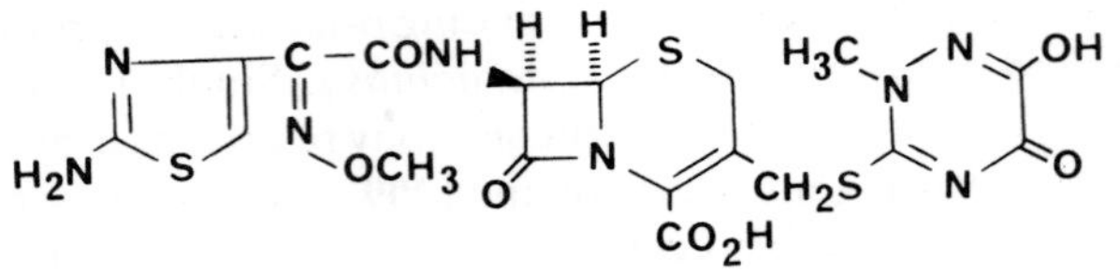

210

(*Basel*), 1981]. Ceftriaxone (**210**) exhibits low MICs against *Haemophilus influenzae*, *Neisseria gonorrhoeae*, *N. meningitis*, *S. pyogenes* and *Serratia marcescens*. It is highly active against non-enterococcal Streptococci, but in general lacks activity against Enterococci and methicillin-resistant Staphylococci (Cleeland and Squires, 1984). Ceftriaxone (**210**) displays a high stability against β-lactamases, and an unique pharmacokinetic profile (Patel and Kaplan, 1984), namely a very long elimination half-life of about 8.5 h in man due to the (2,5-dihydro-6-hydroxy-2-methyl-5-oxo-1,2,4-triazin-3-yl)thio substituent at C-3' (Reiner, 1986). The favourable pharmacokinetic properties (Patel *et al.*, 1981; Gnann *et al.*, 1982) are probably due to a concentration-dependent high plasma protein binding of the drug which exceeds 90%. After i.v. application, about 60% of ceftriaxone (**210**) is recovered unchanged in urine. The remainder is secreted in bile and ultimately found in faeces as microbiologically inactive compounds. One dosage per day has been recommended.

5.1.2.5 Cefuzonam. Cefuzonam (L-105, CL-251 931 (**216**) (*Drugs of the Future*, 1987b), the parent compound of the oral prodrug baccefuzonam, is undergoing clinical evaluation. A special issue on cefuzonam has been published (*Chemotherapy (Tokyo)*, 1986b). The drug is highly active *in vitro* against many pathogens, e.g. *S. pyogenes*, *H. influenza*, *E. coli*, *Klebsiella pneumoniae*, *P. mirabilis*, *P. vulgaris*, *Enterobacter cloacae*, *S. marcescens*, *Staphylococcus aureus* and methicillin-resistant Staphylococci (Arai, 1986). Cefuzonam (**216**) is highly stable towards penicillinases and cephalosporinases, but is slighly hydrolysed by oxyiminocephalosporinase (Hikida *et al.*, 1986). The *in vivo* therapeutic activity of cefuzonam (**216**) in mice

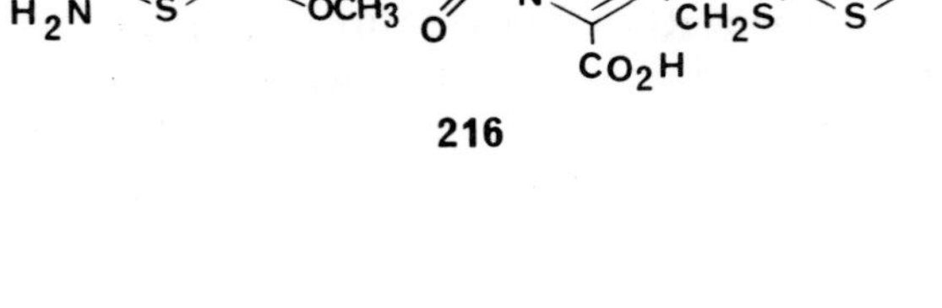

216

against intraperitoneal injected bacteria and lung and kidney infections lies between that of cefotiam (265) and that of ceftazidime (266) (Nishino *et al.*, 1986). In healthy volunteers, the serum half-life is 1.0–1.3 h, and the urinary recovery rate 50–70% (Nakashima *et al.*, 1986a). Cefuzoname (216) did not penetrate well into the CSF of children with meningitis (Fujii *et al.*, 1986).

5.1.2.6 M-14638, M-14643, M-14646, M-14648, and M-14659. Mochida prepared a number of injectable cephalosporins having triazolo-pyrimidinethio substituents at C-3' and an acyl-substituted oxyimino function in the 7-side chain. The title compounds selected on the basis of SAR studies exhibit broad spectrum activity. M-14643 (262b) displays *in vitro* activity against Gram-positive bacteria similar to cefotaxime (207), whereas

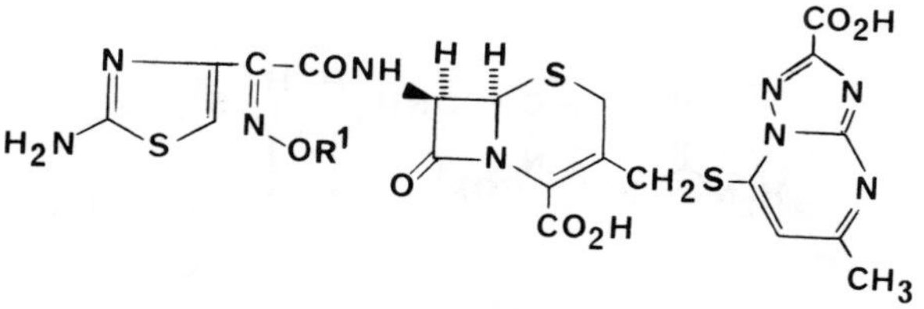

262

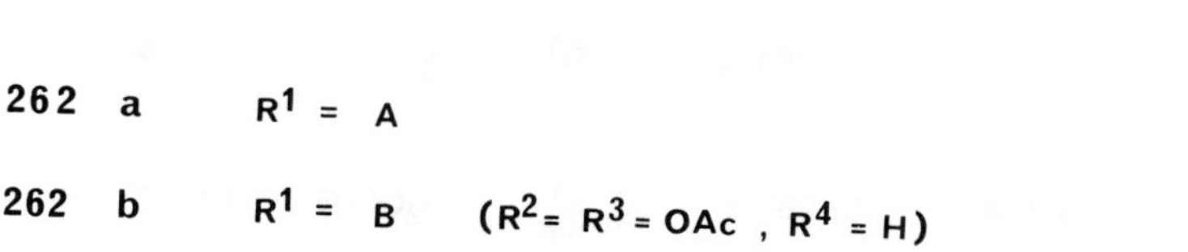

$R^1 = $

A   B   C

262   a $R^1 = $ A

262   b $R^1 = $ B   ($R^2 = R^3 = $ OAc , $R^4 = $ H)

262   c $R^1 = $ B   ($R^2 = R^3 = R^4 = $ OAc)

262   d $R^1 = $ B   ($R^2 = R^3 = $ OAc , $R^4 = $ CH$_3$)

262   e $R^1 = $ C

its activity against *Ps. aeruginosa* and *S. marcescens* is equal to or better than that of cefotaxime (**207**) or ceftazidime (**266**) (Inaba *et al.*, 1985). In experimental mice infection, produced by twelve different strains including methicillin-resistant Staphylococci, M-14 643 (**262b**) is more effective than either cefotaxime (**207**) or ceftazidime (**266**). M-14 638 (**262a**) is very similar to M-14 643 (**262b**) in its *in vitro* and *in vivo* properties. M-14 646 (**262c**), M-14 648 (**262d**), and M-14 659 (**262e**) are also potent broad spectrum antibiotics, active against *Ps. aeruginosa*. M-14 659 (**262e**) is more potent than ceftazidime (**266**) in experimental infections (Kato *et al.*, 1986; Mochizuki *et al.*, 1986).

5.1.2.7 ME-1220, ME-1221, ME-1228, and MT-382. ME-1220 (CP-107) (**263a**), ME-1221 (MT-520) (**263b**), and MT-382 (**225**), possessing quaternary thiopyridinium substituents at C-3′, display broad spectrum activity

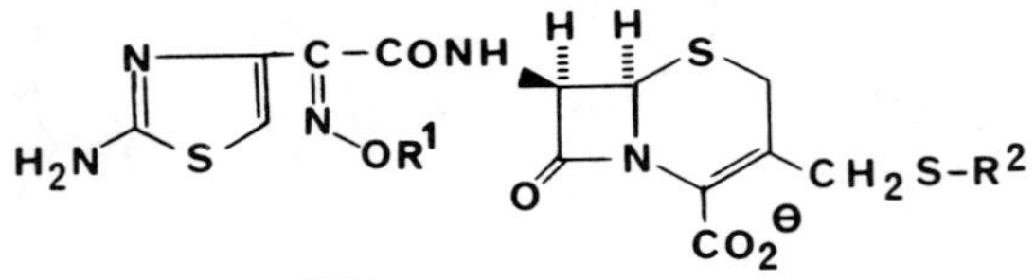

263

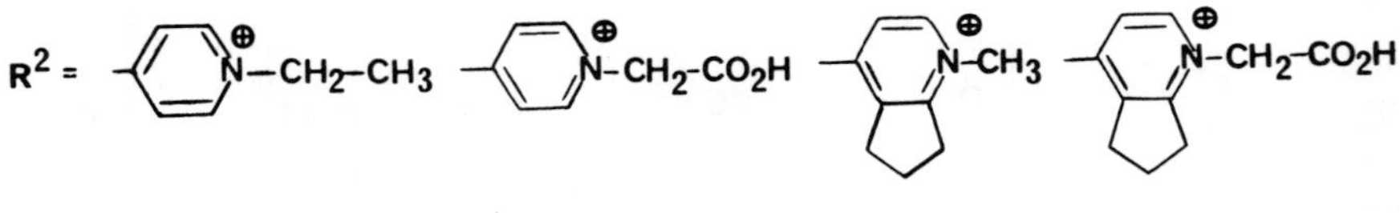

A	B	C	D

263 a	$R^1 = -C_2H_5$	$R^2 = B$
263 b	$R^1 = -CH_2CO_2H$	$R^2 = C$
263 c	$R^1 = -\overset{(S)}{\underset{CH_3}{CH}}-CO_2H$	$R^2 = A$
225	$R^1 = -CH_3$	$R^2 = D$

and are currently being extensively tested (Tsuroaka *et al.*, 1985; Okamoto *et al.*, 1986). Whereas ME-1220 (**263a**) is more active against Gram-positive strains, ME-1221 (**263b**) has better MICs against Gram-negative bacteria including *Ps. aeruginosa*. ME-1220 (**263a**) and ME-1221 (**263b**) seem to be *in vitro* better than ceftazidime (**266**) but less active than cefpirome (**220**) except against *Ps. aeruginosa*, *Ps. cepacia* and *Acinetobacter* spp. ME-1220 (**263a**) and ME-1221 (**263b**) exhibit excellent therapeutic effects in mice infections. They are highly stable to penicillinases and cephalosporinases. After i.v. administration to rats, serum elimination half-lives range between 45 and 66 min. ME-1220 (**263a**) is mainly excreted renally (about 80%), whereas ME-1221 (**263b**) is excreted to about 65% renally and to about 20% via bile. ME-1228 (**263c**) is a new parenteral cephalosporin with broad activity against Gram-positive and Gram-negative bacteria including *Ps. aeruginosa* (Shibahara *et al.*, 1987a). Pharmacokinetics in animals was presented by Yoshida *et al.* (1987).

5.1.2.8 Cefodizime. Cefodizime (HR-221) (**211**) (*Drugs of the Future*, 1987c; Blumbach *et al.*, 1987 and references cited therein) is prepared by displacing the 3′-acetoxy group of cefotaxime (**207**) with a 4-methyl-5-carboxymethyl-1,3-thiazol-2-yl group. It is a bactericidal, β-lactamase stable parenteral cephalosporin which inhibits most of the clinically important Gram-positive and Gram-negative bacteria displaying particularly high activity against Gram-negative species (Limbert *et al.*, 1984a). Cefodizime (**211**) shows much higher antibiotic potency *in vivo* than first and second generation cephalosporins. It exhibits high efficacy in different experimental animal infections, e.g. lung infections due to *K. pneumoniae* (Klesel *et al.*, 1984b,c). The *in vivo* activity of cefodizime (**211**) is comparable to or even higher than that of cefotaxime (**207**) and other third generation cephalosporins, although its MIC values are usually higher than that of cefotaxime (**207**). This surprising property is based on a favourable combination of its antibacterial activity, exceptional pharmacokinetic properties, and a direct effect on the host defence mechanisms. The immune stimulatory effect of cefodizime (**211**) on the host defence system has been evaluated by the mean

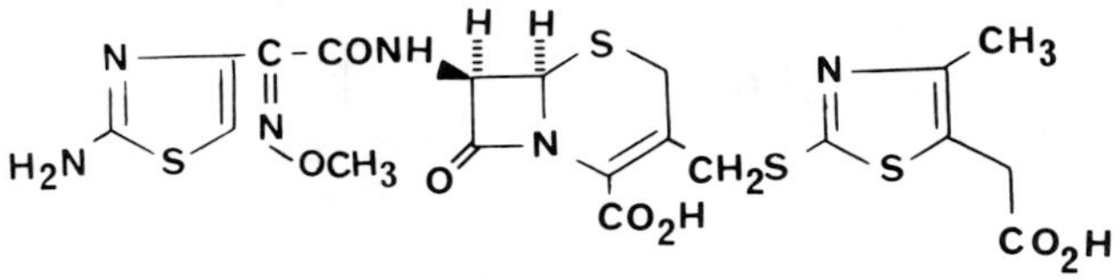

211

survival time of balb/c mice after intravenous infection with *Candida albicans* (Limbert *et al.*, 1984b). Cefodizime (**211**) is highly protein-bound (>80%) and has an elimination half-life of 3.0–3.8 h (Schäfer-Korting *et al.*, 1986; Humbert *et al.*, 1985).

Peritoneal macrophages from NMRI mice treated with cefodizime (**211**) or a variety of its esters prior to harvesting of the cells contained increased levels of lysosomal enzymes and developed enhanced chemoluminescent reaction to stimuli (Limbert *et al.*, 1984b). The clinical relevance of these experimental findings is not yet clear, but could be important in patients with impaired immune functions.

5.1.2.9 YM-13115. YM-13115 (**264**) (Edmiston *et al.*, 1985; Nagano *et al.*, 1987) has better *in vitro* activity against *Pseudomonas* spp. than ceftazidime (**266**). Its pharmacokinetic properties in different animals have been tested and seem to be comparable to ceftriaxone (**210**) and ceftazidime (**266**). YM-13115 (**264**) displays a longer serum half-life in rats than the latter agents.

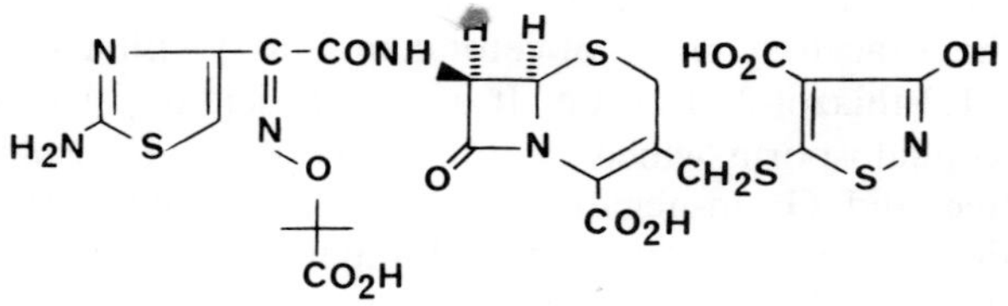

264

5.2.1.10 Ceftiofur. Ceftiofur (U-64279 E) (**212**) (Truesdell *et al.*, 1986; Yancey *et al.*, 1986a,b) displays good *in vitro* antibacterial activity and was effective against mice infections due to *E. coli*, *H. pleuropneumoniae*, *H. somnus*, *Ps. haemolytica*, *Ps. multocida*, *Strep. typhimurium* and *Staph. aureus*. Ceftiofur (**212**) is highly β-lactamase resistant. After i.m. administration to dogs, ceftiofur (**212**) is detectable in the serum even after 24 h,

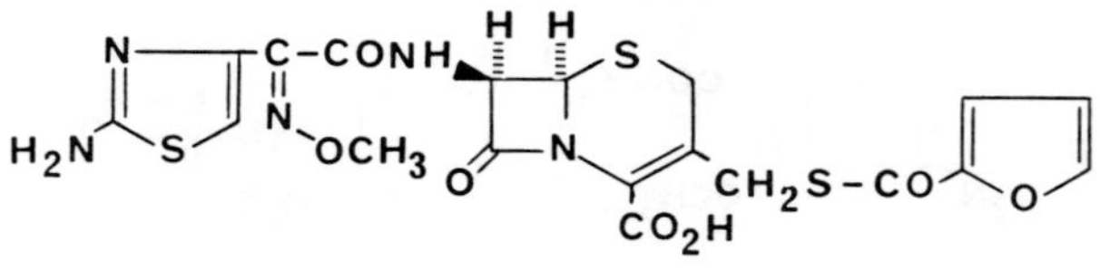

212

indicating a long plasma half-life. It is currently developed for the therapy of serious bacterial infections in domestic animals including bovine and porcine respiratory disease, bovine and swine enteritis and bovine mastitis.

5.1.2.11 Cefotiam. Cefotiam (SCE-963) (**265**), an aminothiazole cephalosporin, was introduced into the market in 1981. It exhibits improved antibacterial properties against Gram-negative pathogens compared to older second generation cephalosporins and is very effective against Streptococci, Staphylococci, Gonococci, Meningococci and *H. influenzae*, but shows no or little activity against *Pseudomonas* spp., Enterococci, and *B. fragilis*. The elimination half-life is dose-dependent, leads to an over-proportional increase of the AUC values, and varies from 0.9–1.6 h in a dosage range from 0.5–2.0 g (Walther and Meyer, 1987, and references cited therein). The CSF levels reach 1–3% of serum concentrations. High biliary

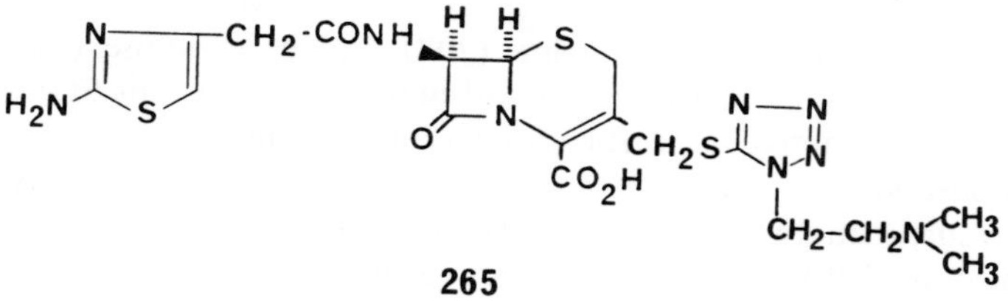

265

levels have been obtained. Cefotiam (**265**) is 40% protein-bound. After i.v. application, about 70% cephalosporin is recovered unchanged in urine. Cefotiam (**265**) is metabolized to about 20%. Clinical experience with cefotiam (**265**) has been summarized by Rouan *et al.* (1985). The local and systemic tolerability is excellent.

5.1.2.12 Ceftiolene. Ceftiolene (RP-42 980) (**213**) (*Drugs of the Future*, 1984d), a 3'-thiovinylcephalosporin, was first presented in 1981. It was claimed to exhibit an antibacterial spectrum similar to those of cefotaxime (**207**) and ceftriaxone (**210**). Ceftiolene (**213**) is poorly active against *Staph.*

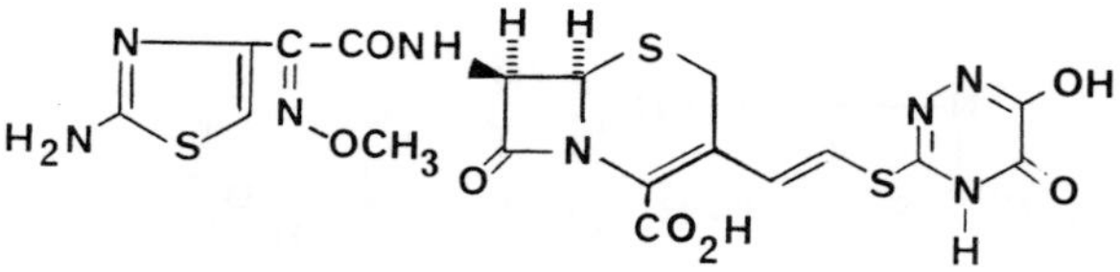

213

aureus, especially against methicillin-resistant strains. The affinities of ceftiolene (**213**) for the PBPs of *E. coli* are comparable to those of ceftriaxone (**210**) and cefotaxime (**207**) (Williamson *et al.*, 1984). Ceftiolene (**213**) is very effective in mice infections produced by a number of pathogens including *Ps. aeruginosa*, as well as in experimental pneumoccocal meningitis.

    5.1.2.13 Cefpirome. Cefpirome (HR-810) (**220**) (*Drugs of the Future*, 1984b, 1985c, 1986a) has been classified as a fourth generation cephalosporin (Neu *et al.*, 1985a) due to its extremely broad spectrum of activity including all relevant Gram-positive and Gram-negative bacteria (Bauernfeind, 1983; Seibert *et al.*, 1983a,b; Wise *et al.*, 1985) and because it retains all the desired antibacterial and pharmacokinetic properties of third generation aminothiazole cephalosporins (Neu *et al.*, 1985a). Table 29 compares the *in vitro* activity of cefpirome (**220**) with the structurally related cephalosporins DN-9550 (**270**), cefepime (**221**) and cefotaxime (**207**). Cefpirome (**220**) is more active than both cefotaxime (**207**) and ceftazidime (**266**) against Gram-positive Cocci, Enterococci and methicillin-resistant Staphylococci. It is almost as active as ceftazidime (**266**) against *Ps. aeruginosa*. The β-lactamase stability of cefpirome (**220**) is very high, the affinity to β-lactamases surprisingly low (Kobayashi *et al.*, 1986). The high *in vitro* activity of cefpirome (**220**) is reflected in excellent *in vivo* activity. In experimental animal infections triggered by *Staph. aureus*, Enterococci and Enterobacteriaceae it was more active than ceftazidime (**266**), cefotaxime (**207**), ceftriaxone (**210**), cefoperazone (**244**), and latamoxef (**273**) (Klesel *et al.*, 1984a). Cefpirome (**220**) was highly effective in experimental mice pneumoniae (Klesel *et al.*, 1986). Excellent penetration into CSF in rabbits with experimental pneumococcal meningitis have been reported (Klesel *et al.*, 1986). The serum half-life in primates exceeds one hour.

    Results of clinical phase I studies have been summarized by Maaß *et al.* (1987a,b), Malerczyk *et al.* (1987) and Verho *et al.* (1987). In healthy volunteers, cefpirome (**220**) has an elimination half-life of 1.9–2.1 h. Urinary recovery is 87% (in 48 h). Clinically relevant urine concentrations are detected for at least 12 h after administration. No metabolites have been detected. Cefpirome (**220**) shows good renal tolerance.

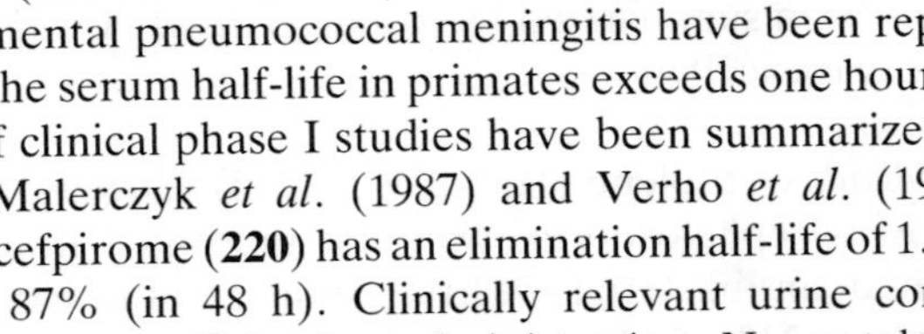

220

TABLE 29

Relative inhibitory antibacterial activities of 3'-quaternary ammonio cephalosporins in comparison with cefotaxime (Dürckheimer et al., 1986)

	Cefpirome 220		DN 9550 270		Cefepime 221		Cefotaxime 207	
	50%	90%	50%	90%	50%	90%	50%	90%
Staph. spp.	++++	++++	+++	++	++	++	+++	+
Staph. spp. (Methicillin resistant)	++	0	0	0	0	0	+	0
Strep. spp. (Serogroup A, B, C)	++++	++	++++	++++	++++	++++	++++	++
Enterococci	++	++	+	0	0	0	++	0
E. coli	++++	++++	++++	+++	++++	+++	++++	+++
Citrobacter spp.	++++	+++	+++	+	+++	+++	++++	+++
Serratia spp.	++++	+++	+++	++	+++	+++	++++	+++
Salmonella spp.	++++	++++	N.D.	N.D.	++++	+++	++++	+++
Klebsiella spp.	++++	+++	++++	+++	++++	+++	++++	++++
Enterobacter spp.	++++	+++	+++	+	+++	+++	+++	++++
Acinetobacter spp.	++++	+++	N.D.	N.D.	++	++	+	0
Ps. aeruginosa	++	++	++	+	++++	+++	+++	++
Prot. mirabilis	++++	+++	+++	+++	++++	+++	++++	+
Prot. indol. pos.	++++	++	+++	++	++++	+++	++++	++++
Bact. fragilis	+	0	0	0	+	0	+	0

++++ ≤ 0.1 µg/ml; +++ ≤ 1.0 µg/ml; ++ 1–8 µg/ml; + 8–32 µg/ml; 0 ≥ 32 µg/ml; N.D., not determined.

5.1.2.14 Ceftazidime. Ceftazidime (**266**) is a third generation cephalo-sporin marketed since 1983. The antibacterial, pharmacological and therapeutic properties of ceftazidime (**266**) have been reviewed by Richards and Brogden (1985). Special issues of *Chemotherapy (Tokyo)* (1981b), *J. Antimicrob. Chemother.* (1981, 1983b), and *Infection* (1987) were dedicated to reports on ceftazidime (**266**). It displays particular activity against *Pseudomonas aeruginosa*, being at least 15 times more active than latamoxef (**273**) or cefotaxime (**207**), but equivalent to cefsulodin (**254**). It is also

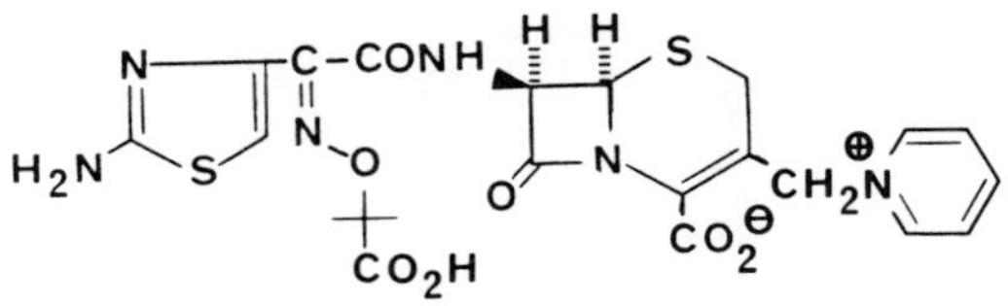

266

active against strains resistant to gentamicin or other aminoglycosides. Ceftazidime (**266**) is highly active against indole-positive *Proteus* spp., whereas the activity against many Enterobacteriaceae is lower than that of cefotaxime (**207**) and latamoxef (**273**). Ceftazidime (**266**) has lower activity against *Staph. aureus* than other third generation cephalosporins and is inactive against *Strep. faecalis* and *B. fragilis*. A high affinity for PBP 3 is found in *Ps. aeruginosa* and *E. coli* (Hayes and Orr, 1983). The half-life of ceftazidime (**266**) in man is about 1.8 h; it is prolonged in patients with renal insufficiency. Ceftazidime (**266**) is eliminated by glomular filtration without tubular secretion. About 80–90% of the drug are excreted in the urine in the first 24 h. No metabolites can be detected. Ceftazidime (**266**) penetrates into CSF in therapeutic concentrations when the meninges are inflamed.

5.1.2.15 Cefepime. Cefepime (BMY-28 142) (**221**) (*Drugs of the Future*, 1985d, 1986k) has been known since 1983 and is undergoing extended biological evaluation. Its *in vitro* antibacterial spectrum was evaluated in comparison with other new cephalosporins (Clarke *et al.*, 1985; Fuchs *et al.*,

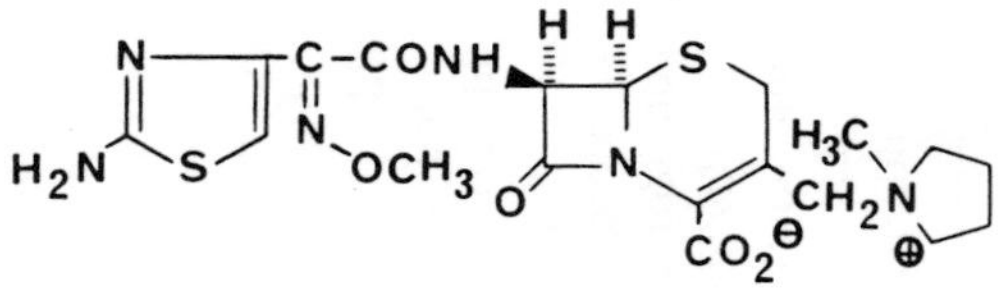

221

1985; Tsuji *et al.*, 1985a,b; Vuye and Pijck, 1985; Bodey *et al.*, 1985; Steele *et al.*, 1985; Tomatsu *et al.*, 1986; Neu *et al.*, 1986b; Naito *et al.*, 1986a). Cefepime (**221**) is in its MICs similar to cefpirome (**220**) for many strains, including *Pseudomonas* spp. (Kessler *et al.*, 1985), whereas its activity against Staphylococci is lower (Norden and Neiderriter, 1987). *Serratia* spp., *Enterobacter* spp., *Klebsiella* spp. and *E. coli* are sensitive, whereas *B. fragilis* and *Strep. faecalis* are resistant. The half-life of cefepime (**221**) in cynomolgus monkeys approximates 1.7 h; more than 90% of the dose is recovered in urine. In mice infections, cefepime (**221**) was as effective as ceftazidime (**266**) against *Ps. aeruginosa* and effective as cefotaxime (**207**) against *Staph. aureus* (Kessler *et al.*, 1985). The urinary recovery in mice is 73%. Cefepime (**221**) binds to human serum proteins to approximately 19%.

5.1.2.16 SG-164. SG-164 (**267**), first presented in 1986, has an unique (2-aminothiazol-4-yl)-2-chloromethylen-acetamido side chain. *In vitro* data reveal a high activity against *Staph. aureus*, in particular against methicillin-resistant *Staph. aureus* and coagulase-negative Staphylococci. The activity of SG-164 (**267**) against Enterobacteriaceae is comparable to that of other

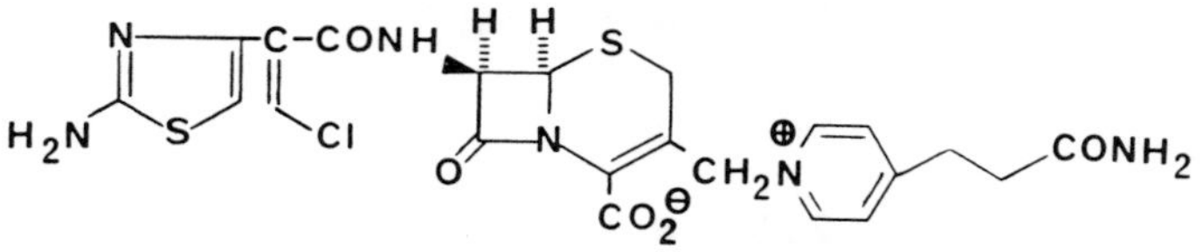

267

third generation cephalosporins. A superior protective effect in MRS infections in mice compared to cefuzonam (**216**) and flomoxef (**260**) has been found (Tunemoto *et al.*, 1986).

5.1.2.17 OCS-575. OCS-575 (**268**) is the most active compound out of a series of 3'-imidazolium-substituted cephalosporins, first presented in 1986.

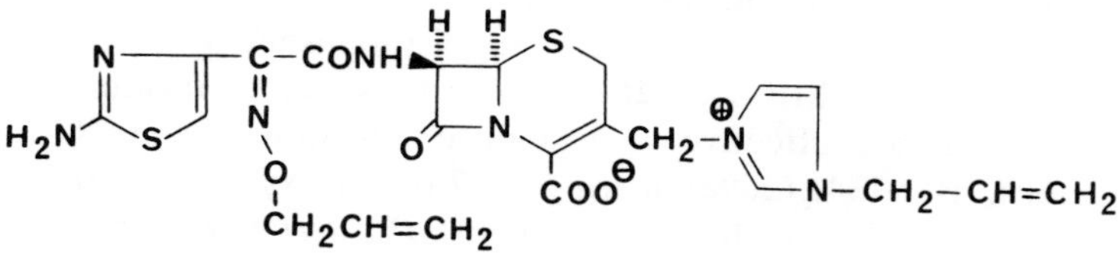

268

OCS-575 (**268**) has a balanced broad antimicrobial activity against Gram-positive and Gram-negative bacteria both *in vitro* and *in vivo*. In mice, OCS-575 (**268**) displays similar pharmacokinetic properties to ceftazidime (**266**). High urinary excretion is observed in rats (Akagi *et al.*, 1986; Suzuki *et al.*, 1986). Its binding to human serum is low.

5.1.2.18 DQ-2522 and DQ-2556. DQ-2522 (**222**) and DQ-2556 (**223**) (Tagawa *et al.*, 1985; Fujimoto *et al.*, 1986; Ejima *et al.*, 1987) are further examples of C-3′ substituted pyridinocephalosporins in preclinical evaluation. Both compounds display similar *in vitro* antibacterial properties. The

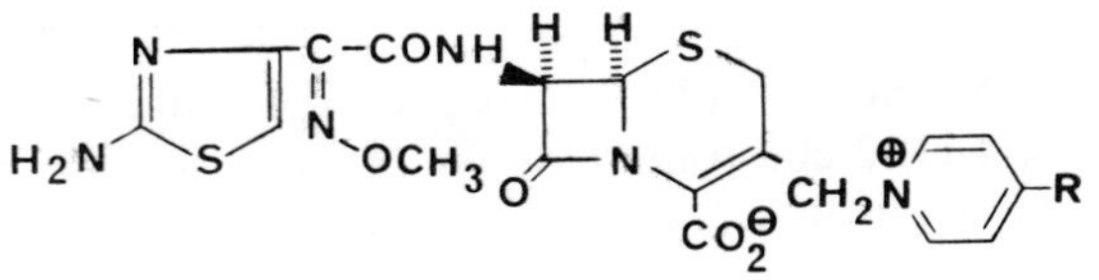

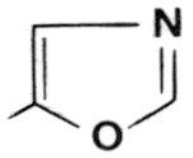

activity of DQ-2556 (**223**) is roughly comparable to that of cefotaxime (**207**) against Enterobacteriaceae. Against *Ps. aeruginosa*, DQ-2556 (**223**) is slightly less active than cefotaxime (**266**). It surpasses both cefotaxime (**207**) and ceftazidime (**266**) in its activity against Staphylococci. *H. influenzae* and *N. gonorrhoeae* are also highly susceptible to DQ-2556 (**223**).

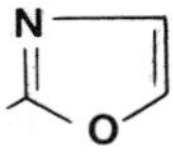

5.1.2.19 BO-1232, BO-1236 and BO-1341. BO-1232 (**269a**) and BO-1236 (**269b**) (Nakagawa *et al.*, 1985, 1987; Sanada *et al.*, 1985), substituted at C-3′ by N-methylisoindolium moieties, are distinguished by good activity against *Ps. aeruginosa*. MICs of **269** exceed those of ceftazidime (**266**). Both compounds are effective against mice infections due to Gram-negative bacteria. BO-1341 (**269c**) bearing a 6,7-dihydroxyisoquinolinium moiety at C-3′ also exhibits high activity against *Ps. aeruginosa*, but weak activity against *Staph. aureus* (Nakagawa *et al.*, 1987).

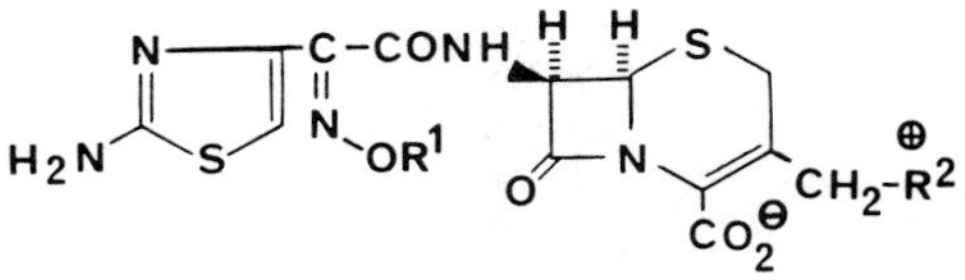

269 a R^1 = $-C_2H_5$ R^2 =

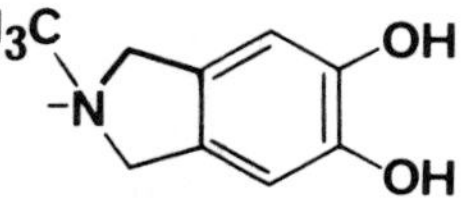

269 b R^1 = $-C(CH_3)_2CO_2H$ R^2 =

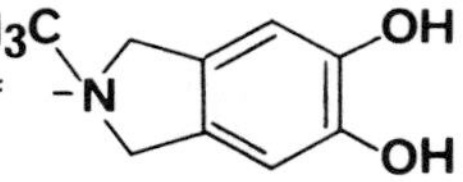

269 c R^1 = $-CH_3$ R^2 =

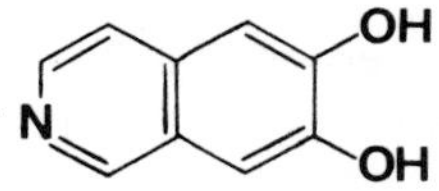

5.1.2.20 DN-9550. DN-9550 (**270**) was presented in 1984 (Une *et al.*, 1984). It seems to be comparable to ceftazidime (**266**) and better than cefoperazone (**244**) in Gram-negative infections. Against Enterobacteriaceae, the activity of DN-9550 (**270**) is slightly less than that of cefotaxime (**207**) (Une *et al.*, 1985).

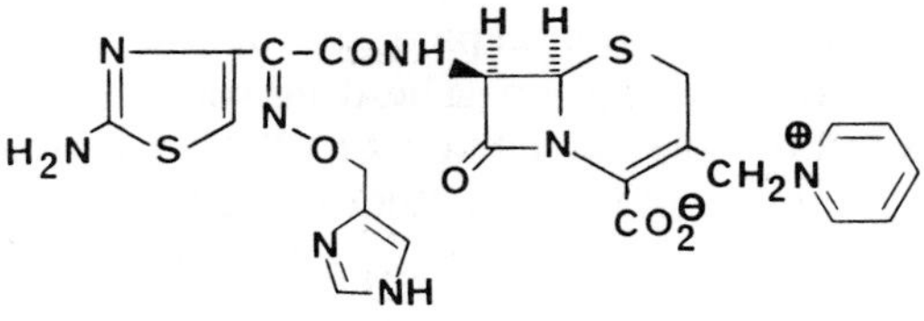

270

5.1.2.21 CM-40874 and CM-40876. CM-40874 (**271a**) (*Drugs of the Future*, 1985b), a 1-(S)-sulphoxide cephalosporin, is currently in clinical trials in France. The antibacterial spectrum to Gram-negative bacteria is

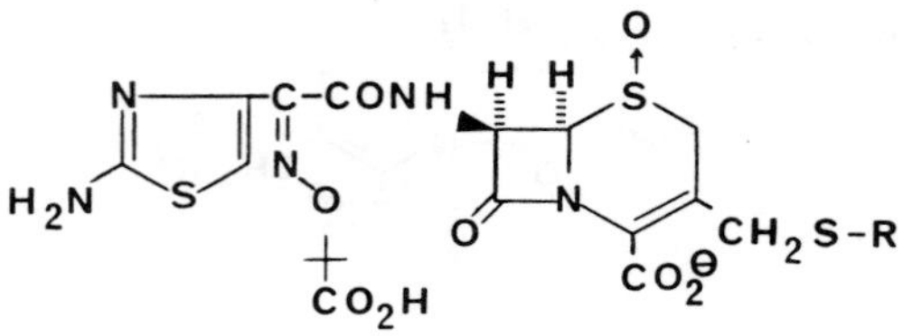

271 a   R =

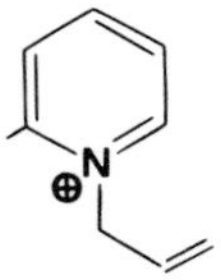

271 b   R =

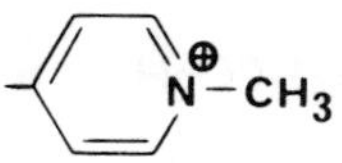

similar to that of ceftazidime (**266**). CM-40874 (**271a**) displays high activity against Streptococci, *S. pneumoniae*, Enterobacteriaceae, *Haemophilus* spp., *Neisseria* spp. and *Pseudomonas* spp. It lacks activity against Staphylococci, *Acinetobacter* spp. and anaerobes. The stability to β-lactamases is very high; the affinity to these enzymes low. Data on the *in vivo* activity are rare. CM-40876 (**217b**) (Salhi *et al.*, 1986; Jarlier *et al.*, 1986; Drigues *et al.*, 1986; Habibi *et al.*, 1986), is a possible successor to CM-40874 (**271a**) and differs by another C-3′ substituent. The antibacterial spectrum is similar to that of CM-40874 (**271a**).

5.1.2.22 CGP-31523 A. CGP-31523 A (**272**) (Wise *et al.*, 1984; Neu *et al.*, 1985b; Tosch *et al.*, 1985b; Zak *et al.*, 1985a; Chin and Neu, 1986) differs from most other third generation cephalosporins by replacement of the oxime group by a formamido group. The drug shows good antistaphylococcal activity exceeding that of latamoxef (**273**) 8–16 fold. Its activity against *B. fragilis* is inferior to that of latamoxef (**273**) or cefoxitin (**104**). It is stable to a wide range of β-lactamases. CGP-31523 A (**272**) is more

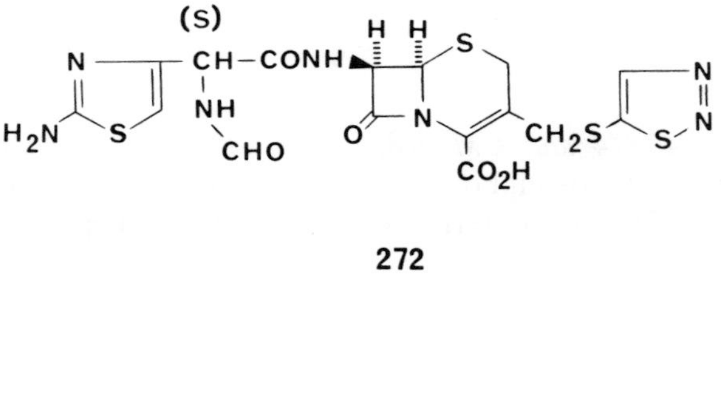

272

effective than cefmenoxime (**208**) against mice infections due to *K. pneumoniae* and *S. pneumoniae*.

5.1.3 N-Acylated Phenylglycine Cephalosporins

5.1.3.1 Cefoperazone. Cefoperazone (T-1551) (**244**) is characterized by an ureido side chain and structurally related to piperacillin. It reached the market in 1981. Antibacterial, pharmacological and therapeutic properties have been extensively reviewed (Brogden *et al.*, 1981; for further references see *Drugs*, 1981 and *Münchener Medizinische Wochenschrift*, 1981). Cefoperazone (**244**) exhibits broad spectrum activity. Its activity against *Pseudomonas* spp. is between that of cefotaxime (**207**) and ceftazidime (**266**). The activity against TEM-β-lactamase-forming *E. coli* is lower than that of other third generation cephalosporins. Cefoperazone (**244**) is about

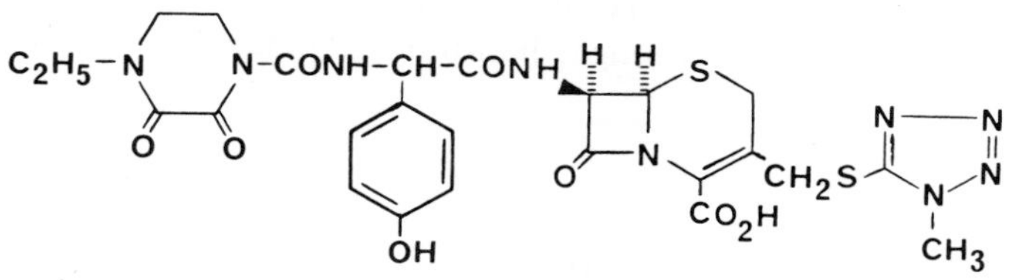

244

90% protein-bound. It is eliminated via bile and kidneys. The serum elimination half-life in adults varies between 1.5 and 2.5 h, in children (up to 2 years) between 1.6 and 5.8 h and 1.3 and 3.0 h (6–16 years) (Walther and Meyer, 1987, ref. cited). Its urinary recovery is between 20 and 25%. In patients with reduced liver function, the half-life is prolonged, the extra-renal clearance reduced and the urinary recovery increased. Bleedings and disulfiram adverse reactions have been observed as with other 3′-1-methyl-tetrazol-5-yl-thio-substituted cephalosporins. Cefoperazone (**244**) combined with the β-lactamase inhibitor sulbactam is developed as sulperazone. This combination showed synergistic antimicrobial activity against several organisms [*Chemotherapy (Tokyo)*, 1984a].

5.1.3.2 Cefpiramide. Cefpiramide (**245**) (Okada *et al.*, 1981) was launched in 1985 in Japan. The clinical efficacy, *in vitro* antibacterial activity and pharmacokinetic properties of cefpiramide have recently been reviewed (Fujimori, 1985). A special issue has been dedicated to clinical experiences

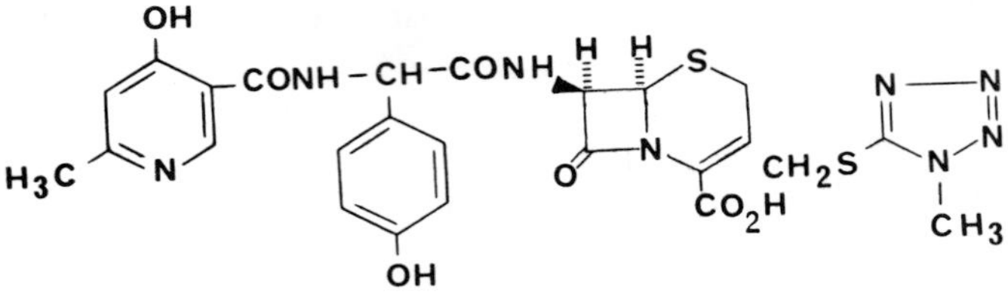

245

with this drug [*Chemotherapy (Tokyo)*, 1983]. It has a half-life of 4.1–5.3 h and UR of 20%.

5.1.3.3 Cefpimizole. The *in vitro* activity of cefpimizole (AC-1370) (**248**) (*Drugs of the Future*, 1984c), which was launched in 1987 in Japan, is similar or inferior to that of cefoperazone (**244**). Against experimental *Pseudomonas* infections in animals it is superior to cefoperazone (**244**), due to higher blood levels and a longer half-life. Cefpimizole (**248**) is mainly

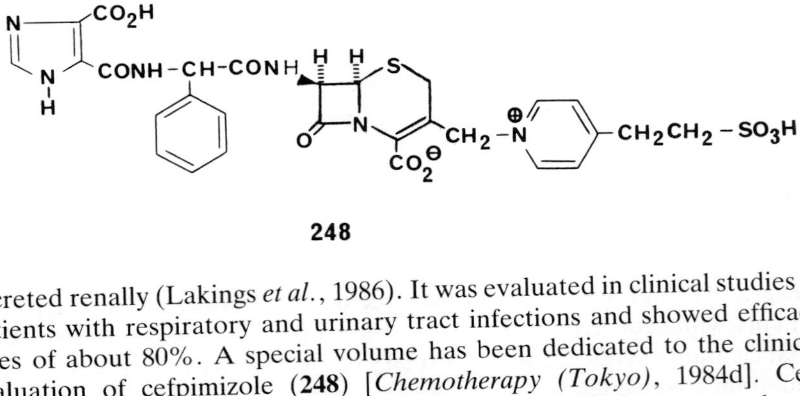

248

excreted renally (Lakings *et al.*, 1986). It was evaluated in clinical studies in patients with respiratory and urinary tract infections and showed efficacy rates of about 80%. A special volume has been dedicated to the clinical evaluation of cefpimizole (**248**) [*Chemotherapy (Tokyo)*, 1984d]. Cefpimizole (**248**) enhances phagocyte function by binding to macrophages (Ohnishi, 1984). Cefpimizole bound macrophages release certain soluble factors which act more potently on neutrophils than the factors released from the resident macrophages.

5.1.3.4 E-0702. E-0702 (**247**) shows high activity against Gram-negative bacteria, especially against *Ps. aeruginosa* [20–110 fold more active than cefoperazone (**244**) or cefotaxime (**207**)] but is less active against *Staph. aureus*. It has remarkable activity against *B. fragilis* [4-fold greater activity

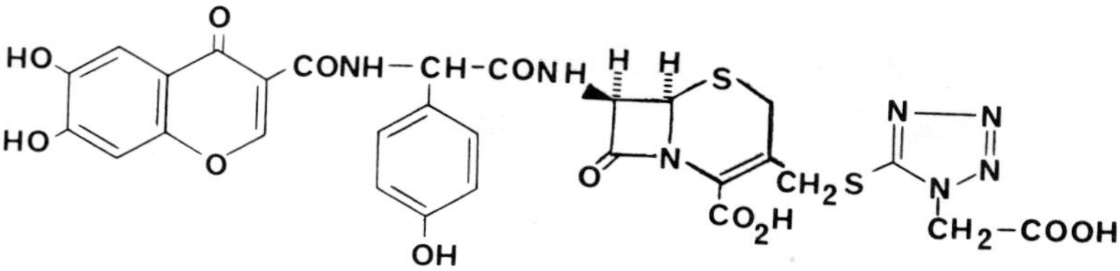

247

than cefoxitin (**104**)] and against many *Acinetobacter* strains (*Drugs of the Future*, 1983a, 1984a).

5.1.3.5 KIT-180. The spectrum of activity of KIT-180 (KI-6269) (**246**) is comparable to that of cefoperazone (**244**), but it possesses faster bactericidal action against *E. coli*, *P. vulgaris* and *Ps. aeruginosa* (**246**) (Takada *et al.*, 1983).

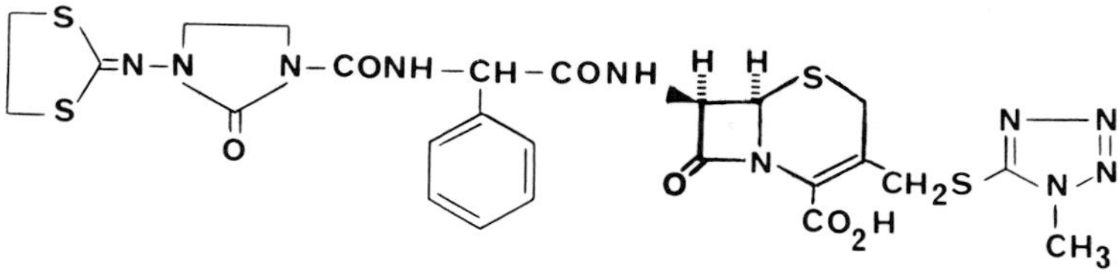

246

5.1.4 Cephalosporins with Different Side Chains at C-7

Cefsulodin. Cefsulodin (SCE-129) (**254**), launched in 1980, was the first narrow spectrum cephalosporin. The drug is markedly active against *Ps. aeruginosa*, being as effective as gentamicin, but has low activity against other Gram-negative strains. The kinetic properties are favourable and enable high serum levels after i.v. or i.m. application. The protein binding is low (about 30%). The serum elimination half-life is 1.5 h, but is prolonged up to several hours in case of disturbed kidney function. The urinary

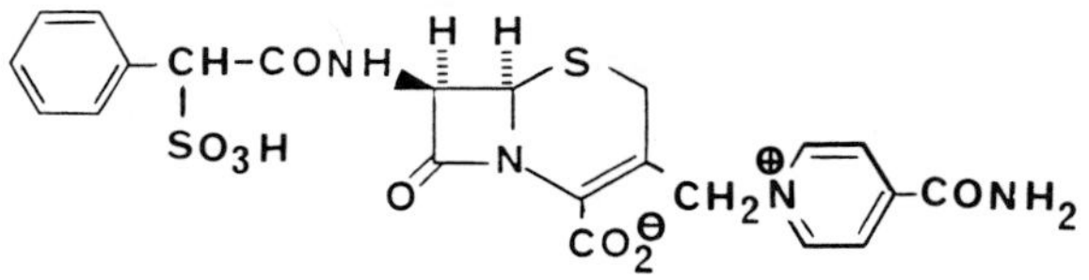

254

recovery rate is high, normally ranging from 60–90%. The antibacterial, pharmacological and clinical properties of cefsulodin (**254**) have been reviewed by Wright (1986).

5.1.5 7α-Substituted Cephalosporins

5.1.5.1 Cefotetan. Cefotetan (YM-09330) (**105**), launched in 1985, is a cephamycin derivative with a unique dithietane side chain. Its antibacterial, pharmacological and therapeutic properties have been reviewed [Ward and Richards, 1985; special issues: *Chemotherapy (Tokyo)*, 1982a; *J. Antimicrob. Chemother.*, 1983a]. Cefotetan (**105**) is less active than cefoxitin (**104**)

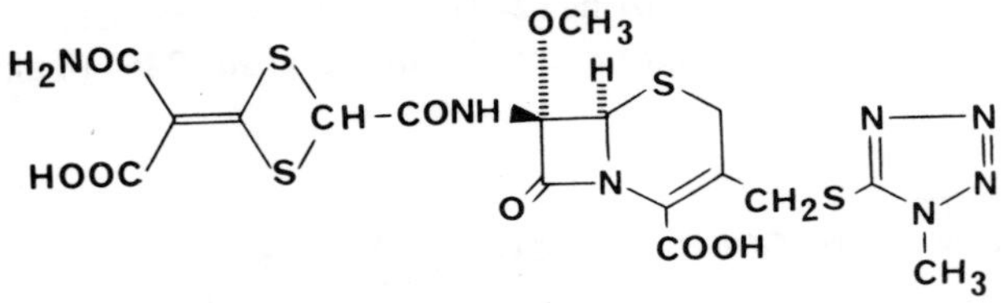

105

against Gram-positive bacteria, but more active against Gram-negative bacteria, e.g. Enterobacteriaceae, *Serratia* spp. and *Proteus* spp. Like other 7α-methoxycephalosporins it is highly β-lactamase resistant and active against β-lactamase forming anaerobes, e.g. *B. fragilis*. Cefotetan (**105**) is inactive against *Pseudomonas* spp. An advantage of cefotetan is its long half-life of 3–4.6 h. It is 88% plasma protein-bound.

5.1.5.2 Cefbuperazone. Cefbuperazone (**106**) [*Drugs of the Future*, 1985a; special issue: *Chemotherapy (Tokyo)*, 1982b], launched in 1985, has

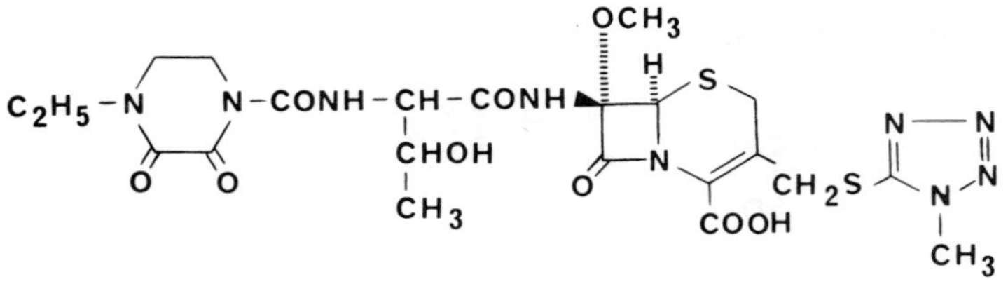

106

a broad spectrum of activity including aerobic, Gram-negative and anaerobic bacteria. It is highly stable to various β-lactamases. The activity against Enterobacteriaceae is higher than that of cefmetazole, cefoxitin (104), cefazolin or cefoperazone (244). After i.v. administration the serum half-life approximates 100 min. The clinical efficacy in respiratory tract, urinary tract and gynaecological infections has been documented (*Drugs of the Future*, 1985a).

5.1.5.3 Cefminox. Cefminox (MT-141) (107), just launched in Japan [special issue: *Chemotherapy (Tokyo)*, 1984b], appears to be effective in the treatment of surgical and urinary tract infections, in particular those involving *B. fragilis*. The overall activity is similar to that of cefotetan (105) and cefbuperazone (106), but slightly or markedly superior to that of cefoxitin (107) or cefmetazole. It lacks activity against *Pseudomonas* spp. Cefminox (107) has a serum half-life of about 2 h, while its urinary recovery rate is in the range of 88% within 24 h.

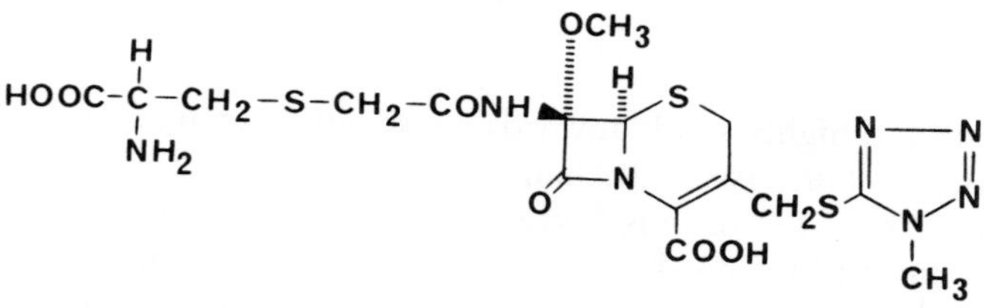

107

5.1.5.4 UG-FA-132. UG-FA-132 (108), presented in 1986, is a cephalosporin with broad spectrum activity including *Pseudomonas* spp. and β-lactamase-producing Gram-negative organisms (Maier *et al.*, 1986).

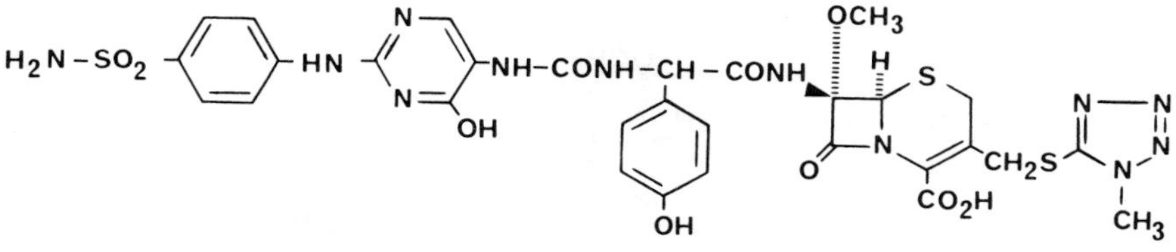

108

5.1.6 1-Oxacephems

5.1.6.1 Latamoxef. Latamoxef (Moxalactam, 6059-S) (**273**), the only oxacephem in clinical practice, was launched in 1982. Antibacterial, pharmacological and therapeutic properties of latamoxef (**273**) have been reviewed (Carmine *et al.*, 1983b). Its spectrum of activity resembles that of cefotaxime (**207**), but latamoxef (**273**) is more active against *B. fragilis*, *E. cloacae* and *C. freundii*, but less active against *Staph. aureus*, *Staph. epidermis* and *S. viridans*. It is also very active against *N. gonorrhoeae* and

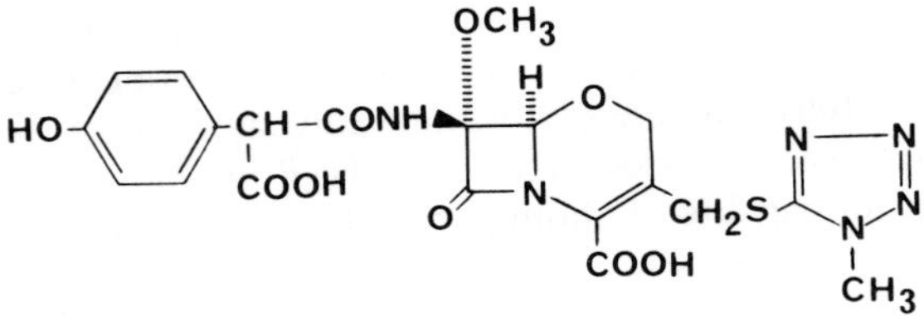

273

H. influenzae and highly stable towards nearly all β-lactamases (Warren *et al.*, 1980; Barry *et al.*, 1980). Its half-life is between 2 and 3 h. After i.v. application, 75% of the drug is excreted unchanged in urine. The protein binding amounts to 43–53%. Latamoxef (**273**) displays a disulfiram-like side effect associated with its 3′-methyltetrazolylthio residue. Acetaldehyde hydrogenase is inhibited, resulting in accumulation of acetaldehyde when ethanol is present. Another adverse reaction connected with the 3′-moiety and limiting the use of latamoxef is the occurrence of bleedings. Therefore, prophylactic administration of vitamin K is recommended.

5.1.6.2 Flomoxef. Flomoxef (6315-S) (**260**) (Goto *et al.*, 1984a; Tsuji *et al.*, 1985a,b; *Drugs of the Future*, 1986e) is currently undergoing clinical trials [special issue: *Chemotherapy (Tokyo)*, 1987]. The *in vitro* antibacterial

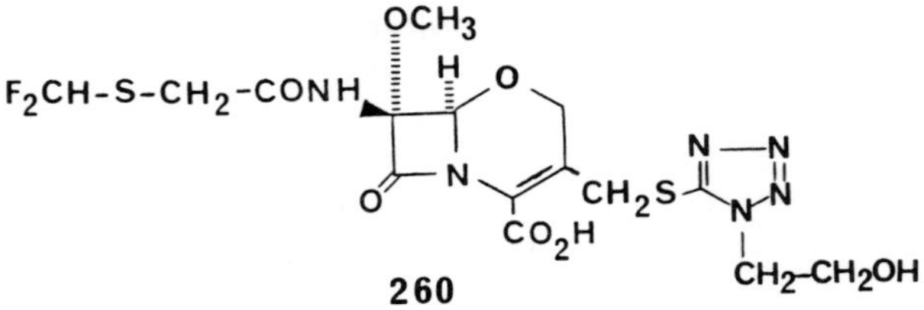

260

spectrum was elucidated in comparison with cefotaxime (**207**), latamoxef (**273**) and cefoperazone (**244**) and other agents (Neu and Chin, 1986). The *in vitro* activity of flomoxef (**260**) against Staphylococci and Streptococci is similar to that of cefazolin, against Enterobacteriaceae to that of latamoxef (**273**). The most remarkable feature of flomoxef (**260**) is its high anti-staphylococcal activity including several clinical isolates of methicillin-resistant Staphylococci. Against anaerobic bacteria, its activity surpasses that of cefotaxime (**207**) and latamoxef (**273**). After i.v. administration, high levels of the drug were assayed in bile and gall bladder, indicating that flomoxef (**260**) may be useful in the treatment of biliary tract infections. The half-life in man is 0.75–1 h after i.v. administration.

5.1.6.3 2355-S. 2355-S (**261**) (Komatsu *et al.*, 1984) is another candidate for further development out of a series of newer oxacephems. It displays similar *in vitro* antibacterial properties to flomoxef (**260**), but superior pharmacokinetic properties.

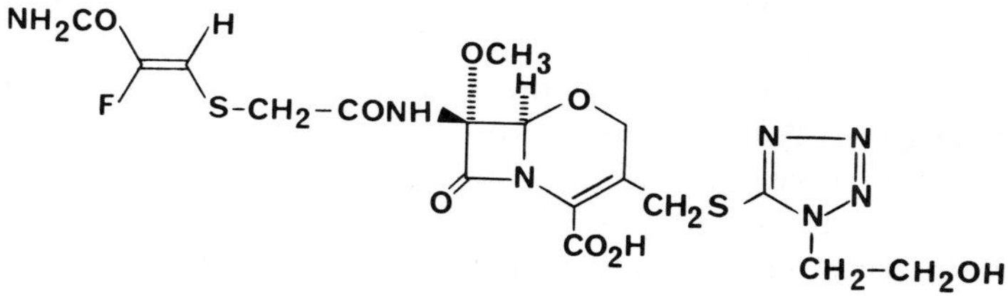

261

5.1.7 1-Carbacephems

Articles on a number of carbacephem derivatives derived from total synthesis have been published in recent years (Mochida *et al.*, 1987). Among them, KT-4380, KT-3767, KT-3937, and KT-4697 display broad spectrum antimicrobial activity *in vitro*. No information about clinical development of these drugs is yet available.

5.1.8 Other Cephalosporins

Other cephalosporin antibiotics which are not reviewed in detail are cefmetazole [for further references see *Chemotherapy (Tokyo)*, 1978b, special issue], cefoxitin [*Chemotherapy (Tokyo)*, 1978a; *J. Antimicrob. Chemother.*, 1978], NY-1675 (Nakayama *et al.*, 1984), ceftezole (Noto *et al.*,

1976), FCE-20 485 (Alpegiani *et al.*, 1983), SKF-80 303 (*Drugs of the Future*, 1980), SKF-88 070 (Grappel *et al.*, 1984), cefonicid (Saltiel and Brogden, 1986), and ceforanide (Karney *et al.*, 1983). The second generation cephalosporins cefonicid, ceforanide, and cefuroxime have been reviewed by Tartaglione and Polk (1985).

5.2 ORAL CEPHALOSPORINS

5.2.1 Introduction

The main objectives in the development of new orally active cephalosporins have been two-fold: firstly, the improvement of older glycylcephalosporins with respect to potency and β-lactamase stability, and secondly the modification of parenteral second and third generation cephalosporins in order to achieve enteral absorption. As a result of these efforts, a new group of oral carboxymethylcephalosporins, structurally derived from aminothiazole cephalosporins, has been found. Progress has also been made to prepare orally active prodrugs of parenteral cephalosporins, especially of cefotaxime analogs. Table 30 shows the structures of cefalexin (**23**), cefixime (**53**) and cefuroxime axetil (**274**) as prototypes for oral cephalosporins. Several drugs of each structural type are currently under extended evaluation or close to introduction into the market.

The main indications for oral cephalosporins are urinary tract, respiratory tract or otorhinolaryngolical infections, with special emphasis in paediatrics. Their therapeutic application for the treatment of severe or life-threatening infections is often not satisfactory, due to widely variable absorption rates depending on the structural type, or to limited antibacterial potency and spectrum. Consequently, a high degree of enteral absorption is desired to reach high serum and tissue levels and to minimize gastrointestinal side effects. Enteral absorption of a drug can be measured by the concentration of the drug in serum and tissues over a period of time and by the urinary recovery. The peak serum level (C_{max}) is a valuable parameter, indicating whether the MICs of the drug against distinct pathogens are reached *in vivo*. The *in vivo* potency of an oral cephalosporin can be assessed by the ratio of curative doses after oral and parenteral application. The urinary recovery rate defines the percentage of a drug which is renally excreted after oral (or parenteral) administration. As far as prodrug esters are concerned, these data are calculated on the basis of the parent compound in animal infection models.

TABLE 30

Oral cephalosporins. One representative example of each group of glycylcephalosporins (cefalexin (**23**)), carboxymethylcephalosporins (cefixime (**53**)) and prodrug cephalosporins (cefuroxime axetil (**274**)) is shown

Glycylcephalosporins

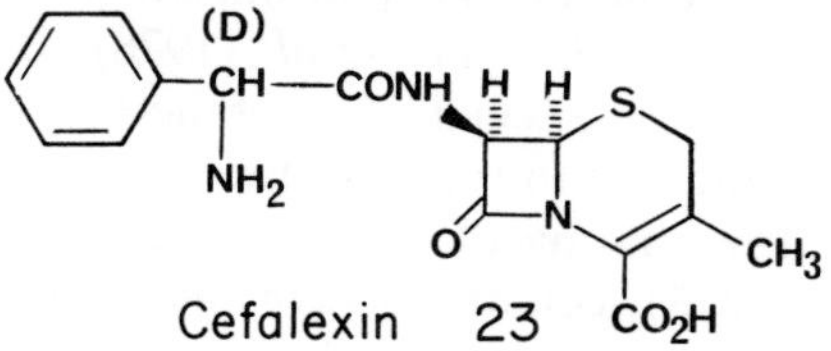

Cefalexin   23

Carboxymethylcephalosporins

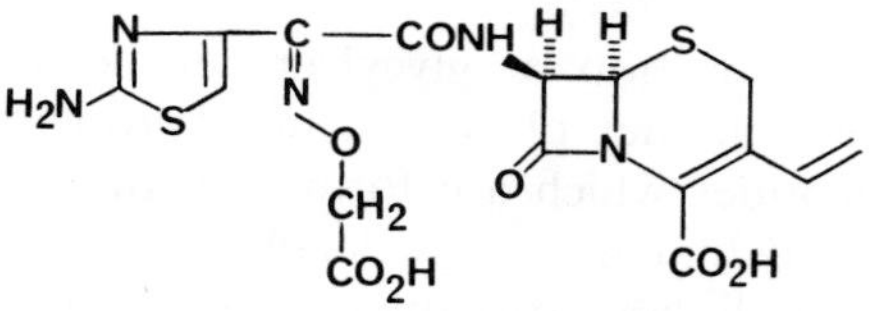

Cefixime   53

Prodrugcephalosporins

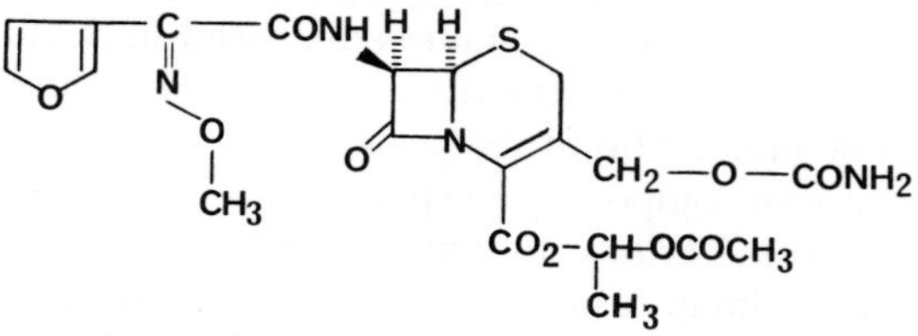

Cefuroxime Axetil   274

5.2.2 Glycylcephalosporins

(D)-Arylglycyl- and (D)-dihydrophenylglycylcephalosporins are a well established group of oral antibiotics with very high enteral absorption. They include structurally similar compounds (Table 31) such as cefalexin (**23**), cefaclor (**275**), cefadroxil (**276**), cefatrizine (**277**), cefradine (**278**) and cefroxadine (**279**), which were all introduced into the market before 1981. Reports on their clinical efficacy and pharmacological and antimicrobial properties were published by Brogard *et al.* (1978), Brogard and Comte (1982), and Riess *et al.* (1982). Special issues of the *Journal of Antimicrobial Chemotherapy* were dedicated to reports on cefalexin **23** (1975) and cefadroxil (**276**) (1982a). The pharmacokinetic properties of cefalexin (**23**) and its congeners cefaclor (**275**), cefadroxil (**276**) and cefroxadine (**279**) have been compared by Lode *et al.* (1979). Compared with second and third generation cephalosporins, glycylcephalosporins are less active against many Gram-negative bacteria and unstable to β-lactamases of these organisms.

The high enteral absorption of glycylcephalosporins is due to their characteristic side chain. In their physicochemical properties, they resemble natural di- and tripeptides which are formed in the intestine from food proteins. It is assumed that most glycylcephalosporins are absorbed by active transport using di- and tripeptide carriers in the intestinal wall (Addison *et al.*, 1975; Kimura *et al.*, 1978; Nakashima *et al.*, 1984a,b; Okano *et al.*, 1986a,b; Sinko and Amidon, 1986). The prototype of glycylcephalosporins, cefalexin (**23**), carries a phenylglycyl side chain known from ampicillin. The synthesis of cefalexin (**23**) is outlined in Section 4.1.3.2, while the chemistry of the glycyl side chain is discussed in Section 4.3.2. Cefalexin (**23**), which was launched as early as 1968, had a worldwide sales volume exceeding one billion DM in 1986.

In the successor compounds the phenyl ring is altered, e.g. by introduction of a *para*-hydroxyl group, by partial hydrogenation or by attachment of aromatic rings. Small residues, especially methyl, are preferred as 3-substituents. Table 32, modified after Riess *et al.* (1982), summarizes important pharmacokinetic data of oral glycylcephalosporins on the market. Cefaclor (**275**), obtained from penicillin by partial synthesis (Section 4.1.3.4), was the first cephem antibiotic with a non-classical substitution pattern at C-3. The advantage of cefaclor (*Drugs of the Future*, 1977a) over cefalexin (**23**) is due to its activity against *H. influenzae*. Drawbacks are the metabolic instability and the lower stability against TEM-β-lactamases compared to cefalexin (**23**). Cefaclor (**275**) has a lower urinary recovery rate than cefalexin (**23**). It

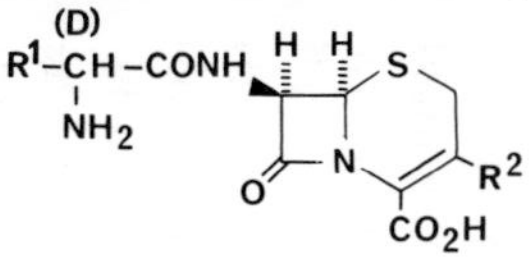

(D)

$$R^1-CH-CONH \quad \text{(cephem nucleus with } R^2, CO_2H)$$
with NH_2

No.	Compound	R^1	R^2
23	Cefalexin	phenyl	$-CH_3$
275	Cefaclor	phenyl	$-Cl$
276	Cefadroxil	HO-phenyl	$-CH_3$
277	Cefatrizine	HO-phenyl	$-CH_2S-$ (triazole, N=N, N-H)
278	Cefradine	cyclohexadienyl	$-CH_3$
279	Cefroxadine	cyclohexadienyl	$-OCH_3$
280	BMY 28100	HO-phenyl	$-CH=CH-CH_3$

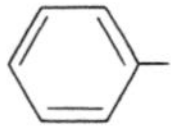

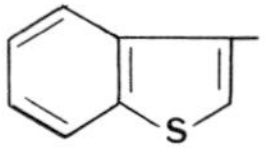

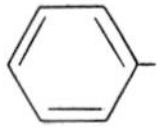

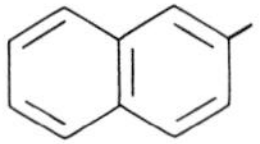

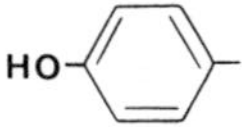

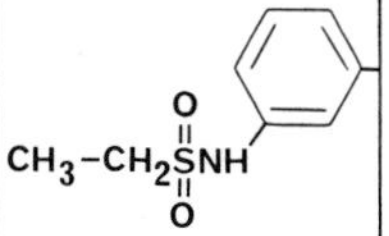

No.	Compound	R^1	R^2
281	LY 164 846	benzothiophene	$-CH_3$
282	LY 171 217	naphthyl	$-CH_3$
283	CGP 19359	phenyl $O=\overset{}{S}=O$ CH_3-CH_2SNH	$-OCH_3$
284	RMI 19592	methylenedioxyphenyl	$-CH_3$
285	Cefedrolor	HO, Cl-phenyl	$-CH_3$
286	Cefsumide	phenyl $CH_3-\overset{O}{\underset{O}{S}}NH$	$-CH_3$
287	SCE 100	cyclohexenyl	$-CH_3$

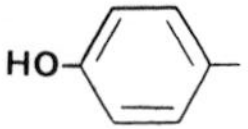

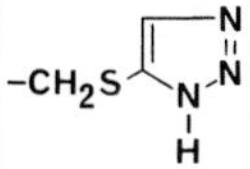

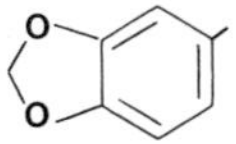

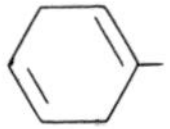

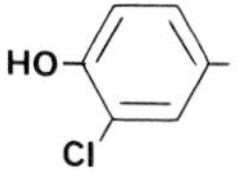

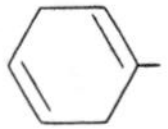

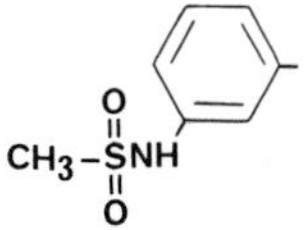

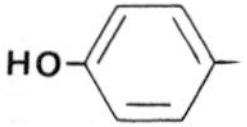

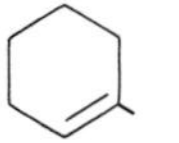

TABLE 32

Pharmacokinetic parameters of oral glycylcephalosporins (modified from Riess et al., 1982)

No.	Compound	AUC^a	Urinary recovery (%)	Half-life (h)	Protein binding
23	Cefalexin	56	88	1.0	15
275	Cefaclor	45	51	0.7	47
276	Cefadroxil	88	79	1.7	17
277	Cefatrizine	39	41	1.5	58
278	Cefradine	56	93	0.7	12
279	Cefroxadine	49	89	0.9	8

AUC^a = AUC referring to a 1 g dose.

is not very stable in solution; but its oral application is not impaired by this fact. A new stable carbacephem analogue of cefaclor, LY-163 892 (KT-3777), was recently presented in several papers (Hirata et al., 1987; Counter et al., 1987; Chin et al., 1987; Sato et al., 1987; Turner et al., 1987; Quay et al., 1987).

Introduction of a para-hydroxyl group in cefalexin (23), as in cefadroxil (276) or cefatrizine (277), leads to a prolonged half-life. The activity of cefadroxil (276) against S. pyogenes is improved and the half-life is nearly doubled (1.7 h). Cefatrizine (277) is the only glycylcephalosporin with a 1,2,3-triazolylthiomethyl group at C-3. In man it is absorbed to a lower extent than cefalexin (23), with an urinary recovery rate of about 41%.

Cefradine (278), formally derived from cefalexin (23) by partial hydrogenation of the aromatic phenyl ring, is comparable to cefalexin (23) in its pharmacokinetic and antibacterial properties. Cefroxadine (CGP-9000) (279) (Drugs of the Future, 1977b), synthesized from penicillin V as outlined in Section 4.1.3.4, exhibits a more favourable pharmacokinetic profile among glycylcephalosporins. Its urinary recovery rate is 89%. The in vitro antibacterial spectrum of cefroxadine (279) is similar to that of cefaclor (275); the MICs against E. coli and Klebsiella spp. are better than those of cefalexin (23), but the β-lactamase stability is somewhat lower. The in vivo activity of cefroxadine (279) is between two and seven times higher than that of cefalexin (23) and cefaclor (275). CGP-19 359 (283) (Zak et al., 1985b; Tosch et al., 1985c), another 3-methoxy derivative, and cefsumide (FR-10 612) (286) (Nishida et al., 1976), have an alkylsulphonylamido group attached to the phenyl ring of the side chain. They possess prolonged kinetics due to retarded absorption. The serum elimination half-life of

CGP-19 359 (**283**) is 4.5 h, the urinary recovery ranges between 67 and 84%. Cefsumide (**286**) has an urinary recovery rate of 89%.

Cefedrolor (BMY-25 154) (**285**) (Leitner *et al*., 1983), a cefadroxil analogue with an additional chlorine atom at the hydroxyphenyl ring, has a favourable activity against Streptococci but decreased potency against Gram-negative bacteria. Other glycylcephalosporins mentioned in the literature are RMI-19 592 (**284**) (*Drugs of the Future*, 1981a) and SCE-100 (**287**) (Yamazaki *et al*., 1976a,b,c). Few new glycylcephalosporins have emerged in recent years. LY-164 846 (**281**) and LY-171 217 (**282**) (Kukolja *et al*., 1985a,b,c) possess benzothienyl and naphthyl residues in the 7-side chain, respectively. Against anaerobic bacteria like *B. fragilis*, LY-164 846 (**281**) (*Drugs of the Future*, 1986f) exhibits good activity and its antibacterial profile resembles that of cefaclor (**275**). The spectrum includes Staphylococci, with the exception of methicillin-resistant strains, Streptococci with the exception of Enterococci, *H. influenzae*, *B. catarrhalis* and some anaerobic strains. LY-164 846 (**281**) lacks activity against Enterobacteriaceae, *Pseudomonas* spp., *Acinetobacter* spp. and *B. fragilis* (Lauderdale *et al*., 1986). It showed favourable pharmacokinetic properties in rats and its oral bioavailability in rhesus monkeys was about 55–60%.

BMY-28 100 (**280**) is a cefadroxil analogue having a (Z)-configurated 3-prop-1-enyl group at C-3. Its preparation is discussed in Section 4.1.3.5. Synthesis and SAR studies of BMY-28 100 (**280**) and related compounds have recently been published (Naito *et al*., 1987). The antibacterial activity of **280** against Gram-positive strains is claimed to exceed that of cefalexin (**23**) and cefaclor (**275**) both *in vitro* and *in vivo* (Chin and Neu, 1987; Eliopoulos *et al*., 1987; Naito *et al*., 1985; Tomatsu *et al*., 1985; Leitner *et al*., 1985, 1987). The activity against Streptococci is enhanced 3- to 5-fold compared with cefaclor (**275**), and 20-fold compared with cefalexin (**23**). Against Staphylococci, BMY-28 100 (**280**) was twice as active as cefaclor (**275**). The MICs against *N. gonorrhoeae* and *B. catarrhalis* or *H. influenzae* are in the range of 4–8 μg/ml. BMY-28 100 (**280**) lacks sufficient activity against *Enterobacter* spp., *Morganella* spp., *Ps. aeruginosa* and *B. fragilis*. After oral administration to mice, bioavailability, peak serum levels and urinary recovery of BMY-28 100 (**280**) are higher than that of cefaclor (**275**) and similar to that of cefalexin (**23**).

5.2.3 Carboxymethylcephalosporins

Cefixime (**53**) is the prototype of carboxymethylcephalosporins which are characterized by an acidic substituent in the 7-amino side chain essential for oral absorption (Table 33). The substituents at C-3 determine the level of absorption (Yamanaka *et al*., 1986). The influence of heterocycles other

TABLE 33

Oral carboxymethylcephalosporins

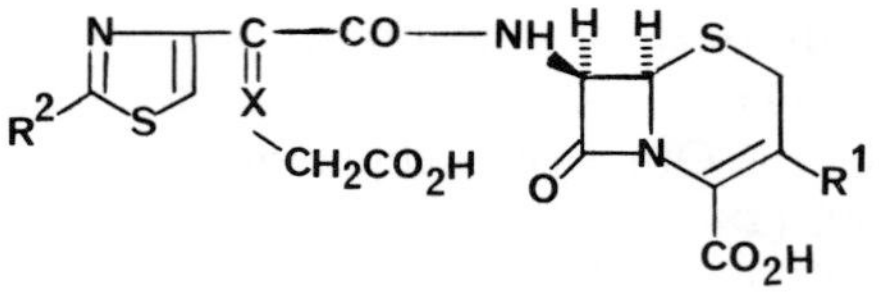

No.	Compound	R^1	R^2	X
53	FK-027, CL-284 635, Cefixime	—CH=CH$_2$	—NH$_2$	=N—O—
288	FK-089	—H	—H	=N—O—
289	7432-S	—H	—NH$_2$	=CH—
290	CGP-33 098 A	—S—(CH$_2$)$_2$NH$_2$	—NH$_2$	=N—O—

than 2-aminothiazolyl in the 7-side chain has also been investigated (Kawabata *et al.*, 1986d). Cefixime (**53**) was launched in Japan in 1987. A special issue was published [*Chemotherapy (Tokyo)*, 1985]. The synthetic routes to **53** are outlined in Section 4.1.3.5. Cefixime (**53**) (*Drugs of the Future*, 1983b, 1984e, 1986h; Yamanaka *et al.*, 1985b) is one of the most active oral cephalosporins against Gram-negative pathogens, including *Enterobacter* spp., *Citrobacter* spp., indol-positive *Proteus* spp. and *Serratia* spp., whereas the activity against Gram-positive bacteria is rather low. Cefixime (**53**) has poor activity against Staphylococci (Kamimura *et al.*, 1984; Brittain *et al.*, 1985), but possesses a high β-lactamase stability. Pharmacokinetic parameters in man were studied by Brittain *et al.* (1985) and Guay *et al.* (1986). The pharmacokinetics in dogs was investigated by Bialer *et al.* (1987). After oral administration, about 20% of the drug is excreted in urine; an equal amount is excreted via the bile. The absorption shows no proportional increase at higher dosage. Due to its high protein binding and tubular reabsorption, cefixime (**53**) has a long half-life of 3.1 h. The incidence of side effects is small; mostly gastrointestinal disorders, bitter taste, heartburn or an occasional rise of serum transaminases are observed. Cefixime (**53**) is absorbed by carrier-mediated active transport processes (Tonelli *et al.*, 1986; Tsuji, 1986; Okano *et al.*, 1987; Tamai *et al.*, 1987; Tsuji *et al.*, 1987a,b,c). *Anti*-cefixime, an isomer possessing an (E)-configurated oxime group, has reduced antimicrobial potency but is highly absorbed (Kawabata *et al.*, 1986a).

FK-089 (**288**) (*Drugs of the Future*, 1986a), a successor compound of cefixime (**53**), lacks both the thiazole amino and the vinyl group. The substitution pattern of the cephem nucleus is similar to ceftizoxime (**209**) (for the synthesis see Section 4.1.3.4). FK-089 (**288**) exhibits a higher *in vitro* activity against Gram-negative bacteria than either cefaclor (**275**) or cefalexin (**23**) (Takaya *et al.*, 1985a). It is stable against plasmid or chromosomally coded β-lactamases. The *in vivo* potency against Gram-negative infections is higher than that of either cefalexin (**23**) or cefaclor (**275**). The absorption mechanism of FK-089 (**288**) corresponds to that of cefixime (**53**) (Tsuji *et al.*, 1987c).

7432-S (**289**) (Nakashima *et al.*, 1986b) is structurally related to cefixime (**53**) and FK-089 (**288**). Synthetic routes to 7432-S (**289**) have recently been published (Yoshioka, 1987). **289** resembles cefixime (**53**) and FK-089 (**288**) in its antibacterial spectrum. Compared with cefaclor (**275**), 7432-S (**289**) is as active against *S. pyogenes* and *S. pneumoniae*, but inactive against Staphylococci and Enterococci. Enterobacteriaceae are extremely susceptible to 7432-S (**289**). The activity against *E. coli*, *Klebsiella* spp., *H. influenzae* and *Neisseria* spp. is also high. The enteral absorption is in the range of 67–75% in healthy volunteers. It is mainly excreted renally. Similarly to cefixime (**53**) and FK-089 (**288**), 7432-S (**289**) is absorbed in the small intestine by the dipeptide transport system (Muranushi *et al.*, 1987; Noshikawa *et al.*, 1987).

CGP-33 098 A (**290**) (Tosch *et al.*, 1985a) is the only member of oral C-3-thiocephems under evaluation. Its spectrum of activity is similar to that of cefixime (**53**) and better than that of older oral cephalosporins, except towards Staphylococci. CGP-33 098 A (**290**) is active against *Ps. aeruginosa*. In mice infection models it displayed greater activity than cefroxadine (**279**) against *S. pyogenes*, *E. coli* and *Ps. aeruginosa*. The urinary recovery rate in mice or rats ranges from 20–25%.

5.2.4 Prodrug Cephalosporins

Many valuable newer cephalosporins with aminothiazolyl side chains are extremely poorly absorbed from the intestine. In order to achieve enteral absorption, similar prodrug concepts as in the penicillin field have been applied (Webber and Wheeler, 1982; Ferres, 1983). By esterification of the cephem carboxylic group the lipid solubility is increased, thus facilitating the diffusion of the prodrugs across the membranes of mucosal epithelial cells. Prodrug esters are mostly acylacetals of formaldehyde or acetaldehyde. By using acetaldehyde as a component, mixtures of diastereomers are obtained. After absorption, rapid hydrolysis is achieved by esterases found in the

TABLE 34

Cleavage pattern of prodrug esters. Primary metabolites of pivaloyloxymethyl-, 1-acetoxyethyl-, phthalidyl-, (5-methyl-2-oxo-1,3-dioxyl-4-yl)methyl- and ethoxy-carbonyloxyethyl esters are shown

Prodrug	Primary Metabolites
$-CH_2-O\overset{O}{\overset{\|}{C}}-\!\!\!+$	HCHO, $+\!\!\!-CO_2H$
$-\underset{CH_3}{\overset{}{CH}}-O\overset{O}{\overset{\|}{C}}CH_3$	CH_3CHO, CH_3CO_2H
	$CH_3\overset{O}{\overset{\|}{C}}-\overset{O}{\overset{\|}{C}}-CH_3$, CO_2
$-\underset{CH_3}{\overset{}{CH}}O\overset{O}{\overset{\|}{C}}OC_2H_5$	CH_3CHO, CO_2, C_2H_5OH

intestinal tissues, liberating the parent drug and prodrug components which can be further metabolized. Table 34 shows the cleavage products of typical prodrug components.

Enteral absorption is considered to be a multistep process, including solvation and distribution of the drug in the gastrointestinal tract, passage across the intestinal walls, enzymatic hydrolysis in the epithelial cells, and transport of the free drug in the blood system. These steps are influenced and limited by a number of parameters, for instance solubility and dispersion of the drug, acid secretion and gastric pH, and activity of luminal esterases (Williams, 1985). Consequently, physicochemical parameters such as molecular weight, pK_a value, partition coefficient, water and lipid solubility, and steric features of distinct substituents, influence the absorption. Several research groups have tried to find quantitative correlations between physicochemical parameters and the bioavailability in animals or with the absorption rates obtained from everted rat intestine models. Yoshimura *et al.* (1986) and Nishimura *et al.* (1987) evaluated optimal ranges for molecular weights, *Hansch*'s parameters of lipophilicity and *Taft*'s steric parameters to optimize bioavailability of cefotiam prodrug esters. Another investigation documented the influence of water solubility and pK_a value on the bioavailability of cephalosporin prodrugs of different structural types (Yoshimura *et al.*, 1985).

Improvement of the bioavailability after food uptake is found for many cephalosporin prodrugs, perhaps due to saturation of luminal esterases, which would otherwise favour the hydrolysis of the prodrugs in the stomach (Williams, 1985).

The prodrug concept meets with limitations if non-proportional dose–bioavailability correlations exist. In such cases, doses in the range of 100–400 mg give linear correlations, whereas beyond 400–500 mg the bioavailability decreases.

The absorption mechanism of cephalosporin prodrugs (Table 35) has not been as thoroughly investigated as has that of penicillin prodrugs (e.g. pivampicillin, bacampicillin, talampicillin and lenampicillin) (Shindo *et al.*, 1978), but it is possible that similar mechanisms are operative. Baccefuzonam (**291**) (Kuck *et al.*, 1985), carrying an ethoxycarbonyloxyethyl ester group known from bacampicillin, was effective in mice septicaemia caused by *E. coli, K. pneumoniae, Staph. aureus* or *S. pyogenes*. No human pharmacokinetic parameters of the compound are available so far. The parent compound cefuzonam (**216**) is under clinical evaluation (see Section 5.1). Cefetamet (deacetoxycefotaxime) (**214**) is the parent compound of cefetamet pivoxyl (Ro 15-8075) (**292**). The *in vitro* antibacterial activity of cefetamet (Ro 15-8074) (**214**) has been evaluated by different groups, sometimes in comparison with other drugs (Fass and Helsel, 1986; Jones *et al.*, 1986; Mittermayer, 1986; Neu *et al.*, 1986a; Thomas and Lang, 1986;

TABLE 35

Oral prodrug cephalosporins with aminothiazolyl side chains and their parenteral parent compounds

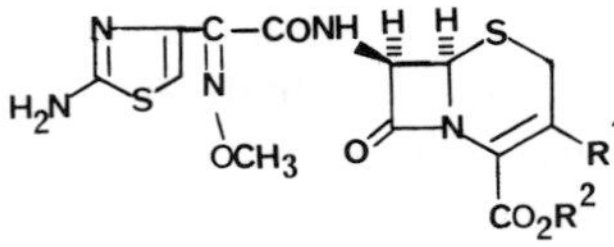

No.	Compound	R^1	R^2	Parent compound $(R^2 = H)$	No.
291	CL 118673 Baccefuzonam	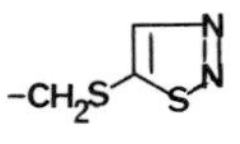 $-CH_2S$-(thiadiazole)	$-CHOCOC_2H_5$, CH_3	L 105 CL 251931 Cefuzonam	216
292	Ro15-8075, Ro 15 Cefetamet Pivoxyl	$-CH_3$	CH_2OC-(O)-(pivaloyl)	Ro 15-8074 Cefetamet	214
293	Ro 19-5248 Ro 19, T 2588 Cefteram Pivoxyl	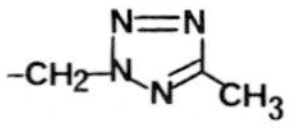 $-CH_2$-N(N=N triazole)CH_3	$-CH_2OC$-(O)-(pivaloyl)	Ro 19-5247 T 2525 Cefteram	215
294	ME 1207	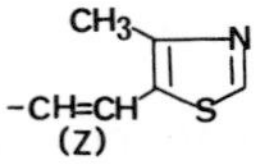 $-CH=CH$-(thiazole CH_3) (Z)	$-CH_2OC$-(O)-(pivaloyl)	ME 1206	218
295	CS 807	$-CH_2OCH_3$	$-CHOCOCH$-(O) CH_3, CH_3, CH_3	R 3763 $(R^2 = H)$	219
				R 3746 $(R^2 = Na)$	296

Chau *et al.*, 1987). The activity of cefetamet (**214**) is restricted mainly to Gram-negative bacteria except *Pseudomonas* spp. In mice infections, cefetamet pivoxyl (**292**) exceeds the activity of cefalexin (**23**) or cefaclor (**275**) by an order of magnitude (serum elimination half-life is about 1.4 h). After oral administration, **292** is absorbed to about 50% in healthy volunteers (Koup *et al.*, 1987).

Cefteram pivoxyl (T-2588, Ro 19-5248) (*Drugs of the Future*, 1986i) (**293**) is the pivaloyloxymethyl ester of cefteram (**215**). The spectrum of the parent compound cefteram (**215**) is, for many bacterial strains, comparable to those of other third generation cephalosporins (Chau *et al.*, 1987; Neu and Chin, 1986; Fass and Helsel, 1986; Okamoto *et al.*, 1987). Compared with cefotaxime (**207**) or cefalexin (**23**), the activity against Staphylococci is reduced. Cefteram (**215**) is not active against *Pseudomonas* spp. It displays good clinical activity against infections of the upper respiratory tract, chronic bronchitis, pyelonephritis, cystitis and urinary tract infections. A summary of reports on the clinical evaluation of **293** has recently been published [*Chemotherapy (Tokyo)*, 1986a]. After oral administration of **293**, 20–35% of the parent drug **215** is recovered in urine. A Δ^2-isomer of **215** is detected in small amounts (Saikawa *et al.*, 1986). Gastrointestinal side effects have been reported in 3% of cases, while a rise of serum transaminases, lactate dehydrogenases or alkaline phosphatases has been observed in 5% of patients.

ME-1206 (**218**), the parent compound of the pivaloyloxymethyl ester ME-1207 (**294**) (Inoue *et al.*, 1985; Komiya *et al.*, 1985), exhibits a higher *in vitro* potency than cefteram (**215**), cefixime (**53**) or cefaclor (**275**) against Gram-positive strains. ME-1206 (**218**) is stable to penicillinases and cephalosporinases. In the treatment of mice septicaemia, **294** was effective against *Staph. aureus*, *E. coli*, *K. pneumoniae* and *P. mirabilis*. The bioavailability in rats is 34%, the half-life 1.8 h, binding to human serum 92%. ME-1206 (**218**) has a high biliary excretion rate.

The parent compound R-3763 (**219**) of the prodrug ester cefpodoxime (CS-807) (**295**) (Komai *et al.*, 1986; Sugawara *et al.*, 1986; Fujimoto *et al.*, 1987) displays broad spectrum activity against Gram-positive bacteria except Enterococci, and also against Gram-negative bacteria except *Pseudomonas* spp. (Utsui *et al.*, 1987). It is highly active against *S. pyogenes*, *S. pneumoniae*, *E. coli*, *K. pneumoniae* and *H. influenzae*. Against *Enterobacter* spp. and indole-positive *Proteus* spp. it surpasses cefalexin (**23**), cefaclor (**275**), and amoxicillin in activity. Cefpodoxime (**295**) displays good therapeutic effects in systemic infections in mice by both Gram-positive and Gram-negative pathogens. After oral administration of **295** to mice, rats, or dogs, approximately 70%, 50%, or 40% of **219** was recovered in urine. In healthy volunteers, urinary recovery was in the range of 40–50% (Kobayashi *et al.*, 1987; Sawae *et al.*, 1987). The absorption was increased after food (Saito, 1987).

Table 36 shows prodrug cephalosporins of different structural types. SCE-2174 (**297**), a prodrug ester of the second generation cephalosporin cefotiam (**265**), has recently been described (Nishimura *et al.*, 1987). It has a bioavailability of about 50% in man (Couet *et al.*, 1987a,b). Cefuroxime (**298**) is a broad spectrum parenteral cephalosporin of the second generation with high β-lactamase stability. Its antibacterial spectrum includes ampicil-

TABLE 36

Oral prodrug cephalosporins with different side chains and their parenteral parent compounds

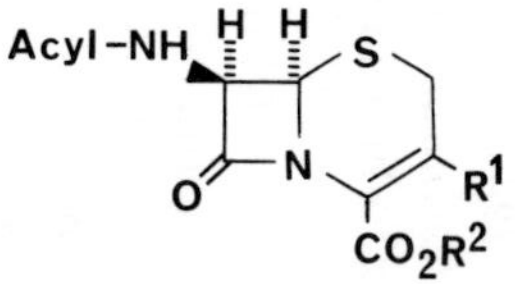

Acyl-NH, H H, S, N, O, R^1, CO$_2$R^2 (cephalosporin core structure)

No.	Compound	R^1	R^2	Acyl	Parent Compound R^2=H	No.
297	SCE 2174	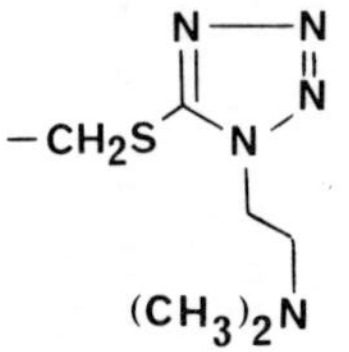 $-CH_2S-$ (tetrazole) $N-(CH_3)_2N$	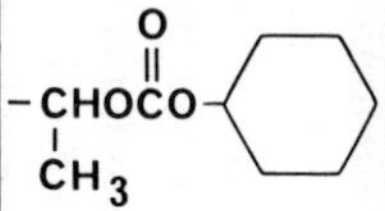 $-CHOCO-$cyclohexyl, CH_3	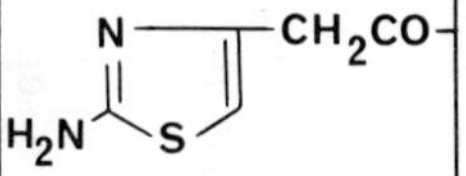 (aminothiazolyl)$-CH_2CO-$, H_2N	Cefotiam	265
274	Cefuroxime Axetil	$-CH_2OCNH_2$ (O)	$-CHOCCH_3$ (O), CH_3	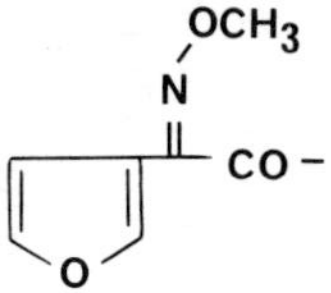 (furanyl) $-C(=N-OCH_3)-CO-$	Cefuroxime	298
299	KY 109	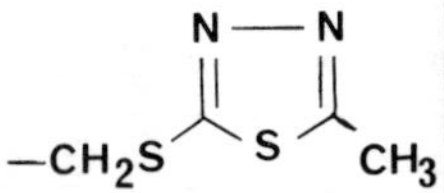 $-CH_2S-$ (thiadiazole) $-CH_3$	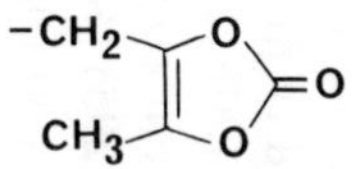 $-CH_2-$ (dioxolone) CH_3	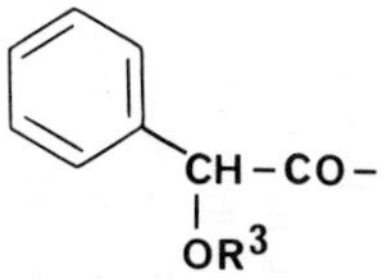 phenyl $-CH-CO-$, OR^3; $R^3 = -COCH_2NH_2$	KY 087 (R^3= H)	249

lin/amoxycillin-resistant *E. coli*, *Klebsiella spp.*, *P. mirabilis*, Staphylococci and *H. influenzae*. Cefuroxime axetil (274) (*Drugs of the Future*, 1986b) is a prodrug ester of 298 with an oral bioavailability of about 50% in healthy volunteers after administration of 250 mg to 1 g. Since the intact prodrug is not detected in the systematic circulation, a rapid ester cleavage during the absorption process is assumed. Cefuroxime axetil (274) is generally well tolerated, although some patients developed severe colitis as well as other gastrointestinal side effects associated with the unabsorbed portion of the drug. Its absorption is enhanced after food uptake, accounting for 40% of urinary recovery and an elimination half-life of 1.4 h. Oral administration in human volunteers produced higher peak serum levels than an equivalent dose of ampicillin and a urinary recovery of 35% (Sommers *et al.*, 1983; Wise *et al.*, 1983). The pharmacokinetic and bacteriological properties of 274 have been evaluated by Ginsburg *et al.* (1985) and Adams *et al.* (1985). A special issue [*Chemotherapy (Tokyo)*, 1986c] summarizes reports on the clinical evaluation of cefuroxime axetil (274).

KY-109 (299), a double prodrug of KY-087 (249), gives high blood levels of 249 after oral administration to rats (Kakeya *et al.*, 1983). KY-087 (249) is a second generation cephalosporin, structurally related to cefamandole, with higher activity than cefalexin (23) or cefaclor (275) against *Staph. aureus*, *S. pneumoniae*, *Micrococcus luteus* and *Bacillus subtilis*, as well as *E. coli*, *P. mirabilis*, *P. vulgaris* and *H. influenzae*.

A new cephalosporin, BMY-28232, bearing a 2-(aminothiazol-4-yl)-2-hydroxyimino side chain and a 3-(2)-propen-1-yl group, was reported recently (Tomatsu *et al.*, 1987). Its pivaloyloxymethyl ester (BMY-28257) and acetoxyethyl ester (BMY-28271) have 60–70% oral bioavailability in mice.

5.2.5 Various Structures

Some oral cephalosporins belonging to different structural types were presented at recent congresses or described in the literature (Table 37). However, only limited data are available. FK-482 (300) (Mine *et al.*, 1987; Sakamoto *et al.*, 1987; Shimada and Soejima, 1987; Takaya *et al.*, 1987) is a 3-vinylcephalosporin which differs from cefixime (53) by the oxime substituent (H instead of CH_2CO_2H). LY-189 972 (301) is a promising candidate from a series of 3-chloro-3-cephem derivatives bearing different side chains (Wright *et al.*, 1986; Kukolja and Wright, 1987; Pfeil *et al.*, 1987). The oral bioavailability in mice is 54%. ICI-156 488 (250) (Bruneau, 1984; Hennessey *et al.*, 1987a) has a unique 7-imidazolylamino substituent combined with the 3′-mercapto triazole residue of cefatrizine (277).

TABLE 37

Oral cephalosporins with different structures

No.	Formula	Code No.
300	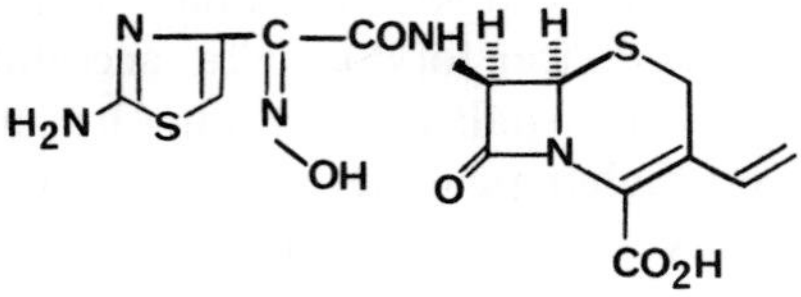	FK 482
301	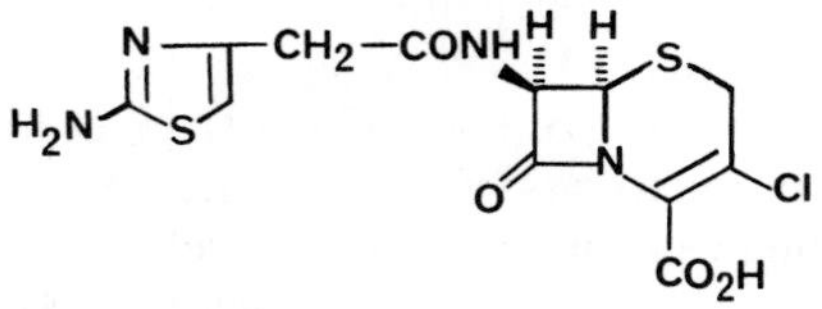	LY 189 972
250	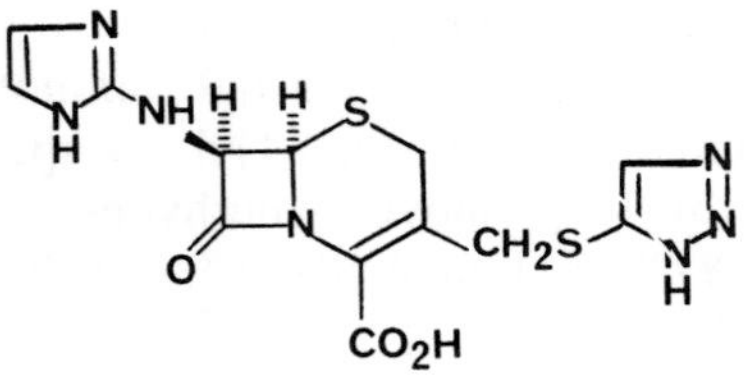	ICI 156 488

6 Mode of Action and Mechanism of Resistance

6.1 MODE OF ACTION

In order to be antibacterially active, cephalosporins, like all other β-lactam antibiotics, require the following basic properties:

- good penetration across the outer layers of the bacterial cell wall;
- high stability against deactivating enzymes, in particular β-lactamases; and
- high affinity for the target enzymes (PBPs) essential for bacterial cell wall biosynthesis.

The combination of these properties, which can be individually evaluated by experimental methods, determines the antibacterial effectiveness. The current knowledge on the roles of various outer membrane components, pathways of penetration, and permeability barriers has been summarized by Nikaido (1985). Studies on Gram-negative bacteria indicate the existence of different pathways by which cephalosporin antibiotics penetrate the outer membrane. Transmembrane diffusion of hydrophobic molecules is largely accomplished by dissolution into the lipophilic hydrocarbon interior of the membrane, followed by partitioning into the aqueous phase on the other side of the membrane. The permeability to hydrophilic cephalosporins is mainly mediated by membrane proteins termed "matrix proteins" or "porins". Specific pathways using receptor proteins and iron-chelator complexes have been suggested. Nikaido (1985) has determined the permeation rates of cephalosporins of different hydrophobicity, size and charge through porin channels.

Zwitterionic compounds like cephaloridine, cefaclor (**275**), or cefalexin (**23**) seem to penetrate much more rapidly than compounds carrying a net negative charge, e.g. cefoxitin (**104**), cefotaxime (**207**), ceftizoxime (**209**), cefoperazone (**244**). Dianionic compounds, like ceftriaxone (**210**), diffuse even slower. Compounds with molecular weights higher than 500 or those with bulky side chains have difficulty in passing the porin channels.

The key to the antimicrobial properties of cephalosporin antibiotics is their covalent binding to penicillin-binding proteins (PBPs) which are located on the bacterial cytoplasmic membrane. Spratt (1975) was the first to describe these target proteins. They are detected by incubation of bacterial membranes with [^{14}C]-penicillin followed by sodium dodecylsulphate gel electrophoresis. A modification of *Spratt*'s method by Schwarz *et al.* (1981), utilizing a ^{125}I-derivative of ampicillin as a marker, allowed a more rapid autoradiographic determination of PBPs and their specific binding to numerous antibiotics of the cefotaxime series.

Bacterial membranes invariably yielded multiple PBPs varying in number (from 3 in Gonococci to 9 or more in Gram-negative bacteria), in molecular weight (from about 30,000 to 100,000), and in quantity. PBPs possess carboxypeptidase, transpeptidase, and transglycosylase activity and perform distinct physiological roles in cell wall peptidoglycan synthesis. The most complete information is available for *E. coli*, whose PBPs are discussed in detail in review articles by Waxman and Strominger (1982), Tipper (1985), and Malouin and Bryan (1986).

Cephalosporins, like all other β-lactam antibiotics, exert their initial antibacterial effect through inhibition of the PBPs as substrate analogues of the acyl-D-alanyl-D-alanino component of peptidoglycan. The binding affinity (I_{50}) of β-lactam antibiotics to the PBPs is defined as the antibiotic concentration required to decrease the binding of the labelled benzylpenicil-lin to a PBP by 50%. Changes in the affinity or quantity of PBPs play a decisive role in development of antibiotic resistance among bacteria. In methicillin-resistant Staphylococci production of altered PBPs with very low affinity to β-lactams or an increase of an altered PBP (PBP 2′) has been described (Ubukata et al., 1985).

Cephalosporins have a considerable affinity to the higher molecular weight PBPs 1–4 and poor affinity to the low molecular weight PBPs 5 and 6. However, introduction of a 7α-methoxy group in cephalosporins decreases the affinity for PBPs 1–4 but favours the binding to 5 and 6 (Seeger et al., 1983). Cefotaxime (207) and many other third generation cephalosporins have the highest affinity in E. coli for PBP 3, followed by PBPs 1A, 1B and 2. Binding to PBP 3 leads to filamentation and prevention of cross wall formation and causes inhibition of cell division. PBP 1 is likely to be the most crucial PBP because inhibition or deletion by genetic mutation leads to cell lysis. In summary, most cephalosporins exert their antibacterial effect by binding to PBPs 1–4, and thereby inactivating enzymes responsible for the biosynthesis of the murein layer. Whether the lysis of bacteria is the direct result of PBP inactivation or whether this primary action leads to secondary effects by "autolysins" (peptidoglycan hydrolases) is a problem discussed by Tomasz (1979).

6.2 MICROBIAL RESISTANCE TO CEPHALOSPORINS

Increasing microbial resistance is a constant threat and a general problem in antibiotic therapy. The interactions between bacteria and β-lactam anti-biotics are very complex and many variables in the microorganisms and the drug can induce this effect. For the design of new cephalosporin antibiotics, it is important to understand the mechanisms of resistance and mode of action. Mechanisms of resistance to cephalosporins can be categorized into the following types (Gootz, 1985; Nikaido, 1985; Wiedemann, 1986):

- inactivation by β-lactamases;
- reduced penetration across the outer membrane, especially in Gram-negative bacteria;
- alteration of the target proteins PBPs; and
- loss of special transport systems.

The β-lactamases are the major determinants of bacterial resistance. They hydrolyse the amide bond of the β-lactam ring and thus inactivate the molecule. Recent reviews on the role of β-lactamases in the resistance of bacteria to β-lactams have been published by Acar and Minozzi (1986),

Wiedemann (1986), and Cole and Nicolas (1986). The production of β-lactamases is due to either chromosomal or plasmid genes, and may be either constitutive or inducible. Plasmid-mediated β-lactamases are important in the spread of bacterial resistance because the genetic material is easily transferred by plasmids.

Chromosome-mediated cephalosporinases in species such as *Serratia* spp., *Citrobacter* spp., *Enterobacter* spp., *Proteus* spp., *Providencia* spp. and *Pseudomonas* spp. are produced in small amounts in bacteria but can be induced at much higher levels in the presence of new β-lactams. Many β-lactams which show high affinity for cephalosporinases but are highly stable to hydrolysis, such as cefoxitin (**104**), latamoxef (**273**) and ceftazidime (**266**), are good inducers of β-lactamases. Poor substrates for inducible enzymes are for instance cefoperazone (**244**) and cefpirome (**220**). β-Lactamases can become packed so tightly in the periplasmatic space that a physical barrier is built up and complexing with β-lactams that are highly stable to β-lactamases neutralizes their antibiotic action (Sanders, 1984; Vuh and Nikaido, 1985). The parameters that contribute to enzyme–substrate interaction have been extensively reviewed.

The inhibition of β-lactamases by simultaneously administered β-lactamase inhibitors or inactivators has become important for cephalosporins and penicillins which are not sufficiently stable against these enzymes. Several potent β-lactamase inhibitors have been described, e.g. clavulanic acid, sulbactam, and YTR 830 (*Drugs of the Future*, 1986g). The synergistic effect of these agents with cephalosporins and penicillins for β-lactamase-forming strains has been demonstrated (Appelbaum *et al.*, 1986 and references cited therein).

The outer membrane of Gram-negative bacteria provides a selective barrier for many cephalosporins; their penetration into the periplasm is dependent on both the size and hydrophobicity of the molecule. Resistance by reduction of protein channels has already been described in this chapter. In enteric bacteria the transcription of the porin genes *omp C* and *omp F* can be regulated or inactivated by mutation. A complex lipopolysaccharide–phospholipid protein structure stabilized by Mg^{2+} ions presents a significant permeability barrier and is responsible for the resistance of the problem pathogens *Ps. aeruginosa* and *Klebsiella* spp. to most cephalosporins.

Modifications of the β-lactam targets, the PBPs, represent another important resistance factor. Mutations conferring cefalexin (**23**) resistance are known for PBP 3 of *E. coli K 12*, and similar changes have been reported for *N. gonorrhoeae* (Hedge and Spratt, 1985; Dougharty, 1984). Resistance by altered PBPs is more common amongst Gram-positive bacteria, e.g. Pneumococci and *Staph. aureus* (Malouin and Bryan, 1986).

A resistance mechanism by loss of special transport systems has been observed in β-lactam antibiotics which contain a catechol group in their molecules and chelate ferric ions. The transport and incorporation of such cephalosporins is accomplished via the *ton B*-dependent ion transport system. An antibiotic of this type is E-0702 (247) (N. Watanabe *et al.*, 1987b).

7 Perspectives

This review has endeavoured to describe the present status of cephem antibiotics from the viewpoint of medicinal chemistry. The last decade has seen considerable progress in improving their antibacterial potency and enhancing their activity spectrum. Semisynthesis has been the most success-ful route, and these efforts will continue. In spite of the almost bewildering number of compounds, the ideal antibiotic has not yet been found. A "therapia magna sterilisans" as Paul Ehrlich had in mind, does not exist. The reasons lie not only in the considerable diversity of bacteria and their subtle defence strategies, but also in the fact that many questions in the pharmaco-logy of antibiotics are not fully answered. Every few years a group of microorganisms achieves prominence as a cause of major resistance. The resistance is an expression of the enormous variability of microorganisms by DNA mutations and recombinations following the principle of move and countermove, as in a game of chess.

The shift in the spectrum of pathogenic organisms is a further factor complicating the advance in antibiotic therapy. The problem of chronic infections, frequently arising from deficiencies of the host defence mechanisms, has not yet been solved.

All advances have been achieved without knowing in detail the molecular structures of the target enzymes, but these disadvantages will be overcome within the next few years. Indeed, an X-ray analysis of a D-ala-D-ala-car-boxypeptidase-transpeptidase from *Streptomyces R 61* is underway and a specific binding site for penicillins and cephalosporins has been located (Knox *et al.*, 1985). It can be assumed that such information, together with advances in molecular modelling by computers, will allow a more rational design of novel cephalosporins and other non-classicial structures with antibacterial properties.

More complicated β-lactam antibiotics demand more sophisticated chemistry. This fact confronts the chemists to elaborate high yielding economic synthesis by using stereoselective or enzymatic reactions. Advanced technology in chemical and microbiological screening systems and gene manipulation techniques give us infinite possibilities of discovering new natural antibiotics which can be used as models for further chemical manipulation.

Finally, the antibiotic market has become much more price-sensitive because the expense of health insurance in most countries has reached the upper limit. It is therefore necessary to define more precisely the position of new antibiotics in therapy and strictly to avoid excessive use.

Acknowledgements

We wish to thank Mrs Gomez-Rosenthal and Mrs Wagner for excellent secretarial assistance, and Mrs Böhm, Mrs Fels and Mrs Palm for preparing the drawings.

References

Abraham, E. P. (1986). *In* "Regulation of Secondary Metabolite Formation" (H. Kleinkauf, H. von Döhren, H. Dornauer and G. Nesemann, eds), pp. 115–132. VCH Verlagsgesellschaft, Weinheim.

Abraham, E. P., and Newton, G. G. F. (1958). "Amino Acids Peptides Antimetabolic Activity." Ciba Foundation Symposium, p. 205.

Abraham, E. P., and Newton, G. G. F. (1961a). *Biochem. J.* **79**, 377–393.

Abraham, E. P., and Newton, G. G. F. (1961b). *Endeavour* **20**, 92–100.

Acar, J. and Minozzi, C. (1986). *Rev. Infect. Dis.* **8** (Suppl. 5), 482–486.

Adam, D., Grobecker, H., and Naber, K. G. (1982). "Fortschritte der Antimikrobiellen und Antineoplastischen Chemotherapie", Vol. 1. Futuramed Verlag, München.

Adams, D. H., Wood, M. J., Farrell, I. D., Fox, C., and Ball, A. P. (1985). *J. Antimicrob. Chemother.* **16**, 359–366.

Addison, J. M., Burston, D., Dalrymple, J. A., Matthews, D. A., Payne, J. W., Sleisenger, M. H., and Wilkinson, S. (1975). *Clin. Sci. Molec. Med.* **49**, 313–322.

Akagi, H., Matsumura, K., Suzuki, D., and Shimabayashi, A. (1986). *In* "Program and Abstracts of the 26th Interscience Conference on Antimicrobial Agents and Chemotherapy", New Orleans. Abstr. 1299.

Alpegiani, M., Casabuona, F., Giorgi, R., Nannini, G., Perrone, E., Meinardi, G., Bianchi, A., and Monti, G. (1983). *J. Antibiot.* **36**, 1013–1019.

Alpegiani, M., Bedeschi, A., Foglio, M., and Perrone, E. (1984). *Gazz. Chim. Italiana* **114**, 391–393.

Amsterdam, D., Jones, R., Ven, H., Thornsberry, C., and Lowells, Y. (1985). *Antimicrobial Newsletter* **2**, 33–40.

Angerbauer, R., Boberg, M., Metzger, K. G., and Zeiler, H. J. (1985a). Ger. Offen. DE 3,343,208, 5 June.

Angerbauer, R., Boberg, M., Metzger, K. G., and Zeiler, H. J. (1985b). Ger. Offen. DE 3,419,012, 28 November.

Angerbauer, R., Boberg, M., Kinast, G., and Metzger, K. G. (1987). *In* "Abstracts of the 15th International Congress of Chemotherapy", Istanbul. Abstr. 465.

Animati, F., Botta, M., DeAngelis, F., Dorigo, A., Grgurina, I., and Nicoletti, R. (1983). *J. Chem. Soc. Perkin Trans.* I, 2281–2286.

Appelbaum, P. C., Jacobs, M. R., Spangler, S. K., and Yamabe, S. (1986). *Antimicrob. Agents Chemother.* **30**, 789–791.

Applegate, H. E., Cimarusti, C. M., Dolfini, J. E., Funke, P. T., Koster, W. H., Puar, M. S., Slusarchyk, W. A., and Young, M. G. (1979). *J. Org. Chem.* **44**, 811–818.

Arai, T. (1986). *Jap. J. Antibiotics* **39**, 1237–1240.

Aratani, M., and Hashimoto, M. (1980). *J. Am. Chem. Soc.* **102**, 6171–6172.

Arimoto, M., Ejima, A., Watanabe, T., Tagawa, H., and Furukawa, M. (1986a). *J. Antibiot.* **39**, 1236–1242.

Arimoto, M., Hayano, T., Soga, T., Yoshioka, T., Tagawa, H., and Furukawa, M. (1986b). *J. Antibiot.* **39**, 1243–1256.

Atsumi, K., Sakagami, K., Yamamoto, Y., Yoshida, T., Nishita, K., Kondo, S., and Fukabu, S. (1986). Eur. Pat. Appl. EP 175,610, 26 March.

Balant, L., Dayer, P., and Auckenthaler, R. (1985). *Clin. Pharmacokinetics* **10**, 101–143.

Baldwin, J. E. (1984). *In* "Selectivity—A Goal for Synthetic Efficiency" (W. Bartmann and B. M. Trost, eds), pp. 391–409. Verlag Chemie, Weinheim.

Baldwin, J. E. (1985). *In* "Recent Advances in the Chemistry of β-Lactam Antibiotics" (A. G. Brown and S. M. Roberts, eds), Special Publication No. 52, pp. 62–85. The Royal Society of Chemistry, London.

Baldwin, J. E., Bahadur, G. A., Usher, J. J., Abraham, E. P., Jayatilake, G. S., and White, R. L. (1981). *J. Am. Chem. Soc.* **103**, 7650–7651.

Baldwin, J. E., Adlington, R. M., Domayne-Hayman, B. P., Ting, H. H., and Turner, N. J. (1986a). *J. Chem. Soc., Chem. Comm.*, 110–113.

Baldwin, J. E., Adlington, R. M., Basak, A, Flitsch, S. L., Forrest, A. K., and Ting, H. H. (1986b). *J. Chem. Soc., Chem. Comm.*, 273–275.

Baldwin, J. E., Adlington, R. M., Robinson, N. G., and Ting, H. H. (1986c). *J. Chem. Soc., Chem. Comm.*, 409–411.

Baldwin, J. E., Adlington, R. M., Basak, A., Flitsch, S. L., Petersson, S., Turner, N. J., and Ting, H. H. (1986d). *J. Chem. Soc., Chem. Comm.*, 975–976.

Baldwin, J. E., Adlington, R. M., Basak, A., and Ting, H. H. (1986e). *J. Chem. Soc., Chem. Comm.*, 1280–1281.

Baldwin, J. E., Adlington, R. M., Flitsch, S. L., Ting, H. H., and Turner, N. J. (1986f). *J. Chem. Soc., Chem. Comm.*, 1305–1308.

Baldwin, J. E., Killin, S. J., Pratt, A. J., Sutherland, J. D., Turner, N. J., Crabbe, J. C., Abraham, E. P., and Willis, A. C. (1987). *J. Antibiot.* **40**, 652–659.

Balsamo, A., Epifani, E., Giorgi, I., Lapucci, A., Maccia, B., and Maccia, F. (1981). *Il Farmaco—Ed. Sc.* **36**, 705–710.

Barriere, S. L., and Flaherty, J. F. (1984). *Clin. Pharmacol.* **3**, 351–373.

Barry, A. L., Thornsberry, C., and Jones, R. N. (1980). *J. Antimicrob. Chemother.* **6**, 775–784.

Basker, J. M., Branch, C. L., Finch, S. C., Guest, A. W., Milner, P. H., Pearson, M. J., Ponsford, R. J., and Smale, T. X. (1986). *J. Antibiot.* **39**, 1788–1791.

Bauernfeind, A. (1983). *Z. Antimikr. Antineoplast. Chemother.* **1**, 67–72.

Bell, R., Hallam, P. D., and Foxton, M. W. (1985). Ger. Offen. DE 3,516,777, 14 November.

Bell, R., Foxton, M. W., and Looker, B. E. (1986), Eur. Pat. Appl. EP 181,172, 14 May.

Bentley, P. H., Brooks, G., and Zomaya, I. (1976). *Tetrahedron Lett.* **41**, 3739–3742.

Bergan, T. (1984). *Scand. J. Infect. Dis.* (Supp. 42), 83–98.

Bergogne-Berezin, E. (1984). *Drugs Exp. Clin. Res.* **10**, 821–825.

Bialer, M., Batra, K., Morrison, J. A., Silber, B. M., Look, Z. M., and Yacobi, A. (1987). *Pharm. Res.* **4**, 33–37.

Blumbach, J., Fleischmann, K., Kirrstetter, R., Klesel, W., Lattrell, R., Ross, B., Schrinner, E., and Schwab, W. (1983). *In* "Proceedings of the 13th International Congress of Chemotherapy" (K. Spitzy and K. Karrer, eds), Vol. 4, PS 4.2/11-4. Egermann, Wien.

Blumbach, J., Dürckheimer, W., Ehlers, E., Fleischmann, K., Klesel, N., Limbert, M., Mencke, B., Reden, J., Scheunemann, K. H., Schrinner, E., Seibert, G., Wieduwilt, M., and Worm, M. (1987). *J. Antibiot.* **40**, 29–42.

Bodey, G. P., Ho, D. H., and Leblanc, B. (1985). *Antimicrob. Agents Chemother.* **27**, 265–269.

Böhme, E. H. W., Applegate, H. E., Toeplitz, B., Dolfini, J. E., and Gougoutas, J. Z. (1971). *J. Am. Chem. Soc.* **93**, 4324–4326.

Bonetti, A. (1981). *Schweiz. Apoth.-Ztg.* **119**, 411–436.

Bonjouklian, R. (1981). Eur. Pat. Appl. EP 39,924, 2 September.

Bonjouklian, R., and Philipps, M. L. (1981). *Tetrahedron Lett.* **22**, 3915–3918.

Bormann, D., Dürckheimer, W., and Schrinner, E. (1979). Ger. Offen. DE 2,822,860, 29 November.

Boswell, G. A. Jr, and Brittelli, D. R. (1975). US Patent 3,919, 204, 11 November.

Botta, M., DeAngelis, F., Grgurina, I., Marzi, M., and Nicoletti, R. (1985). *J. Heterocyclic Chem.* **22**, 1001–1007.

Boyd, D. B. (1982). In "Chemistry and Biology of β-Lactam-Antibiotics" (R. B. Morin and M. Gorman, eds), Vol. 1, pp. 437–545. Academic Press, New York and London.

Boyd, D. B. (1983). *J. Med. Chem.* **26**, 1010–1013.

Boyd, D. B. (1984). *J. Med. Chem.* **27**, 63–66.

Boyd, D. B. (1985). *J. Org. Chem.* **50**, 886–888.

Bradbury, R. H., Jung, F. H., Lohmann, J. J., Marsham, P. R., and Pasquet, G. (1985). Eur. Pat. Appl. EP 164,944, 18 December.

Branch, C. L., Basker, M. J., and Pearson, M. J. (1986). *J. Antibiot.* **39**, 1792–1795.

Branch, C. L., Basker, M. J., Finch, S. C., Guest, A. W., Harrington, F. P., Kaura, A. C., Knott, S. J., Milner, P. H., and Pearson, M. J. (1987). *J. Antibiot.* **40**, 646–651.

Brandt, A., Cerquetti, M., Corsi, B., Pascucci, G., Simeoni, A., Martelli, P., and Valcavi, U. (1987). *J. Med. Chem.* **30**, 764–767.

Brittain, D. C., Scully, B. E., Hirose, T., and Neu, H. C. (1985). *Clin. Pharmacol. Ther.* **38**, 590–594.

Brocalli, G., DePascale, A., and Dorigotti, L. (1983). In "Proceedings of the 13th International Congress of Chemotherapy" (K. Spitzy and K. Karrer, eds), Vol. 4, SE 4.2/15–14. Egermann, Wien.

Brogard, J. M. and Comte, F. (1982). In "Antibiotics and Chemotherapy", Vol. 31: Pharmaco-kinetic II (H. Schoenfeld, ed.), pp. 145–210. Karger-Verlag, Basel.

Brogard, J. M., Comte, F., and Pinget, H. (1978). In "Antibiotics and Chemotherapy", Vol. 25: Pharmacokinetic I (H. Schoenfeld, ed.), pp. 123–162. Karger-Verlag, Basel.

Brogden, R. N., Carmine, A., Heel, R. C., Morley, P. A., Speight, T. M., and Avery, G. S. (1981). *Drugs* **22**, 423–460.

Brown, A. G., and Roberts, S. M. V. (eds) (1985). "Recent Advances in the Chemistry of β-Lactam Antibiotics". Special Publication No. 52, The Royal Society of Chemistry, London.

Bruneau, P. (1984). Eur. Pat. Appl. EP 117,651, 5 September.

Bucourt, R., Heymes, R., Lutz, A., Penasse, L., and Perronnet, J. (1977). *C. R. Acad. Sci. Paris, Ser. D* **284**, 1847–1849.

Bucourt, R., Heymes, R., Lutz, A., Penasse, L., and Perronnet, J. (1978). *Tetrahedron* **34**, 2233–2243.

Bucourt, R., Heymes, R., Perronnet, J., Lutz, A., and Penasse, L. (1981). *Eur. J. Med. Chem.—Chimia Therapeutica* **16**, 307–316.

Cama, L. D., and Christensen, B. G. (1974). *J. Am. Chem. Soc.* **96**, 7582–7584.

Cama, L. D., and Christensen, B. G. (1978). *Ann. Rep. Med. Chem.* **13**, 149–158.

Cama, L. D., Leanza, W. J., Beattie, T. R., and Christensen, B. G. (1972). *J. Am. Chem. Soc.* **94**, 1408–1410.

Campoli-Richards, D. M., and Todd, P. A. (1987). *Drugs* **34**, 188–221.

Carmine, A. A., Brogden, R. N., Heel, R. C., Speight, T. M., and Avery, G. S. (1983a). *Drugs* **25**, 223–289.

Carmine, A. A., Brogden, R. N., Heel, R. C., Romankiewicz, J. A., Speight, T. M., and Avery, G. S. (1983b). *Drugs* **26**, 279–333.

Chau, P. Y., Leung, Y. K., Ng, W. W. S., and Arnold, K. (1987). *Antimicrob. Agents Chemother.* **31**, 473–476.

Chauvette, A., and Chauvette, R. R. (1981). US Pat. 4,281,117, 28 July.

Chauvette, R. R., and Pennington, P. A. (1975). *J. Med. Chem.* **18**, 403–408.

Chemotherapy (Basel) (1981). **27**, Suppl. 1.

Chemotherapy (Tokyo) (1978a). **26**, Suppl. 1.

Chemotherapy (Tokyo) (1978b). **26**, Suppl. 5.

Chemotherapy (Tokyo) (1980a). **28**, Suppl. 1.

Chemotherapy (Tokyo) (1980b). **28**, Suppl. 5.

Chemotherapy (Tokyo) (1981a). **29**, Suppl. 1.

Chemotherapy (Tokyo) (1981b). **29**, Suppl. 3.

Chemotherapy (Tokyo) (1982a). **30**, Suppl. 1.

Chemotherapy (Tokyo) (1982b). **30**, Suppl. 3.

Chemotherapy (Tokyo) (1983). **31**, Suppl. 1.

Chemotherapy (Tokyo) (1984a). **32**, Suppl. 4.

Chemotherapy (Tokyo) (1984b). **32**, Suppl. 5.

Chemotherapy (Tokyo) (1984c). **32**, Suppl. 7.

Chemotherapy (Tokyo) (1984d). **32**, Suppl. 9.

Chemotherapy (Tokyo) (1985). **33**, Suppl. 6.

Chemotherapy (Tokyo) (1986a). **34**, Suppl. 2.

Chemotherapy (Tokyo) (1986b). **34**, Suppl. 3.

Chemotherapy (Tokyo) (1986c). **34**, Suppl. 5.

Chemotherapy (Tokyo) (1987). **35**, Suppl. 1.

Chin, N. X., and Neu, H. C. (1986). *Chemioterapia* **5**, 92–100.

Chin, N. X., and Neu, H. C. (1987). *Antimicrob. Agents Chemother.* **31**, 480–483.

Chin, N. X., Cao, C., and Neu, H. C. (1987). *In* "Program and Abstracts of the 27th Interscience Conference on Antimicrobial Agents and Chemotherapy", New York. Abstr. 1192.

Chou, T.-S. (1977). Ger. Offen. DE 2,726,394, 29 December.

Christensen, B. G., Firestone, R. A., Fahey, J. L., Maciejewicz, N. S., and Patel, G. S. (1977). *J. Med. Chem.* **20**, 551–556.

Clarke, A. M., Zemcov, S. J. V., and Wright, J. M. (1985). *J. Antimicrob. Chemother.* **15**, 305–310.

Cleeland, R., and Squires, E. (1984). *Am. J. Med.* **77**, 3–11.

Coene, B., Schanck, A., Dereppe, J.-M., and Van Meerssche, M. (1984). *J. Med. Chem.* **27**, 694–700.

Cole, S. T., and Nicolas, M. H. (1986). *Microbiol. Sci.* **3**, 334–339.

Comereski, C. R., Bregman, C. L., and Buroker, R. A. (1987). *Fund. Appl. Toxicol.* **8**, 280–289.

Cooper, R. D. G., and Koppel, G. A. (1982). *In* "Chemistry and Biology of β-Lactam-Antibiotics" (R. B. Morin and M. Gorman, eds), Vol. 1, pp. 2–92. Academic Press, New York and London.

Cooper, R. D. G., and Spry, D. O. (1972). *In* "Cephalosporins and Penicillins. Chemistry and Biology" (E. H. Flynn, ed.), pp. 183–254. Academic Press, New York and London.

Cooper, R. D. G., DeMarco, P. V., Cheng, J. C., and Jones, N. D. (1969). *J. Am. Chem. Soc.* **91**, 1408–1415.

Cooper, R. D. G., DeMarco, P. V., Murphy, C. F., and Spangle, L. A. (1970). *J. Chem. Soc.* (*C*), 341–344.

Couet, W., Lefebvre, M.-A., Girault, A., Mignot, A., Bizouard, J., and Fourtillan, J. B. (1987a). *In* "Abstracts of the 15th International Congress of Chemotherapy", Istanbul. Abstr. 243.

Couet, W., Lefebvre, M.-A., Millerioux, L., Mignot, A., Bizouard, J., and Fourtillan, J. B. (1987b). *In* "Abstracts of the 15th International Congress of Chemotherapy", Istanbul. Abstr. 244.

Counter, F. T., Ensminger, P. W., Alborn, W. E., Preston, D. A., and Turner, J. R. (1987). *In* "Program and Abstracts of the 27th Interscience Conference on Antimicrobial Agents and Chemotherapy", New York. Abstr. 1188.

Cowley, B. R., Humber, D. C., Laundon, B., and Long, A. G. (1983a). *Tetrahedron* **39**, 337–342.

Cowley, B. R., Humber, D. C., Laundon, B., Long, A. G., and Lynd, A. L. (1983b). *Tetrahedron* **39**, 461–467.

Crowfoot-Hodgkin, D., and Malen, E. N. (1961). *Biochem. J.* **79**, 393–402.

Csendes, I. (1985). Ger. Offen. DE 3,518,848, 28 November.

Csendes, I., Müller, B. W., Scartazzini, R., and Tosch, W. (1983a). *In* "Proceedings of the 13th International Congress of Chemotherapy" (K. Spitzy and K. Karrer, eds), Vol. 5, PS 4.6/7-14. Egermann, Wien.

Csendes, I., Müller, B. W., and Tosh, W. (1983b). *J. Antibiot.* **36**, 1020–1033.

Csendes, I., Tosch, W., and Zak, O. (1985). *In* "Proceedings of the 4th Mediterranean Congress of Chemotherapy" (G. K. Daikos and H. Giamarellio, eds), *Chemioterapia* **4** (Suppl. 2), 261–262.

Cunha, B. A., Ristuccia, A. M., Jonas, M., Ristuccia, P. A., and Janelli, D. E. (1982). *J. Antimicrob. Chemother.* **10** (Suppl. C), 117–120.

Dagrosa, E. E., Hajdu, P., Malerczyk, V., de Looze, S., Seeger, K., and Grötsch, H. (1987). *Clin. Therap.* **10**, 18–31.

De Koning, J. J., Marx, A. F., Poot, M. M., Smid, P. M., and Verweij, J. (1977). *In* "Recent Advances in the Chemistry of β-Lactam Antibiotics" (J. Elks, ed.), pp. 161–166. The Royal Society of Chemistry, London.

Demain, A. L. (1963). *Biochem. Biophys. Res. Commun.* **10**, 45–48.

Demain, A. L., and Brana, A. F. (1986). *In* "Regulation of Secondary Metabolite Formation" (H. Kleinkauf, H. von Döhren, H. Dornauer and G. Nesemann, eds), pp. 77–88. VCH Verlagsgesellschaft, Weinheim.

Demain, A. L., and Wolfe, S. (1987). *Dev. Ind. Microbiol.* **27**, 175–182.

Dette, G. A. (1986). *Z. Antimikr. Antineoplast. Chemother.* **4**, 95–101.

Doherty, J. B., Ashe, B. M., Argenbright, L. W., Barker, P. L., Bonney, R. J., Chandler, G. O., Dahlgren, M. E., Dorn, C. P. Jr, Finke, P. E., Firestone, R. A., Fletcher, D., Hagmann, W. K., Mumford, R., O'Grady, L., Maycock, A. L., Pisano, J. M., Shah, S. K., Thompson, K. R., and Zimmerman, M. (1986). *Nature* **322**, 192–194.

Dougharty, T. J. (1984). *In* "Microbiology" (D. Schlesinger, ed.), pp. 398–401. The American Society for Microbiology, Washington.

Doyle, T. W., Douglas, J. L., Belleau, B., Conway, T. T., Ferrari, C. F., Horning, D. E., Lim,

G., Luh, B. Y., Mortel, A., Menard, M., and Morris, L. R. (1980). *Can. J. Chem.* **58**, 2508–2523.

Drigues, P., Roche, G., Combes, T., and Salhi, A. (1986). *In* "Program and Abstracts of the 26th Interscience Conference on Antimicrobial Agents and Chemotherapy", New Orleans. Abstr. 1313.

Drugs (1981). Suppl. 1.

Drugs (1987). Suppl. 2.

Drugs of the Future (1977a). **2**, 368–371.

Drugs of the Future (1977b). **2**, 574–578.

Drugs of the Future (1980). **5**, 252–253.

Drugs of the Future (1981a). **6**, 38–39.

Drugs of the Future (1981b). **6**, 132–134.

Drugs of the Future (1981c). **6**, 569–572.

Drugs of the Future (1983a). **8**, 102–104.

Drugs of the Future (1983b). **8**, 682–683.

Drugs of the Future (1984a). **9**, 140.

Drugs of the Future (1984b). **9**, 252–255.

Drugs of the Future (1984c). **9**, 460.

Drugs of the Future (1984d). **9**, 572–574.

Drugs of the Future (1984e). **9**, 928–929.

Drugs of the Future (1985a). **10**, 14–16.

Drugs of the Future (1985b). **10**, 193–195.

Drugs of the Future (1985c). **10**, 332.

Drugs of the Future (1985d). **10**, 805–808.

Drugs of the Future (1986a). **11**, 103–105.

Drugs of the Future (1986b). **11**, 141.

Drugs of the Future (1986c). **11**, 324–325.

Drugs of the Future (1986d). **11**, 417–418.

Drugs of the Future (1986e). **11**, 452–455.

Drugs of the Future (1986f). **11**, 570–572.

Drugs of the Future (1986g). **11**, 588–592.

Drugs of the Future (1986h). **11**, 706–708.

Drugs of the Future (1986i). **11**, 732–736.

Drugs of the Future (1986k). **11**, 880–882.

Drugs of the Future (1987a). **12**, 91.

Drugs of the Future (1987b). **12**, 110–112.

Drugs of the Future (1987c). **12**, 286–289.

Drugs of the Future (1987d). **12**, 581.

Dürckheimer, W. (1986). *In* "Frontiers of Antibiotic Research", p. 33. Takeda Science Foundation Symposium on Bioscience, Kyoto.

Dürckheimer, W., and Schrinner, E. (1985). *In* "Proceedings of the 14th International Congress of Chemotherapy" (J. Ishigami, ed.), Vol. 1, pp. 51–53. University of Tokyo Press, Tokyo.

Dürckheimer, W., and Seliger, H. (1982). *In* "Proceedings of the 12th International Congress of Chemotherapy" (P. Periti and G. G. Grassi, eds), Vol. 1, pp. 592–594. The American Society for Microbiology, Washington.

Dürckheimer, W., Klesel, N., Limbert, M., Schrinner, E., Seeger, K., and Seliger, H. (1981). *In* "Recent advances in the Chemistry of β-Lactam Antibiotics" (G. J. Gregory, ed.), pp. 46–56. The Royal Society of Chemistry, London.

Dürckheimer, W., Blumbach, J., Heymes, P., Schrinner, E., and Seeger, K. (1982). *In* "New β-Lactam Antibiotics from Chemistry to Clinical Efficacy of the New Cephalosporins"

(H. C. Neu, ed.), Vol. 1, pp. 3–21. Francis Clark Wood Institute for the History of Medicine, College of Physicians of Philadelphia, Philadelphia.

Dürckheimer, W., Lattrell, R., and Seeger, K. (1984). Ger. Offen. DE 3,247,613, 5 July.

Dürckheimer, W., Blumbach, J., Lattrell, R., and Scheunemann, K. H. (1985). Angew. Chem. Int. Ed. Engl. **24**, 180–202, and references cited therein.

Dunn, G. L. (1982). J. Antimicrob. Chemother. **10** (Suppl. C), 1–10.

Dunn, G. L. (1986). Ann. Rep. Med. Chem. **21**, 131–138, and references cited therein.

Ebbinghaus, C. F., Morrissey, P., and Rosati, R. L. (1979). J. Org. Chem. **44**, 4697–4699.

Edmiston, C., Scarry, R., and Matsui, H. (1985). In "Program and Abstracts of the 25th Interscience Conference on Antimicrobial Agents and Chemotherapy", Minneapolis. Abstr. 358.

Edwards, M. L., and Erickson, R. C. (1979). J. Med. Chem. **22**, 1416–1418.

Ejima, A., Hayano, T., Ebata, T., Nagahara, T., Koda, H., Tagawa, H., and Furukawa, M. (1987). J. Antibiot. **40**, 43–48.

Eliopoulos, G. M., Reiszner, E., Wennersten, C., and Moellering, R. C. (1987). Antimicrob. Agents Chemother. **31**, 653–656.

English, A. R., Retsema, J. A., and Lynch, J. E. (1976). Antimicrob. Agents Chemother. **10**, 132–138.

Ernest, I. (1979). Helv. Chim. Acta **62**, 2681–2694.

Ernest, I. (1980). Helv. Chim. Acta **63**, 201–213.

Evans, D., and Sjogren, E. B. (1985). Tetrahedron Lett. **26**, 3787–3790.

Faraci, W. S., and Pratt, R. F. (1984). J. Am. Chem. Soc. **106**, 1489–1490.

Farina, V. (1986). Synthetic Comm. **16**, 1029–1035.

Fass, R. J., and Helsel, V. L. (1986). Antimicrob. Agents Chemother. **30**, 429–434.

Fechtig, B., Peter, H., Bickel, H., and Vischer, E. (1968). Helv. Chim. Acta **51**, 1108–1119.

Ferres, J. (1983). Drugs of Today **19**, 499–538.

Feyen, P., and Schröck, W. (1981). Angew. Chem. **93**, 814–815.

Firestone, R. A., and Christensen, B. G. (1973). J. Org. Chem. **38**, 1436–1437.

Fleischmann, K., Blumbach, J., Dürckheimer, W., Lattrell, R., Scheunemann, K. H., and Klesel, N. (1985). Ger. Offen. DE 3,330,605, 14 March.

Fletton, R. A., Humber, D. C., Roberts, S. M., and Wright, J. L. (1985). J. Chem. Soc. Perkin Trans. **I**, 1523–1526.

Fortschritte der Antimikrobiellen, Antineoplastischen Chemotherapie (1982). **1**.

Fourtillan, J.-B., Bryskier, A., Mignot, A., Borso, F., and Humbert, G. (1984). Am. J. Med. **77**, 28–31.

Fuchs, P., Jones, R., Barry, A., and Thornsberry, C. (1985). Antimicrob. Agents Chemother. **27**, 679–682.

Fujii, R., Meguro, H., Arimasu, O., Mashiko, J., Kobayashi, M., and Nakazawa, S. (1986). Jap. J. Antibiot. **39**, 2601–2619.

Fujimori, I. (1985). Jap. J. Antibiot. **38**, 7–48.

Fujimoto, K., Ishihara, S., Yanagisawa, H., Ide, J., Nakayama, E., Nakao, H., Sugawara, S.-I., and Iwata, M. (1987). J. Antibiot. **40**, 370–384.

Fujimoto, K., Otani, T., Nakajima, R., Une, T., and Osada, Y. (1986). Antimicrob. Agents Chemother. **30**, 611–613.

Fujisawa Pharmaceutical Co. Ltd (1982). Jpn. Kokai Tokkyo Koho JP 8270,893, 1 May.

Fujisawa Pharmaceutical Co. Ltd (1983). Jpn. Kokai Tokkyo Koho JP 58,222,092, 23 December.

Fujisawa Pharmaceutical Co. Ltd (1985). Jpn. Kokai Tokkyo Koho JP 60,226,886, 12 November.

Furlanut, M., Montanari, G., Padrini, R., Meinardi, G., Tamassia, V., and Bruno, R. (1983). Drugs Exp. Clin. Res. **98**, 657–659.

Furukawa, M., Arimoto, M., Nakamura, S., Ejima, A., Higashi, Y., and Tagawa, H. (1986). *J. Antibiot.* **39**, 1225–1235.

Ganzinger, U. (1987). *Int. J. Clin. Pharmacol. Ther. Toxicol.* **25**, 262–278.

Garzone, P., Lyon, J., and Yu, V. L. (1983). *Drug. Intell. Clin. Pharmacy* **17**, 507–515.

Geddes, A. M., Acar, J. F., and Knothe, H. (1980). *J. Antimicrob. Chemother.* **6** (Suppl. A), 63–161.

Ginsburg, C. M., McCracken, G. M. Jr, Petruska, M., and Olson, K. (1985). *Antimicrob. Agents Chemother.* **28**, 504–507.

Gleason, J. G., Bryan, D. B., and Holden, K. (1980). *Tetrahedron Lett.* **21**, 3947–3950.

Gnann, J. W. Jr., Goetter, W. E., Elliott, A. M., and Cobbs, C. G. (1982). *Antimicrob. Agents Chemother.* **22**, 1–9.

Goerdeler, J. (1954). *Chem. Ber.* **87**, 57–67.

Goldstein, E. J. C., and Citron, D. M. (1985). *Antimicrob. Agents Chemother.* **28**, 160–162.

Gootz, T. D. (1985). *Ann. Rep. Med. Chem.* **20**, 137–144.

Gordon, E. M., and Sykes, R. B. (1982). *In* "Chemistry and Biology of β-Lactam Antibiotics (R. B. Morin and M. Gorman, eds), Vol. 1, pp. 199–370. Academic Press, New York and London.

Gordon, E. M., Chang, H. W., Cimarusti, C. M., Toeplitz, B., and Gougoutas, J. Z. (1980). *J. Am. Chem. Soc.* **102**, 1690–1702.

Gordon, E. M., Chang, H. W., Cimarusti, C. M. (1977). *J. Am. Chem. Soc.* **99**, 5504–5505.

Gorman, M., and Ryan, C. W. (1972a). *In* "Cephalosporins and Penicillins" (E. H. Flynn, ed.), pp. 532–582. Academic Press, New York and London.

Gorman, M., and Ryan, C. W. (1972b). *In* "Cephalosporins and Penicillins" (E. H. Flynn, ed.), pp. 554–569. Academic Press, New York and London.

Goto, S., Ogawa, M., Miyazaki, S., Kaneko, Y., and Kuwahara, S. (1984a). *In* "Program and Abstracts of the 24th Interscience Conference on Antimicrobial Agents and Chemotherapy", Washington. Abstr. 644.

Goto, J., Sakane, N., Nakai, Y., Teraji, T., and Kamiya, T. (1984b). *J. Antibiot.* **37**, 532–545.

Goto, J., Sakane, K., Nakai, Y., Teraji, T., and Kamiya, T. (1984c). *J. Antibiot.* **37**, 546–556.

Goto, J., Sakane, K., and Teraji, T. (1984d). *J. Antibiot.* **37**, 557–571.

Grabowski, E. J. J., Douglas, A. W., and Smith, G. B. (1985). *J. Am. Chem. Soc.* **107**, 267–268.

Grappel, S. F., Phillips, L., Dunn, G. L., Jakas, D. R., Pitkin, D., and Actor, P. (1984). *Antimicrob. Agents Chemother.* **25**, 694–700.

Greene, T. W. (1981). "Protective Groups in Organic Synthesis". Wiley, New York.

Guay, D. R. P., Meatherall, R. C., Harding, G. K., and Brown, G. R. (1986). *Antimicrob. Agents Chemother.* **30**, 485–490.

Guest, A. W., Branch, C. L., Finck, S. C., Kaura, A. C., Milner, P. H., Pearson, M. J., Ponsford, R. J., and Smale, C. T. (1987). *J. Chem. Soc., Perkin Trans.* **I**, 45–55.

Habibi, E. H., Roche, G., and Salhi, A. (1986). *In* "Program and Abstracts of the 26th Intelligence Conference on Antimicrobial Agents and Chemotherapy", New Orleans. Abstr. 1314.

Hagiwara, D., Aratani, M., Hemmi, K., and Hashimoto, M. (1981). *Tetrahedron* **37**, 703–707.

Hamashima, Y. (1985). Eur. Pat. Appl. EP 136,721, 10 April.

Hamashima, Y., and Nagata, W. (1980). Ger. Offen. DE 2,937,868, 3 April.

Hamashima, Y., Ishikura, K., Ishitobi, H., Itani, H., Kubota, T., Minami, K., Murakami, M., Nagata, W., Narisada, M., Nishitani, Y., Okada, T., Onoue, H., Satoh, H., Sendo, Y., Tsuji, T., and Yoshioka, M. (1976). *In* "Recent Advances in the Chemistry of β-Lactam Antibiotics" (J. Elks, ed.), Special Publication No. 28, pp. 243–251. The Royal Society of Chemistry, London.

Hashimoto, T., Kawano, Y., Natsume, S., and Tanaka, T. (1978). *Chem. Pharm. Bull.* **26**, 1803–1811.

Hashimoto, Y., Takasawa, S., Ogasa, T., Saito, H., Hirata, T., and Kimura, K. (1984). *Ann. N.Y. Acad. Sci.* **434**, 206–209.

Hatanaka, M., Yamamoto, Y., Ishimaru, T., and Takai, Y. (1985). *Chem. Lett.* 183–186. .

Hatanaka, M., Nitta, H., and Ishimaru, T. (1987). *J. Chem. Soc., Chem. Comm.* 51–52.

Hatfield, L. D., Blaszak, L. C., Fisher, J. W., and Bunnel, C. A. (1980a). Eur. Pat. Appl. EP 14,567, 8 August.

Hatfield, L. D., Fisher, J. W., Dunigan, J. M., Burchfield, R. W., Greene, J. M., Webber, J. A., Vasileff, R. T., and Kinnick, M. D. (1980b). *Phil. Trans. R. Soc. Lond. B* **289**, 173–179.

Hayes, M. V., and Orr, D. C. (1983). *J. Antimicrob. Chemother.* **12**, 119–126.

Hedge, J., and Spratt, B. (1985). *Eur. J. Biochem.* **151**, 111–121.

Hennessey, T. D., Edwards, J. R., and Williams, S. (1987a). *In* "Program and Abstracts of the 27th Interscience Conference on Antimicrobial Agents and Chemotherapy", New York. Abstr. 805.

Hennessey, T. D., Edwards, J. R., and Curtis, N. A. C. (1987b). *In* "Program and Abstracts of the 27th Interscience Conference on Antimicrobial Agents and Chemotherapy", New York. Abstr. 811.

Hikida, M., Mitsuhashi, S., and Inoue, M. (1986). *Chemotherapy (Tokyo)* **34** (Suppl. 3), 1–16.

Hirata, T., Matsukuma, I., Mochida, K., and Sato, K. (1987). *In* "Program and Abstracts of the 27th Interscience Conference on Antimicrobial Agents and Chemotherapy", New York. Abstr. 1187.

Hoffler, D., Koeppe, P., and Williams, K. J. (1983). *J. Antimicrob. Chemother.* **12** (Suppl. A), 241–245.

Holden, K. G., Gleason, J. G., Hoffman, W. F., and Perchonek, C. D. (1979). *In* "Drug Action and Design" (T. Kalman, ed.), pp. 225–248. Elsevier, North Holland, New York.

Horii, S., Fukase, H., and Mizokami, N. (1979). Jpn. Kokai Tokkyo Koho JP 79,92,986, 23 July.

Hrytsak, M., and Durst, T. (1987). *Heterocycles* **26**, 2393–2409.

Hoshide, Y., and Ogawa, H. (1982). *J. Pharm. Soc. Jpn.* **102**, 816–822.

Hoshide, Y., Ogawa, H., Suzuki, K., Seki, T., and Tasaka, S. (1982a). *J. Pharm. Soc. Jpn.* **102**, 823–843.

Hoshide, Y., Hashimoto, Y., Ogawa, H., Suzuki, K., Segi, T., and Tasaka, S. (1982b). *J. Pharm. Soc. Jpn.* **102**, 844–853.

Huang, H. T. (1963). *Appl. Microbiol.* **11**, 1–6.

Humber, D. C., and Roberts, S. M. (1985). *Synth. Commun.* **15**, 681–687.

Humber, D. C., Laing, S. B., and Weingarten, G. G. (1981). *In* "Recent Advances in the Chemistry of β-Lactam Antibiotics" (G. I. Gregory, ed.), Special Publication No. 38, pp. 38–45. The Royal Society of Chemistry, London.

Humbert, G., Bryskier, A., Borsa, F., Tremblay, D., Fourtillan, J. B., and Leroy, A. (1985). *In* "Proceedings of the 14th International Congress of Chemotherapy" (J. Ishigami, ed.), pp. 937–938. University of Tokyo Press, Tokyo.

Inaba, H., Mochizuki, H., Kato, K., Kosuzume, H., and Ohnishi, H. (1985). *In* "Proceedings of the 14th International Congress of Chemotherapy" (J. Ishigami, ed.), Vol. 2, pp. 879–880. University of Tokyo Press, Tokyo.

Indelicato, J. M., Engel, G. L., and Occolowitz, J. L. (1985). *J. Pharm. Sci.* **74**, 1162–1166.

Infection (1985). **13** (Suppl. 1).

Infection (1987). **15** (Suppl. 4).

Inoue, M., Tamura, A., Yoshida, T., Okamoto, R., Atsumi, K., Nishihata, K., and Mitsuhashi, S. (1985). *In* "Program and Abstracts of the 25th Interscience Conference on Antimicrobial Agents and Chemotherapy", Minneapolis. Abstr. 582.

Inouye, S., Tsurnoka, T., Goi, H., Iwamatsu, K., Miyanchi, K., Ishii, T., Tamura, A., Kazimo, Y. and Matsuhashi, M. (1984). *J. Antibiot.* **37**, 1403–1413.

Iorio, M. A., and Nicoletti, M. (1986). *Il Farmaco—Ed. Sc.* **41**, 801–807.

Ishimaru, H. (1983). Jpn. Kokai Tokkyo, Koho, JP 5865,296, 18 April.

Ishimaru, H. (1984). Jpn. Kokai Tokkyo, Koho, JP 5965,095, 13 April.

J. Antimicrob. Chemother. (1975). **1** (Suppl.).

J. Antimicrob. Chemother. (1978). **4** (Suppl. B).

J. Antimicrob. Chemother. (1980). **6** (Suppl. A).

J. Antimicrob. Chemother. (1981). **8** (Suppl. B).

J. Antimicrob. Chemother. (1982a). **10** (Suppl. B).

J. Antimicrob. Chemother. (1982b). **10** (Suppl. C).

J. Antimicrob. Chemother. (1983a). **11** (Suppl. A).

J. Antimicrob. Chemother. (1983b). **12** (Suppl. A).

J. Antimicrob. Chemother. (1984). **14** (Suppl. B).

Jarlier, V., Philippon, A., Nicolas, M. H., and Bismuth, R. (1986). *In* "Program and Abstracts of the 26th Interscience Conference on Antimicrobial Agents and Chemotherapy", New Orleans. Abstr. 1312.

Jaszberenyi, J. C., Petrikovics, I., Gunda, E. T., and Hosztafi, S. (1982). *Acta Chim. Acad. Sci. Hung.* **110**, 81–84.

Jones, R. N., and Wilson, H. W. (1982). *Infection* **10**, 303–306.

Jones, R. N., Fuchs, P. C., Barry, A. L., Ayers, L. W., Gerlach, E. H., and Gavan, T. L. (1986). *Antimicrob. Agents Chemother.* **30**, 961–963.

Jung, F. A., Pilgrim, W. R., Poyser, J. P., and Siret, P. J. (1980). *In* "Topics in Antibiotic Chemistry" (P. G. Sammes, ed.), Vol. 4, pp. 173–179. Ellis Horwood Limited, New York, Chichester, Brisbane, Toronto.

Kadurugamuwa, J. L., Anwar, H., Brown, M. R. W., and Zak, O. (1985). *Antimicrob. Agents Chemother.* **27**, 220–223.

Kaiser, G. V., Cooper, R. D. G., Koehler, R. E., Murphy, C. F., Webber, J. A., Wright, I. G., and Van Heyningen, E. M. (1970). *J. Org. Chem.* **35**, 2430–2433.

Kakeya, N., Nishimura, K., Yoshimi, A., Nakamura, S., Tamaki, S., Matsui, H., Kawamura, T., Kasai, M., Tachi, T., and Kitao, K. (1983). *In* "Program and Abstracts of the 23rd Interscience Conference on Antimicrobial Agents and Chemotherapy", Las Vegas. Abstr. 257.

Kakeya, N., Nishimura, K., Yoshimi, A., Nakamura, S., Nishizawa, S., Tamaki, S., Matsui, H., Kawamura, T., Kasai, M., and Kitao, K. (1984). *Chem. Pharm. Bull.* **32**, 692–698.

Kamei, C., Sugimoto, Y., Muroi, N., and Tasaka, K. (1986). *J. Pharm. Pharmacol.* **38**, 823–828.

Kamimura, T., Kojo, H., Matsumoto, Y., Mine, Y., Croto, S., and Kuwahara, S. (1984). *Antimicrob. Agents Chemother.* **25**, 98–104.

Karney, W., Correa-Corononas, R., Zajtchuk, R., Schwartz, J., Smith, L. P., and Tramont, E. (1983). *Antimicrob. Agents Chemother.* **24**, 85–88.

Katner, A. S. (1985). Eur. Pat. Appl. EP 138,552, 24 April.

Kato, K., Murakami, K., Yamamoto, I., Ohashi, M., Tomiguchi, A., Mochizuki, H., and Mochida, E. (1986). *In* "Program and Abstracts of the 26th Interscience Conference on Antimicrobial Agents and Chemotherapy", New Orleans. Abstr. 1303.

Kawabata, K., Miyai, K., Takasugi, H., and Takaya, T. (1986a). *Chem. Pharm. Bull.* **34**, 3458–3464.

Kawabata, K., Masugi, T., and Takaya, T. (1986b). *J. Antibiot.* **39**, 384–393.
Kawabata, K., Masugi, T., and Takaya, T. (1986c). *J. Antibiot.* **39**, 394–403.
Kawabata, K., Yamanaka, H., Takasugi, H., and Takaya, T. (1986d). *J. Antibiot.* **39**, 404–414.
Kawano, Y., Watanabe, T., Sakai, J., Watanabe, H., Nagano, M., Nishimura, T., and Miyadera, T. (1980). *Chem. Pharm. Bull.* **28**, 70–79.
Kessler, R. E., Bies, M., and Buck, R. E. (1985). *Antimicrob. Agents Chemother.* **27**, 207–216.
Kim, C. U., Misco, P. F., and McGregor, D. N. (1979). *J. Med. Chem.* **22**, 743–745.
Kim, C. U., Misco, P. F., Haynes, U. J., and McGregor, D. N. (1984). *J. Med. Chem.* **27**, 1225–1229.
Kimura, T., Endo, H., Yoshida, M., Muranishi, S., and Sezaki, H. (1978). *J. Pharmacobio. Dynamics* **1**, 262–267.
Kinast, G., Boberg, M., Metzger, K. G., and Zeiler, H. J. (1984). Ger. Offen. DE 3,239,365, 26 April.
Kirrstetter, R., Dürckheimer, W., Lattrell, R., Mencke, B., Scheunemann, K., Schwab, W., Seeger, K., and Winkler, I. (1983). In "Proceedings of the 13th International Congress of Chemotherapy" (K. Spitzy and K. Karrer, eds), Vol. 4, PS 4.2/11-3. Egermann, Wien.
Kirrstetter, R., Dürckheimer, W., Lattrell, R., and Schwab, W. (1984). Ger. Offen. DE 3,316,797, 8 November.
Kishi, M., Ishitobi, H., Nagata, W., and Tsuji, T. (1979). *Heterocycles* **13**, 197–202.
Klastersky, M. D. (ed.) (1983). "Nosocomial Infections: Current Problems and Role of the New Cephalosporins, 1983 Update". Reports on a Symposium held in Brussels on 22 April, 1983. Europrint, Brussels.
Klasterky, J., Regnier, B., and Acar, J. F. (1986). In "The Antimicrobial Agents, Ann. 1" (P. K. Peterson and J. Verhoef, eds), pp. 538–544. Elsevier, New York and Oxford.
Klesel, N., Limbert, M., Schrinner, E., Seeger, K., Seibert, G., and Winkler, I. (1984a). *Infection* **12**, 286–292.
Klesel, N., Limbert, M., Seeger, K., Seibert, G., Winkler, I., and Schrinner, E. (1984b). *J. Antibiot.* **37**, 901–909.
Klesel, N., Limbert, M., Seibert, G., Winkler, I., and Schrinner, E. (1984c). *J. Antibiot.* **37**, 1712–1718.
Klesel, N., Isert, D., Limbert, M., Seibert, G., Winkler, I., and Schrinner, E. (1986). *J. Antibiot.* **39**, 971–977.
Knothe, H., and Dette, G. A. J. (1981). *J. Antimicrob. Chemother.* **8** (Suppl. B), 33–41.
Knothe, H. (1984). In "Transferable Antibiotic Resistance" (S. Mitsuhashi and V. Krcmery, eds), pp. 37–41. Springer-Verlag, Berlin.
Knox, J. R., Bartolone, J. B., Hite, G. J., and Kelly, J. A. (1985). In "Recent Advances in the Chemistry of β-Lactam Antibiotics" (A. G. Brown and S. M. Roberts, eds), Special Publication No. 52, pp. 318–327. The Royal Society of Chemistry, London.
Kobayashi, T., Iino, K., and Hiraoka, T. (1979). *Chem. Pharm. Bull.* **27**, 2727–2734.
Kobayashi, S., Arai, S., Hayashi, S., and Fujimoto, K. (1986). *Antimicrob. Agents Chemother.* **30**, 713–718.
Kobayashi, S., Oguchi, K., Uchida, E., Yasuhara, H., Sakamoto, K., Sekine, J., and Sasahara, K. (1987). In "Program and Abstracts of 27th Interscience Conference on Antimicrobial Agents and Chemotherapy", New York. Abstr. 664.
Komai, T., Fujimoto, K., Sekine, M., and Masuda, H. (1986). In "Program and Abstracts of the 26th Interscience Conference on Antimicrobial Agents and Chemotherapy", New Orleans. Abstr. 593.
Komatsu, Y., Nagata, W., Matsuura, S., Harada, Y., Yoshida, T., and Kuwahara, S. (1984). In "Program and Abstracts of the 24th Interscience Conference on Antimicrobial Agents and Chemotherapy", Washington. Abstr. 645.

Komiya, I., Yoshida, T., Matsumoto, T., Yamamoto, Y., Sakagami, K., Atsumi, K., Nishio, M., Kazuno, Y., Fukatsu, S., and Mitsuhashi, S. (1985). *In* "Program and Abstracts of the 25th Interscience Conference on Antimicrobial Agents and Chemotherapy", Minneapolis. Abstr. 583.

König, H. B., and Metzger, K. G. (1981). Ger. Offen. DE 3,021,373, 17 December.

Koppel, G. A., and Koehler, R. E. (1973). *J. Am. Chem. Soc.* **95**, 2403–2404.

Koppel, G. A., Kinnick, M. D., and Nummy, L. J. (1977). *J. Am. Chem. Soc.* **99**, 2821–2822.

Koup, J. R., Stoeckel, K., Kneer, J., and Dubach, U. C. (1987). *In* "Abstracts of the 15th International Congress of Chemotherapy", Istanbul. Abstr. 445.

Koupal, L. R., Weissberger, B., Shungu, L. D., Weinberg, E., and Gadebusch, H. H. (1987). *J. Antibiot.* **40**, 354–362.

Kuck, N. A., Curran, W. V., and Testa, R. T. (1985). *In* "Proceedings of the 14th International Congress of Chemotherapy" (J. Ishigami, ed.), Vol. 2, pp. 1137–1138. University of Tokyo Press, Tokyo.

Kuhlmann, J. (1981). *Deutsche Apotheker Zeitung* **121**, 1765–1771.

Kukolja, S. (1976). *In* "Recent Advances in the Chemistry of β-Lactam Antibiotics" (J. Elks, ed.), Special Publication No. 28, pp. 181–188. The Royal Society of Chemistry, London.

Kukolja, S., and Chauvette, R. R. (1982). *In* "Chemistry and Biology of β-Lactam Antibiotics" (R. B. Morin and M. Gorman, eds), Vol. 1, pp. 93–198. Academic Press, New York and London.

Kukolja, S., and Wright, E. (1987). Eur. Pat. Appl. EP 211,526, 25 February.

Kukolja, S., Lammert, S. P., Gleissner, M. R. B., and Ellis, A. I. (1976). *J. Am. Chem. Soc.* **98**, 5040–5041.

Kukolja, S., Draheim, S. E., Pfeil, J. L., Cooper, R. D. G., Graves, B. J., Holmes, R. E., Neel, D. A., Huffman, G. W., Webber, J. A., Kinnick, M. D., Vasileff, R. T., and Foster, B. J. (1985a). *J. Med. Chem.* **28**, 1886–1896.

Kukolja, S., Draheim, S. E., Graves, B. J., Hunden, D. C., Pfeil, J. L., Cooper, R. D. G., Ott, J. L., and Counter, F. T. (1985b). *J. Med. Chem.* **28**, 1896–1903.

Kukolja, S., Pfeil, J. L., Draheim, S. E., and Ott, J. L. (1985c). *J. Med. Chem.* **28**, 1903–1906.

Kühn, K., and Zimmermann, R. (1986). *Deutsche Apotheker Zeitung* **126**, 1991–1999, and references cited therein.

Lakings, D. B., Novak, E., Friis, J. M., *et al.* (1986). *Antimicrob. Agents Chemother.* **29**, 271–277.

Lam, C., Laber, G., Hildebrandt, J., Wenzel, A., Turnowsky, F., and Schütze, E. (1984). *Drugs Exp. Clin. Res.* **10**, 703–711.

Lattrell, R., Wieduwilt, M., Dürckheimer, W., Blumbach, J., and Seeger, K. (1982). Eur. Pat. Appl. EP 64,740, 17 November.

Lattrell, R., Dürckheimer, W., Klesel, N., Kirrstetter, R., Seibert, G., and Wieduwilt, M. (1983a). *In* "Proceedings of the 13th International Congress of Chemotherapy" (K. Spitzky and K. Karrer, eds), Vol. 4, PS 4.2/11-1. Egermann, Wien.

Lattrell, R., Kirrstetter, R., Schwab, W., Dürckheimer, W., and Seibert, G. (1983b). Ger. Offen. DE 3,207,840, 15 September.

Lattrell, R., Kirrstetter, R., Dürckheimer, W., Schwab, W., and Klesel, N. (1984). Ger. Offen. DE 3,247,614, 5 July.

Lattrell, R., Blumbach, J., Dürckheimer, W., Schwab, W., and Seeger, K. (1985). Eur. Pat. Appl. EP 137,442, 17 April.

Lattrell, R., Dürckheimer, W., Kirrstetter, R., and Seibert, G. (1987). Ger. Offen. DE 3,539,901, 5 May.

Lauderdale, B. L., Yu, P. K. W., and Washington, J. A. (1986). *Antimicrob. Agents Chemother.* **29**, 560–564.

LeFrock, J. L., Prince, R. A., and Leff, R. D. (1982). *Pharmacother.* **2**, 174–184.

Leitner, F., Pursiano, T. A., Chisholm, D. R., Tsai, Y. H., Buck, R. E., and Misiek, M. (1983). *In* "Program and Abstracts of the 23rd Interscience Conference on Antimicrobial Agents and Chemotherapy", Las Vegas. Abstr. 575.

Leitner, F., Buck, R. E., Pursiano, T. A., Misiek, M., Kessler, R. E., and Price, K. E. (1985). *In* "Proceedings of the 14th International Congress of Chemotherapy" (J. Ishigami, ed.), Vol. 2, pp. 1153–1154. University of Tokyo Press, Tokyo.

Leitner, F., Pursiano, T. A., Buck, R. E., Tsai, Y. H., Chisholm, D. R., and Kessler, R. E. (1987). *Antimicrob. Agents Chemother.* **31**, 238–243.

Leone, C. A., Mosca, F., Borghese, M., and Cione, P. (1982). *Otorinolaringologia* **32**, 391–398.

Limbert, M., and Seibert, G. (1986). *In* "Protein Binding and Drug Transport" (J.-P. Tillement and E. Lindenlaub, eds), pp. 249–252. Schattauer Verlag, Stuttgart and New York.

Limbert, M., Seibert, G., and Schrinner, E. (1982). *Infection* **10**, 97–101.

Limbert, J., Klesel, N., Seeger, G., Seibert, G., Winkler, I., and Schrinner, E. (1984a). *J. Antibiot.* **37**, 892–900.

Limbert, M., Bartlett, R. R., Dickneite, G., Klesel, N., Schorlemmer, H. U., Seibert, G. Winkler, I., and Schrinner, E. (1984b). *J. Antibiot.* **37**, 1719–1726.

Lode, H., Stahlmann, R., and Koeppe, P. (1979). *Antimicrob. Agents Chemother.* **16**, 1–6.

Looker, B. E., and Paternoster, I. L. (1985). *In* "Recent Advances in the Chemistry of β-Lactam Antibiotics" (A. G. Brown and S. M. Roberts, eds), Special Publication No. 52, pp. 346–349. The Royal Society of Chemistry, London.

Lunn, W. H. W. (1983). Ger. Offen. DE 3,233,376, 24 March.

Lunn, W. H. W., and Shadle, J. K. (1982). Eur. Pat. Appl. EP 60,144, 15 September.

Lunn, W. H. W., and Shadle, J. K. (1983). Ger. Offen. DE 3,233,377, 24 March.

Lunn, W. H. W., and Vasileff, R. T. (1983). Eur. Pat. Appl. EP 74,268, 16 March.

Lunn, W. H. W., and Wheeler, W. J. (1983). US Pat. Appl. US 4,379,787, 12 April.

Maaß, L., Malerczyk, V., Verho, M., Hajdu, P., Seeger, K., and Klesel, N. (1987a). *Infection* **15**, 202–206.

Maaß, L., Malerczyk, V., and Verho, M. (1987b). *Infection* **15**, 207–210.

Maier, R., Wetzel, B., Woitun, E., Reuter, W., Lechner, U., and Appel, K.-R. (1986). *Arzneim. Forsch.* **36** (II), 1297–1300.

Malerczyk, V., Maaß, L., Verho, M., Hajdu, P., Klesel, N., and Rangoonwala, R. (1987). *Infection* **15**, 211–214.

Malouin, F., and Bryan, L. E. (1986). *Antimicrob. Agents Chemother.* **30**, 1–5.

Martin, J. F., Lopez-Nieto, M. J., Castro, J. F., Cortes, J., Romero, J., Ramos, F. R., Cantoral, J. M., Alvarez, E., Dominguez, M. G., Barredo, J. L., and Liras, P. (1986). *In* "Regulation of Secondary Metabolite Formation" (H. Kleinkauf, H. von Döhren, H. Dornauer and G. Nesemann, eds), pp. 41–75. VCH Verlagsgesellschaft, Weinheim.

Mastalerz, H., and Vinet, V. (1987). *J. Chem. Soc., Chem. Commun.*, 1283–1284.

Matsuda, A., and Ichikomaton, K. (1985). *J. Bacteriol.* **163**, 1222–1228.

Matsumura, K., Akagi, H., Suzuki, D., and Shimbayashi, A. (1987). Eur. Pat. Appl. EP 214,600, 18 March.

Mazzeo, P., and Romeo, A. (1972). *J. Chem. Soc. Perkin* I, 2532.

McCombie, S. W., Metz, W. A., and Afonso, A. (1986). *Tetrahedron Lett.* **27**, 305–308.

McShane, L. J. (1985). Eur. Pat. Appl. EP 132,394, 30 January.

McShane, L. J., and Dunigan, J. M. (1986). *Synth. Comm.* **16**, 649–652.

Micetich, R. G., Singh, R., and Maiti, S. N. (1984). *Heterocycles* **22**, 531–535.

Milner, P. H. (1984). PCT Int. Appl. WO 8402, 911, 2 August.

Minami, I., Akimoto, H., Kondo, M., and Nomura, H. (1983). *Chem. Pharm. Bull.* **31**, 482–489.

Mine, Y., Yokota, Y., Kamimura, T., Tawara, T., and Shibayama, F. (1987). *In* "Program and Abstracts of the 27th Interscience Conference on Antimicrobial Agents and Chemotherapy", New York. Abstr. 653.

Miskolczi, I., Sztaricskai, F., and Bognar, R. (1981). *Org. Prep. Proc. Int.* **13**, 315–322.

Mitsuhashi, S. (ed.) (1981). "β-Lactam Antibiotics", Japanese Scientific Society Press, Tokyo.

Mitsuhashi, S., and Ochiai, M. (1985). *Chemotherapy (Tokyo)* **33**, 519–527.

Mittermayer, H. (1986). *Eur. J. Clin. Microbiol.* **5**, 530–534.

Miyake, A., Kondo, M., and Fujino, M. (1985). Eur. Pat. Appl. EP 164,113, 11 December.

Mizokami, N., Fukase, H., Horii, S., and Kuwada, Y. (1983). *Chem. Pharm. Bull.* **31**, 1482–1493.

Mobashery, S., and Johnston, M. (1986a). *J. Org. Chem.* **51**, 4723–4726.

Mobashery, S., and Johnston, M. (1986b). *Tetrahedron Lett.* **27**, 3333–3336.

Mobashery, S., Lerner, S. A., and Johnston, M. (1986). *J. Am. Chem. Soc.* **108**, 1685–1686.

Mochida, K., Ono, Y., Yamasaki, M., Shiraki, C., and Hirata, T. (1987). *J. Antibiot.* **40**, 182–189.

Mochizuki, H., Oikawa, Y., Inaba, H., Kato, K., Murakami, K., and Mochida, E. (1986). *In* "Program and Abstracts of the 26th Interscience Conference on Antimicrobial Agents and Chemotherapy", New Orleans. Abstr. 1304.

Monguzzi, R., Pinza, M., Pifferi, G., Visconti, M., and Broccali, G. (1985). *Il Farmaco-Ed. Sci.* **40**, 956–969.

Morin, R. B., and Gorman, M. (eds) (1982), "Chemistry and Biology of β-Lactam Antibiotics", Vols 1–3. Academic Press, New York and London.

Morin, J. M. Jr, and Leonard, N. J. (1986). Eur. Pat. Appl. EP 186,463, 2 July.

Morin, R. B., Jackson, B. G., Flynn, E. H., and Roeske, R. W. (1962a). *J. Am. Chem. Soc.* **84**, 3400–3401.

Morin, R. B., Jackson, B. G., Mueller, R. A., Lavagnino, E. R., Scanlon, W. B., and Andrews, S. L. (1962b). *J. Am. Chem. Soc.* **85**, 1896–1897.

Müller, B. (1981). Eur. Pat. Appl. EP 37,797, 14 October.

Müller, B., and Csendes, I. (1982). Eur. Pat. Appl. EP 47,977, 24 March.

Müller, B., Heinrich, P., Schneider, P., and Bickel, H. (1975). *Helv. Chim. Acta* **58**, 2469–2473.

Münchener Medizinische Wochenschrift (1981). **123** (Suppl. 2).

Muranushi, N., Yoshikawa, T., Nishiuchi, M., Oguma, T., Hirano, K., and Yamada, H. (1987). *J. Pharmacobiodyn.* **10**, s-72.

Murphy, C. F., and Webber, J. A. (1972). *In* "Cephalosporins and Penicillins" (E. H. Flynn, ed.), pp. 134–182. Academic Press, New York and London.

Nagano, K., Murakami, Y., Hara, R., Nakano, K., Koda, A., Maeda, T., Shibanuma, T., Yamazaki, A., and Matsui, H. (1986a). Jpn. Kokai Tokkyo Koho, JP 61,106,580, 24 May.

Nagano, K., Murakami, Y., Hara, R., Nakano, K., Koda, A., Maeda, T., Shibanuma, T., Yamazaki, A., and Matsui, H. (1986b). Jpn. Kokai Tokkyo Koho, JP 61,176,592, 8 August.

Nagano, N., Nakano, K., Shibanuma, T., Murakami, Y., and Hara, R. (1987). *J. Antibiot.* **40**, 173–181.

Nagarajan, R., Boeck, L. D., Gorman, M., Hamill, R. L., Higgins, C. E., Hoehn, M. M., Stark, W. M., and Whitney, J. G. (1971). *J. Am. Chem. Soc.* **93**, 2308–2310.

Nagakura, I. (1981). *Heterocycles* **16**, 1495–1498.

Nagata, W., Otsuka, H., Narisada, M., Yoshida, T., Horada, Y., and Yamada, H. (1981). *Med. Res. Rev.* **1**, 217–248.

Nagata, W. (1982). *In* "Current Trends in Organic Synthesis" (H. Nozaki, ed.), pp. 83–100. Pergamon Press, Oxford and New York (and references cited therein).

Naito, T., Hoshi, H., Abe, Y., Aburaki, S., Okumura, J., and Kawaguchi, H. (1985). *In* "Proceedings of the 14th International Congress of Chemotherapy" (J. Ishigami, ed.), Vol. 2, pp. 1149–1150. University of Tokyo Press, Tokyo.

Naito, T., Aburaki, S., Kamachi, H., Narita, Y., Okumura, J., and Kawaguchi, H. (1986a). *J. Antibiot.* **39**, 1092–1107.

Naito, T., Yokoyama, M., Sasaki, K., Yamamoto, M., and Amemiya, K. (1986b). Eur. Pat. Appl. EP 178,527, 23 April.

Naito, T., Hoshi, H., Aburaki, S., Abe, Y., Okumura, J., Tomatsu, K., and Kawaguchi, H. (1987). *J. Antibiot.* **40**, 991–1005.

Nakabayashi, S., Akita, E., Iwamatsu, K., Shudo, K., and Okamoto, T. (1982). *Tetrahedron Lett.* **23**, 4267–4268.

Nakagawa, S., Ushijima, R., Nakano, F., Ban, N., Yamada, K., and Asai, A. (1985). *In* "Program and Abstracts of the 25th Interscience Conference on Antimicrobial Agents and Chemotherapy", Minneapolis. Abstr. 363.

Nakagawa, S., Sanada, M., Matsuda, K., Hazumi, N., and Tanaka, N. (1987). *Antimicrob. Agents Chemother.* **31**, 1100–1105.

Nakano, H. (1981). *Med. Res. Rev.* **1**, 127–157.

Nakashima, E., Tsuji, A., Kagatani, S., and Yamana, T. (1984a). *J. Pharmacobio. Dynamics* **7**, 452–464.

Nakashima, E., Tsuji, A., Mizuo, H., and Yamana, T. (1984b). *Biochem. Pharmac.* **33**, 3345–3352.

Nakashima, M., Hashimoto, H., Takiguchi, Y., Mizuno, A., Watanabe, K., and Ueno, K. (1986a). *Chemotherapy (Tokyo)* **34** (Suppl. 3), 133–148.

Nakashima, M., Iida, M., Yoshida, T., Kitagawa, T., Oguma, T., and Ishi, H. (1986b). *In* "Program and Abstracts of the 26th Interscience Conference on Antimicrobial Agents and Chemotherapy", New Orleans. Abstr. 591.

Nakashima, M., Uematsu, T., Mizuno, A., Takiguchi, Y., and Kanamaru, M. (1987). *In* "Program and Abstracts of the 27th Interscience Conference on Antimicrobial Agents and Chemotherapy", New York. Abstr. 642.

Nakayama, I., Nagano, N., Nakano, K., Shibanuma, T., Murakami, Y., and Susaki, S. (1984). *In* "Program and Abstracts of the 24th Interscience Conference on Antimicrob. Agents and Chemotherapy", Washington. Abstr. 737.

Nannini, G., Perrone, E., Severino, D., Bedeschi, A., and Biasoli, G. (1981a). *J. Antibiot.* **34**, 412–426.

Nannini, G., Perrone, E., Severino, D., Casabuona, F., Bedeschi, A., Buzzetti, F., Giraldi, P. N., Meinardi, G., Monti, G., Ceriani, A., and De Carneri, I. (1981b). *J. Antibiot.* **34**, 1456–1468.

Narisada, M., Yoshida, T., Onoue, H., Ohtani, M., Okada, T., Tsuji, T., Kikkawa, I., Haga, N., Satoh, H., Itani, H., and Nagata, W. (1979). *J. Med. Chem.* **22**, 757–759.

Narisada, M., Hamashima, Y., Matsumura, H., Matsuma, S., Nagata, W., and Yoshida, T. (1981). *In* "Recent Advances in the Chemistry of β-Lactam Antibiotics" (G. I. Gregory, ed.), Special Publication No. 38, pp. 57–79. The Royal Society of Chemistry, London.

Narisada, M., Nishikawa, J., Watanabe, F., and Terui, Y. (1987). *J. Med. Chem.* **30**, 514–522.

Narita, Y., Iimura, S., Okumura, J., Naito, T. and Aburaki, S. (1984). Ger. Offen. DE 3,404,615, 16 August.

Neu, H. C. (1982a). *Ann. Int. Med.* **97**, 408–419.

Neu, H. C. (1982b). *Ann. Rev. Pharmacol. Toxicol.* **22**, 599–642

Neu, H. C. (1982c). *Lancet* **2/8292**, 252–255.

Neu, H. C. (ed.) (1982d). "New β-Lactam Antibiotics: A Review from Chemistry to Clinical Efficacy of the New Cephalosporins", Symposia on Frontiers of Pharmacology Vol. I.

Francis Clark Wood Institute for the History of Medicine, College of Physicians of Philadelphia, Philadelphia.

Neu, H. C. (1984a). *Bull. N.Y. Acad. Med.* **60**, 327–339.

Neu, H. C. (1984b). *Pharmacotherapy* **4**, 47–60.

Neu, H. C. (1984c). *Scand. J. Infect. Dis.* (Suppl.) **42**, 7–16.

Neu, H. C. (1984d). *J. Antimicrob. Chemother.* **14** (Suppl. B), 1–12.

Neu, H. C. (1985). *Am. J. Med.* **79** (Suppl. 2A), 2–13.

Neu, H. C., and Chin, N.-X. (1986). *Antimicrob. Agents Chemother.* **30**, 638–644.

Neu, H. C., Chin, N. X., and Labthavikul, P. (1985a). *Infection* **13**, 146–155.

Neu, H. C., Labthavikul, P., and Chin, N. X. (1985b). *In* "Program and Abstracts of the 25th Interscience Conference on Antimicrobial Agents and Chemotherapy", Minneapolis. Abstr. 357.

Neu, H. C., Chin, N. X., and Labthavikul, P. (1986a). *Antimicrob. Agents Chemother.* **30**, 423–428.

Neu, H. C., Chin, N. X., Jules, K., and Labthavikul, P. (1986b). *J. Antimicrob. Chemother.* **17**, 441–452.

Newall, C. E. (1985). *In* "Recent Advances in the Chemistry of β-Lactam Antibiotics" (A. G. Brown and S. M. Roberts, eds), Special Publication No. 52, pp. 1–17. The Royal Society of Chemistry, London.

Newall, C. E., and Tonge, A. P. (1982). *J. Antibiot.* **35**, 1404–1406.

Newman, N. (1985). *Drugs Exp. Clin. Res.* **11**, 421–426.

Nikaido, H. (1985). *Pharmac. Ther.* **27**, 197–231.

Nishida, M., Murakawa, T., Kamimura, T., Okada, N., Sakamoto, H., Fukuda, S., Nakamoto, S., Yokata, Y., and Miki, K. (1976). *J. Antibiot.* **29**, 444–459.

Nishide, K., Kobori, T., Tunemoto, D., and Kondo, K. (1987). *Heterocycles* **26**, 633–640.

Nishikawa, J., and Tori, K. (1984). *J. Med. Chem.* **27**, 1657–1663.

Nishikawa, J., Watanabe, F., Shudou, M., Terui, Y., and Narisada, M. (1987). *J. Med. Chem.* **30**, 523–527.

Nishimura, H. (1986). Jpn. Kokai Tokkyo Koho JP 1053-289-A, 17 March.

Nishimura, T., Yoshimura, Y., Miyake, A., Yamaoka, M., Takanohashi, K., Hamaguchi, N., Hirai, S., Yashiki, T., and Numata, M. (1987). *J. Antibiot.* **40**, 81–90.

Nishino, T., Obana, Y., Gotoh, T., Ohtsuki, M., Kitagawa, H., and Tanaka, K. (1986). *Chemotherapy (Tokyo)* **34** (Suppl. 3), 79–95.

Noble, J. T., and Barza, M. (1985). *Drugs* **30**, 175–181.

Norden, C. W., and Neiderriter, K. (1987). *Chemotherapy (Basel)* **33**, 15–17.

Noshikawa, T., Muranushi, N., Yoshida, M., Oguma, T., Hirano, K., and Yamada, H. (1987). *J. Pharmacobiodyn.* **10**, s-142.

Noto, T., Nehashi, T., Endo, H., Saito, M., Matsubara, S., Harada, Y., Suzuki, S., Ogawa, H., and Koyama, K. (1976). *J. Antibiot.* **29**, 1058–1070.

Nozaki, Y., Okonogi, K., Katayama, N., Ono, H., Harada, S., Kondo, M., and Okazaki, H. (1984). *J. Antibiot.* **37**, 1555–1565.

Nozaki, Y., Katayama, N., Tsubotani, S., Ono, H., and Okazaki, H. (1985). *J. Antibiot.* **38**, 1141–1151.

O'Callaghan, C. H., and Harper, P. B. (1985). *Fortschr. Antimikrob. Antineopl. Chemotherapie* **4**, 555–564.

Ochiai, M., Morimoto, A., Matsushita, Y., Kaneko, T., and Kida, M. (1980a). *J. Antibiot.* **33**, 1005–1013.

Ochiai, M., Morimoto, A., Okada, T., Matsushita, Y., Yamamoto, H., Aki, O., and Kida, M. (1980b). *J. Antibiot.* **33**, 1022–1030.

Ochiai, M., Morimoto, A., Matsushita, Y., and Okada, T. (1981a). *J. Antibiot.* **34**, 160–170.

Ochiai, M., Morimoto, A., Miyawaki, T., Matsushita, Y., Okada, T., Natsugari, H., and Kida, M. (1981b). *J. Antibiot.* **34**, 171–185.

Ochiai, M., Morimoto, A., and Miyawaki, T. (1981c). *J. Antibiot.* **34**, 186–192.

Ohi, N., Aoki, B., Shinozaki, T., Moro, K., Kuroki, T., Noto, T., Nehashi, T., Matsumoto, M., Okazaki, H., and Matsunaga, I. (1987). *Chem. Pharm. Bull.* **35**, 1903–1909.

Ohkawa, M., Nakashima, T., Shoda, R., Ikeda, A., Orito, M., and Sawaki, M. (1984). *Chemotherapy (Tokyo)* **32**, 811–818.

Ohnishi, H. (1984). *Antimicrob. Agents Chemother.* **25**, 88–92.

Oka, M., Yamashita, H., Naito, T., and Okumura, J. (1985). Ger. Offen. DE 3,512,225, 17 October.

Okada, K., Murakami, Y., and Kinoshita, H. (1981). *Chemotherapy (Tokyo)* **31** (Suppl. 1), 516–527.

Okamoto, R., Tamura, A., Inoue, M., Kondo, S., and Mitsuhashi, S. (1986). *In* "Program and Abstracts of the 26th Interscience Conference on Antimicrobial Agents and Chemotherapy", New Orleans. Abstr. 1301.

Okamoto, S., Hamana, Y., Inoue, M., and Mitsuhashi, S. (1987). *Antimicrob. Agents Chemother.* **31**, 1111–1116.

Okano, T., Inui, K., Takano, M., and Hori, R. (1986a). *Biochem. Pharmac.* **35**, 1781–1786.

Okano, T., Inui, K., Maegawa, H., Takano, M., and Hori, R. (1986b). *J. Biol. Chem.* **261**, 14,130–14,134.

Okano, T., Maegawa, H., Takano, M., Inui, T., and Hori, R. (1987). *J. Pharmacobiodyn.* **10**, s-141.

Okubadejo, O., and Bax, R. P. (1982). *J. Antimicrob. Chemother.* **9**, 86.

Omura, S. (1986). *Microbiol. Rev.* **50**, 259–279.

Ono, H., Nozaki, Y., Katamaya, N., and Okazaki, H. (1984). *J. Antibiot.* **37**, 1528–1535.

Page, M. I. (1984). *Acc. Chem. Res.* **17**, 144–151.

Page, M. I., and Proctor, P. (1984). *J. Am. Chem. Soc.* **106**, 3820–3825.

Palomo-Coll, A., Palomo-Coll, A. L., and Palomo-Nicolau, C. (1985). *Tetrahedron* **41**, 5133–5139.

Patel, I. H., Chen, S., Parsonnet, M., Hackman, M. R., Brooks, M. A., Konikoff, J., and Kaplan, S. A. (1981). *Antimicrob. Agents. Chemother.* **20**, 634–641.

Patel, I. H., and Kaplan, S. A. (1984). *Am. J. Med.* **77**, 17–25.

Pearson, M. J., and Branch, C. L. (1982). *Tetrahedron Lett.* **23**, 3003–3006.

Pearson, M. J., and Branch, C. L. (1983). *Tetrahedron Lett.* **24**, 1649–1652.

Pearson, M. J., and Branch, C. L. (1986). *J. Chem. Soc., Perkin Trans.* **I**, 1097–1100.

Pearson, M. J., Branch, C. L., and Finch, S. C. (1982). *Tetrahedron Lett.* **23**, 4381–4384.

Pelak, B. A., Gilfillan, E. C., Weissberger, B., and Gadebusch, H. H. (1987). *J. Antibiot.* **40**, 354–362.

Perlman, D. (ed.) (1977). "Structure–Activity Relationships among the Semisynthetic Antibiotics". Academic Press, New York and London.

Perrone, E., Alpegiani, M., Giudici, F., Buzzetti, F., and Nannini, G. (1984a). *J. Antibiot.* **37**, 1423–1440.

Perrone, E., Alpegiani, M., Giudici, F., Bedeschi, A., Pelazzato, R., and Nannini, G. (1984b). *J. Heterocyclic Chem.* **21**, 1097–1111.

Perrone, E., Alpegiani, M., Bedeschi, A., and Franceschi, G. (1984c). *Tetrahedron Lett.* **25**, 4167–4170.

Perrone, E., Alpegiani, M., Bedeschi, A., and Franceschi, G. (1986). *Tetrahedron Lett.* **27**, 3041–3044.

Peter, H., and Bickel, H. (1974). *Helv. Chim. Acta* **57**, 2044–2054.

Peterson, P. K., and Verhoef, J. (eds) (1986). "The Antimicrobial Agents Annual/1", Elsevier, Amsterdam, New York and Oxford.

Peyronel, J. F., Moutonnier, C., and Plau, B. (1985). *In* "Recent Advances in the Chemistry of β-Lactam Antibiotics" (A. G. Brown and S. M. Roberts, eds), Special Publication No. 52, pp. 336–341. The Royal Society of Chemistry, London.

Pfeil, J. L., Draheim, S. E., Counter, F. T., Kukolja, S., and Ott, J. L. (1987). *In* "Program and Abstracts of the 27th Interscience Conference on Antimicrobial Agents and Chemotherapy", New York. Abstr. 804.

Phillips, I., Warren, C., Shannon, K., King, A., and Hanslo, D. J. (1981). *J. Antimicrob. Chemother.* **8** (Suppl. B), 23–31.

Polacek, I., and Starke, B. (1980). *J. Antibiot.* **33**, 1031–1036.

Prager, B. C., and Sturm, H. (1986). Eur. Pat. Appl. EP 204,657, 5 May.

Presslitz, I. E. (1978). *Antimicrob. Agents Chemother.* **14**, 144–150.

Price, K. E., and McGregor, D. N. (1984). *Scand. J. Infect. Dis.* **42** (Suppl.), 50–63.

Quay, J. F., Coleman, D. L., Finch, L. S., Indelicato, J. M., Pasini, C. E., Shoufler, J. R., Sullivan, H. R., and Turner, J. C. (1987). *In* "Program and Abstracts of the 27th Interscience Conference on Antimicrobial Agents and Chemotherapy", New York. Abstr. 1205.

Quintiliani, R., French, M., and Nightingale, C. H. (1982). *Med. Clin. North Am.* **66**, 183–197.

Reiner, R. (1986). *Drugs Exp. Clin. Res.* **12**, 299–302.

Reiner, R., and Weiss, U. (1982). Eur. Pat. Appl. EP 49,855, 21 April.

Riess, W., Meyer-Brunot, H. G., and Brechbuehler, S. (1982). *Fortschr. Antimicrob. Antineoplast. Chemother.* **1**, 115–131.

Richards, D. M., and Brogden, R. N. (1985). *Drugs* **29**, 105–161.

Richards, D. M., and Heel, R. C. (1985). *Drugs* **29**, 281–329.

Richards, D. M., Heel, R. C., Brogden, R. N., Speight, T. M., and Avery, G. S. (1984). *Drugs* **27**, 469–527.

Rolinson, G. N. (1986). *J. Antimicrob. Chemother.* **17**, 5–36.

Rosati, R. L., Kapili, L. V., and Morrissey, P. (1982). *J. Am. Chem. Soc.* **104**, 4262–4264.

Ross, B. C., Daniels, N. J., Johnson, G., and Yeomans, M. A. (1982). *J. Chem. Soc., Chem. Comm.*, 3373–3377.

Rouan, M.-C., Lecaillon, J.-B., Guibert, J., Modai, J., and Schoeller, J. P. (1985). Antimicrob. Agents Chemother. **27**, 177–180.

Ruf, B. (1982). *Infection* **10**, 76–80.

Sadaki, H., Narita, H., Imaizumi, H., Konishi, Y., Inaba, T., Hirakawa, T., Taki, H., Tai, M., Watanabe, Y., and Saikawa, I. (1982). Ger. Offen. DE 3,137,854, 15 April.

Sadaki, H., Imaizumi, H., Inaba, T., Hirakawa, T., Murrotani, Y., and Saikawa, I. (1986a). *J. Pharm. Soc. Jpn* **106**, 117–122.

Sadaki, H., Imaizumi, H., Inaba, T., Hirakawa, T., Murrotani, Y., Watanabe, Y., Minami, S., and Saikawa, I. (1986b). *J. Pharm. Soc. Jpn* **106**, 129–146.

Sadaki, H., Imaizumi, H., Inaba, T., Hirakawa, T., Murotani, Y., Watanabe, Y., Minami, S., and Saikawa, I. (1986c). *J. Pharm. Soc. Jpn* **106**, 147–153.

Saikawa, I., Takano, S., Momonoi, K., Takamura, I., Tanaka, K., and Kutani, C. (1985). *Chem. Pharm. Bull.* **33**, 5534–5538.

Saikawa, I., Nakajima, Y., Tai, M., Sakai, H., Demachi, K., Kajita, T., Hayakawa, H., Onoda, M., Fukuda, H., and Sadaki, H. (1986). *J. Pharm. Soc. Jpn* **106**, 478–490.

Saito, A. (1987). *In* "Program and Abstracts of the 27th Interscience Conference on Antimicrobial Agents and Chemotherapy", New York. Abstr. 665.

Sakagami, K., Mishina, T., Kuroda, T., Hatanaka, M., and Ishimaru, T. (1983). *J. Antibiot.* **36**, 1205–1210.

Sakagami, K., Atsumi, K., Nishihata, K., Yoshida, T., and Fukatsu, S. (1986). Eur. Pat. Appl. EP 168 327, 15 January.

Sakane, K., Kamimura, T., Yokota, Y., Matsumoto, Y., Mine, Y., Kikuchi, H., Goto, J., and Kuwahara, S. (1984). In "Abstracts of the 24th Interscience Conference on Antimicrobial Agents and Chemotherapy", Washington. Abstr. 731.

Sakane, K., Goto, J., Takasugi, H., Teraji, T., and Takaya, T. (1985). J. Pharmacobiodyn. 8, 170.

Sakamoto, H., Shibayama, F., and Mine, Y. (1987). In "Program and Abstracts of the 27th Interscience Conference on Antimicrobial Agents and Chemotherapy", New York. Abstr. 654.

Salhi, A., Combes, T., Labeuw, B., Drigues, P., and Roche, G. (1986). In "Program and Abstracts of the 26th Interscience Conference on Antimicrobial Agents and Chemotherapy", New Orleans. Abstr. 1311.

Saltiel, E., and Brogden, R. N. (1986). Drugs 32, 222–259.

Salton, M., and Shockman, G. D. (eds) (1981). "β-Lactam-Antibiotics—Mode of Action, New Developments and Future Prospects". Academic Press, New York.

Sammes, P. G. (1976). Chem. Rev. 1, 113–155.

Sammes, P. G. (ed.) (1980). "Topics in Antibiotic Chemistry", Vol. 4, pp. 13–100. Ellis Horwood, Chichester.

Sanada, M., Hazumi, N., Matuda, K., and Nakagawa, S. (1985). In "Program and Abstracts of the 25th Interscience Conference on Antimicrobial Agents and Chemotherapy", Minneapolis. Abstr. 364.

Sanada, M., Matsuda, K., and Tanaka, N. (1987). In "Program and Abstracts of the 27th Interscience Conference on Antimicrobial Agents and Chemotherapy", New York. Abstr. 646.

Sanders, C. C. (1984). J. Antimicrob. Chemother. 13, 1–3.

Sanders, C. C., and Sanders, W. E. Jr (1986a). In "The Antimicrobial Agents Annual/1" (P. K. Petersen and J. Verhoef, eds), pp. 66–90. Elsevier, Amsterdam, New York and Oxford.

Sanders, C. C., and Sanders, W. E. Jr (1986b). In "The Antimicrobial Agents Annual/1" (P. K. Peterson and J. Verhoef, eds), pp. 72–73. Elsevier, Amsterdam, New York and Oxford.

Sassiver, M. L., and Shepherd, R. G. (1969). Tetrahedron Lett., 3993–3996.

Sassiver, M. L., and Lewis, A. (1977). In "Structure–Activity Relationships among the Semisynthetic Antibiotics" (D. Perlman, ed.), p. 129. Academic Press, New York, San Francisco and London.

Satoh, H., and Tsuji, T. (1984). Tetrahedron Lett. 25, 1737–1740.

Sattler, F. R., Weitekamp, M. R., and Ballard, J. O. (1986). Ann. Intern. Med. 105, 924–931.

Sawae, Y., Eto, K., and Ueda, S. (1987). In "Program and Abstracts of the 27th Interscience Conference on Antimicrobial Agents and Chemotherapy", New York. Abstr. 666.

Scartazzini, R., Schneider, P., and Bickel, H. (1975). Helv. Chim. Acta 58, 2437–2450.

Scartazzini, R., and Bickel, H. (1977). Heterocycles 7, 1165–1188.

Scartazzini, R. (1983). Eur. Pat. Appl. EP 76,452, 13 April.

Scartazzini, R., and Bickel, H. (1983). US Patent 4,405,778, 20 September.

Schäfer-Korting, M., Korting, H. C., Maaß, L., Klesel, N., Grigoleit, H.-G., and Mutschler, E. (1986). Eur. J. Clin. Pharmacol. 30, 295–298.

Schröck, W., and Kinast, G. (1983). Tetrahedron Lett. 24, 283–286.

Schwab, W., Dürckheimer, W., Lattrell, R., Limbert, M., Seibert, G., and Wieduwilt, M. (1983). In "Proceedings of the 13th International Congress of Chemotherapy" (K. Spitzy and K. Karrer, eds), Vol. 4, PS 4.2/11-2. Egermann, Wien.

Schwarz, U., Seeger, K., Wengenmayer, F., and Strecker, H. (1981). *FEMS Microbiol. Lett.* **10**, 107.

Seeger, K., Dürckheimer, W., Wengenmeyer, F., and Strecker, H. (1983). *Drugs Exp. Clin. Res.* **9**, 427–431.

Seibert, G., Klesel, N., Limbert, M., Schrinner, E., Seeger, K., Winkler, I., Lattrell, R., Blumbach, J., Dürckheimer, W., Fleischmann, K., Kirrstetter, R., Mencke, B., Ross, B. C., Scheunemann, K.-H., Schwab, W., and Wieduwilt, M. (1983a). *Arzneim. Forsch./ Drug Res.* **33**, 1084–1086.

Seibert, G., Limbert, M., Winkler, I., and Dick, T. (1983b). *Infection* **11**, 275–279.

Shibanuma, T., Nakano, K., Nagano, N., Murakami, Y., and Hara, R. (1984). Eur. Pat. Appl. EP 112,164, 27 June.

Shibanuma, T., Nagano, N., Hara, R., Nakano, K., Koda, A., Yamazaki, A., and Murakami, Y. (1985). Eur. Pat. Appl. EP 142,274, 22 May.

Shibahara, S., Okonogi, T., Murai, Y., Kudo, T., Yoshida, T., Nishihata, K., and Kondo, S. (1987a). *In* "Program and Abstracts of the 27th Interscience Conference on Antimicrobial Agents and Chemotherapy", New York. Abstr. 643.

Shibahara, S., Okonogi, T., Murai, Y., Yoshida, T., Kondo, S., and Christensen, B. G. (1987b). *In* "Program and Abstracts of the 27th Interscience Conference on Antimicrobial Agents and Chemotherapy", New York. Abstr. 647.

Shibuya, Y., Matsumoto, K., and Fuji, T. (1981). *Agric. Biol. Chem.* **45**, 1561–1567.

Shimada, K., and Soejima, R. (1987). *In* "Program and Abstracts of the 27th Interscience Conference on Antimicrobial Agents and Chemotherapy", New York. Abstr. 655.

Shindo, H., Fukuda, K., Kawai, K., and Tamaka, K. (1978). *J. Pharm. Dyn.* **1**, 310–323.

Shoji, J., Kato, T., Sakazaki, R., Nagata, W., Terni, Y., Nakagawa, Y., Shiro, M., Matsumoto, K., Hattori, T., Yoshida, T., and Kondo, E. (1984). *J. Antibiot.* **37**, 1486–1490.

Simon, C., and Stille, W. (1985). "Antibiotika-Therapie in Klinik und Praxis." Schattauer Verlag, Stuttgart.

Singh, P. D., Young, M. G., Johnson, J. H., Cimarusti, C. M., and Sykes, R. B. (1984). *J. Antibiot.* **37**, 773–780.

Sinko, P. J., and Amidon, G. L. (1986). *Pharm. Res.* **3** (Suppl.), 93S.

Skotnicki, J. S., and Steinbaugh, B. A. (1986). *J. Antibiot.* **39**, 372–379.

Skotnicki, J. S., and Strike, D. P. (1986). *J. Antibiot.* **39**, 380–383.

Smith, B. R., and Lefrock, J. L. (1982). *Hosp. Pharm.* **17**, 176–183.

Smith, G. C. D. (1983). Eur. Pat. Appl. EP 70,706, 26 January.

Sommers, D. K., Van Wyk, M., Williams, P. E. O., and Harding, S. M. (1983). *In* "Program and Abstracts of the 23rd Interscience Conference on Antimicrobial Agents and Chemotherapy", Las Vegas, Abstr. 720.

Southgate, R., and Elson, S. (1985). *In* "Progress in the Chemistry of Organic Natural Products" (L. Zechmeister, ed.), Vol. 43, pp. 1–106. Springer Verlag, New York.

Spencer, J. L., Siu, F. Y., Jackson, B. G., Higgins, H. M., and Flynn, E. H. (1967). *J. Org. Chem.* **32**, 500–501.

Spratt, B. G. (1975). *Proc. Nat. Acad. Sci.* **72**, 2999–3003.

Spry, D. O. (1980a). *Tetrahedron Lett.* **21**, 1289–1292.

Spry, D. O. (1980b). *Tetrahedron Lett.* **21**, 1293–1296.

Spry, D. O. (1985). US Patent US 4,560,749, 24 December.

Spry, D. O. (1986). Eur. Pat. Appl. EP 168,222, 15 January.

Spry, D. O., and Bhala, A. R. (1984). *Heterocycles* **22**, 2487–2490.

Spry, D. O., and Bhala, A. R. (1985). *Heterocycles* **23**, 1901–1905.

Spry, D. O., and Bhala, A. R. (1986a). *Heterocycles* **24**, 1653–1661.

Spry, D. O., and Bhala, A. R. (1986b). *Heterocycles* **24**, 1799–1806.

Spry, D. O., Bhala, A. R., Spitzer, W. A., Jones, N. D., and Swartzendruber, J. K. (1984). *Tetrahedron Lett.* **25**, 2531–2534.

Stamm, J. M., Girolami, R. L., Shipkowitz, N. I., and Bower, R. R. (1981). *Antimicrob. Agents Chemother.* **19**, 454–460.

Stapley, E. O., Jackson, M., Hernandez, S., Zimmerman, S. B., Currie, S. A., Mochales, S., Mata, J. M., Woodruff, H. B., and Hendlin, D. (1972). *Antimicrob. Agents Chemother.* **2**, 122–131.

Steele, J. C. H., Edwards, B. H., and Rissing, J. P. (1985). *J. Antimicrob. Chemother.* **16**, 463–468.

Stoodley, R. J., Pant, C. M., Whiting, A., and Williams, D. J. (1984). *J. Chem. Soc., Chem. Comm.* 1289–1291.

Sugawara, T., Masuya, H., Matsuo, T., and Miki, T. (1979a). *Chem. Pharm. Bull.* **27**, 2544–2546.

Sugawara, T., Masuya, H., Matsuo, T., and Miki, T. (1979b). *Chem. Pharm. Bull.* **27**, 3095–3100.

Sugawara, T., Masuya, H., Kawano, Y., Matsuo, T., and Kuwada, Y. (1980a). *Chem. Pharm. Bull.* **28**, 1339–1341.

Sugawara, T., Masuya, H., Matsuo, T., and Miki, T. (1980b). *Chem. Pharm. Bull.* **28**, 2116–2118.

Sugawara, T., Iwata, M., Tajima, M., Magaribuchi, T., Yanagisawa, H., Nakao, H., and Kuwahara, J. (1986). *In* "Program and Abstracts of the 26th Interscience Conference on Antimicrobial Agents and Chemotherapy", New Orleans. Abstr. 592.

Sugimura, Y., Jino, K., Iwano, Y., Saito, T., and Hiraoka, T. (1976). *Tetrahedron Lett.* **17**, 1307–1310.

Suzuki, E., Akai, K., and Yokota, T. (1986). *In* "Program and Abstracts of the 26th Interscience Conference on Antimicrobial Agents and Chemotherapy", New Orleans. Abstr. 1300.

Sweet, R. M. (1972). *In* "Cephalosporins and Penicillins" (E. H. Flynn, ed.), pp. 280–309. Academic Press, New York and London.

Sykes, R. B., Bonner, D. P., and Swabb, E. A. (1985). *Pharm. Ther.* **29**, 321–352.

Szwajcer, E., and Mosbach, K. (1985). *Biotechnol. Lett.* **7**, 1–7.

Tagawa, H., Hayano, T., Ejima, A., Une, T., Fujimoto, T., Osada, Y., and Furukawa, M. (1985). *In* "Program and Abstracts of the 25th Interscience Conference on Antimicrobial Agents and Chemotherapy", Minneapolis. Abstr. 361.

Takada, K., Shitori, Y., Fujii, T., Sato, N., and Aoyama, T. (1983). *In* "Proceedings of the 13th International Congress of Chemotherapy" (K. Spitzy and K. Karrer, eds), Vol. 4, SE 4.2/15-9. Egermann, Wien.

Takao, T., and Chiba, T. (1980). Ger. Offen. DE 3,005,888. 28 August.

Takao, T., Takashi, M., Takashi, O., Hisashi, T., and Hideaki, Y. (1984). Eur. Pat. Appl. EP 111,281, 20 June.

Takao, T., Hisashi, T., and Hideaki, Y. (1985). US Pat. 4,499,088, 12 February.

Takasugi, H., Tozuka, Z., and Takaya, T. (1983a). *J. Antibiot.* **36**, 36–41.

Takasugi, H., Kochi, H., Masugi, T., Nakano, H., and Takaya, T. (1983b). *J. Antibiot.* **36**, 846–854.

Takatani, T., Araya, M., and Ishe, M. (1986). Jpn. Kokai Tokkyo Koho JP 6133,190, 17 February.

Takaya, T., Kawanishi, K., Hiromu, S., Masugi, T. (1978). Ger. Offen. DE 2824004, 14 December.

Takaya, T., Takasugi, H., Murakawa, T., and Nakano, H. (1981a). *J. Antibiot.* **34**, 1300–1310.

Takaya, T., Takasugi, H., Masugi, T., Kochi, H., and Nakano, H. (1981b). J. Antibiot. 34, 1357–1359.

Takaya, T., Tozuka, Z., Takasugi, H., Kamiya, T., and Nakano, H. (1982). J. Antibiot. 35, 585–588.

Takaya, T., Takasugi, H., Chiba, T., and Tsuji, K. (1983). Eur. Pat. Appl. EP 88,385, 14 September.

Takaya, T., Takasugi, H., Yamanaka, H., Miyai, K., and Inoue, Y. (1984). Eur. Pat. Appl. EP 103,264, 21 March.

Takaya, T., Kamimura, T., Yokota, Y., Mine, Y., Kikuchi, H., Goto, S., and Kuwahara, S. (1985a). In "Proceedings of the 14th International Congress of Chemotherapy" (J. Ishigami, ed.), Vol. 2, pp. 1143–1144. University of Tokyo Press, Tokyo.

Takaya, T., Sakane, K., and Yamanaka, H. (1985b). Eur. Pat. Appl. EP 149,487, 24 July.

Takaya, T., Sakana, K., Yamanaka, H., and Miyai, K. (1985c). Eur. Pat. Appl. EP 154,354, 11 September.

Takaya, T., Tozuka, Z., Yasuda, N., and Kawabata, K. (1985d). Belg. Pat. Appl. BE 900,230, 28 January.

Takaya, T., Kamimura, T., Watanabe, Y., Matsumoto, Y., Tawara, S., Shibayama, F., and Mine, Y. (1987). In "Program and Abstracts of the 27th Interscience Conference on Antimicrobial Agents and Chemotherapy", New York. Abstr. 652.

Tamai, I., Hirooka, H., Kin, Y., Terasaki, T., and Tsuji, A. (1987). J. Pharmacobiodyn. 10, s-140.

Tartaglione, T. A., and Polk, R. E. (1985). Drug Intell. Clin. Pharmacy 19, 188–189.

Taylor, E. C., and Davies, H. M. L. (1986). J. Org. Chem. 51, 1537–1540.

Terachi, T., Sakane, K., and Goto, J. (1985). Jpn. Kokai Tokkyo Koho, JP 60,132,992, 16 July.

Teraji, T., Sakane, K., and Goto, J. (1981). Eur. Pat. Appl. EP 27,599, 29 April.

Teraji, T., Sakane, K., and Goto, J. (1982). Eur. Pat. Appl. EP 62,321, 13 October.

Teraji, T., Sakane, K., and Goto, J. (1983). Eur. Pat. Appl. EP 74,653, 23 March.

Teraji, T., Sakane, K., and Goto, J. (1984). Eur. Pat. Appl. EP 99,553, 1 February.

Teutsch, J. G., Bonnet, A., and Aszodi, J. (1987). Eur. Pat. Appl. EP 214,029, 11 March.

Tipper, D. J. (1985). Pharmac. Ther. 27, 1–35.

Thomas, M. G., and Lang, S. D. R. (1986). Antimicrob. Agents Chemother. 29, 945–947.

Thornsberry, C. (1985). Am. J. Med. 79 (Suppl. 2A), 14–20.

Tomasz, A. (1979). Ann. Rev. Microbiol. 33, 113–137.

Tomatsu, K., Hoshiya, T., Ando, S., and Miyahi, T. (1985). In "Proceedings of the 14th International Congress of Chemotherapy" (J. Ishigami, ed.), Vol. 2, pp. 1151–1152. University of Tokyo Press, Tokyo.

Tomatsu, K., Ando, S., Masuyoshi, S., Hirano, M., Miyaki, T., and Kawaguchi, H. (1986). J. Antibiot. 39, 1584–1591.

Tomatsu, K., Masuyoshi, S., Hirano, M., Kamachi, H., Narita, Y., Naito, T., Oki, T., and Kawaguchi, H. (1987). In "Program and Abstracts of the 27th Interscience Conference on Antimicrobial Agents and Chemotherapy", New York. Abstr. 806.

Tonelli, A. P., Bialer, M., Zook, Z. M., Carson, S., and Yacobi, A. (1986). Pharmaceut. Res. 3, 150–155.

Toothaker, R. D., Wright, D. S., and Pachla, A. P. (1987). Antimicrob. Agents Chemother. 31, 1157–1163.

Torii, S., Tanaka, H., Siroi, T., and Sasaoka, M. (1983a). J. Org. Chem. 48, 3551–3553.

Torii, S., Tanaka, H., Siroh, T., Madono, T., Saitoh, N., Sasaoka, M., and Nokami, J. (1983b). Bull. Chem. Soc. Jpn 56, 1567–1568.

Torii, S., Tanaka, H., Saitoh, N., Sirodi, T., Sasaoka, M., Tada, N., and Nokami, J. (1983c). Bull. Chem. Soc. Jpn 56, 2185–2186.

Torii, S., Tanaka, H., Ohshima, T., and Sasaoka, M. (1986). *Bull. Chem. Soc. Jpn* **59**, 3975–3976.

Tosch, W., Csendes, I., Zak, O., and Scartazzini, R. (1985a). *In* "Program and Abstracts of the 25th Interscience Conference on Antimicrobial Agents and Chemotherapy", Minneapolis. Abstr. 595.

Tosch, W., Frei, J., Konopka, E. A., Scartazzini, R., and Zak, O. (1985b). *In* "Proceedings of the 14th International Congress of Chemotherapy" (J. Ishigami, ed.), Vol. 2, pp. 883–884. University of Tokyo Press, Tokyo.

Tosch, W., Vischer, W., Wiederkehr, R., Imhof, P., and Zak, O. (1985c). *In* "Proceedings of the 14th International Congress of Chemotherapy" (J. Ishigami, ed.), Vol. 2, pp. 1141–1142. University of Tokyo Press, Tokyo.

Toyama Chemical Co., Ltd (1985a). Jpn. Kokai Tokkyo Koho JP 60,06,694, 14 January.

Toyama Chemical Co., Ltd (1985b). Jpn. Kokai Tokkyo Koho JP 60,04,191, 10 January.

Trown, P. W., and Sharp, M. (1963). *Biochem. J.* **86**, 280–284.

Truesdell, S. E., Winterrowd, C. A., Gilbertson, T. J., Zurenko, G. E., and Laborde, A. L. (1986). *In* "Program and Abstracts of the 26th Interscience Conference on Antimicrobial Agents and Chemotherapy", New Orleans. Abstr. 1315.

Tsubotani, S., Hida, T., Kasahara, F., Wada, Y., and Harada, S. (1984). *J. Antibiot.* **37**, 1546–1554.

Tsubotani, S., Hida, T., Kasahara, F., Wada, Y., and Harada, S. (1985). *J. Antibiot.* **38**, 1152–1165.

Tsuji, T., Satoh, H., Narisada, M., Hamashima, Y., and Yoshida, T. (1984). *J. Antibiot.* **38**, 466–476.

Tsuji, A., Maniatis, A., Bertram, M. A., and Young, L. S. (1985a). *Antimicrob. Agents Chemother.* **27**, 515–519.

Tsuji, T., Satoh, H., Narisada, M., Hamashima, Y., and Yoshida, T. (1985b). *J. Antibiot.* **38**, 466–476.

Tsuji, A. (1986). *In* "Frontiers of Antibiotic Research", p. 43. Takeda Science Foundation Symposium on Bioscience, Kyoto.

Tsuji, A., Hirooka, H., Tamai, I., and Teresaki, T. (1986). *J. Antibiot.* **39**, 1592–1597.

Tsuji, A., Tamai, I., Hirooka, H., and Terasaki, T. (1987a). *Biochem. Pharmacol.* **36**, 565–567.

Tsuji, A., Terasaki, T., Tamai, I., and Hirooka, H. (1987b). *J. Pharmacol. Exp. Ther.* **241**, 594–601.

Tsuji, A., Hirooka, H., Terasaki, T., *et al.* (1987c). *J. Pharm. Pharmacol.* **39**, 272–277.

Tsuroaka, T., Yoshida, T., Katano, K., Nakabayashi, S., Iwamatsu, K., Ogino, H., Okonogi, T., Murai, Y., Komiya, I., Nishio, M., Kazuno, Y., and Inouye, S. (1985). *In* "Proceedings of the 14th International Congress of Chemotherapy" (J. Ishigami, ed.), Vol. 2, pp. 877–878. University of Tokyo Press, Tokyo.

Tsushima, S., Sendai, M., Shiraishi, M., Kato, M., Matsumoto, N., Naito, K., and Numata, M. (1979). *Chem. Pharm. Bull.* **27**, 696–702.

Tunemoto, D., Kobori, T., Nishide, K., Kondo, K., Toshioka, T., Takanashi, M., Ohno, A., and Goto, S. (1986). *In* "Program and Abstracts of the 26th Interscience Conference on Antimicrobial Agents and Chemotherapy", New Orleans. Abstr. 1302.

Turner, J. C., Sullivan, H. R., Quay, J. F., Finch, L. S., and Stucky, J. F. (1982). *In* "Program and Abstracts of the 27th Interscience Conference on Antimicrobial Agents and Chemotherapy", New York. Abstr. 1204.

Ubukata, K., Yamashita, N., and Konno, M. (1985). *Antimicrob. Agents Chemother.* **27**, 851–857.

Une, T., Ikeuchi, T., Osada, Y., Ogawa, H., Sato, K., and Mitsuhashi, S. (1984). *In* "Program and Abstracts of the 24th Interscience Conference on Antimicrobial Agents and Chemotherapy", Washington. Abstr. 729.

Une, T., Otani, T., Sato, M., Ikeuchi, T., Osada, Y., and Ogawa, H. (1985). *Antimicrob. Agents Chemother.* **27**, 473–478.

Utsui, Y., Inoue, M., and Mitsuhashi, S. (1987). *Antimicrob. Agents Chemother.* **31**, 1085–1092.

Uyeo, S., and Ona, H. (1980). *Chem. Pharm. Bull.* **28**, 1563–1577.

Vanderhaeghe, H., Herdewijn, P., and Claes, P. J. (1986). *J. Med. Chem.* **29**, 661–664.

Van Krimpen, P. C., Van Bennekom, W. P., and Bult, A. (1987). *Pharmaceut. Weekblad Scient. Ed.* **9**, 1–23.

Verho, M., Maaß, L., Malerczyk, V., and Grötsch, M. (1987). *Infection* **15**, 215–219.

Vignau, M., and Heymes, R. (1981). Ger. Offen. DE 3,027,281, 12 February.

Vuh, V., and Nikaido, H. (1985). *Antimicrob. Agents Chemother.* **27**, 393–398.

Vuye, A., and Pijck, J. (1985). *Antimicrob. Agents Chemother.* **27**, 574–577.

Walther, H., and Meyer, F. P. (eds) (1987). "Klinische Pharmakologie Antibakterieller Arzneimittel", Ch. 3, pp. 139–196. Verlag Urban & Schwarzenberg, München.

Ward, A., and Richards, D. M. (1985). *Drugs* **30**, 382–426.

Warren, C. A., King, B. A., Shannon, K. P., Eykyn, S. J., and Philips, I. (1980). *J. Antimicrob. Chemother.* **6**, 607–615.

Watanabe, N., Katsu, K., Moriyama, M., Sugiyama, I., Kitoh, K., and Yamauchi, H. (1987a). *In* "Program and Abstracts of the 27th Interscience Conference on Antimicrobial Agents and Chemotherapy", New York. Abstr. 636.

Watanabe, N., Nagasu, T., Katsu, K., and Kitoh, K. (1987b). *Antimicrob. Agents Chemother.* **31**, 497–504.

Watanabe, T., Kawano, Y., Tanaka, T., Hashimoto, T., and Miyadera, T. (1980). *Chem. Pharm. Bull.* **28**, 62–69.

Watanabe, Y., Yokoo, C., Goi, M., Onodera, A., Murata, M., Fukushima, H., and Sota, K. (1987a). Eur. Pat. Appl. EP 210,078, 28 January.

Watanabe, Y., Yokoo, C., Goi, M., Onodera, A., Murata, M., Fukushima, H., and Sota, K. (1987b). Eur. Pat. Appl. EP 212,923, 3 March.

Watanabe, Y., Yokoo, C., Goi, M., Onodera, A., Murata, M., Fukushima, H., Taguchi, M., and Sota, K. (1987c). Eur. Pat. Appl. EP 228,906, 15 July.

Waxman, D. J., and Strominger, J. L. (1982). *In* "Chemistry and Biology of β-Lactam Antibiotics" (R. B. Morin and M. Gorman, eds), Vol. 3, pp. 209–285. Academic Press, New York and London.

Webber, J. A., Huffman, G. W., Koehler, R. E., Murphy, C. F., Ryan, C. W., Van Heyningen, E. M., and Vasileff, R. T. (1971). *J. Med. Chem.* **14**, 113–116.

Webber, J. A., and Ott, J. L. (1977). *In* "Structure–Activity Relationships among the Semisynthetic Antibiotics" (D. Perlman, ed.), p. 161. Academic Press, New York and London.

Webber, J. A., and Wheeler, W. J. (1982). *In* "Chemistry and Biology of β-Lactam Antibiotics" (R. B. Morin and M. Gorman, eds), Vol. 1, pp. 371–442. Academic Press, New York and London.

Weinstein, A. J. (1980). *Drugs* **20**, 137–154.

Wetzel, B., Woitun, E., Maier, R., Reuter, W., and Lechner, K. (1985). *J. Antibiot.* **38**, 740–745.

Wheeler, W. J., Deeter, J. B., Finley, D. R., Kinnick, M. D., Koehler, R., Osborne, H. E., and Ott, J. T. (1986a). *J. Antibiot.* **39**, 111–120.

Wheeler, W. J., Finley, D. R., Messenger, R. J., Köhler, R., and Ott, J. T. (1986b). *J. Antibiot.* **39**, 121–127.

Wiedemann, J. (1986). *J. Antimicrob. Chemother.* **18** (Suppl. B), 31–38.

Williams, J. D. (1983). *In* "Proceedings of the 13th International Congress of Chemotherapy" (K. Spitzy and K. Karrer, eds), Vol. 1, SY 41-1. Egermann, Wien.

Williams, P. E. O. (1985). *Biochem. Soc. Trans.* **13**, 511–513.

Williamson, R., Gutman, L., Kitzis, M.-D., and Acar, J. F. (1984). *J. Antimicrob. Chemother.* **14**, 581–593.

Wilson, E. M. (1984). *Chem. Ind. (London)*, 217–221.

Wise, R. (1982). *Lancet* **2/8290**, 140–143.

Wise, R., Andrews, J. M., and Bennett, S. (1983). *In* "Program and Abstracts of the 23rd Interscience Conference on Antimicrobial Agents and Chemotherapy", Las Vegas. Abstr. 721.

Wise, R., Cross, C., and Andrews, J. M. (1984). *Antimicrob. Agents Chemother.* **26**, 876–880.

Wise, R., Andrews, J. M., Cross, C., and Piddock, L. J. V. (1985). *J. Antimicrob. Chemother.* **15**, 449–456.

Wojtkowski, P. W., Dolfini, J. E., Kocy, O., and Cimarusti, C. (1975). *J. Am. Chem. Soc.* **97**, 5628–5630.

Woodward, R. B. (1966). *Angew. Chem.* **78**, 557–564.

Woodward, R. B., Heusler, K., Gosteli, J., Naegeli, P., Oppolzer, W., Ramage, R., Ranganathan, S., and Vorbrüggen, H. (1966). *J. Am. Chem. Soc.* **88**, 852–853.

Wright, D. B. (1986). *Drug Intell. Clin. Pharm.* **20**, 845–849.

Wright, W. E., Quay, J. F., Kukolja, S. P., Eudaly, J. A., Stucky, J. R., Johnson, R. J., Pfeil, J. L., Draheim, S. E., Ott, J. L., Counter, F. T., Cooper, R. D. G., Shoufler, J. R., and Johnson, J. A. (1986). *In* "Program and Abstracts of the 26th Interscience Conference on Antimicrobial Agents and Chemotherapy", New Orleans. Abstr. 594.

Yamada, H., Masai, N., Ueda, S., Okuda, T., Fukasawa, M., Kato, M., and Fukumura, M. (1985). Eur. Pat. Appl. EP 150,458, 7 August.

Yamamoto, Y., Yoshida, T., Fukatsu, S., and Ishimaru, T. (1986). Eur. Pat. Appl. EP 186,586, 2 July.

Yamanaka, H., Takasugi, H., Masugi, T., Kochi, H., Miyai, K., and Takaya, T. (1985a). *J. Antibiot.* **38**, 1068–1076.

Yamanaka, H., Chiba, T., Kawabata, H., Masugi, T., and Takaya, T. (1985b). *J. Antibiot.* **38**, 1738–1751.

Yamanaka, H., Kawabata, K., Miyai, K., Takasugi, H., Kamimura, T., Mine, Y., and Takaya, T. (1986). *J. Antibiot.* **39**, 101–110.

Yamazaki, T., and Tsuchiya, K. (1976a). *J. Antibiot.* **29**, 559–565.

Yamazaki, T., and Tsuchiya, K. (1976b). *J. Antibiot.* **29**, 566–570.

Yamazaki, T., and Tsuchiya, K. (1976c). *J. Antibiot.* **29**, 571–578.

Yanagisawa, H., Fukushima, M., Ando, A., and Nakao, H. (1975). *Tetrahedron Lett.* **16**, 2705–2708.

Yancey, R. J., Lallinger, A. J., Baird, G. M., Frecker, J. K., and Ford, C. W. (1986a). *In* "Program and Abstracts of the 26th Interscience Conference on Antimicrobial Agents and Chemotherapy", New Orleans. Abstr. 1316.

Yancey, R. J., Kinney, M. L., Roberts, B. J., Goodenough, K. R., Hamel, J. C., and Ford, C. W. (1986b). *In* "Program and Abstracts of the 26th Interscience Conference on Antimicrobial Agents and Chemotherapy", New Orleans. Abstr. 1317.

Yoshida, T. (1980). *Phil. Trans. R. Soc. Lond. B* **289**, 231–237.

Yoshida, T., Shibahara, S., Yamamoto, H., Niizato, T., Matsumoto, T., Komiya, I., Kai, F., Kurebe, M., Inone, S., and Kondo, S. (1987). *In* "Program and Abstracts of the 27th Interscience Conference on Antimicrobial Agents and Chemotherapy", New York. Abstr. 645.

234   W. DÜRCKHEIMER *et al.*

Yoshimura, Y., Hamaguchi, N., and Yashiki, T. (1985). *Int. J. Pharmaceut.* **23**, 117–129.
Yoshimura, Y., Hamaguchi, N., and Yashiki, T. (1986). *J. Antibiot.* **39**, 1329–1342.
Yoshioka, M. (1987). *Pure Appl. Chem.* **59**, 1041–1046.
Zak, O., Konopka, E. A., Kunz, J., Frei, J., Tosch, W., and Scartazzini, R. (1985a). *In* "Proceedings of the 14th International Congress of Chemotherapy" (J. Ishigami, ed.), Vol. 2, pp. 885–886. University of Tokyo Press, Tokyo.
Zak, O., Tosch, W., Wiederkehr, R., Batt, E., Kunz, S., Konopka, E. A., and Scartazzini, R. (1985b). *In* "Proceedings of the 14th International Congress of Chemotherapy" (J. Ishigami, ed.), Vol. 2, pp. 1139–1140. University of Tokyo Press, Tokyo.

Recent Experimental and Conceptual Advances in Drug Receptor Research in the Cardiovascular System

ROBERT R. RUFFOLO, JR., and ANDREW J. NICHOLS

Department of Pharmacology, Smith Kline & French Laboratories, King of Prussia, Pennsylvania, USA

ADVANCES IN DRUG RESEARCH, VOL. 17
ISBN 0-12-013317-2

The following abbreviations are used in this article: DA, dopamine; EDRF, endothelium-derived relaxing factor; 5HT, 5-hydroxytryptamine; NANC, non-adrenergic, non-cholinergic; PBDA, N-n-propyl,N-n-butyldopamine; PGI$_2$, prostacyclin; SHRSP, stroke-prone spontaneously hypertensive rats; SIADH, syndrome of inappropriate secretion of antidiuretic hormone; TXA$_2$, thromboxane A$_2$.

1 Control of the Cardiovascular System

1.1 ORGANIZATION OF THE AUTONOMIC NERVOUS SYSTEM

The cardiovascular system is under the control and regulation of the autonomic nervous system. While effector organs of the cardiovascular system (heart, vasculature, kidneys) function in the absence of autonomic nerves, the sympathetic and parasympathetic divisions of the autonomic nervous system provide a delicate balance involving closed reflex loops to maintain these organs in their optimal functional state.

The autonomic nervous system is composed of the parasympathetic division, in which the neurotransmitter at the effector organ is acetylcholine, and the sympathetic division, in which the neurotransmitter is norepinephrine. The parasympathetic division exits the central nervous system from the brain stem (vagus) and the sacral region of the spinal cord. These nerves are characterized by long preganglionic neurons and short postganglionic neurons, the latter innervating the effector organs. The neurotransmitter in the parasympathetic ganglia is acetylcholine. The heart receives a dense cholinergic innervation from the vagus, and cholinergic "tone" in the heart predominates over adrenergic tone. In general, there is no significant parasympathetic innervation to the vasculature, although blood vessels nonetheless contain muscarinic cholinergic receptors that are stimulated by acetylcholine and mediate vasodilation through release of an endothelial derived relaxing factor (Furchgott and Zawadzki, 1980).

The sympathetic division of the autonomic nervous system originates from the intermediolateral cell column of the thoracic and lumbar portions of the spinal cord. The relatively short preganglionic fibres characteristic of sympathetic nerves terminate in the sympathetic ganglia arranged in a paravertebral chain, where again the neurotransmitter is acetylcholine. The postganglionic sympathetic neurons are long and liberate norepinephrine which interacts postsynaptically with adrenoceptors in the heart, vasculature, and kidney. The innervation to the vasculature is almost exclusively sympathetic where the end organ response is vasoconstriction.

Although the sympathetic and parasympathetic components of the autonomic nervous system originate in the spinal cord and are considered peripheral nerves, both divisions are under the control of nuclei located in the brain stem which in turn receive input from higher centres in the brain. Most of the cardiovascular reflex loops consist of afferent nerves from various chemoreceptors and baroreceptors in the periphery, which travel to these regulatory nuclei in the brain stem where the information is integrated. The efferent component of the reflex loop involves descending pathways originating from the brain stem nuclei, which ultimately recruit the sympathetic and parasympathetic divisions of the autonomic nervous system to make the necessary alterations in the functional state of the various effector organs of the cardiovascular system.

1.2 CARDIOVASCULAR REFLEXES

Cardiovascular reflexes maintain cardiovascular function, in particular blood pressure, within a relatively narrow optimal range. A sensitive and highly efficient series of positive and negative feedback loops detect deviations from normal cardiovascular function and then "up-regulate" or "down-regulate" the function of peripheral organs of the cardiovascular system after integration in the central nervous system. Pressure receptors in the carotid sinus and aortic arch sense changes in peripheral arterial blood pressure and initiate the cardiovascular reflex. Afferents from the carotid sinus and aortic arch enter the central nervous system through cranial nerves IX (glossopharyngeal) and X (vagus), respectively, and form, in part, the solitary tract in the medulla. The first synapse in the cardiovascular reflex loops occurs in the nucleus tractus solitarii where the neurotransmitter appears to be L-glutamate (Reis, 1984). Synapses are made within the nucleus tractus solitarii with inhibitory neurons that course to the ventrolateral medulla which ultimately regulates sympathetic outflow, and with excitatory neurons that send connections to the dorsal motor nucleus of the vagus, which in turn regulates parasympathetic outflow.

Increases in systemic arterial blood pressure elicit the afferent component of the cardiovascular reflex loop. As a result, the inhibitory neurons originating in the nucleus tractus solitarii and terminating in the ventro-lateral medulla are activated, reducing sympathetic outflow to the heart, vasculature, and kidney. As a direct consequence, heart rate, stroke volume (and therefore cardiac output), and total peripheral vascular resistance are reduced, and blood pressure subsequently reurns to within normal limits. In addition, the excitatory neurons that originate from the nucleus tractus solitarii and terminate in the dorsal motor nucleus of the vagus are activated and cholinergic outflow is increased, further decreasing heart rate and cardiac output (Kobinger, 1978) and thus augmenting the reduction of arterial blood pressure.

2 α-Adrenoceptors

α-Adrenoceptors exist in many organs of the body, and the functions they mediate are only now beginning to be understood. Because of the prominent role that α_2-adrenergic receptors play in the cardiovascular system, their distribution and function in this important system will be discussed separately.

2.1 CENTRAL MEDULLARY α-ADRENOCEPTORS

Stimulation of central α_2-adrenergic receptors in the ventrolateral medulla induces a reduction in sympathetic outflow to the periphery, manifested as a reduction in arterial blood pressure accompanied by bradycardia. This response has been studied extensively over the past two decades and several comprehensive reviews are available (Schmitt, 1971; Kobinger, 1978; van Zwieten et al., 1983; Ruffolo, 1984a). Quantitative structure–activity studies have shown excellent correlation between the α_2-adrenergic receptor agonist potency of a series of clonidine analogues, and blood pressure reduction, provided a lipophilicity term is included to correct for penetration through the blood–brain barrier which is required in order to gain access to the site of action within the central nervous system (Timmermans et al., 1980, 1981; Ruffolo et al., 1982c,d).

The characteristic response to intravenous administration of an α_2-adrenergic receptor agonist in a normotensive or hypertensive animal is an immediate pressor response, due to stimulation of peripheral arterial post-junctional α_2-adrenergic receptors (Ruffolo et al., 1982c). The same response is also seen in human subjects following intravenous administration of clonidine (Onesti et al., 1971). This pressor response is relatively short-lived, and is followed by a slow decline in arterial blood pressure to levels lower than those observed prior to drug administration. This long-lasting depressor/antihypertensive response is a result of central α_2-adrenergic receptor stimulation. Heart rate declines immediately following administration, and continues to be reduced for the duration of drug action. If the α_2-adrenergic receptor agonist is administered directly into the central nervous system, or via the vertebral artery which allows for easy access to the central nervous system, the initial pressor response is not observed (Ruffolo et al., 1982c,d; Timmermans et al., 1980). High oral doses of centrally acting α_2-adrenergic receptor agonists, such as clonidine or guanfacine, can also increase blood pressure via peripheral arterial α-adrenergic receptor stimulation (Davis et al., 1977), and provide an explanation for the "therapeutic window" seen with clonidine in antihypertensive therapy (Frisk-Holmberg et al., 1984).

Although the peripheral prejunctional action of α_2-adrenergic receptor agonists does not appear to make a major contribution to the antihypertensive activity of these compounds, a peripheral neuroinhibitory action of clonidine can be demonstrated in the cat on the cardiovascular response to electrical stimulation of sensory fibres in vivo (Walland, 1978). This peripheral action has been postulated to contribute to the antihypertensive effects of clonidine under conditions where blood pressure escapes baroreceptor-mediated homeostatic control. A similar peripheral presynaptic contribution to blood pressure effects in human subjects has been proposed by Gunnar Wallin and Frisk-Holmberg (1981). Furthermore, the bradycardia associated with α_2-adrenergic receptor agonists may result, in part, from a peripheral presynaptic action at prejunctional α_2-adrenergic receptors on sympathetic nerves in the heart, since heart rate can be reduced in pithed rats (Drew, 1976), and, in contrast to hypotension, α_2-adrenergic receptor agonist-induced bradycardia in the anesthetized rat does not require penetration into the central nervous system (de Jonge et al., 1981).

The antihypertensive action of α_2-adrenergic receptor agonists is likely to result from stimulation of postsynaptic α_2-adrenergic receptors in the brainstem. Animal experiments have shown that catecholamine depletion with reserpine, or destruction of sympathetic neurons by treatment with 6-hydroxydopamine, does not generally attenuate the ability of α_2-adrenergic receptor stimulation to decrease sympathetic outflow (Haeusler, 1974; Kobinger and Pichler, 1976), although Dollery and Reid (1973) showed a slight attenuation by 6-hydroxydopamine. This would indicate that the central α_2-adrenergic receptor involved in this response is not located prejunctionally on a catecholaminergic neuron. A brainstem site is indicated, based on the inability of transection at the intercollicular level or at the pontomedullary junction to attenuate the antihypertensive activity of clonidine (Schmitt and Schmitt, 1969). Many experiments have been performed in an attempt to locate more precisely the site of action of α_2-adrenergic receptor agonists within the brainstem. Although the nucleus tractus solitarius has been often considered as the principal site of action of central α_2-adrenergic receptor agonists (Schmitt, 1971), recent studies using microinjections of clonidine suggest the lateral reticular nucleus in the ventrolateral medulla as a more likely candidate (Gillis et al., 1985). This nucleus is readily accessible from the ventral surface of the medulla, where α_2-adrenergic receptor agonists have been shown to be effective following local application (Bousquet and Guertzenstein, 1973; Scholtysik et al., 1975; Srimal et al., 1977; Gillis et al., 1985). Although guanfacine has been reported to be ineffective via this route (Scholtysik et al., 1975), the body of experimental evidence would suggest that all α_2-adrenergic receptor agonists are acting at this same central locus.

In addition to a reduction in sympathetic outflow, central α_2-adrenergic receptor stimulation can enhance parasympathetic outflow. This has usually been demonstrated as a potentiation of the reflex bradycardia induced by intravenous injection of a pressor agent such as angiotensin II (Kobinger, 1978; Connor et al., 1982). This action requires penetration of the α_2-adrenergic receptor agonist into the central nervous system (Kobinger, 1978), but the precise site of action has not yet been determined (Gillis et al., 1985).

Central α_2-adrenergic receptor stimulation has been utilized clinically as antihypertensive therapy. In addition to the directly acting central α_2-adrenergic receptor agonists discussed above, α-methyldopa, which has been extensively employed for over a decade, is now known to stimulate central α_2-adrenergic receptors following metabolic conversion to α-methyl-norepinephrine (van Zwieten, 1980), which has much greater α_2-adrenergic receptor selectivity than norepinephrine (Ruffolo et al., 1982b; Jarrott et al., 1984). Following chronic treatment with α-methyldopa in rats, medullary norepinephrine stores are almost completely replaced by α-methyl-norepinephrine (Conway et al., 1979) which is available for interaction with medullary α_2-adrenergic receptors to inhibit sympathetic outflow. The therapeutic and side-effect profile of α-methyldopa is similar to that observed with the directly acting central α_2-adrenergic receptor agonists (van Zwieten et al., 1983).

In addition to clonidine and α-methyldopa, guanfacine (BS 100–141) is now in general use as an antihypertensive drug. This compound has a similar *in vitro* pharmacological profile to clonidine (Scholtysik, 1980), but appears to have a longer duration of action (Jain *et al.*, 1985; Farsang *et al.*, 1984; Reid *et al.*, 1983b). Clinical trials have been conducted with several other α_2-adrenergic receptor agonists, including St-600 (Kho *et al.*, 1975), tiamenidine (Campbell *et al.*, 1980; Clifton *et al.*, 1981), monoxidine (Planitz, 1984), lofexidine (Schultz *et al.*, 1981; Wilkins *et al.*, 1981; Lopez and Mehta, 1984) and B-HT 933 (azepexole) (Reid *et al.*, 1983b). The latter compound is more selective than clonidine for α_2- *vis-à-vis* α_1-adrenergic receptors (van Meel *et al.*, 1981c), and its antihypertensive activity confirms an α_2-adrenergic receptor-mediated mechanism. As in animal studies, the clinical cardiovascular profiles of the various α_2-adrenergic receptor agonists is similar (Reid, 1985). Besides their antihypertensive indication, the sympatholytic action of the centrally active α_2-adrenergic receptor agonists may offer clinical benefit in congestive heart failure and angina pectoris, again through a centrally mediated reduction in sympathetic outflow. Although extensive evaluation for efficacy in these conditions has not yet been performed, preliminary trials in patients are encouraging (Giles *et al.*, 1985).

While the antihypertensive activity of clonidine and clonidine-like imidazolidines results from their pharmacological selectivity for central α_2-adrenergic receptors, it is also known that the physicochemical properties of clonidine-like imidazolidines are critical in determining the antihypertensive efficacy of such compounds (for review see Timmermans *et al.*, 1980). Highly lipophilic imidazolidines, such as clonidine, which readily cross the blood–brain barrier and gain access to their site(s) of action in the brain stem, are potent antihypertensive agents. Conversely, many imidazolidines with similar selectivities as clonidine for α_2-adrenergic receptors, but with low lipophilicity, do not readily cross the blood–brain barrier and are either weak antihypertensive agents, or completely devoid of all antihypertensive activity. Such compounds are still effective in lowering blood pressure when injected beyond the blood–brain barrier into specific brain regions, such as the ventrolateral medulla, or when injected into the cerebral ventricles or cisterna magna (see Ruffolo, 1984a; Ruffolo *et al.*, 1982c,d). Because these α_2-adrenergic receptor agonists with low lipophilicity are still active when the blood–brain barrier is bypassed, it has been concluded that one major factor affecting the antihypertensive activity of clonidine-like imidazolidines following systemic administration is their ability to cross the blood–brain barrier, and this, in turn, is highly dependent upon overall lipophilicity.

Many properties of a molecule will determine overall lipophilicity which, as indicated above, is critical for antihypertensive efficacy of clonidine-like imidazolidines. For these particular compounds, the most important determinant of lipophilicity is the extent of ionization occurring at physiological pH and this property is governed by the ionization constant (K_a) (Timmermans and van Zwieten, 1978; Timmermans et al., 1977, 1981; Ruffolo et al., 1982c,d). Imidazolidines in the ionized species possess low lipophilicity and will permeate the blood–brain barrier slowly, whereas the un-ionized form is highly lipophilic and will cross the blood–brain barrier rapidly. Thus, the ratio of the un-ionized:ionized species is a major determinant of the antihypertensive efficacy and potency of many clonidine-like imidazolidines. Table 1 shows that there exists an excellent correlation between the antihypertensive potencies of a series of clonidine-like imidazolidines and their pK_a (Ruffolo et al., 1982d), such that those compounds with low pK_a values, and which are therefore significantly un-ionized at physiological pH, will cross the blood–brain barrier rapidly and be potent antihypertensive agents, whereas those imidazolidines with high pK_a values, and which are extensively ionized at physiological pH, will penetrate the blood–brain barrier to a lesser extent (or at a slower rate) and be weaker antihypertensive agents (Ruffolo et al., 1982d).

Clonidine is not metabolized to a great extent in humans (Lowenthal, 1980), and the limited metabolism that does occur does not take place in the brain. As a result, termination of the central antihypertensive effects of clonidine and clonidine-like imidazolidines is likely to be by diffusion out of the central nervous system. It has recently been demonstrated that the pK_a of clonidine-like imidazolidines, and therefore their ratios of un-ionized:ionized species, also governs the diffusion of these compounds out

TABLE 1

Summary of the pharmacological effects and ionization constants of clonidine and a series of structural analogues (from Ruffolo et al., 1982d)

Compound	pK_a	Antihypertensive[a] (intravenous) ED_{30} ($\mu g/kg$)	Pressor[b] (intracisternal) ED_{20} ($\mu g/kg$)
Clonidine	7.7	3.3	24
St-363	8.3	19	56
St-93	9.2	37	62
St-375	9.2	34	76
St-608	9.2	63	66
St-600	9.5	380	135
St-91	10.8	—	210

[a]Antihypertensive activity in spontaneously hypertensive rats.
[b]Pressor activity in reserpinized rats (a measure of diffusion through the blood–brain barrier).

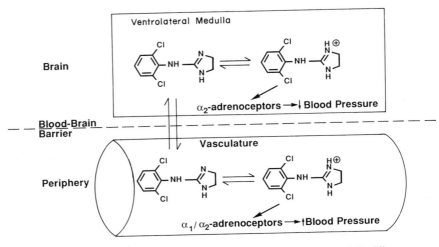

FIG. 1. Schematic representation of the pharmacological activities of clonidine.

of the brain (Ruffolo *et al.*, 1982d). As expected, high proportions of the un-ionized species with high lipophilicity are associated with a more rapid exit from the central nervous system by diffusion through the blood–brain barrier in the reverse direction (Ruffolo *et al.*, 1982d).

Based on the importance of the physicochemical properties of imidazolidines in governing their pharmacological activity at central α_2-adrenergic receptors, the following scheme, shown diagrammatically in Fig. 1, has been proposed to explain the antihypertensive effects of clonidine (Ruffolo, 1984c). Following systemic administration, clonidine will exist in the blood in an equilibrium between the ionized and un-ionized species, with the relative proportions of each species being determined by the pK_a and physiological pH. The ionized form will interact with postsynaptic vascular α_1- and α_2-adrenergic receptors (Ruffolo *et al.*, 1982c) to mediate a transient pressor response, which is particularly apparent following intravenous administration. The un-ionized form (mainly) will cross the blood–brain barrier to gain access to the site(s) of action in the ventrolateral medulla. Again, a new equilibrium between the ionized and un-ionized form will be established within the central nervous system, the extent of which also being determined by the pK_a and the pH of cerebrospinal fluid. The ionized form (Ruffolo *et al.*, 1982c) is believed to be the species responsible for activation of central α_2-adrenergic receptors to mediate the decrease in sympathetic outflow and the increase in parasympathetic outflow which ultimately produces the antihypertensive and bradycardic response. While the ionized species appears to interact with the central α_2-adrenergic receptor, it is the un-ionized species which will permeate the blood–brain barrier in the reverse direction and exit from the central nervous system to terminate the antihypertensive response. Once in the periphery, the drug is subsequently removed from the blood by metabolism and/or excretion.

In contrast to the imidazolidines, the physicochemical properties of α-methyldopa play a lesser role in the antihypertensive activity of this compound. α-Methyldopa gains access to the central nervous system via the aromatic amino acid transport system. In the brain, α-methyldopa is sequentially decarboxylated and β-hydroxylated to form (1R,2S)-(−)-*erythro-α*-methylnorepinephrine which then activates medullary α_2-adrenergic receptors to inhibit sympathetic outflow and enhance parasympathetic outflow.

One of the concerns associated with antihypertensive therapy with centrally acting α_2-adrenergic receptor agonists is the "rebound hypertension" or "withdrawal" phenomenon that often occurs when treatment is abruptly terminated (Reid *et al.*, 1977; Hansson *et al.*, 1973). This phenomenon is characterized by tachycardia and abrupt rises in blood pressure, sometimes to levels greater than that observed before initiation of therapy (Hansson, 1983; Weber, 1980). Studies in animals have confirmed the presence of a hyper-adrenergic state following abrupt termination of chronic clonidine therapy (Lewis *et al.*, 1981; Engberg *et al.*, 1982; Thoolen *et al.*, 1983; Jarrott *et al.*, 1984). Administration of an α_2-adrenergic receptor antagonist, such as yohimbine, can also precipitate this withdrawal phenomenon (Thoolen *et al.*, 1983).

The withdrawal phenomenon observed following abrupt cessation of α_2-adrenergic receptor agonist therapy bears some similarity to opiate withdrawal (Hansson *et al.*, 1973; Engberg *et al.*, 1982; Jarrott *et al.*, 1984), and appears to involve overactivity of locus coeruleus neurons (Engberg *et al.*, 1982). This may represent a rebound phenomenon following chronic suppression of the firing rate of these neurons during chronic antihypertensive treatment. In view of the similarities and possible receptor interactions between α_2-adrenergic and opiate receptors (see below), it is not surprising that morphine can suppress, via a naloxone sensitive mechanism, some of the cardiovascular rebound effects observed following termination of clonidine infusion in rats (Thoolen *et al.*, 1983).

2.2 PERIPHERAL α-ADRENOCEPTORS

2.2.1 Presynaptic α-Adrenoceptors

The first physiological action described for α_2-adrenoceptors, and the reason for postulating the existence of α_2-adrenoceptors, is the inhibition of neurotransmitter release mediated by α_2-adrenoceptors located on, or near, nerve terminals. The α_2-adrenoceptor mediates inhibition of norepinephrine release from sympathetic nerves, acetylcholine release from parasympathetic nerves, as well as the release of various central neurotransmitters [for review, see Starke (1981)].

The prejunctional α_2-adrenoceptor serves as a key element in a local feedback system modulating neurotransmitter release. Activation of these α_2-adrenoceptors by either norepinephrine or epinephrine, the natural physiological ligands, or by synthetic molecules having α_2-adrenoceptor agonist activity, such as B-HT 920, B-HT 933, UK-14,304 and clonidine, will inhibit stimulation-evoked neurotransmitter release from nerve terminals. Conversely, α_2-adrenoceptor antagonists, such as idazoxan, yohimbine, rauwolscine and SK&F 86466, will potentiate stimulation-evoked norepinephrine release. This potentiation shows that the prejunctional α_2-adrenoceptor is normally under active tone as a result of endogenously released norepinephrine. The results of activation or blockade of prejunctional α_2-adrenoceptors can be demonstrated *in vivo* in both animals (Langer *et al.*, 1985) and in humans (Brown *et al.*, 1985), as well as in isolated tissues. Since prejunctional α_2-adrenoceptors have been found in all sympathetically innervated tissues thus far examined, this neuromodulatory system appears to play an important role in the control of sympathetic tone.

The magnitude of prejunctional α_2-adrenoceptor mediated effects are dependent upon the pattern of neuronal activity. As the amount of norepinephrine in the synaptic cleft is increased by a higher frequency and/or duration of nerve stimulation, the prejunctional α_2-adrenoceptor is activated to greater degree by the neuronally released norepinephrine. Hence, the ability of an exogenously administered α_2-adrenoceptor agonist to inhibit sympathetic neurotransmission will decrease as stimulation frequency or duration is increased, since the prejunctional α_2-adrenoceptor mediated autoinhibition system will already be maximally activated. Conversely, potentiation by an α_2-adrenoceptor antagonist will be enhanced as stimulation parameters are increased to yield a more intense stimulation of prejunctional α_2-adrenoceptors (Auch-Schwelk *et al.*, 1983). In this regard, an α_2-adrenoceptor antagonist would not be expected to potentiate the release of neurotransmitter induced by a single pulse of nerve stimulation, since there would be no tone at the prejunctional α_2-adrenoceptor under such conditions. Studies have suggested that a minimum interval of a few seconds between pulses is required for activation of the prejunctional α_2-adrenoceptor (Auch-Schwelk *et al.*, 1983; Story *et al.*, 1981).

It is generally assumed that prejunctional α-adrenoceptors are solely of the α_2-subtype. However, recent evidence has cast some doubt on this hypothesis. Studies of the effect of α_1-adrenoceptor agonists on cardiac sympathetic neurotransmission in the pithed rat have suggested that α_1-

adrenoceptors may coexist with α_2-adrenoceptors on sympathetic nerve varicosities, and that, similar to α_2-adrenoceptors, they mediate an inhibition of norepinephrine release (Kobinger and Pichler, 1982; Docherty, 1983a). However, it has recently been demonstrated that α_1-adrenoceptor agonists are also capable of inhibiting cardiac sympathetic neurotransmission in pithed rats via a postjunctional mechanism (de Jonge et al., 1986). Thus, the data from pithed rats do not provide conclusive evidence for the existence of prejunctional inhibitory α_1-adrenoceptors. On the other hand, α_1-adrenoceptor agonists inhibit nerve stimulated [^{3}H]-norepinephrine release from rat atria in vitro, an effect which is antagonized by α_1-adrenoceptor antagonists (Story et al., 1985). These data provide stronger evidence for the existence of prejunctional inhibitory α_1-adrenoceptors. Furthermore, Story et al. (1985) have shown that α_1-adrenoceptor antagonists potentiate nerve stimulation-evoked [^{3}H]-norepinephrine release, thus suggesting that prejunctional α_1-adrenoceptors may be activated by endogenous norepinephrine during sympathetic nerve activity. Additional in vivo evidence for the presence of prejunctional α_1-adrenoceptors at the cardiac neuroeffector junction in the dog has been provided by Uchida et al. (1984) who found similar functional effects of α_1-adrenoceptor agonists and antagonists on sympathetic neurotransmission. Docherty and coworkers have also demonstrated the presence of prejunctional α_1-adrenoceptors which inhibit neurotransmitter release in the rat vas deferens in vitro (Docherty, 1983b; Warnock et al., 1985). Thus, the currently available evidence strongly suggests that there are, indeed, prejunctional α_1-adrenoceptors on sympathetic neurons which act to inhibit neurotransmitter release, and that these receptors may be activated during sympathetic nerve activity. However, the importance of these receptors in the modulation of neurotransmitter release under physiological and pathophysiological conditions is unknown.

In contrast to sympathetic neurons, chromaffin cells in the adrenal medulla which release epinephrine do not appear to possess inhibitory α_2-adrenoceptors (Powis and Baker, 1986). The α_2-adrenoceptor agonist, clonidine, does inhibit epinephrine release from bovine adrenal chromaffin cells evoked by nicotinic receptor stimulation, but this has recently been shown not to result from α_2-adrenoceptor stimulation. Rather, this effect of clonidine is mediated by an action at the nicotinic receptor, resulting in inhibition of the depolarizing Na^+ influx produced by nicotinic receptor stimulation (Powis and Baker, 1986).

α-Adrenoceptor activation inhibits stimulation-evoked acetylcholine release from parasympathetic neurons in guinea-pig ileum (Paton and Vizi, 1969), rabbit intestine (Vizi and Knoll, 1971) and from isolated superior cervical ganglia (Dawes and Vizi, 1973). These studies were performed before the α_1/α_2-adrenoceptor subdivision was established; hence the nature of the prejunctional α-adrenoceptor on cholinergic nerve terminals was not determined. More recently, several investigators have compared the prejunctional α-adrenoceptors on sympathetic and parasympathetic nerve terminals, and have concluded that both of these α-adrenoceptors were of the α_2-subtype (Starke, 1981; Drew, 1978).

Prejunctional α-adrenoceptors are also present at the skeletal neuromuscular junction. In contrast to autonomic neuroeffector junctions, activation of these receptors causes an enhancement of acetylcholine release (Malta et al., 1979). However, based on the pharmacological characterization of this receptor, it cannot be considered as an α_2-adrenoceptor since the α_1-adrenoceptor agonists, methoxamine and phenylephrine, also produce similar effects (Malta et al., 1979).

2.2.2 Postsynaptic Vascular α-Adrenoceptors in the Arterial Circulation

a. Systemic Arterial Circulation. Postjunctional α_2-adrenergic receptors are present on arterial smooth muscle, as demonstrated by the pressor response produced by α_2-adrenergic receptor agonists in the pithed rat. This response fulfills all the criteria for an α_2-adrenergic receptor-mediated response, in that it is produced by highly selective α_2-adrenergic receptor agonists, such as B-HT 920, B-HT 933 and UK 14,304, and is blocked competitively by selective α_2-adrenergic receptor antagonists, such as rauwolscine and idazoxan, and almost completely insensitive to α_1-adrenergic receptor blockade with prazosin. Since the discovery of arterial α_2-adrenergic receptors in the pithed rat (Bentley et al., 1977; Docherty et al., 1979; Drew and Whiting, 1979; Timmermans et al., 1979), this preparation has been used extensively to characterize the postjunctional arterial α_2-adrenergic receptor. An added advantage to this preparation is the ability to compare pre- and postjunctional α_2-adrenergic receptor function in the same animal. Subsequent experiments have been performed to show the presence of postjunctional arterial α_2-adrenergic receptors in dogs (Constantine et al., 1980), cats (Timmermans et al., 1983), rabbits (McGrath et al., 1982; van Meel et al., 1982) and humans (Elliott and Reid, 1983).

α_2-Adrenergic receptor-mediated pressor responses can be demonstrated in intact animals, although centrally mediated sympathoinhibition produced by those α_2-adrenergic receptor agonists that cross the blood–brain barrier may complicate the interpretation of results. The pressor response to intravenous administration of guanabenz, a selective α_2-adrenergic receptor agonist, to conscious rabbits is blocked by low doses of idazoxan (Hannah et al., 1983). In the conscious rabbit, rauwolscine or yohimbine are more effective in blocking the pressor response induced by norepinephrine than that elicited by phenylephrine, a selective α_1-adrenergic receptor agonist. Conversely, prazosin is more potent in blocking the pressor response of phenylephrine (Hamilton and Reid, 1982). Similar experiments have been performed in normal human volunteers, using epinephrine as a nonselective α-adrenergic receptor agonist, and phenylephrine to activate only the α_1-adrenergic receptor. Prazosin and yohimbine were most effective in blocking the phenylephrine and epinephrine responses, respectively (Goldberg and Robertson, 1984).

In addition to pressor responses in intact or decentralized animals, arterial α_2-adrenergic receptors can be demonstrated in a variety of perfused vascular beds. Langer et al. (1981) have demonstrated that the increases in blood pressure induced by intra-arterial administration of norepinephrine in the canine autoperfused hind limb are relatively resistant to prazosin blockade. Prazosin, at a dose that significantly attenuated the response to phenylephrine, has no effect on the response to guanabenz; in contrast, the response to guanabenz can be selectively inhibited by rauwolscine. Similar results have been obtained in Elsner et al. (1984).

Direct injection of clonidine into the femoral artery of an anaesthetized dog produced a decrease in femoral arterial blood flow which was completely insensitive to blockade by prazosin, but sensitive to antagonism by yohimbine (Horn et al., 1982). Conversely, methoxamine and phenylephrine produced effects which were blocked by prazosin, but not by yohimbine. Similar experiments in the renal vascular bed showed less of an α_2-adrenergic receptor-mediated contribution (see below), suggesting that the density of arterial α_2-adrenergic receptors may vary in different vascular beds (Horn et al., 1982).

Experiments in the rabbit autoperfused hind limb have demonstrated the presence of arterial α_2-adrenergic receptors, based on a significant vasoconstrictor response produced by the selective α_2-adrenergic receptor agonist, xylazine, which could be blocked by rauwolscine, but not by prazosin (Madjar et al., 1980).

In their initial studies with the isolated perfused rat hindquarters, Kobinger et al. (1980) did not detect an α_2-adrenergic receptor-mediated pressor response to B-HT 920, although the preparation remained responsive to α_1-adrenergic receptor agonists. The principal difference between this preparation and the other perfused vascular beds described above is that a physiologic salt solution was used by Kobinger et al. (1980) to perfuse the tissue, as opposed to whole blood. Additional experiments from this group (Kobinger and Pichler, 1981) and others (van Meel et al., 1983) have shown that an α_2-adrenergic receptor-mediated vasoconstrictor response to B-HT 920 could be produced in hindquarters isolated from rats pretreated with reserpine. This observation is consistent with a report (Hicks and Waldron, 1982) showing supersensitivity to α_2-adrenergic receptor agonists in the pithed rat following reserpine pretreatment. This effect may reflect post-receptor changes as opposed to a true denervation supersensitivity, since chemical sympathectomy with 6-hydroxydopamine combined with adrenal demedullectomy did not mimic the reserpine-induced supersensitivity changes in α_2-adrenergic receptor-mediated vascular response.

Despite the demonstration of arterial α_2-adrenergic receptors in a variety of *in vivo* models, and in autoperfused vascular beds, *in vitro* studies have not been able to provide conclusive evidence of α_2-adrenergic receptor-mediated arterial vasoconstriction. Although certain tissues, such as the rat aorta, are sensitive to clonidine-induced contraction, this effect has been shown to be mediated by α_1-adrenergic receptors, although these α_1-adrenergic receptors may differ somewhat from those found in other commonly studied arterial tissues (Ruffolo, 1985a). A norepinephrine-induced vasoconstrictor response that is insensitive to prazosin has been observed in certain human arteries, such as the palmar digital artery (Jauernig *et al.*, 1978); however, further studies of this tissue suggest the presence of an atypical α_1-adrenergic receptor, rather than an arterial α_2-adrenergic receptor (Stevens and Moulds, 1982). An *in vitro* study of isolated human arteries from several vascular beds has failed to demonstrate responsiveness to the highly selective α_2-adrenergic receptor agonist, UK 14,304 (Calvette *et al.*, 1984).

Almost all other isolated arterial tissues studied respond only to higher concentrations of selective α_2-adrenergic receptor agonists, and this effect is generally sensitive to blockade by α_1-adrenergic receptor antagonists (see Langer and Hicks, 1984). One notable exception seems to be the canine basilar artery, in which clonidine produces contraction that is insensitive to blockade by corynanthine (Sakakibara *et al.*, 1982), but is sensitive to inhibition by yohimbine. Similar conclusions in this tissue were obtained by Toda (1983), who found the response to norepinephrine to be insensitive to blockade by prazosin; however, the failure of this selective α_1-adrenergic receptor antagonist to block the response to phenylephrine (Toda, 1983) suggests that the response seen in the canine basilar artery may not be a typical α_2-adrenergic receptor-mediated response. A report by Ito and Chiba (1985) describes an α_2-adrenergic receptor-mediated contraction in the perfused ear artery of the dog. Xylazine, a moderately selective α_2-adrenergic receptor agonist, induced contraction that was preferentially antagonized by yohimbine. Conversely, phenylephrine-induced contraction was preferentially antagonized by prazosin. However, these experiments were not conducted under equilibrium conditions, since both the agonists and antagonists were administered as bolus injections into the perfusion flow; hence receptor dissociation constants for the antagonists used could not be obtained to compare to other established systems in order to verify α_2-adrenergic receptor activity.

Despite the failure to demonstrate convincing contractile responses to α_2-adrenergic receptor agonists in most isolated arteries, studies with antagonists often suggest a contribution of α_2-adrenergic receptors in the vasoconstrictor response to nonselective agonists, such as norepinephrine (Skarby et al., 1983; Hieble and Woodward, 1984).

There are two possible explanations for the apparent paradox of arterial α_2-adrenergic receptors being clearly demonstrable in vivo but not in vitro: (1) the α_2-adrenergic receptors are present only on very small resistance arteries or arterioles which are not routinely studied in vitro; or (2) some factor present under in vivo, but not in vitro conditions is required for expression of the response to arterial α_2-adrenergic receptors.

If α_2-adrenergic receptors are present only on smaller resistance arteries, α_2-adrenergic receptor-mediated increases in perfusion pressure should be evident in isolated perfused organs or vascular beds, since the entire arterial/arteriolar system is intact. As indicated above, the initial studies of Kobinger et al. (1980) could not demonstrate α_2-adrenergic receptor-mediated vasoconstriction in isolated rat hindquarters perfused with Tyrode's solution. The few other reported studies using saline-perfused organs report either only α_1-adrenergic receptor-mediated responses (perfused rat kidney), or a mixture of α_1- and α_2-adrenergic receptor-mediated responses (perfused cat spleen) (Langer and Hicks, 1984).

Changes in α-adrenergic receptor characteristics with decreasing arterial size have not been studied extensively, but there is evidence for abrupt changes in receptor characteristics, and adrenergic receptor function in general, as lumen diameter decreases (Owen and Bevan, 1985; Oriowo et al., 1985). These changes may relate to anatomical differences in the walls of large and small blood vessels (Bevan et al., 1985). Further studies on α_2-adrenergic receptor responsiveness in both saline-perfused vascular beds and in isolated small arteries are warranted.

It is well known that α_2-adrenergic receptor-mediated contraction of the canine saphenous vein is dependent on extracellular calcium concentration, and that removal of extracellular calcium will abolish the response (Jim and Matthews, 1985). In addition, it has also been reported that partial blockade of calcium channels with a relatively low concentration of nifedipine alters the B-HT 920 concentration–response curve in the canine saphenous vein by eliminating the abrupt increase in tension that occurs when a "threshold" concentration of the α_2-adrenergic receptor agonist is reached (Sulpizio and Hieble, 1985). Since α_2-adrenergic receptor-mediated contractile responses are highly dependent on extracellular calcium, the effects of activation of the calcium channel on the expression of an α_2-adrenergic receptor-mediated contraction in arterial tissue was studied. It has recently been observed that the plantar branch of canine saphenous artery contracted in a concentration-dependent manner to B-HT 920 *in vitro* only in the presence of a relatively low concentration of the calcium channel activator, BAY k 8644, and the response was blocked selectively by rauwolscine, but not by prazosin (Sulpizio and Hieble, 1987). These findings indicate that the response to B-HT 920 in this arterial tissue is mediated by postjunctional vascular α_2-adrenergic receptors. These results may suggest that *in vivo*, circulating factors that increase the probability of the calcium channel opening may be necessary for the expression of arterial responses to postjunctional α_2-adrenergic receptor stimulation, and that partial calcium channel activation may be necessary for the *in vitro* expression of postjunctional arterial α_2-adrenergic receptor-mediated responses.

It is now widely accepted that arterial vasoconstriction may be mediated by a mixed population of postsynaptic vascular α_1- and α_2-adrenergic receptors. The physiological function and/or distribution of these receptors is beginning to be understood. By using a variety of α_1-selective, α_2-selective and nonselective α-adrenergic receptor antagonists, Yamaguchi and Kopin (1980) observed that the pressor responses to exogenously administered catecholamines were selectively antagonized by α_2-adrenergic receptor blockers. Conversely, the pressor response evoked by sympathetic nerve stimulation was selectively antagonized by α_1-adrenergic receptor blockers. These authors postulated that postsynaptic vascular α-adrenergic receptors located at the neuroeffector junction (i.e., junctional receptors) were of the α_1-subtype, while those located away from the neuroeffector junction (i.e., extrajunctional receptors) were of the α_2-subtype.

Support of the concept of junctional α_1- and extrajunctional α_2-adrenergic receptors in the arterial circulation has been obtained in perfused cat spleen, where increases in perfusion pressure elicited by nerve stimulation, norepinephrine and phenylephrine were found to be differentially inhibited by selective α_1- and α_2-adrenergic receptor antagonists (Langer and Shepperson, 1982a). The responses to nerve stimulation and phenylephrine were abolished by the selective α_1-adrenergic receptor antagonist, prazosin, with the response to norepinephrine being only partially inhibited. Based on the known α_1-adrenergic receptor selectivity of phenylephrine, and the nonselective activity of norepinephrine, the results were compatible with the notion that neuronally released norepinephrine interacted with junctional α_1-adrenergic receptors, which could also be activated by exogenously administered phenylephrine and norepinephrine. Postsynaptic vascular α_2-adrenergic receptors in this model were proposed to reside extrajunctionally since they were not activated by norepinephrine released from sympathetic nerves, but could be stimulated by exogenously administered norepinephrine. In further studies using neuronal uptake inhibitors, Langer and Shepperson (1982a,b) have shown that postjunctional vascular α_1-adrenergic receptors are located in the vicinity of the neuronal uptake pump (uptake$_1$), and that postjunctional vascular α_2-adrenergic receptors are positioned away from this site. These results, and those obtained by Wilffert *et al.* (1982), strongly suggest the existence of junctional α_1- and extrajunctional α_2-adrenergic receptors located postsynaptically in the arterial circulation.

The physiological role of the postsynaptic junctional α_1-adrenergic receptors appears to be in maintaining resting vascular tone. Presumably, these receptors, which are located in the vicinity of the neurovascular junction, would interact with endogenous norepinephrine liberated from sympathetic nerves. The physiological role of the extrajunctional α_2-adrenergic receptors is not fully understood. It has been suggested that the extrajunctional α_2-adrenergic receptors would not normally interact with liberated norepinephrine since they are located some distance from the adrenergic nerve terminal, and the highly efficient neuronal uptake pump keeps synaptic levels of norepinephrine sufficiently low and thereby prevents diffusion of the neurotransmitter to the extrajunctional sites (Langer and Shepperson, 1982a). It has been proposed that the extrajunctional α_2-adrenergic receptors may respond to circulating epinephrine acting as a blood-borne hormone (Langer and Shepperson, 1982b). Although circulating catecholamines may be below the levels required to exert a physiological effect, it has been suggested that in times of stress, these levels may be raised to threshold levels where postsynaptic vascular α_2-adrenergic receptors are activated (Cutter *et al.*, 1980). It has also been suggested that the contribution made by arterial extrajunctional α_2-adrenergic receptors to total peripheral vascular resistance may be greater in certain hypertensive states than in normotensive patients (Bolli *et al.*, 1984; Jie *et al.*, 1986), implying that postsynaptic vascular α_2-adrenergic receptors may play an important role in pathophysiological states such as hypertension and possibly congestive heart failure, where circulating catecholamine levels are high (Levine *et al.*, 1982). It is unclear whether epinephrine is, in fact, responsible for stimulating the extrajunctional α_2-adrenergic receptors in these states, since circulating levels of norepinephrine are also particularly high and could account, at least in part, for their activation in disease states such as hypertension and congestive heart failure.

Although α_1- and α_2-adrenergic receptors coexist postjunctionally in arteries, and both subtypes mediate vasoconstriction, recent evidence suggests that α_1- and α_2-adrenergic receptors may be coupled differently to their respective vasoconstrictor processes (Ruffolo and Yaden, 1984). The nature of this difference between α_1- and α_2-adrenergic receptor coupling to arterial vasoconstriction may be reflected in quantitatively different "occupancy–vasoconstriction response" relationships, as well as qualitatively different mechanisms for the translation of stimuli into vasoconstrictor responses.

The relationship between α_1-adrenergic receptor occupancy by agonists and vasoconstrictor response has been studied *in vitro* for many years (Besse and Furchgott, 1976; Purdy and Stupecky, 1984; Ruffolo *et al.*, 1979a,b). In general, non-linear occupancy–response relationships have been obtained in most arterial vessels studied, with approximately 6% α_1-adrenergic receptor occupancy by full agonists being required for a half-maximal vasoconstrictor response to be obtained. "Spare" α_1-adrenergic receptors are commonly found. A direct comparison of the occupancy–response relationships for α_1- and α_2-adrenergic receptor-mediated arterial vasoconstriction has not been performed *in vitro* due to the difficulty in demonstrating α_2-adrenergic receptor-mediated vasoconstriction in isolated arterial preparations (see above). However, from studies *in vivo* where α_2-adrenergic receptor-mediated arterial vasoconstriction is easily quantified, evidence for differences in α_1- and α_2-adrenergic receptor occupancy–response relationships has been accumulated. Irreversible alkylation of postsynaptic vascular α_1-adrenergic receptors by phenoxybenzamine *in vivo* produces marked rightward shifts in the dose–response curves of α_1-adrenergic receptor agonists with no depression of the maximum response, whereas α_2-adrenergic receptor alkylation by higher doses of phenoxybenzamine is associated with depressed maximum vasoconstrictor responses with only small rightward shifts in the dose–response curves to α_2-adrenergic receptor agonists (Hamilton *et al.*, 1983; Reid *et al.*, 1983a; Ruffolo and Yaden, 1984). It appears, therefore, that a more favourable relationship exists between α_1-adrenergic receptor occupancy and vasoconstrictor response than between α_2-adrenergic receptor occupancy and vasoconstrictor response, and that the degree of "receptor reserve" is greater for postjunctional vascular α_1-adrenergic receptors, at least for the particular agonists used in these studies (Hamilton *et al.*, 1983; Reid *et al.*, 1983a; Ruffolo and Yaden, 1984).

Recently, it has been shown that the pressor response mediated by postjunctional vascular α_1-adrenergic receptors is resistant to antagonism by calcium slow channel blocking agents, suggesting that α_1-adrenergic receptors do not rely heavily upon extracellular calcium to produce arterial vasoconstriction. In contrast, vasoconstriction elicited by postjunctional arterial α_2-adrenergic receptors appears to be critically dependent upon extracellular calcium, as shown by the extreme sensitivity of this response to inhibition by the calcium channel blocking agents (Cavero *et al.*, 1983; van Meel *et al.*, 1981a,b).

The proposal that α_1- and α_2-adrenergic receptor-mediated arterial vaso-constriction results from utilization of different calcium pools has met with some criticism (Ruffolo *et al.*, 1984c; Hamilton *et al.*, 1983), and is inconsistent with *in vitro* studies in which α_1-adrenergic receptor-mediated vaso-constriction is also found to be highly sensitive to antagonism by calcium channel blockers (Awad *et al.*, 1983; Beckeringh *et al.*, 1984; van Breeman *et al.*, 1982). As a possible explanation for the resistance of the α_1-adrenergic receptor-mediated vasoconstrictor process *in vivo* to antagonism by calcium channel blockers, it has been argued (Reid *et al.*, 1983a; Ruffolo *et al.*, 1984c) that the large receptor reserve known to exist for postsynaptic vascular α_1-adrenergic receptors (Ruffolo and Yaden, 1984) would "buffer" this process from antagonism by any noncompetitive antagonist, including calcium channel blockers, in accord with receptor theory (Ariëns and van Rossum, 1957). When the large α_1-adrenergic receptor reserve is removed by pretreatment with phenoxybenzamine (Ruffolo *et al.*, 1984c) or benex-tramine (Nichols and Ruffolo, 1986), or when α_1-adrenergic receptor partial agonists are investigated for which no receptor reserve exists (Ruffolo *et al.*, 1984c), α_1-adrenergic receptor-mediated arterial vasoconstriction appears to be just as sensitive as α_2-adrenergic receptor-mediated arterial vaso-constriction to inhibition by calcium channel antagonists. It appears, there-fore, that both α_1- and α_2-adrenergic receptor-mediated arterial vaso-constrictor processes are highly dependent upon the mobilization of extracellular calcium (Ruffolo *et al.*, 1984c). It has recently been proposed that α_1-adrenergic receptor-mediated arterial vasoconstriction produced by full agonists may also depend, in part, on the mobilization of intracellular stores of calcium in addition to the translocation of extracellular calcium (Chiu *et al.*, 1986), whereas α_2-adrenergic receptor-mediated vasoconstric-tion involves only the translocation of extracellular calcium (Timmermans and Thoolen, 1987).

The biochemical correlates of α_1- and α_2-adrenergic receptor-mediated arterial vasoconstriction are poorly understood. While both α-adrenergic receptor subtypes may utilize predominantly extracellular calcium to evoke vasoconstrictor responses, it is unlikely that the steps leading up to calcium translocation are the same for both the postsynaptic vascular α_1- and α_2-adrenergic receptors. In most α_1-adrenergic receptor-mediated systems (Michell, 1979), including the vasculature (Villalobos-Molina *et al.*, 1982), calcium translocation is secondary to enhanced turnover of inositol phos-pholipids, the latter induced as a direct consequence of agonist interaction with α_1-adrenergic receptors. In contrast, although vasoconstriction mediated by postjunctional vascular α_2-adrenergic receptors is equally dependent (or more so) upon mobilization of extracellular calcium, this process appears not to be secondary to increases in phosphatidylinositol turnover (Reese and Matthews, 1986). In many systems, α_2-adrenergic receptor-mediated responses are closely coupled to the inhibition of adenylate cyclase. However, it is not known at present whether pressor responses elicited by postjunctional vascular α_2-adrenergic receptor agonists result from α_2-adrenergic receptor-mediated inhibition of vascular adenylate cyclase.

    b. Coronary Arterial Circulation. While the precise role of α_2-adrenergic receptor stimulation in the dynamic regulation of coronary blood flow is still unclear, it has been known for some time that following β-adrenergic receptor blockade, α-adrenergic receptor agonists or cardiac sympathetic nerve stimulation can produce coronary artery vasoconstriction leading to an increase in coronary arterial resistance and a decrease in coronary artery blood flow. α-Adrenergic receptor agonists, such as phenylephrine (Pitt *et al.*, 1967; Williams and Most, 1981), methoxamine (Hashimoto *et al.*, 1960), and norepinephrine (Berne, 1958; Hashimoto *et al.*, 1960; Gaal *et al.*, 1967; Lioy, 1967; Malindzak *et al.*, 1978), produce coronary artery vasoconstriction in the dog as well as in other species (Proctor, 1968; Glomstien *et al.*, 1967; Broadley, 1970; Parratt, 1969). In animals pretreated with β-adrenergic receptor-blocking agents, cardiac sympathetic nerve stimulation produces a fall in coronary artery blood flow that can be blocked by α-adrenergic receptor antagonists, demonstrating that α-adrenergic receptors can mediate vasoconstriction to both endogenous and exogenous norepinephrine in the coronary circulation (Feigl, 1967, 1975; Hamilton and Feigl, 1976; Malindzak *et al.*, 1978).

    It has recently been suggested that α_2-adrenergic receptors may play a role in the α-adrenergic receptor-mediated regulation of coronary artery blood flow. In the presence of β-adrenergic receptor blockade, intracoronary administration of the selective α_1-adrenergic receptor agonist, phenylephrine, and the selective α_2-adrenergic receptor agonist, B-HT 933, produce a rapid decrease in coronary artery blood flow, and these effects are blocked by the α_1- and α_2-adrenergic receptor agonists, prazosin and rauwolscine, respectively (Holtz *et al.*, 1982). These same investigators have demonstrated that the reduction in coronary artery blood flow elicited by exogenously administered norepinephrine is antagonized to a greater degree by rauwolscine than by prazosin, thus suggesting a more prominent role of α_2-adrenergic receptors in the regulation of coronary artery blood flow. The presence of α_1-adrenergic receptors on the large, epicardial coronary arteries has recently been demonstrated (Heusch *et al.*, 1984), while α_2-adrenergic receptors appear to be located primarily on the smaller subendocardial resistance vessels of the coronary vascular bed (Kopia *et al.*, 1986). In addition, it has been found that the presence of a flow-limiting coronary artery stenosis can unmask a vasoconstrictor response mediated by sympathetic nerve stimulation, and that this response can be antagonized by the nonselective α-adrenergic receptor antagonist, phentolamine, as well as by the selective α_2-adrenergic receptor antagonist, rauwolscine, but not by the selective α_1-adrenergic receptor antagonist, prazosin (Heusch and Deussen, 1983). These results suggest that α-adrenergic receptor-mediated coronary artery vasoconstriction may occur in the coronary circulation under pathological circumstances (i.e., coronary artery disease, angina or coronary artery vasospasm), and that α_2-adrenergic receptors might therefore represent a novel therapeutic target.

It has recently been shown (Kopia *et al.*, 1986) that equieffective blocking doses of the α_1-adrenergic receptor antagonist, prazosin, and the α_2-adrenergic receptor antagonist, idazoxan, produce a rightward shift in the left circumflex coronary artery blood flow–frequency response curve, with idazoxan producing greater blockade than prazosin. A similar result is also obtained when a more prolonged period of stimulation is used. The results indicate that α_1- and α_2-adrenergic receptors coexist in the coronary circulation, and that both α-adrenergic receptor subtypes mediate coronary artery vasoconstriction. Furthermore, the data suggest that postjunctional vascular α_2-adrenergic receptors may play a more important functional role than postjunctional vascular α_1-adrenergic receptors in the canine coronary circulation, and that α_2-adrenergic receptors may be preferentially innervated (i.e., junctional), since they may be selectively activated by endogenous norepinephrine liberated from sympathetic nerves upon electrical stimulation. These results are consistent with the observations of Holtz *et al.* (1982) which show that the α_2-adrenergic receptor-blocking agent, rauwolscine, produced a greater degree of inhibition of the coronary vasoconstrictor response to exogenously administered norepinephrine than did an equieffective blocking dose of prazosin.

In total, the results allow the following conclusions to be drawn regarding the coronary arterial circulation:

(1) that postjunctional vascular α_1- and α_2-adrenergic receptors coexist in the coronary circulation;

(2) both α-adrenergic receptor subtypes have the capacity to produce coronary artery vasoconstriction;

(3) the postjunctional vascular α_2-adrenergic receptor may be more important than the postjunctional vascular α_1-adrenergic receptor in the regulation of coronary artery blood flow;

(4) that neuronally released norepinephrine may selectively activate postjunctional vascular α_2-adrenergic receptors rather than α_1-adrenergic receptors;

(5) that postjunctional vascular α_2-adrenergic receptors may have pre-

dominantly a junctional or synaptic distribution, with the postjunctional vascular α_1-adrenergic receptors residing extrajunctionally to a greater extent; and

(6) that α_2-adrenergic receptors may be located on subendocardial resistance vessels in the coronary arterial circulation, whereas the α_1-adrenergic receptors may be located predominantly in the larger epicardial conduit vessels.

c. *Pulmonary Arterial Circulation.* Postjunctional vascular α_1- and α_2-adrenergic receptors mediate vasoconstriction in the pulmonary circulation of the dog (Shebuski *et al.*, 1986). This is shown by the dose-related increases in pulmonary perfusion pressure observed following the administration of the selective α_1-adrenergic receptor agonist, methoxamine, which is highly sensitive to blockade with the α_1-adrenergic receptor antagonist, prazosin, and resistant to the α_2-adrenergic receptor antagonist, rauwolscine. Accordingly, the pulmonary pressor effects mediated by the selective α_2-adrenergic receptor agonist, B-HT 933, were sensitive to blockade by rauwolscine and were resistant to prazosin. The results indicate that postjunctional vascular α_1- and α_2-adrenergic receptors coexist in the pulmonary circulation of the dog, and that both α-adrenergic receptor subtypes mediate vasoconstriction. Similar results have also been reported in the pulmonary vasculature of the cat (Hyman and Kadowitz, 1985). The maximal pulmonary pressor response attainable is greater with methoxamine than with B-HT 933, indicating that under conditions of normal pulmonary vascular tone, α_1-adrenergic receptor-mediated responses may predominate over α_2-adrenergic receptor-mediated responses.

The greatest increase in pulmonary perfusion pressure is achieved with the non-selective α-adrenergic receptor agonist, norepinephrine. Prazosin and rauwolscine both antagonize the increases in pulmonary perfusion pressure elicited by exogenously administered norepinephrine, indicating that norepinephrine has the capacity to stimulate both postjunctional α_1- and α_2-adrenergic receptors in the pulmonary vascular bed of the dog (Shebuski *et al.*, 1986). Pulmonary pressor responses to endogenous norepinephrine released from sympathetic nerves by administration of the indirectly acting sympathomimetic amine, tyramine, are antagonized primarily by prazosin, with little or no effect of rauwolscine. It appears, therefore, that endogenous norepinephrine acts primarily on α_1-adrenergic receptors in the pulmonary vascular bed of the dog (Shebuski *et al.*, 1986), and that endogenously released norepinephrine stimulates predominantly intrasynaptic α_1-adrenergic receptors, whereas exogenously administered norepinephrine stimulates both intrasynaptic α_1- as well as extrasynaptic α_2-adrenergic receptors in the canine pulmonary vascular bed. Similar conclusions have been made regarding the peripheral arterial circulation of the dog, in which preferential innervation of postjunctional vascular α_1-adrenergic receptors has been demonstrated (Langer et al., 1981).

The ability of selective α_2-adrenergic receptor agonists and exogenously administered norepinephrine to elicit increases in pulmonary perfusion pressure may indicate that, under some conditions, circulating catecholamines may play a role in maintaining or elevating pulmonary vascular tone by a mechanism involving, at least in part, postsynaptic vascular α_2-adrenergic receptors. Hyman et al. (1985) have infused epinephrine into the perfused pulmonary circulation of the cat (after propranolol treatment) to elicit a large rise in pulmonary perfusion pressure (10–20 mm Hg). Recently, Sawyer et al. (1985) have demonstrated that circulating catecholamines are responsible for α_2-adrenergic receptor-mediated pressor effects in the spontaneously hypertensive rat. Therefore, it may be postulated in certain disease states, such as congestive heart failure, in which pulmonary pressure is elevated and circulating catecholamine levels are high (Cohn et al., 1984), that α_2-adrenergic receptor-mediated increases in pulmonary vascular resistance may be secondary to the elevated circulating catecholamines.

It appears, therefore, that α_1- and α_2-adrenergic receptors can be identified in the pulmonary circulation of the dog and cat, and both α-adrenergic receptor subtypes mediate vasoconstriction. Norepinephrine released from sympathetic nerves activates primarily α_1-adrenergic receptors, whereas exogenously administered norepinephrine may activate both α_1- and α_2-adrenergic receptors under conditions of normal pulmonary vascular tone. Based on these observations, it has been suggested that postjunctional vascular α_1-adrenergic receptors in the pulmonary circulation are located at the vascular neuroeffector junction, whereas postjunctional vascular α_2-adrenergic receptors may be located extrajunctionally (Shebuski et al., 1986).

Under conditions of normal pulmonary vascular tone, postjunctional vascular α_1- and α_2-adrenergic receptors mediate vasoconstriction in the pulmonary circulation of the dog (Shebuski et al., 1986) and cat (Hyman and Kadowitz, 1985). Under these conditions (basal pressure = 10 ± 1 mm Hg), α_1-adrenergic receptor-mediated responses predominate over α_2-adrenergic receptor-mediated responses (Hyman and Kadowitz, 1985; Shebuski et al., 1986). However, when pulmonary vascular tone is elevated, even slightly, with a vasoconstrictor agent, responses to the selective α_2-adrenergic receptor agonist, B-HT 933, are markedly enhanced (Shebuski et al., 1987; Hyman and Kadowitz, 1986). Furthermore, the enhanced responsiveness of α_2-adrenergic receptors is tone-dependent and highly selective for α_2-adrenergic receptors, since responses to the α_1-

adrenergic receptor agonist, methoxamine, or to angiotensin II were not enhanced by elevating pulmonary vascular tone (Shebuski et al., 1987). The nature of the vasoconstrictor agent used to elevate pulmonary vascular tone does not influence the enhanced α_2-adrenergic receptor responsiveness, although the manner in which pulmonary vascular pressure is elevated is critically important. When pulmonary perfusion pressure is elevated by increased pulmonary blood flow as opposed to pulmonary vasoconstriction, responses to B-HT 933 are not enhanced as they are when vasoconstrictor agents are utilized to elevate pulmonary pressure (Shebuski et al., 1987). This observation indicates that pulmonary vascular smooth muscle tone, and not pulmonary pressure per se, is the major determinant of enhanced α_2-adrenergic receptor responsiveness in the pulmonary vasculature.

Thus, under conditions of elevated pulmonary vascular tone, α_2-adrenergic receptor-mediated responsiveness is markedly enhanced. Enhancement of pulmonary α_2-adrenergic receptor responsiveness is tone-dependent and selective for postjunctional vascular α_2-adrenergic receptors. Enhanced responsiveness of α_2-adrenergic receptors in the pulmonary circulation at high tone does not appear to be due to generalized improvement in vascular excitation–contraction coupling, but may be due to improved function of voltage-dependent calcium channels linked to pulmonary vascular α_2-adrenergic receptors.

d. Renal Arterial Circulation. The kidneys receive approximately 20% of the cardiac output and provide a significant contribution to total systemic vascular resistance. Their dense noradrenergic innervation extends to both the afferent and efferent arterioles (Barajas and Wang, 1979). Stimulation of the renal nerves, and administration of α-adrenergic receptor agonists, produce an increase in renal vascular resistance with redistribution of blood flow from the cortical to the medullary areas. This response is blocked by phenoxybenzamine or phentolamine (Cooke et al., 1972; Oswald and Greven, 1981), indicating the activation of α-adrenergic receptors. Initial in vivo studies of the α-adrenergic receptor subtype mediating renal vascular responses to exogenously administered agonists suggested an almost exclusive role of α_1-adrenergic receptors in the renal vasculature of the rat (Schmitz et al., 1981), cat (Drew and Whiting, 1979) and dog (Horn et al., 1982). More recent studies show that the α_2-adrenergic receptor agonist, B-HT 933, produces renal vasoconstriction in the dog, and this response is blocked by the selective α_2-adrenergic receptor antagonist, rauwolscine (A. J. Nichols and R. R. Ruffolo, in prep.), indicating the presence of postjunctional arterial α_2-adrenergic receptors in the renal vasculature of the dog. It should be emphasized, however, that the renal vasoconstriction produced by B-HT 933 is much less than that observed in the hindlimb vasculature and is less than that produced by the α_1-adrenergic receptor agonist, cirazoline, in the renal arterial circulation. Significant renal vaso-constrictor responses are also produced by postjunctional α_2-adrenergic receptor activation in the rabbit *in vivo* (Hesse and Johns, 1984). In contrast, studies on isolated rabbit perfused afferent and efferent arterioles have identified vasoconstriction mediated by α_1-adrenergic receptors, but not by α_2-adrenergic receptors, with no significant difference in the sensitivity of afferent and efferent arterioles being observed (R. M. Edwards, pers. comm.). This lack of α_2-adrenergic receptor-mediated vasoconstriction *in vitro* may result from the relatively low density of postjunctional α_2-adrenergic receptors that exist in the renal arterial vasculature as suggested by the *in vivo* studies. Efferent renal nerve stimulation in the dog produces vasoconstriction via activation of α_1-adrenergic receptors (Osborn *et al.*, 1983). However, it has been suggested that in the rabbit, α_2-adrenergic receptors may play a role in neurogenic vasoconstrictor responses (Hesse and Johns, 1984). Thus, despite evidence demonstrating the presence of postjunctional α_2-adrenergic receptors in the renal arterial vasculature and suggestions of slight species differences, postjunctional α_1-adrenergic receptors predominate.

e. Mesenteric Arterial Circulation. The splanchnic circulation receives approximately 20–25% of the cardiac output, and contains a similar propor-tion of the blood volume. The major part of the splanchnic blood supply is received by the mesenteric circulation which supplies the small intestine and the upper two-thirds of the large intestine via the superior mesenteric artery. Consequently, the mesenteric circulation has the potential to play a major role in the determination of total systemic vascular resistance. Sympathetic nerve stimulation and exogenous norepinephrine administration produce mesenteric arteriolar vasoconstriction via activation of α-adrenergic recep-tors (Granger *et al.*, 1980). Studies using the *in situ* autoperfused superior mesenteric arterial bed of the rat suggest that only α_1-adrenergic receptors are present in the mesenteric vasculature, since vasoconstrictor responses to norepinephrine are blocked exclusively by low doses of prazosin and are relatively unaffected by yohimbine (Nichols and Hiley, 1985; Nichols, 1985). Similarly, the α_1-adrenergic receptor agonists, phenylephrine, amidephrine and cirazoline, produce mesenteric arterial vasoconstriction, whereas the α_2-adrenergic receptor agonists, xylazine, B-HT 920 and B-HT 933, do not (Nichols, 1985). However, Hiley and Thomas (1987), using the microsphere technique in the pithed rat, have shown that the mesenteric vasculature of the rat does indeed possess postjunctional vascular α_2-adrenergic receptors in addition to the previously identified α_1-subtype, with an apparent greater density of α_1-adrenergic receptors relative to α_2-adrenergic receptors. Similarly, studies in the cat (Drew and Whiting, 1979) and the dog (Shepperson et al., 1982) have demonstrated a significant population of postjunctional vascular α_2-adrenergic receptors in the superior mesenteric arterial bed. In the cat, it appears that α_2-adrenergic receptors are less prominent in the mesenteric vasculature than in the hindlimb skeletal muscle vasculature (Drew and Whiting, 1979). No studies have been specifically designed to determine whether or not α_1- and α_2-adrenergic receptors are differentially distributed within the intestinal wall. However, neuronally released norepinephrine, which presumably acts exclusively on α_1-adrenergic receptors in the resistance vessels, does not produce a significant redistribution of blood flow within the intestinal wall. Thus, it would appear that α_1-adrenergic receptors are relatively uniformly distributed throughout the arterial circulation in the gut wall. No information is available regarding the distribution of postjunctional vascular α_2-adrenergic receptors in the mesenteric arterial circulation.

 f. Cerebral Arterial Circulation. The arteries supplying blood to the brain clearly have different pharmacological characteristics compared to peripheral arteries. If the reactivity of the vertebral or carotid artery of the rabbit to norepinephrine is determined sequentially, a marked decrease in sensitivity is seen just prior to the entry of the vessel into the subarachnoid space (Bevan, 1979). The point of transition corresponds to the change in embryological origin of the proximal and distal portions of each of these blood vessels. Although most studies have been performed on the relatively large cerebral arteries, such as the basilar artery or the middle cerebral artery, these may be the most important sites for an α_2-adrenergic receptor-mediated effect, since, as in other vascular beds, such as the pulmonary circulation, the contribution of α-adrenergic receptors may decrease with decreasing vascular diameter (Bevan et al., 1985).

Although cerebral blood vessels have extensive and active sympathetic innervation (Duckles, 1980), the α-adrenergic receptor-mediated responses of these vessels to sympathetic nerve stimulation is small compared to peripheral vessels (McCalden, 1981). This may be related either to insensitivity of the α-adrenergic receptor, or to a reduced α-adrenergic receptor number (Bevan, 1984). Nevertheless, there is evidence that the sympathetic nervous system can modulate cerebral blood flow in the conscious animal through an α-adrenergic receptor-mediated effect as measured by hypothalamic washout of radioactive xenon in the rabbit (Rosendorff et al., 1976).

In vitro characterization of α-adrenergic receptors on cerebral blood vessels has not yet yielded a uniform picture. Radioligand binding studies show the presence of both [³H]-prazosin and [³H]-yohimbine binding sites in membranes from human and monkey cerebral arteries. In contrast, only [³H]-yohimbine sites could be detected in canine and bovine cerebral arteries. Furthermore, the B_{max} for [³H] yohimbine was higher in canine (450 fmol/mg protein) and bovine (670 fmol/mg) cerebral arteries compared to human (240 fmol/mg) and monkey (200 fmol/mg) cerebral arteries (Usui et al., 1985). This suggests an increased α_2-adrenergic receptor contribution in the canine and bovine cerebral vessels.

Physiological support for this hypothesis has been provided by the observations that clonidine produces a yohimbine-sensitive contraction in the isolated canine basilar artery (Sakakibara et al., 1982). Yohimbine inhibits the contractile response to norepinephrine in canine, but not in monkey and human cerebral arteries. Conversely, the contractile response to norepinephrine in monkey and human cerebral arteries are sensitive to prazosin (Sakakibara et al., 1982; Toda, 1983). However, the vascular α-adrenergic receptor of the canine cerebral artery may be atypical, since phenylephrine will produce a response in this tissue that is insensitive to blockade by prazosin (100 nM), but is antagonized by a moderate concentration of yohimbine (K_b < 50 nM) (Toda, 1983). The magnitide of contraction in the canine cerebral artery induced by norepinephrine and other α_1-adrenergic receptor agonists is also lower than that seen in human and monkey cerebral arteries (Usui et al., 1985). This is also consistent with a relatively small number of α_1-adrenergic receptors observed in radioligand binding studies in the canine cerebral artery.

The cat cerebral artery also has predominantly α_2-adrenergic receptors located postjunctionally, since rauwolscine is approximately 100-fold more potent than prazosin in blocking vasoconstriction responses elicited by norepinephrine (Skarby, 1984).

In addition to the α_1- and α_2-adrenergic receptors, rabbit cerebral arteries also show a vasoconstrictor response to high concentrations (> 100 μM) of norepinephrine, and this response is insensitive to blockade by phenoxybenzamine and other α-adrenergic receptor antagonists (Duckles et al., 1976). It has been proposed that this response may not be mediated by specific receptors, since the effect produced by norepinephrine at these concentrations is not stereospecific. Nevertheless, the response to high concentrations of norepinephrine has been postulated to play a role in cerebrovascular neurotransmission, due to the limited number of α-adrenergic receptors present on these vessels (Bevan et al., 1985). This type of response has also been reported in peripheral blood vessels following phenoxybenzamine treatment.

Much information regarding the role of the α-adrenergic receptor subtypes in mediating vasoconstriction of cerebral arteries still remains to be elucidated. Nevertheless, at least in certain species, the α_2-adrenergic receptor appears to be demonstrable in radioligand binding studies, by vasoconstriction induced by α_2-adrenergic receptor agonists, and by blockade of the response to the physiological neurotransmitter, norepinephrine, by selective α_2-adrenergic receptor antagonists.

g. *Endothelium*. It has recently been demonstrated that vascular endothelial cells mediate relaxation of arterial smooth muscle in response to certain vasodilators, such as acetylcholine, bradykinin and substance P, by the release of the so-called endothelium-derived relaxing factor (EDRF) (Furchgott, 1983). It has been proposed that activation of α_2-adrenergic receptors on endothelial cells stimulates the release of EDRF (Egleme *et al.*, 1984; Cocks and Angus, 1983; Matsuda *et al.*, 1985), an action which would tend to antagonize vasoconstriction produced by activation of postjunctional vascular α-adrenergic receptors. Thus, removal of endothelial cells from rat aorta produces an increase in responsiveness to α-adrenergic receptor agonists (Egleme *et al.*, 1984). However, the mechanism by which endothelium removal enhances α-adrenergic receptor responsiveness in this tissue may not result from the removal of α_2-adrenergic receptor-stimulated release of EDRF, since enhancement of α-adrenergic receptor-mediated vasoconstriction by removal of the endothelium in rat aorta is not related to the α-adrenergic subtype specificity of the agonist used, inasmuch as both α_1- and α_2-adrenergic receptor agonists produce this effect (Malta *et al.*, 1986; Martin *et al.*, 1986). Furthermore, removal of the α_1-adrenergic receptor reserve for phenylephrine markedly enhances the potentiating effect of endothelium removal (Martin *et al.*, 1986). Combined with the failure of clonidine to produce relaxation of precontracted endothelium-intact rat aorta (Martin *et al.*, 1986), these data suggest that spontaneous release of EDRF from rat aortic endothelium depresses contractility of the vascular smooth muscle by functional antagonism of the response to α_1-adrenergic receptor activation, with the depression of responsiveness being inversely related to agonist efficacy (Malta *et al.*, 1986; Martin *et al.*, 1986). However, in other vascular preparations, there is convincing evidence that endothelial cells lining arteries do possess α_2-adrenergic receptors which mediate the release of EDRF. Cocks and Angus (1983) demonstrated that removal of endothelium enhanced the contractile response produced by norepinephrine in canine and porcine circumflex coronary artery, and that after blockade of α_1-adrenergic receptors, norepinephrine could produce yohimbine- and idazoxan-sensitive relaxation of precontracted arteries only in the presence of an intact endothelium. Additional studies have shown that α_2-adrenergic receptors mediated release of EDRF from carotid, mesenteric, renal and femoral arteries from dogs and pigs, although there do appear to be species differences in the magnitude of this response (Angus *et al.*, 1986). Furthermore, it has been suggested that endothelial α_2-adrenergic receptors mediate release of EDRF in coronary microvessels (Angus *et al.*, 1986). Thus, α_2-adrenergic receptor agonists do indeed appear to have the capability of modulating vascular responsiveness via stimulation of the release of EDRF in both large arteries and the microcirculation, but this effect does not occur in all vessels.

    h. Occupancy–Response Coupling in the Arterial Circulation. The relationship between α_1-adrenoceptor occupancy by agonists and receptor activation has been studied extensively in cardiovascular tissues *in vitro*. Full α_1-adrenoceptor agonists commonly have a non-linear occupancy–response relationship in most arterial vessels, and most full agonists (e.g., norepinephrine, epinephrine, phenylephrine and cirazoline) produce half-maximal responses at approximately 5–10% α_1-adrenoceptor occupancy in large blood vessels such as rat aorta (Ruffolo *et al.*, 1979a,b), guinea-pig aorta (Ruffolo and Waddell, 1982), canine aorta (Sastre *et al.*, 1984), rabbit aorta (Besse and Furchgott, 1976; Purdy and Stupecky, 1984) and rabbit ear artery (Purdy and Stupecky, 1984). Because of the difficulty in obtaining α_2-adrenoceptor-mediated contractile responses in arterial vessels *in vitro* (see above), no direct comparison of the α_1- and α_2-adrenoceptor occupancy–response relationships has been made in arterial blood vessels.

    On the other hand, α_2-adrenoceptor-mediated arterial vasoconstriction may be readily demonstrated *in vivo* (see Section 2.2.2.*a*) where comparisons between the occupancy–response relationships for α_1- and α_2-adrenoceptor mediated vasopressor effects can be made. Irreversible alkylation of postsynaptic vascular α_1-adrenoceptors by phenoxybenzamine in conscious rabbits and pithed rats produces marked rightward shifts in the pressor dose–response curves to α_1-adrenoceptor agonists before depressions of the maximum response are observed. In contrast, alkylation of α_2-adrenoceptors by phenoxybenzamine is associated with depressed maximum vasoconstrictor responses with only small rightward shifts in the dose–response curves to α_2-adrenoceptor agonists (Hamilton *et al.*, 1983; Reid *et al.*, 1983a; Ruffolo and Yaden, 1984). These results are highly suggestive of a more favourable occupancy–response relationship for α_1-adrenoceptors than for α_2-adrenoceptors in the arterial circulation. This differential pattern of α_1- and α_2-adrenoceptor responses following alkylation of vascular α-adrenoceptors was analyzed further in the pithed rat using cirazoline as an α_1-adrenoceptor agonist and B-HT 933 as an α_2-adrenoceptor agonist (Ruffolo and Yaden, 1984). Cirazoline possesses a hyperbolic relationship between the maximum pressor effect that can be obtained, and the fraction of α_1-adrenoceptors remaining available for interaction with cirazoline after phenoxybenzamine treatment, suggesting the existence of a large α_1-adrenoceptor reserve. In contrast, for the α_2-adrenoceptor agonist, B-HT 933, a linear relationship was found to exist between the maximum pressor response obtainable and the proportion of intact α_2-adrenoceptors available for interaction with the agonist (Ruffolo and Yaden, 1984), a situation highly characteristic of a system with no receptor reserve (Ruffolo, 1982). The α_1-adrenoceptor-mediated vasopressor effect of cirazoline had a five-fold more favourable occupancy–response relationship than was found for the α_2-adrenoceptor-mediated vasopressor effect of B-HT 933, which is consistent with the hypothesis that there may be spare α_1-adrenoceptors, but not α_2-adrenoceptors, in the arterial circulation for these agonists *in vivo*. This apparent large difference between the α_1- and α_2-adrenoceptor occupancy–response relationships in the arterial circulation may partly explain the difficulty in studying postjunctional vascular α_2-adrenoceptors in arteries *in vitro*, compared to the ease with which α_1-adrenoceptors can be studied (Ruffolo, 1986).

2.2.3 Postsynaptic Vascular α-Adrenoceptors in the Venous Circulation

a. *Saphenous Vein*. In contrast to arterial α_2-adrenergic receptors, vascular α_2-adrenergic receptors in isolated veins can be studied easily *in vitro*, at least in certain tissues; indeed most of the characterization of venous α_2-adrenergic receptors has been performed *in vitro*.

The most commonly studied vein is the canine saphenous vein. DeMey and Vanhoutte (1981a,b) first reported the potent vasoconstrictor activity of clonidine in this tissue. Additional studies have shown that highly selective α_2-adrenergic receptor agonists, such as B-HT 920, B-HT 933 and UK 14,304, will produce a vasoconstrictor response that is resistant to antagonism by prazosin and sensitive to blockade by rauwolscine (Fowler *et al.*, 1984; Alabaster *et al.*, 1985; Ruffolo and Zeid, 1985). Receptor dissociation constants calculated for α_2-adrenergic receptor antagonists in the canine saphenous vein correlate well with the values obtained at prejunctional α_2-adrenergic receptors (Fowler *et al.*, 1984; Hieble *et al.*, 1986).

Although α_1-adrenergic receptors are also present in canine saphenous vein, the use of selective agonists and/or antagonists allows the postsynaptic vascular α_2-adrenergic receptor to be studied without interference from the α_1-adrenergic receptor. In the canine saphenous vein, norepinephrine, which can activate both α_1- and α_2-adrenergic receptors, appears to activate preferentially the α_2-subtype. Fowler *et al.* (1984) found the response to low concentrations of norepinephrine to be relatively unaffected by prazosin. Flavahan *et al.* (1984) observed qualitatively similar results, with the lower portion of the dose–response curve to norepinephrine being blocked by prazosin to a lesser extent than the higher concentration range. In contrast, Alabaster et al. (1985) and Sullivan and Drew (1980) observed competitive blockade of the norepinephrine response by prazosin at both the lower and higher concentration ranges. The inconsistencies between these observations have yet to be resolved.

Saphenous veins from other species also show α_2-adrenergic receptor responsiveness. Alabaster et al. (1985) suggest that the rabbit saphenous vein represents a more useful model tissue to study postsynaptic vascular α_2-adrenergic receptors than the canine saphenous vein, based on a proposed smaller contribution of α_1-adrenergic receptor-mediated responses. However, Levitt and Hieble (1985), although observing potent blockade of B-HT 933 induced vasoconstriction by rauwolscine ($K_b = 3.6$ nM), found the response to norepinephrine to be sensitive to both prazosin ($K_b = 13$ nM) and rauwolscine ($K_b = 7$ nM), suggesting a significant contribution from both α_1-adrenergic receptors and α_2-adrenergic receptors in this tissue.

Experiments in isolated human saphenous vein (Muller-Schweinitzer, 1984) show similar results to those reported by Fowler et al. (1984) in the canine saphenous vein. The response to low concentrations of norepinephrine were essentially unaffected by prazosin, but potently antagonized by yohimbine ($K_b = 25$ nM).

Inhibition of the vasoconstrictor response to field stimulation of adrenergic nerve terminals in both canine (Sullivan and Drew, 1980; Flavahan et al., 1984) and human (Docherty and Hyland, 1984; Göthert et al., 1984) saphenous vein is mediated via prejunctional α_2-adrenergic receptors, based on blockade of this response by yohimbine, but not by prazosin.

The venous circulation, in particular the canine saphenous vein, resembles the arterial circulation in that postsynaptic vascular α_1- and α_2-adrenergic receptors coexist, with each α-adrenergic receptor subtype mediating vasoconstriction (Constantine et al., 1982; DeMey and Vanhoutte, 1981a,b; Flavahan et al., 1984; Docherty and Hyland, 1984). However, in contrast to the arterial circulation, postsynaptic vascular α_2-adrenergic receptors in the canine saphenous vein appear to be preferentially innervated, with postsynaptic vascular α_1-adrenergic receptors being innervated to a lesser degree and possibly located predominantly extrajunctionally (Flavahan et al., 1984).

In the canine saphenous vein, the α_1-adrenergic receptor occupancy–response relationship (obtained for cirazoline) is approximately four-fold more favourable than the α_2-adrenergic receptor occupancy–response relationship (obtained for B-HT 933), although both agonists are associated with a significant receptor reserve (Ruffolo and Zeid, 1985). Both the α_1-adrenergic receptor occupancy–response relationship of cirazoline and the α_2-adrenergic receptor occupancy–response relationship of B-HT 933 are rectangular hyperbolas, which suggests that both compounds have high intrinsic efficacy at their respective α-adrenergic receptor subtypes (Ruffolo and Zeid, 1985). The results indicate that the α-adrenergic receptor reserve may be significantly larger for postsynaptic vascular α_1-adrenergic receptors than for postsynaptic vascular α_2-adrenergic receptors in canine saphenous vein, as also appears to be the case in the peripheral arterial circulation (Ruffolo and Zeid, 1985).

The maximum contractile response observed to B-HT 933 is significantly less than that obtained with cirazoline in the canine saphenous vein (Ruffolo and Zeid, 1985). This observation has been made previously for a number of α_2-adrenergic receptor agonists that routinely produce lower maximum responses than α_1-adrenergic receptor agonists in the canine saphenous vein (Flavahan et al., 1984). The lower maximum responses commonly observed with α_2-adrenergic receptor agonists in the canine saphenous vein could result from four factors:

(1) the α_2-adrenergic receptor agonists studied to date could be partial agonists (i.e., low intrinsic efficacy characterized by relatively linear occupancy–response relationships);
(2) a relative deficiency in α_2-adrenergic receptor number;
(3) poor coupling between α_2-adrenergic receptor activation and vaso-constrictor response; or
(4) limitations in the α_2-adrenergic receptor excitation–contraction coupling mechanism.

The first possibility may be eliminated because the α_2-adrenergic receptor occupancy–response relationship of B-HT 933 in canine saphenous vein is hyperbolic, characteristic of a full agonist. In fact, the α_2-adrenergic receptor occupancy–response relationship for B-HT 933 is as favourable for α_2-adrenergic receptors as cirazoline is for α_1-adrenergic receptors (Ruffolo and Zeid, 1985). In other words, B-HT 933 has as high an efficacy at α_2-adrenergic receptors as cirazoline has at α_1-adrenergic receptors, at least in canine saphenous vein. The second and third possibilities of limited α_2-adrenergic receptor number, or poor coupling between α_2-adrenergic receptor occupancy and vasoconstrictor response, may be eliminated because in the canine saphenous vein there exists an α_2-adrenergic receptor reserve for B-HT 933, and this could not occur if the number of α_2-adrenergic receptors was low, or if coupling was poor. This reserve exists because of the high efficacy of the agonist, such that only 60% of the α_2-adrenergic receptor population is required by B-HT 933 to produce a maximum response (Ruffolo and Zeid, 1985). It is unlikely, therefore, that with 40% of the α_2-adrenergic receptor population representing excess or spare α_2-adrenergic receptors, that limited α_2-adrenergic receptor number could contribute to the lower maximum response observed for B-HT 933 relative to the α_1-adrenergic receptor agonist, cirazoline, in canine saphenous vein. In addition, if there were poor coupling between α_2-adrenergic receptor occupancy and vasoconstrictor response, there would not exist a reserve in α_2-adrenergic receptors, and the occupancy–response relationship for B-HT 933 would be linear. At present, evidence supports the contention that the lower maximum response observed with α_2-adrenergic receptor agonists relative to α_1-adrenergic receptor agonists in the canine saphenous vein results from fundamental differences in the excitation–contraction coupling mechanisms utilized by α_1- and α_2-adrenergic receptors, such that α_2-adrenergic receptor-mediated vasoconstriction is not capable of producing the degree of vasoconstriction observed with α_1-adrenergic receptor agonists. Although not completely understood, the excitation–contraction coupling mechanisms for postsynaptic vascular α_1- and α_2-adrenergic receptors in the canine saphenous vein appear to be different in terms of electrophysiological activity (Matthews et al., 1984b), and possibly calcium utilization (Langer and Shepperson, 1982a,b), and these factors may selectively limit the degree of vasoconstriction that can be produced by an α_2-adrenergic receptor agonist in this tissue.

It is interesting to note that cirazoline produces a half-maximal response in the canine saphenous vein by occupying approximately 4–5% of the available α_1-adrenergic receptor pool. (Ruffolo and Zeid, 1985). It has been reported that cirazoline produces a half-maximal response in guinea-pig aorta by occupancy of approximately 6% of the α_1-adrenergic receptor pool (Ruffolo and Waddell, 1982), and is identical to norepinephrine in this regard (Ruffolo and Waddell, 1982). It appears, therefore, that the relationship between α_1-adrenergic receptor occupancy and response is similar in the canine saphenous vein and the guinea-pig aorta. Inasmuch as most full α_1-adrenergic receptor agonists, such as norepinephrine, epinephrine, phenylephrine, and cirazoline, produce half-maximal responses at approximately 5–10% α_1-adrenergic receptor occupancy in large blood vessels such as rat aorta (Ruffolo et al., 1979b), guinea-pig aorta (Ruffolo et al., 1982b), canine aorta (Sastre et al., 1984), rabbit aorta (Besse and Furchgott, 1976), and rabbit ear artery (Purdy and Stupecky, 1984), it has been proposed that the coupling between α_1-adrenergic receptor occupancy and response is similar in most large blood vessels, regardless of arterial or venous origin (Ruffolo, 1984b).

There is one important difference between α_2-adrenergic receptor reserves in arteries and veins that must be emphasized. In the arterial circulation of the rat, there is no reserve in α_2-adrenergic receptors, the latter being characterized by a linear occupancy–response relationship for B-HT 933 (Ruffolo and Yaden, 1984). In contrast, in the canine saphenous vein, there is a significant α_2-adrenergic receptor reserve, such that a non-linear, hyperbolic occupancy–response relationship is obtained for B-HT 933. The fact that there exists an α_2-adrenergic receptor reserve in the canine saphenous vein, but not in the arterial circulation of the rat, may have profound implications concerning fundamental differences between arteries and veins. As indicated previously, it has been suggested that the venous circulation is significantly more dependent on postsynaptic vascular α_2-adrenergic receptors than is the arterial circulation (Flavahan et al., 1984; Ruffolo, 1985b), and that this may be a direct consequence of the presence of spare α_2-adrenergic receptors in veins (at least the canine saphenous vein) but not arteries (Ruffolo and Yaden, 1984). In fact, it may be argued that the difficulty in studying the postsynaptic vascular α_2-adrenergic receptor in isolated arteries in vitro, and the ease with which these receptors may be studied in isolated venous preparations (such as the canine saphenous vein), may also be attributed to the greater number of spare α_2-adrenergic receptors found in larger veins but not in larger arteries. Indeed, studies in vivo also tend to indicate that the postsynaptic vascular α_2-adrenergic receptor may play a more prominent role in venous capacitance vessels than in arterial resistance and conduit vessels (see below; Appleton et al., 1984; Greenway and Innes, 1981; Patel et al., 1981; Segstro and Greenway, 1986).

As indicated previously, in the canine saphenous vein, the lower portion of the dose–response curve to norepinephrine is mediated predominantly by α_2-adrenergic receptors, whereas responses at higher concentrations are mediated predominantly by α_1-adrenergic receptors (Matthews et al., 1984a). The α_1-adrenergic receptor-mediated vasoconstrictor response in the canine saphenous vein results from electromechanical coupling in which the contractile response parallels electrophysiologic changes in membrane potential (Matthews et al., 1984b). In contrast, the α_2-adrenergic receptor-mediated response in the canine saphenous vein results from pharmacomechanical coupling, in which the contractile response is not paralleled by electrophysiological changes.

Vasoconstriction in canine saphenous vein mediated by both the postsynaptic vascular α_1- and α_2-adrenergic receptors appears to be critically dependent on the translocaion of extracellular calcium. In the canine saphenous vein, vasoconstrictor responses mediated by the α_1-adrenergic receptor agonist, phenylephrine, and by the α_2-adrenergic receptor agonist, M-7, are both inhibited by calcium slow-channel antagonists, such as diltiazem and verapamil (Langer and Shepperson, 1981). Although α_1- and α_2-adrenergic receptor-mediated vasoconstriction of the canine saphenous vein is predominantly dependent upon the translocation of extracellular calcium, evidence exists to suggest that in this tissue, α_1-adrenergic receptor agonist may also trigger, to a smaller and limited extent, the release of intracellular calcium (Langer and Shepperson, 1981; Matthews *et al.*, 1984a).

b. Pulmonary Vein. Assessment of postjunctional α-adrenergic receptor activity in the pulmonary vasculature *in vitro* provides some interesting correlates to what is observed in canine saphenous vein. Intralobar pulmonary veins have been reported to contract to the selective α_2-adrenergic receptor agonist, B-HT 933, and this response is sensitive to inhibition by the selective α_2-adrenergic receptor antagonist, rauwolscine (Shebuski *et al.*, 1987; Ohlstein *et al.*, 1986). In contrast, intralobar pulmonary arteries are relatively unresponsive to B-HT 933 *in vitro*. These results indicate that postjunctional vascular α_2-adrenergic receptors may be preferentially located on the venous side of the pulmonary circulation, as also appears to be the case in the peripheral circulation (Ruffolo, 1985a).

c. Hepatic Portal System. A similar situation to that described in the canine saphenous vein also exists *in vivo* in the intestinal venous circulation (Patel *et al.*, 1981). In addition, in the hepatic venous circulation of the cat *in vivo*, blood volume responses to norepinephrine are mediated by post-synaptic vascular α_2-adrenergic receptors, as is the hepatic venous response to sympathetic nerve stimulation (Segstro and Greenway, 1986). These results are suggestive of a dominance of α_2- over α_1-adrenergic receptors in the hepatic venous circulation, as well as a preferential, if not exclusive, junctional location of postsynaptic vascular α_2-adrenergic receptors (Segstro and Greenway, 1986). Furthermore, α_2-adrenergic receptor-mediated responses in the venous circulation appear to be more marked than those in the arterial circulation, consistent with the notion that postsynaptic vascular α_2-adrenergic receptors may play a more important functional role in venous than in arterial blood vessels (Ruffolo, 1985a).

d. Other Veins. Most other veins have less of an α_2-adrenergic receptor contribution relative to that observed in the saphenous vein. Shoji *et al.* (1983) compared the responsiveness of many canine veins to norepinephrine, phenylephrine and clonidine. The saphenous and cephalic veins have the greatest response to clonidine, followed by the femoral vein. Analysis of the response to clonidine confirmed the presence of both α_1- and α_2-adrenergic receptors in the saphenous vein. Interestingly, longitudinal, but not helical, strips of portal vein, mesenteric vein and vena cava readily respond to clonidine. However, analysis of the response in the portal vein revealed only α_1-adrenergic receptor activation. Evidence for postjunctional α_2-adrenergic receptors in human femoral vein has been provided by the failure of prazosin to antagonize the response to low concentrations of norepinephrine in this tissue, and by the potent contractile effect observed with guanfacine, a moderately selective α_2-adrenergic receptor agonist (Glusa and Markwardt, 1983).

In a quantitative analysis of α_1- and α_2-adrenergic receptor characteristics in femoral and saphenous veins, the selective α_2-adrenergic receptor agonist, UK 14,304, was much less effective in inducing contraction in the femoral vein (22% of norepinephrine maximum) compared to the saphenous vein (86% of norepinephrine maximum) (Flavahan and Vanhoutte, 1986a). As seen in some arteries, the response to norepinephrine in certain veins, such as the canine splenic vein, may be sensitive to blockade by both rauwolscine and prazosin, even though the tissue is unresponsive to highly selective α_2-adrenergic receptor agonists (Hieble and Woodward, 1984).

e. Physiological Significance of Venous α_2-Adrenergic Receptors. The physiological significance of venous α_2-adrenergic receptors is unclear. *In vivo* studies with α_2-adrenergic receptor agonists in the rat (Gerold and Haeusler, 1983) or dog (Zandberg *et al.*, 1984) cannot demonstrate a significant haemodynamic effect clearly attributable to effects on venous capacitance vessels. Since venous α_2-adrenergic receptors are sensitive to temperature changes (McAdams and Waterfall, 1984; Flavahan and Vanhoutte, 1986b), and α_2-adrenergic receptors are most prominent in cutaneous tissue (Flavahan *et al.*, 1984), the venous α_2-adrenergic receptor may be involved in blood flow redistribution to optimize the thermoregulatory process. It has been reported (Kalkman *et al.*, 1984) that α_2-adrenergic receptor-mediated venoconstriction can significantly reduce venous capacitance and thereby increase venous return to the heart, resulting in an increase in cardiac output.

f. Occupancy–Response Coupling in the Venous Circulation. It is only fairly recently that α-adrenoceptor occupancy–response relationships have been studied in venous preparations, and such studies have been confined to the femoral and saphenous veins maintained *in vitro*. Similar to canine aorta (Sastre *et al.*, 1984), canine saphenous vein possesses a large α_1-adrenoceptor reserve for full agonists, such as cirazoline (Ruffolo and Zeid, 1985; Flavahan and Vanhoutte, 1986a) and phenylephrine (Flavahan and Vanhoutte, 1986a). Thus, the non-linear relationship between α_1-adrenoceptor occupancy and vascular contractile response is similar in canine aorta and saphenous vein. In contrast to the saphenous vein, the femoral vein of the dog possesses a very small or no α_1-adrenoceptor reserve for phenylephrine (Flavahan and Vanhoutte, 1986a). Thus, it is apparent that the degree of coupling between α_1-adrenoceptor occupancy and response can vary between vessels of different anatomic location and serving different functions. Flavahan and Vanhoutte (1986b) have suggested that this difference in α_1-adrenoceptor density between femoral and saphenous veins may result from the thermoregulatory role of these vessels. Cooling, which acts as a functional antagonist, reduces α_1-adrenoceptor-mediated vasoconstriction in the femoral vein since there is little α_1-adrenoceptor reserve. However, the α_1-adrenoceptor-mediated responses of the saphenous vein are buffered from the effect of cooling because of the large α_1-adrenoceptor reserve and thus, canine saphenous vein can still constrict in response to α_1-adrenoceptor agonists when cooled. This leads to maintained constriction of the saphenous vein, but markedly reduced constriction of the femoral vein which, *in vivo*, will divert blood from the superficial areas to the deeper layers of the leg and thus retard heat loss.

In contrast to the arterial circulation *in vivo*, it has been reported that the canine saphenous vein *in vitro* possesses an α_2-adrenoceptor reserve for B-HT 933, such that a hyperbolic occupancy–response relationship is observed for this agonist (Ruffolo and Zeid, 1985). However, in these experiments there was also found to be a four-fold larger α_1-adrenoceptor reserve for cirazoline than α_2-adrenoceptor reserve for B-HT 933 (Ruffolo and Zeid, 1985), which is similar to the five-fold difference in the occupancy–relationships observed for these agonists in the arterial circulation of the pithed rat (Ruffolo and Yaden, 1984). In contrast to the findings of Ruffolo and Zeid (1985), Flavahan and Vanhoutte (1986a) found no α_2-adrenoceptor reserve in canine saphenous vein for UK-14,304, a potent, full α_2-adrenoceptor agonist. At present, it is not understood why the studies of Ruffolo and Zeid (1985) and Flavahan and Vanhoutte (1986a) have yielded different estimates of α_2-adrenoceptor reserve for full α_2-adrenoceptor agonists in the canine saphenous vein. Nevertheless, it is obvious that α_1-adrenoceptors predominate over α_2-adrenoceptors, and are associated with a larger receptor reserve, in both venous and arterial vascular smooth muscle.

2.2.4 Postsynaptic Myocardial α-Adrenoceptors

The cardiac adrenergic neuroeffector junction is in many respects similar to neuroeffector junctions in other peripheral tissues as far as α-adrenergic receptors are concerned. Presynaptic α_2-adrenergic receptors on postganglionic sympathetic nerve terminals have been identified in isolated hearts from many species. As in other organs, the presynaptic α_2-adrenergic receptors in myocardium, when activated, mediate an inhibitory effect on neurotransmitter release (Doxey and Roach, 1980; Drew, 1976; Hieble and Pendleton, 1979). As such, α-adrenergic receptor antagonists that are non-selective, or selective α_2-adrenergic receptor antagonists, have the capacity to produce positive inotropic and chronotropic responses (Benfey and Varma, 1962) by enhancing neurotransmitter liberation resulting from loss of the autoinhibition mediated by presynaptic α_2-adrenergic receptors (Starke *et al.*, 1971a,b).

The predominant adrenergic receptor located postsynaptically in the heart is the β_1-adrenergic receptor, which mediates a positive inotropic and chronotropic response (Broadley, 1982). However, postsynaptic α-adrenergic receptors also exist in the hearts of many mammalian species, including humans, and mediate a positive inotropic response with little or no change in heart rate (Govier, 1967; Osnes, 1976; Schumann and Brodde, 1978; Schumann and Endoh, 1976). Most physiological and radioligand binding data indicate that the postsynaptic α-adrenergic receptor in myocardium is exclusively of the α_1-subtype (Hoffman and Lefkowitz, 1980; Raisman *et al.*, 1979; Schumann and Brodde, 1979). The mechanism by which cardiac α_1-adrenergic receptors increase force of myocardial contraction has not been established, but it appears not to be associated with the accumulation of cAMP or stimulation of adenylate cyclase (Brodde *et al.*, 1978), and in this respect, α_1-adrenergic receptors differ from β_1-adrenergic receptors in the myocardium. Other differences between α_1- and β_1-adrenergic receptor-mediated effects in the heart include the rate of onset and duration of action, which are particularly long for α_1-adrenergic receptor-mediated inotropic effects (Schumann *et al.*, 1975). Furthermore, while β_1-adrenergic receptor-mediated inotropic responses occur at all frequencies of stimulation, the effect mediated by myocardial α_1-adrenergic receptors is apparent only at low frequencies (Broadley, 1982).

2.2.5 Renal α-Adrenoceptors Involved in Fluid and Electrolyte Balance

The existence of α-adrenergic receptors in the kidney has been known for many years, since α-adrenergic drugs produce a variety of renal effects. The functions and locations of the renal α-adrenergic receptors are only now beginning to be understood. Radioligand binding studies indicate that α_1- and α_2-adrenergic receptors coexist in the kidneys of a variety of mammalian species including humans; however, the number, proportion, and distribution of each α-adrenergic receptor subtype may vary from one species to another (McPherson and Summers, 1981; Summers and McPherson, 1982; Summers, 1984).

The kidney receives a dense noradrenergic innervation which extends not only to the afferent and efferent arterioles (Barajas and Wang, 1979), but also to all portions of the nephron including the collecting duct (Barajas *et al.*, 1984). In addition, α-adrenergic receptors are known to be present with an approximate two-fold greater density of α_2- over α_1-adrenergic receptors in crude membrane fractions of rat kidney (Sanchez and Pettinger, 1981). While it is generally accepted that α_1-adrenergic receptors are most important in mediating vasoconstriction (Schmitz et al., 1981) and tubular sodium reabsorption (Obsorn et al., 1982, 1983), the precise functional role of the predominant α_2-adrenergic receptors is less clearly understood. In the rat, α_2-adrenergic receptors of the juxtaglomerular apparatus have been proposed to inhibit renin release (Pettinger, 1987). Both α_1- and α_2-adrenergic receptors have been proposed to alter electrolyte and fluid balance, but their exact roles are not fully understood.

Radioligand binding studies in rat kidney reveal that the major concentration of phentolamine displaceable [^{3}H]-rauwolscine binding sites is found in the renal cortex, with a particularly high density associated with the proximal tubules, blood vessels and glomeruli (Stephenson and Summers, 1985). In contrast to this predominant proximal tubular location of α_2-adrenergic receptors as assessed by radioligand binding techniques, physiological studies suggest a more important functional role for renal α_2-adrenergic receptors in the distal tubule and collecting duct. α_2-Adrenergic receptor activation weakly attenuates parathyroid hormone-induced activation of adenylate cyclase in isolated rat proximal convoluted tubule, but more effectively inhibits vasopressin-evoked stimulation of adenylate cyclase in the medullary and cortical collecting tubules with no effect in the medullary and cortical thick ascending limb (Umemura et al., 1985). In addition, α_2-adrenergic receptor stimulation antagonizes the vasopressin-induced reduction in sodium and water excretion in isolated rat perfused kidney (Smyth et al., 1985a) and water reabsorption in rabbit isolated cortical collecting tubules (Krothapalli et al., 1983).

The effects of the selective α_1-adrenergic receptor agonist, cirazoline, and the selective α_2-adrenergic receptor agonist, B-HT 933, were assessed on renal haemodynamics and on water and solute excretion in conscious, chronically instrumented rats (Gellai and Ruffolo, 1987). Infusion of equipressor doses of cirazoline and B-HT 933 decreased renal plasma flow without changing glomerular filtration rate. Cirazoline infusion did not affect urinary excretion of water, electrolytes or total solutes. In marked contrast, B-HT 933 increased urine flow and sodium excretion significantly, but did not significantly alter potassium and urea excretion. Urine osmolality decreased to hyposmotic levels (from 613 ± 86 to 172 ± 8 mOsm/kg H_2O) during the infusion of B-HT 933, suggesting a possible interaction between the α_2-adrenergic receptor and the vasopression system. This unique diuretic action of the selective α_2-adrenergic receptor agonist was also observed following the infusion of subpressor doses of B-HT 933 (Gellai and Ruffolo, 1987). In rats treated with the ganglionic blocker, hexamethonium (10 mg/kg, i.v.), the B-HT 933-induced diuresis was not affected, confirming an action in the periphery, most likely at the level of the kidney. These results suggest that stimulation of renal α_2-adrenergic receptors mediates the inhibition of water and sodium reabsorption at the site of the distal renal nephron, most likely the cortical collecting duct, and is thereby responsible for producing diuresis and natriuresis (Gellai and Ruffolo, 1987).

As indicated above, the diuretic action of B-HT 933 is associated with sustained low levels of urine osmolality, maintained at 200 mOsm/kg H_2O or less, substantially less than plasma osmolality (290 mOsm/kg H_2O) (Gellai and Ruffolo, 1987). The formation of urine that is hypotonic to plasma is indicative of a reduction in vasopressin-associated renal water reabsorption. Infusions of other α_2-adrenergic receptor agonists (clonidine or guanabenz) have been reported to decrease secretion of vasopressin in anaesthetized rats and dogs (Reid et al., 1979; Roman et al., 1979; Strandhoy et al., 1982). However, Olsen (1976) did not observe inhibition of vasopressin secretion by clonidine in conscious dogs. Strandhoy and coworkers (1982) emphasized that although infusion of guanabenz in anaesthetized dogs decreased the plasma concentration of vasopressin, this alone could not account for the diuretic effect of guanabenz. Inhibition of the tubular action of vasopressin on water reabsorption by stimulation of tubular α_2-adrenergic receptors was suggested. Such inhibition has been demonstrated in studies of isolated rabbit cortical collecting tubules (Krothapalli et al., 1983; Chabardes et al., 1984), and in studies of isolated toad urinary bladder (Kinter et al., 1985). In these studies, α_2-adrenergic receptor stimulation inhibited vasopressin-dependent increases in water permeability by attenuating vasopressin-stimulated adenylate cyclase activity. Whether B-HT 933 impairs the secretion of vasopressin, or inhibits its tubular action, or both, cannot be inferred at present. However, the formation of hypotonic urine strongly implicates inhibition of vasopressin-dependent epithelial functions in the mechanism of action of B-HT 933, and supports the proposed collecting tubule/collecting duct site of action.

Smyth et al. (1985b) have proposed separate roles of the α-adrenergic receptor subtypes in the handling of water and electrolytes. These authors suggest that renal nerve stimulation potentiates tubular water and sodium reabsorption via α_1-adrenergic receptor stimulation, a concept that is generally accepted. In contrast, due to their extrajunctional location, renal α_2-adrenergic receptors may not be activated by renal nerve stimulation. Thus, renal α_2-adrenergic receptors may be stimulated by circulating catecholamines, and play an important role in the regulation of water and sodium excretion, possibly by modulating the actions of vasopressin and other hormones in the distal nephron. Although this proposal by Smyth et al. (1985b) suggests a delicately balanced interaction of the two α-adrenergic receptor subtypes with neuronally released and circulating catecholamines, respectively, in the handling of water and electrolytes by the kidneys, the role of the α_2-adrenergic receptor in modulating sodium reabsorption under basal conditions has not been fully addressed. Smyth *et al.* (1985b) propose a relatively minor role for renal α_2-adrenergic receptors based on experimental data showing opposite effects by epinephrine on sodium reabsorption in α_1-adrenergic receptor-blocked, furosemide- or vasopressin-infused isolated rat kidneys, and no effect at all when epinephrine was infused under basal conditions in the same preparation (Smyth *et al.*, 1984, 1985a). In contrast, under normal physiological conditions, renal α_2-adrenergic receptors may play an important role in the control of sodium and fluid reabsorption. It has been proposed that in a state of normal fluid balance (at least in the rat), the well-demonstrated role of α_1-adrenergic receptors to stimulate the increase in sodium reabsorption in the proximal tubule and thick ascending limb is balanced by the proposed action of the extrajunctional α_2-adrenergic receptor, to inhibit sodium and water reabsorption in the collecting tubules and ducts. Accordingly, changing the activity of one of the α-adrenergic receptor subtypes, or changing the balance in supply of catecholamine (i.e., neuronal vs circulating), could unmask the actions of the other subtype or source of catecholamine. Thus, the natriuresis observed during the decrease in renal efferent sympathetic nerve activity, as would also occur upon stimulating the cardiopulmonary vagal afferent limb (left atrial stretch receptor stimulation), could result, at least partially, from the stimulating effect of circulating catecholamines on the extrajunctional α_2-adrenergic receptors; a selective α_2-adrenergic receptor antagonist would therefore be expected to attenuate the natriuresis. This scheme is summarized in Fig. 2. Application of highly selective α_1- and α_2-adrenergic

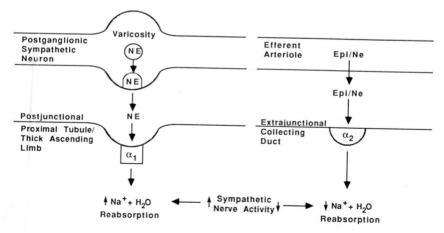

FIG. 2. Diagrammatic representation of the effect of α_1- and α_2-adrenoceptor activation on renal tubular function.

receptor agonists and antagonists should assist in further elucidation of the potentially important role of the α_2-adrenergic receptor in the control of body fluid balance by the kidneys.

To summarize, it appears that the major function of α_2-adrenergic receptors in the kidney is to mediate the inhibition of vasopressin-induced sodium and water reabsorption in the cortical, and possibly medullary, collecting tubule and duct, leading to a natriuresis and diuresis while possibly sparing potassium. The diuresis is characterized by a hyposmotic urine. The role, if any, of the dense population of α_2-adrenergic receptors associated with the proximal convoluted tubule remains to be elucidated.

2.3 CARDIOVASCULAR EFFECTS OF α-ADRENERGIC DRUGS

2.3.1 Central α_2-Adrenoceptor Agonists in Hypertension

As indicated earlier, reductions in blood pressure and heart rate may be elicited by stimulation of α_2-adrenoceptors in the brain stem with the subsequent interruption of the cardiovascular reflex loop. Clonidine, when administered systemically, will cross the blood–brain barrier and activate α_2-adrenoceptors in the nucleus of the solitary tract to inhibit sympathetic and enhance the parasympathetic outflows which ultimately produces vasodilation and bradycardia. α-Methyldopa works in much the same manner as clonidine, but it uses an amino acid transport system to gain access to the brain where it is subsequently converted to α-methylnorepinephrine by the same enzymes responsible for the biosynthesis of the neurotransmitter, norepinephrine. α-Methylnorepinephrine, like clonidine, is a highly selective α_2-adrenoceptor agonist which is responsible for the antihypertensive and bradycardic effects of α-methyldopa.

Both clonidine and α-methyldopa are highly effective antihypertensive agents. However, both are also extremely sedative, which somewhat limits their utility. Behavioural studies indicate that a different population of central α_2-adrenoceptors from those responsible for the cardiovascular effects of these agents may mediate their marked sedative effects (Timmermans and van Zwieten, 1982).

2.3.2 Peripheral α-Adrenoceptor Antagonists in Hypertension

Since vascular tone is mediated predominantly by α-adrenoceptors, it is logical to assume that pharmacological antagonists of α-adrenoceptors would abate hypertension. Indeed, the α-adrenoceptor antagonists, tolazoline and phentolamine, were introduced as clinical antihypertensive agents many years ago. These competitive α-adrenoceptor antagonists do, in fact, lower blood pressure, but their clinical efficacy has been unaccountably low. One explanation that has been proposed for the ineffectiveness of these agents in hypertension is their ability to potentiate neuronal norepinephrine release (Stokes and Marwood, 1984). Both tolazoline and phentolamine are non-selective α-adrenoceptor antagonists and therefore have potent antagonist activity at prejunctional α_2-adrenoceptors in addition to their postjunctional α-adrenolytic effects. Their prejunctional α_2-adrenoceptor antagonist activity appears to interrupt the inhibitory negative feedback loop that regulates neurotransmitter release, thereby increasing norepinephrine release which may partially overcome the postjunctional α_1-adrenoceptor antagonist effects and thus limit antihypertensive efficacy. This hypothesis has been widely accepted, primarily in light of the high antihypertensive efficacy observed with prazosin, a highly selective α_1-adrenoceptor antagonist (Davey, 1980). Since prazosin possesses only weak antagonist activity at the presynaptic α_2-adrenoceptors, the neuronal negative feedback loop remains intact to prevent synaptic concentrations of norepinephrine from becoming elevated (Davey, 1980).

In the human forearm, yohimbine, a selective α_2-adrenoceptor antagonist, produces arterial vasodilation and increases blood flow (Bolli *et al.*, 1983). This finding suggests that, at least in this vascular bed, the postsynaptic extrajunctional α_2-adrenoceptor may also play a significant role, along with the junctional α_1-adrenoceptor, in maintaining vascular tone. Vasoconstrictor activity mediated by postsynaptic extrajunctional α_2-adrenoceptors may play more of a role in the hypertensive state, as shown both in animal studies (Majewski *et al.*, 1981; Medgett *et al.*, 1984) and in clinical studies in which increased vasodilatory activity of yohimbine and increased pressor potency to epinephrine have been observed in patients with essential hypertension (Bolli *et al.*, 1984).

Circulating catecholamines are known to be elevated in a major sub-population of patients with essential hypertension (Goldstein, 1983), and these high plasma catecholamine levels have been proposed to contribute to the increased vascular resistance characteristic of essential hypertension (Amann *et al.*, 1981). The fact that circulating catecholamines appear to be the endogenous agonists for the extrajunctional vascular α_2-adrenoceptors suggests that in this subgroup of patients, postjunctional α_2-adrenoceptors may, in fact, contribute to the elevated peripheral vascular resistance. As such, α_2-adrenoceptor blockade may prove to be beneficial in clinical antihypertensive therapy. To date, α_2-adrenoceptor-blocking drugs given orally have been poorly absorbed or are only of short duration of action. Phentolamine administered orally produces only very low plasma levels in humans (Sioufi *et al.*, 1981) and short-lived antihypertensive activity in DOCA-salt hypertensive rats (Hieble *et al.*, 1985). Improved α_2-adrenoceptor antagonists showing a superior profile to phentolamine in animal models have been identified (Hieble *et al.*, 1985; Roesler *et al.*, 1986) and are currently being evaluated in humans to determine whether α_2-adrenoceptor blockade may also be a useful therapeutic approach in hypertension.

2.3.3 α-Adrenoceptor Antagonists in Congestive Heart Failure

Vasodilators have assumed a more prominent role in the treatment of congestive heart failure over the past decade, in part because technical advances have shown their desirable haemodynamic effect (Breckenridge, 1982). In most patients with congestive heart failure the optimal vasodilator is one that acts relatively equally on both the arterial and venous beds. Sodium nitroprusside does so, but must be administered intravenously. Prazosin, an orally active selective α_1-adrenoceptor antagonist, has been shown to mimic the haemodynamic effects of nitroprusside in congestive heart failure, increasing cardiac output, decreasing left ventricular filling pressure and systemic and pulmonary vascular resistance, and maintaining heart rate (Awan *et al.*, 1977, 1978). Although acute tolerance has been observed after multiple doses of prazosin over a period of 24–72 h (Arnold *et al.*, 1979), the beneficial effect often returns with continued therapy, and long-term clinical trials with prazosin show chronic efficacy in patients with congestive heart failure (Stanaszek *et al.*, 1983). Prazosin improves symptoms most during exercise (Rubin *et al.*, 1979).

Since there is evidence that the degree of sympathetic tone is proportional to the severity of heart failure (Ogasawara *et al.*, 1983; Thomas and Marks, 1978), and the level of plasma catecholamines has been implicated as a primary risk factor in patients with congestive heart failure (Cohn *et al.*, 1984), the use of α-adrenoceptor antagonists in low output cardiac failure may have a rational advantage over other vasodilators. An additional benefit may be that anginal frequency decreases with reduced afterload, and cardiac oxygen needs may be diminished (Bertel *et al.*, 1981).

The factor that correlates best with mortality in patients with heart failure is a high level of circulating catecholamines (Cohn *et al.*, 1984). Since, as discussed earlier, circulating catecholamines may be the natural substrates for postsynaptic extrajunctional α_2-adrenoceptor in the arterial circulation, and since high plasma catecholamine levels may contribute to the increased total peripheral vascular resistance characteristic of congestive heart failure (Bristow, 1984; Ogasawara *et al.*, 1981), the evaluation of an α_2-adrenoceptor antagonist in low output cardiac failure is indicated.

3 β-Adrenoceptors

3.1 CENTRAL β-ADRENOCEPTORS

β-Adrenoceptors have been identified on many neurons in the central nervous system (Iversen, 1977), but their role in cardiovascular regulation is unclear. Activating central β-adrenoceptors has been shown to elevate blood pressure and heart rate (Day and Roach, 1974). This observation is supported by the fact that injecting β-adrenoceptor antagonists into the central nervous system decreases blood pressure and heart rate (Day and Roach, 1974). In addition, systemically administering β-adrenoceptor antagonists produces decreases in resting splanchnic sympathetic nerve discharge that correlates with reductions in arterial blood pressure (Lewis and Haeusler, 1975). Intravenously administered propranolol has been reported to interrupt the cardiovascular reflex loop in the central nervous system and inhibit sympathetic outflow (Dorward and Korner, 1978). Increases in blood pressure and heart rate evoked by sino-aortic denervation may be attenuated by injecting small doses of propranolol into the central nervous system (Montastruc and Montastruc, 1980). These results are highly suggestive of a centrally mediated tonic β-adrenergic influence to increase blood pressure, and of a possible central mechanism for the antihypertensive effects of β-blockers (Korner and Angus, 1981). However, those β-adrenoceptor antagonists that do not permeate the blood–brain barrier, such as atenolol, are also highly effective antihypertensive agents, suggesting that the peripheral antihypertensive effects of β-adrenoceptor antagonists are also significant.

3.2 PERIPHERAL β-ADRENOCEPTORS

3.2.1 Presynaptic β-Adrenoceptors

The best understood presynaptic adrenoceptor is the α_2-adrenoceptor which inhibits neurotransmitter liberation. More recently, presynaptic β_2-adrenoceptors have been identified and shown to facilitate neurotransmitter release. It has been shown that presynaptic β_2-adrenoceptors enhance stimulus-evoked norepinephrine release, suggesting that prejunctional β_2-adrenoceptors mediate a positive feedback on sympathetic neuro-transmission. The prejunctional β_2-adrenoceptor has been found in a variety of species, including humans (Brown and Macquin, 1981; Majewski et al., 1982a,b).

Most experiments characterizing the prejunctional β_2-adrenoceptor have used either epinephrine or isoproterenol as agonists. Norepinephrine is not a potent presynaptic β_2-adrenoceptor agonist (Majewski *et al.*, 1981), acting instead on the presynaptic α_2-adrenoceptor to inhibit neurotransmitter release. It is therefore logical to assume that epinephrine is the physiological ligand for the presynaptic β_2-adrenoceptor. This has led to the "epinephrine hypothesis" of essential hypertension, which suggests that activation of prejunctional β_2-adrenoceptors by neuronally released epinephrine may initiate the disease process.

3.2.2 Epinephrine Hypothesis of Essential Hypertension

Epinephrine synthesized and released by the adrenal gland has a short half-life in the systemic circulation. Although circulating epinephrine levels during stress are equivalent to the threshold concentration for *in vitro* activation of prejunctional β_2-adrenoceptors (Langer, 1977), β_2-adrenoceptor-mediated effects of circulating epinephrine on neuronal norepinephrine release should be transient. However, circulating epinephrine is readily accumulated by sympathetic nerve terminals via the neuronal uptake pump for sympathomimetic amines (uptake$_1$). In the sympathetic nerve terminal, epinephrine can be co-stored and co-released with norepinephrine (Majewski *et al.*, 1981). Increases in the epinephrine content of tissues with dense sympathetic innervation are observed after stimulation-induced adrenal epinephrine secretion (Raab and Gigee, 1953). Since epinephrine, but not norepinephrine, will activate the prejunctional β_2-adrenoceptor, epinephrine co-released with norepinephrine will shift the balance toward increased β_2- relative to α_2-adrenoceptor-mediated prejunctional effects, thus increasing the net efficiency of sympathetic neurotransmission. Increased norepinephrine release in response to neuronally released epinephrine has been demonstrated both *in vitro* in guinea-pig and rat atrial tissue (Majewski *et al.*, 1982b), as well as *in vivo* in humans (Brown and Macquin, 1981).

Continuous infusion of low doses of epinephrine induces hypertension in rats (Majewski *et al.*, 1982b; Tung *et al.*, 1981). This effect is not mimicked by norepinephrine infusion and can be blocked by propranolol, suggesting an action on prejunctional β_2-adrenoceptors. Tachycardia is often an additional consequence of epinephrine infusion; this tachycardia is attenuated by neuronal uptake blockade and is much more persistent after epinephrine infusion than after isoproterenol, the latter not being a substrate for neuronal uptake (Brown *et al.*, 1983).

The results of a large-scale clinical study in Great Britain correlating blood pressure and plasma catecholamines in hypertensive and prehypertensive subjects support a role of epinephrine in the development of the hypertensive state (Brown, 1985). While the mechanism(s) of the antihypertensive activity of β-adrenoceptor blocking agents has not been established, the blockade of presynaptic facilitory β-adrenoceptors and the resulting inhibition of neurotransmitter liberation must be considered.

3.2.3 Myocardial β-Adrenoceptors

The postsynaptic β-adrenoceptor of the heart that mediates an increase in both the rate and force of contraction is predominantly the β_1-subtype (Broadley, 1982). Biochemical studies indicate that the positive inotropic and chronotropic responses to catecholamines are mediated by β_1-adrenoceptor activation of adenylate cyclase, with the ultimate generation and accumulation of cyclic-AMP (Broadley, 1982).

It has been shown that there also may exist myocardial β_2-adrenoceptors in the sinoatrial node in some mammalian species. The functional significance of these β_2-adrenoceptors is not known and they appear not to be innervated (Broadley, 1982). It has been proposed that non-innervated extrajunctional β_2-adrenoceptors in the heart may represent "hormonal" adrenoceptors that are responsive to circulating blood-borne epinephrine (Ariëns, 1981; Broadley, 1982).

3.2.4 Vascular β-Adrenoceptors

Postsynaptic vascular β_2-adrenoceptors mediate vasodilation. It appears that the vascular β_2-adrenoceptors, like the vascular α_2-adrenoceptors, are not innervated (i.e., are located extrajunctionally) (Ariëns, 1981). It has been proposed, therefore, that extrajunctional vascular β_2-adrenoceptors are "hormonal" receptors that mediate vasodilation in response to circulating epinephrine in certain vascular beds at times of stress, when plasma levels of epinephrine are elevated. It has recently been shown that the vasodilatory response mediated by vascular β_2-adrenoceptors after ganglionic stimulation is abolished by bilateral adrenalectomy, indicating that this response results from the action of circulating epinephrine liberated by the adrenal glands (Ariëns, 1981).

a. Coronary Circulation. If coronary vascular resistance is elevated, stimulation of sympathetic nerves produces coronary artery vasodilation, and this effect is mediated by β-adrenoceptors in coronary resistance vessels (Cohen *et al.*, 1984). Although most vascular β-adrenoceptors in the peripheral circulation are of the β_2-subtype (see above), those present in the resistance vessels of the coronary circulation appear to be predominantly of the β_1-subtype. This accounts for the fact that exogenously or neuronally-released norepinephrine, which is markedly selective for β_1-adrenoceptors, elicits a vasodilator response in the coronary circulation (Cohen *et al.*, 1984).

There is also evidence, obtained from *in vitro* studies of large epicardial coronary arteries, for the existence of β_2-adrenoceptors, which, like the β_1-adrenoceptors in the resistance coronary vessels, mediate vasodilation (Gross and Feigl, 1975). These β_2-adrenoceptors are likely to be extrajunctional in distribution and may respond to circulating epinephrine acting as a blood-borne hormone, thereby augmenting coronary blood flow.

   b. Pulmonary Circulation. β-Adrenoceptors are present in the pulmonary circulation and mediate a vasodilator response, decreasing pulmonary vascular resistance and pulmonary arterial pressure. The β-adrenoceptor-mediated pulmonary vasodilator response is especially marked when pulmonary vascular resistance is high. Pharmacological studies indicate that the β-adrenoceptor present in the pulmonary circulation is of the β_2-subtype (Hyman *et al.*, 1981). There is evidence to suggest that the β_2-adrenoceptors mediating vasodilation in the pulmonary circulation may be innervated by the sympathetic nervous system (Hyman *et al.*, 1981), in contrast to other systemic vascular beds in which β_2-adrenoceptors are non-innervated and located extrajunctionally (see above).

   c. Cerebral Circulation. When vascular tone is high, stimulating β-adrenoceptors by isoproterenol or norepinephrine dilates cerebral arteries *in vitro*. This vasodilation is mediated by β_1-adrenoceptors (Winquist *et al.*, 1982). *In vivo* studies on the effects of β-adrenoceptor stimulation on pial arterial resistance have produced conflicting results (Sercombe *et al.*, 1977; Wahl *et al.*, 1974), hence the role of the β-adrenoceptor in regulating cerebral blood flow in the intact animal has not been firmly established.

   In addition to β_1-adrenoceptors, β_2-adrenoceptors have been identified in rat cerebral microvessels (Kobayashi *et al.*, 1981). This may have some physiological relevance to the human cerebral circulation, particularly since this receptor subtype may be involved with oxygen consumption and cerebral glucose uptake (Magnoni *et al.*, 1983). It may also be important in the pathology of malignant hypertension, since it has been shown that the density of β_2-adrenoceptors in the rat cerebral microvasculature is decreased in rats with hypertension (Magnoni *et al.*, 1983).

   d. Renal Circulation. Renal vascular β-adrenoceptors mediate vasodilation and consequently a decrease in renal vascular resistance (Insel and

Snavely, 1981). However, α-adrenoceptors appear to greatly outnumber β-adrenoceptors, and β-adrenoceptor-mediated vasodilation occurs to a lesser degree in the kidney than in other vascular beds (Insel and Snavely, 1981). Perhaps the most important known role of β-adrenoceptors in the kidney is in the regulation of renin release from the juxtaglomerular apparatus (DiBona, 1982). Stimulation of renal nerves under conditions that do not affect renal perfusion pressure, renal blood flow, glomerular filtration rate, or sodium excretion, causes renin release (Osborn et al., 1981). This response can be blocked by β_1-, but not by β_2-adrenoceptor antagonists (Osborn et al., 1981). β-Adrenoceptor agonists also stimulate fluid absorption by approximately 60% in the proximal convoluted tubule in vitro and double the rate of net chloride reabsorption in the cortical collecting tubule in vitro.

e. Splanchnic Circulation. Stimulation of β-adrenoceptors with iso-proterenol results in a vasodilatory response in all organs supplied by the splanchnic circulation (Chou and Kvietys, 1981). This response is inhibited by the β-adrenoceptor antagonist, propranolol (Immink et al., 1976; Richardson, 1984). However, propranolol alone does not significantly alter blood flow in any of the organs supplied by the splanchnic circulation (Richardson, 1984), suggesting that β-adrenoceptors are not involved in the maintenance of normal vascular tone in this circulatory bed. It appears that the β-adrenoceptor subtype mediating splanchnic vasodilation is β_2 (Richardson, 1984).

3.2.5 Renal β-Adrenoceptors

The kidney is also heavily under adrenergic control. Probably the most important adrenergic effect in the kidney is the regulation of renin release from the juxtaglomerular apparatus (Keeton and Campbell, 1980). Renin release from the juxtaglomerular cells is enhanced by β_1-adrenoceptor stimulation and/or stimulation of renal adrenergic nerves (Keeton and Campbell, 1980). The increase in renin release evoked by the exogenous administration of β-adrenoceptor agonists or by adrenergic nerve stimulation is antagonized by β-adrenoceptor blocking agents such as propranolol. It appears that the juxtaglomerular cells are under a constant adrenergic tone since β-adrenoceptor blocking agents also inhibit basal renin release (Keeton and Campbell, 1980). It has been suggested that the magnitude of the antihypertensive response to β-adrenoceptor antagonists depends on the initial plasma renin activity and the degree of its suppression by β-adrenoceptor blockade (Buhler et al., 1972). However, the relevance of the decrease in renin release mediated by β-adrenoceptor antagonists to the antihypertensive effects of these compounds has been questioned, since the reduction in blood pressure does not always parallel the reduction in renin release. In addition, some β-adrenoceptor blockers with intrinsic sympathomimetic activity may themselves promote renin release by their inherent β-adrenoceptor agonist properties (Keeton and Campbell, 1980), yet these compounds nonetheless are effective antihypertensive agents in humans.

Renal β-adrenoceptors also appear to regulate renal blood flow at the vascular level. β-Adrenoceptors in the vasculature have been identified pharmacologically and mediate the expected vasodilatory response resulting in an increase in renal blood flow.

β-Adrenoceptors may also affect renal salt and water metabolism, but these effects are controversial and the results are often contradictory (Keeton and Campbell, 1980).

3.3 CARDIOVASCULAR EFFECTS OF β-ADRENERGIC DRUGS

3.3.1 β-Adrenoceptor Antagonists in Hypertension

Table 2 shows the β-adrenoceptor blocking agents that are commonly used to treat hypertension and their principal pharmacological actions. Several β-adrenoceptor antagonists are available and they are significantly different. Certain β-adrenoceptor antagonists, such as propranolol, are non-selective

TABLE 2

Pharmacological properties of β-adrenoceptor antagonists

Drug	β-Adrenoceptor selectivity	Intrinsic sympathomimetic activity	Membrane stabilizing activity
Acebutolol	$\beta_1 > \beta_2$	+	+
Alprenolol	$\beta_1 = \beta_2$	+	+
Atenolol	$\beta_1 \gg \beta_2$	−	−
Metoprolol	$\beta_1 \gg \beta_2$	−	−
Oxprenolol	$\beta_1 = \beta_2$	++	+
Pindolol	$\beta_1 = \beta_2$	+++	−
Practolol	$\beta_1 \gg \beta_2$	++	−
Propranolol	$\beta_1 = \beta_2$	−	+
Sotalol	$\beta_1 = \beta_2$	−	−
Timolol	$\beta_1 = \beta_2$	−	−

in that they antagonize both β_1- and β_2-adrenoceptors. Other β-adrenoceptor antagonists, such as atenolol, are termed "cardioselective" in as much as they may preferentially antagonize myocardial β_1-adrenoceptors. Finally, a class of β-adrenoceptor antagonists with intrinsic sympathomimetic activity is now available, the prototype being pindolol. These different classes of β-adrenoceptors antagonists produce qualitatively and quantitatively distinct haemodynamic responses in humans and therefore should not be considered to be one homogeneous class of drugs possessing similar pharmacological activities.

As indicated earlier, the mechanism of action of β-adrenoceptor antagonists in hypertension is still a matter of controversy. On the basis of the previously discussed effects that may be attributed to central β-adrenoceptors, and peripheral presynaptic and postsynaptic β-adrenoceptors in the heart, vasculature, and kidney, four logical mechanisms for the antihypertensive activity of β-blocking agents may be postulated:

(1) an action within the central nervous system to antagonize the central β-adrenoceptor-mediated increases in blood pressure and heart rate;

(2) presynaptic β-adrenoceptor blockade to inhibit the β-adrenoceptor-mediated positive feedback mechanism on neurotransmitter (norepinephrine) liberation in the heart and vasculature;

(3) blockade of postsynaptic cardiac β_1-adrenoceptors to decrease the rate and force of myocardial contraction and thereby decrease cardiac output; and

(4) inhibition of renin release, which is stimulated by β_1-adrenoceptor activation (in humans).

All classes of β-adrenoceptor antagonists lower blood pressure regardless of β-adrenoceptor subtype selectivity or the presence of intrinsic sympathomimetic activity. Furthermore, no one mechanism will adequately account for the antihypertensive activity of β-adrenoceptor antagonists in general. Thus, some β-adrenoceptor blockers do not cross the blood–brain barrier whereas others with intrinsic sympathomimetic activity may enhance renin release. In addition, β-adrenoceptor antagonists decrease heart rate and cardiac output acutely, yet the antihypertensive effect of β-adrenoceptor blockers may take days to develop. It is likely, therefore, that several of these mechanisms may contribute to the antihypertensive activity of any one β-adrenoceptor blocker.

When β-adrenoceptor antagonists (without intrinsic sympathomimetic activity) are first administered, there is an acute decrease in heart rate and cardiac output and a reflex increase in total peripheral vascular resistance, such that no net change in blood pressure results. After a period of latency, total peripheral vascular resistance begins to decrease towards initial values in the face of continued reduced cardiac output, and the net effect is a decrease in blood pressure (Korner, 1976). At times, total peripheral resistance may only return to normal levels, but cardiac output remains low and the net effect is still a reduction in blood pressure (Meier *et al.*, 1980).

In spite of the initial elevation in total peripheral vascular resistance, it has been shown that the antihypertensive effect of propranolol follows closely the secondary fall in peripheral resistance that occurs with time, even when there is some restoration in cardiac output.

3.3.2 β-Adrenoceptor Antagonists in Angina

The β-adrenoceptor blocking agents are useful in angina pectoris because they decrease myocardial oxygen demand. There are three determinants of myocardial oxygen demand:

(1) myocardial wall tension, which is a function of ventricular pressure and the radius of the ventricle;
(2) heart rate; and
(3) contractility.

β-Adrenoceptor antagonists produce a decrease in heart rate and contractile force, resulting simply from β-adrenoceptor blockade. The chronic antihypertensive effect of β-adrenoceptor blockers will also serve to reduce myocardial wall tension by decreasing ventricular systolic developed pressure and by decreasing the size of the hypertrophied left ventricle. Therefore, the utility of β-adrenoceptor antagonists in treating angina pectoris results from the ability of these compounds to decrease the demand made by the myocardium for oxygen by each of the three factors known to create an oxygen demand (Gross and Urquilla, 1982).

3.3.3 β-Adrenoceptor Agonists in Congestive Heart Failure

In heart failure, the goal of therapy is usually to increase cardiac output, and this is often done by increasing the contractile state of the myocardium. One mechanism that may be used to augment cardiac function is by activating myocardial β_1-adrenoceptors, which increases heart rate and contractility and therefore increases cardiac output. The increase in heart rate that occurs with isoproterenol may be undesirable since it increases myocardial work and oxygen demand. With certain inotropic agents, it is possible to increase selectively myocardial contractility while producing little or no increase in heart rate.

Intravenous infusion of dobutamine generally increases cardiac output by augmenting stroke volume, the latter occurring directly from enhanced left ventricular contractility (dp/dt max) (Jewitt et al., 1974). Total peripheral vascular resistance (afterload) is reduced in part by reflex withdrawal of sympathetic tone (Liang and Hood, 1979) and in part by direct arterial vasodilation (Ruffolo and Morgan, 1984). The reduction in afterload produced by dobutamine further increases left ventricular stroke volume by reducing the impedance to left ventricular ejection. Furthermore, the decrease in total peripheral vascular resistance offsets the contribution made by cardiac output to blood pressure such that mean arterial pressure is only minimally affected while cardiac output is significantly increased (Leier and Unverferth, 1983).

Dobutamine infusion is generally associated with decreases in central venous pressure, right and left atrial pressures, pulmonary artery pressure and resistance and pulmonary capillary wedge pressure (Leier and Unverferth, 1983). Consequently, left ventricular end diastolic volume (preload, represented by left ventricular end-diastolic pressure) is lowered, allowing the hypertrophied myocardium characteristic of congestive heart failure to reduce to a more efficient size (Sonnenblick et al., 1979). The decrease in left ventricular end-systolic volume also decreases myocardial wall tension, an important determinant of myocardial oxygen consumption (Gross and Urquilla, 1982).

With doses of isoproterenol and dobutamine that produce comparable increases in cardiac output, larger decreases in total peripheral vascular resistance, and hence greater reductions in blood pressure, are observed with isoproterenol (Sonnenblick et al., 1979). In addition, tachycardia is more pronounced with isoproterenol (Jewitt et al., 1974), resulting from a greater direct positive chronotropic effect of isoproterenol as well as from an additional reflex increase in cardiac rate secondary to the greater reduction in vascular tone. The more profound increase in cardiac rate observed with isoproterenol relative to dobutamine at doses that produce equivalent increases in cardiac output indicates that a smaller contribution to cardiac output is derived from augmentation of stroke volume with isoproterenol relative to dobutamine.

When dopamine and dobutamine are infused at doses that produce equivalent increases in cardiac output, dobutamine is generally associated with greater reductions in left ventricular filling pressure and pulmonary capillary wedge pressure (Leier and Unverferth, 1983). Quite commonly, dopamine is associated with no change or even an increase in pulmonary artery pressure, pulmonary capillary wedge pressure, and left ventricular end-diastolic pressure. Whereas dobutamine tends to have minimal effects on blood pressure, dopamine has been shown to produce a selective increase in total peripheral vascular resistance and mean arterial blood pressure (Leier and Unverferth, 1983). At low doses, dopamine has been shown to produce a selective increase in renal blood flow, secondary to a decrease in renal vascular resistance (Goldberg *et al.*, 1977). This action of dopamine, which is lacking with dobutamine, has been ascribed to selective renal vasodilation resulting from activation of renal DA_1-dopamine receptors. In contrast, the improvement in renal function observed with dobutamine appears to be secondary to an increase in cardiac output and a reflex decrease in total peripheral vascular resistance (Leier and Unverferth, 1983).

At doses that produce comparable increases in cardiac output, epinephrine and norepinephrine tend to cause more tachycardia and greater increases in total peripheral vascular resistance than dobutamine. Consequently, dobutamine tends to increase stroke volume while not greatly affecting blood pressure or heart rate, whereas epinephrine and norepinephrine may cause a smaller increase in stroke volume due to the increased impedance to left ventricular ejection resulting from elevation of afterload, the latter serving to limit increases in stroke volume elicited by improved myocardial contractility.

4 Dopamine Receptors

4.1 CENTRAL DOPAMINE RECEPTORS

Administration of dopamine or other dopamine receptor agonists into various brain regions may elicit a hypotensive and bradycardic response that is antagonized by dopamine receptor antagonists (Barrett and Lokhand-wala, 1982). It has also been reported that dopamine administered directly into the brain produces an increase in blood pressure and heart rate (Day and Roach, 1976). However, in the latter studies, only dopamine was used, and it is established that dopamine will produce effects on α- and β-adrenoceptors (Ruffolo and Morgan, 1984) as well as dopamine receptors, making the results of such studies difficult to interpret. In spite of the complexities in studying the central cardiovascular regulatory effects of dopamine, the use of selective and relatively specific dopamine receptor agonists suggests a minor inhibitory effect mediated by dopamine receptors on blood pressure and heart rate, although a much less significant effect than the one elicited by norepinephrine and α_2-adrenoceptors.

4.2 PERIPHERAL DOPAMINE RECEPTORS

4.2.1 Subclassification of Dopamine Receptors

As observed with α- and β-adrenoceptors, dopamine receptors have been identified both on sympathetic nerve terminals (presynaptic or DA_2), and on smooth muscle cells of certain vascular beds (postsynaptic or DA_1). The presynaptic DA_2 dopamine receptors mediate an inhibition of neurotransmitter release, whereas the postsynaptic DA_1 dopamine receptors on vascular smooth muscle mediate a vasodilatory response. Although the presence of specific receptors for dopamine has been conclusively established, the presence of dopamine-releasing neurons in the periphery is still controversial, except for the interneurons in sympathetic ganglia. Table 3 shows the commonly used agonists and antagonists with selectivity for either the DA_1 or DA_2 receptor.

4.2.2 Presynaptic Dopamine (DA_2) Receptors

Neurotransmission at the vascular and cardiac sympathetic neuroeffector junctions can be modulated via presynaptic DA_2 receptors which exert an inhibitory influence on stimulus-evoked neurotransmitter release from sympathetic nerve terminals (Cavero et al., 1982; Lokhandwala and Barrett, 1982). In the vasculature, which is under a dominant adrenergic control, stimulation of presynaptic DA_2 receptors on sympathetic neurons leads to inhibition of norepinephrine release, thereby producing passive vasodilation. This passive vasodilation results in a decrease in total peripheral resistance and a concomitant reduction in blood pressure.

In the heart, a similar response to presynaptic dopamine receptor activation occurs; however, the heart, unlike the vasculature, is under both cholinergic inhibitory and adrenergic facilitory neurogenic tone, and the cholinergic input dominates. Stimulation of presynaptic DA_2 receptors on postganglionic sympathetic nerve terminals produces the expected inhibition of norepinephrine release and subsequent decrease in adrenergic tone to the heart, with bradycardia resulting from an even further dominance of cholinergic tone. This effect has been demonstrated in vivo as inhibition of the chronotropic response to electrical stimulation of the cardioaccelerator nerve (Bhatnagar et al., 1982; Hamed et al., 1981) or as inhibition of reflex tachycardia resulting from nitroglycerin-induced hypotension (Blumberg et al., 1985).

TABLE 3

Receptor subtype selectivities of various dopamine receptor agonists and antagonists

	Vascular DA$_1$ receptors	Neuronal DA$_2$ receptors
Agonists	Fenoldopam > dopamine = 6,7-ADTN = DP-5,6-ADTN ≥ DP-6,7-ADTN > SK&F 38393 > DPDA ≫ DEDA	DP-5,6-ADTN > DP-6,7-ADTN > 6,7-ADTN > dopamine ≥ DPDA > DEDA ≫ fenoldopam > SK&F38393
Antagonists	SCH 23390 > (+)-butaclamol > cis-α-flupenthixol > fluphenazine > sulpiride ≫ domperidone = haloperidol	Domperidone = (+)-butaclamol = fluphenazine = haloperidol ≫ cis α-flupenthixol = sulpiride > SCH 23390

Stimulation of DA_2 receptors on sympathetic nerve terminals removes the input that these nerves provide to their effector organs by inhibiting norepinephrine release. The consequent loss of vascular and cardiac sympathetic tone results in an antihypertensive response and bradycardia.

4.2.3 Postsynaptic Vascular Dopamine (DA_1) Receptors

Postsynaptic vascular dopamine receptors mediate an active vasodilatory response in renal, mesenteric, hepatic, coronary and cerebral vascular beds in a variety of species, including humans (Furster and Whalley, 1981; Goldberg et al., 1968; Veda et al., 1982). The use of selective dopamine agonists and antagonists have shown this receptor to be of the DA_1 subtype. The presence of vascular DA_1 receptors mediating an active postsynaptic (versus passive presynaptic) vasodilatory response in some, but not all, vascular beds offers a potentially important opportunity for selective drug action, especially since the vascular beds containing these DA_1 receptors include those most involved in cardiovascular disorders.

a. Coronary Circulation. Dopamine receptors have recently been identified in the coronary circulation, where they mediate a vasodilatory response. These receptors, which are of the DA_1 subtype, are associated with the smooth muscle layer of coronary arteries, where they produce direct vascular smooth muscle relaxation (Brodde, 1982), decreasing coronary vascular resistance.

b. Cerebral Circulation. Stimulation of dopamine receptors by dopamine or selective dopamine receptor agonists mediates relaxation of cerebral blood vessels (Brodde, 1982). Results from pharmacological studies on isolated human cerebral blood vessels suggest that these dopamine receptors are of the dopamine DA_1-subtype (Edvinsson et al., 1978; Forster et al., 1983), similar to those receptors which are linked to adenylate cyclase and that are located postsynaptically in selected peripheral vasculature beds (Brodde, 1982). The existence of DA_1-receptors in the cerebral vasculature is supported by recent studies that have shown that dopamine selectively increases cAMP levels in pial arteries (Amenta et al., 1984).

c. Renal Circulation. Dopamine receptors of both the DA_1 and DA_2 subtypes have been identified in the kidney (Felder et al., 1984a,b). Low concentrations of dopamine infused directly into the renal artery induce vasodilation that is inhibited by dopamine receptor antagonists (Goldberg et al., 1978). In addition, dopamine relaxes glomerular arterioles *in vitro*

(Edwards, 1985). The vasodilatory effect of dopamine in the renal circula-tion is mediated by dopamine-DA_1 receptors linked to adenylate cyclase (Murthy et al., 1973). Although a physiological role for dopamine in regulating renal haemodynamics is not yet conclusive, evidence suggests there is dopaminergic innervation to the kidney that is capable of mediating renal vasodilation (DiBona, 1982).

Dopamine receptors of the DA_1 subtype have also been found in renal cortical tubules (Felder et al., 1984a,b), whereas glomeruli appear to possess dopamine DA_2 receptors (Felder et al., 1984a). Although the role of dopamine in the glomerulus is unknown, dopamine has been shown to inhibit fluid absorption in the straight portion of the proximal tubule (Kaneda and Bello-Reuss, 1983), which may, in part, explain the natriuresis observed following dopamine infusions.

d. *Splanchnic Circulation.* The splanchnic circulation contains dopamine receptors which, when stimulated, produce vasodilation (Richardson, 1984; Yeh et al., 1969). At high doses, dopamine causes vasoconstriction through stimulation of α-adrenoceptors (Pawlik et al., 1976; Yeh et al., 1969). The hepatic vascular responses are variable. Low doses of dopamine adminis-tered directly into the hepatic artery produce vasodilation (Richardson and Withrington, 1978) in experimental animals. Similar doses of dopamine administered into the portal vein cause venoconstriction. Higher doses cause hepatic artery constriction and portal vein vasodilation. It is doubtful whether the actions of dopamine on the splanchnic circulation have physio-logical significance (Richardson, 1984).

4.2.4 Dopamine Receptors in Sympathetic Ganglia

Dopamine-containing neurons have been identified in sympathetic ganglia (Libet and Tosaka, 1970). These dopaminergic neurons are postulated to be short interneurons between preganglionic and postganglionic sympathetic nerves (Greengard and Kebabian, 1974). When activated by preganglionic sympathetic neurons, these interneurons release dopamine, which produces a long-lasting inhibitory postsynaptic potential of the postganglionic sym-pathetic neuron to inhibit efferent sympathetic outflow (Willems, 1973). This neuroinhibitory action is thought to be mediated via a dopamine-sensi-tive adenylate cyclase (Kebabian and Greengard, 1971).

Recent evidence suggests that DA_1 receptors may be involved in the ganglia to inhibit sympathetic outflow, since the selective DA_1 agonist, fenoldopam, inhibits ganglionic neurotransmission (Alkhadhi et al., 1984; Lokhandwala et al., 1984; Sabouni and Lokhandwala, 1984). Further evidence for DA_1-mediated inhibition in sympathetic ganglia has been provided by the observation that the neuroinhibitory effect of fenoldopam could not be blocked by the S-enantiomer of sulpiride, which has high DA_2 receptor selectivity, but was attenuated by R,S-sulpiride, an antagonist of both DA_1 and DA_2 receptors (Lokhandwala et al., 1984). The ability of fenoldopam to produce cutaneous and skeletal vasodilation in the canine forelimb has been ascribed to DA_1 receptor mediated inhibition of neurotransmission in the sympathetic ganglia (Grega et al., 1984).

The possible therapeutic significance of the ganglionic dopamine receptor is unclear. Since activation of the ganglionic dopamine receptor inhibits neuronal activity of postganglionic sympathetic nerve fibres to the vasculature and heart (Horn et al., 1981), a DA_1 agonist such as fenoldopam could produce a sympathoinhibitory effect similar to that seen upon activation of presynaptic DA_2 receptors on postganglionic nerve terminals. Hence, DA_1 receptor activation may have both direct (postsynaptic) and indirect (ganglionic) vasodilator effects, and such drugs may prove to be effective antihypertensive agents in humans.

4.3 DOPAMINERGIC DRUGS USED IN THE TREATMENT OF CARDIOVASCULAR DISORDERS

4.3.1 Dopamine in the Treatment of Shock

Dopamine is an agonist at presynaptic and postsynaptic dopamine receptors, DA_2 and DA_1, respectively, in the cardiovascular system. In addition, dopamine is also a potent indirectly-acting sympathomimetic amine that is capable of entering the sympathetic nerve terminal and releasing endogenous stores of norepinephrine into the synapse. As such, some of the effects of the liberated norepinephrine (e.g., α_1-, α_2- and β_1-adrenoceptor activation) also are observed following dopamine administration. In addition, dopamine itself will stimulate α- and β-adrenoceptors directly. It is now clear that this multitude of activities of dopamine contributes to the mostly beneficial effects of the compound in shock of multiple etiologies (McCannel et al., 1966). Thus, the dopaminergic effects of dopamine result in increases in renal, cerebral and coronary perfusion by an action on postsynaptic vascular DA_1-dopamine receptors to produce vasodilation in these critical vascular beds. The presynaptic DA_2 receptor effects of dopamine also inhibit norepinephrine release from nerves innervating the vasculature, and may further contribute to vasodilation in the renal, cerebral and coronary beds. Vasoconstriction produced by dopamine in the less vital skeletal muscle and skin vascular beds, which is mediated by stimulation of α_1- and

α_2-adrenoceptors, as well as the positive inotropic effect of dopamine mediated by myocardial β_1-adrenoceptors, all contribute to the redistribution of blood to the kidney, brain and heart. These multiple effects of dopamine tend to sustain cardiac function while enhancing distribution of blood flow to vital organs.

4.3.2 Presynaptic DA₂ Dopamine Receptor Agonists in Hypertension and Congestive Heart Failure

Presynaptic DA_2-dopamine receptors that inhibit norepinephrine release from adrenergic nerve terminals innervating the vasculature and heart are logical targets for drug action. Activation of these presynaptic dopamine receptors will decrease sympathetic tone to the vasculature and heart, leading to a decrease in blood pressure and heart rate (Lokhandwala and Barrett, 1982). In a preliminary clinical trial, N-n-propyl,N-n-butyl-dopamine (PBDA), a selective dopamine agonist, has been shown to be effective in lowering blood pressure in patients with essential hypertension at doses that were well tolerated (Taylor et al., 1984). The reduction in blood pressure was proposed to be mediated by stimulation of presynaptic DA_2 receptors. The observed increase in renal blood flow most likely results from stimulation of renal vascular DA_1 receptors.

Presynaptic dopamine DA_2 receptor agonists may also be useful in managing severe congestive heart failure as a direct consequence of their ability to reduce afterload by inhibiting norepinephrine release, and thereby reducing total peripheral vascular resistance. In a recent study of risk factors in patients with congestive heart failure, plasma catecholamine level was the only variable to correlate significantly with mortality; higher plasma catecholamine levels were associated with a poor prognosis (Cohn et al., 1984). The sympatholytic effect of a prejunctional DA_2 agonist may be especially beneficial in low output cardiac failure by producing peripheral arterial vasodilation and reduction in afterload without lowering inotropic state. Although the clinical efficacy of a DA_2 agonist in heart failure has not been established conclusively, PBDA has been shown to have a beneficial effect in the haemodynamic profiles of patients with low output cardiac failure, producing dose-dependent reductions in mean arterial pressure, left ventricular filling pressure, pulmonary vascular resistance, and systemic vascular resistance, accompanied by an increase in stroke volume and cardiac index (Fennell et al., 1983). Heart rate and stroke work index were unchanged (Fennell et al., 1983). Furthermore, it has recently been shown that the administration of levodopa, a precursor to dopamine, in the periphery, will increase cardiac index and stroke volume, and decrease total peripheral vascular resistance with no change in blood pressure or heart rate in patients with congestive heart failure (Rajfer *et al.*, 1984).

4.3.3 *Postsynaptic DA₁ Dopamine Receptor Agonists in Hypertension and Renal Insufficiency*

Agonists of postsynaptic DA_1-receptors produce active vasodilation of certain vascular beds, among the most important of which is the renal vasculature. Such compounds produce an antihypertensive response in humans, which may be secondary to diuresis resulting from enhanced renal blood flow, as well as from a possible tubular action of DA_1-receptors to inhibit sodium and water reabsorption. Currently, no selective postsynaptic DA_1-dopamine receptor agonists are clinically available. However, fenoldopam, a potent and selective DA_1 receptor agonist, has been shown to be effective in reducing blood pressure in patients with essential hypertension (Carey *et al.*, 1983; Harvey *et al.*, 1986; Ventura *et al.*, 1983) and increasing renal plasma flow in normal volunteers (Carey *et al.*, 1983; Stote *et al.*, 1983), and is currently under additional clinical evaluation as an antihypertensive drug.

5 Serotonin (5HT) Receptors

5.1 CENTRAL 5HT RECEPTORS

Low doses of serotonin injected into the rat brain produce an increase in blood pressure and heart rate (Korner and Angus, 1981). Centrally administered 5HT also increases the firing rate of peripheral preganglionic sympathetic nerves, an effect that is presumably responsible for the observed hypertension and tachycardia (Korner and Angus, 1981). Centrally administered 5,6-dihydroxytryptamine, which destroys serotonin-containing nerves and thereby releases 5HT, produced tachycardia and hypertension (Korner and Angus, 1981). Some data indicate that the tachycardia observed following stimulation of 5HT receptors in the brain results from inhibition of cholinergic outflow, whereas the increase in blood pressure appears to coincide with an increase in sympathetic outflow to the vasculature (Korner and Angus, 1981).

5.2 PERIPHERAL POSTSYNAPTIC VASCULAR 5HT RECEPTORS

The peripheral effects of serotonin are complex, sometimes increasing and at other times decreasing blood pressure. It appears that the occasional decrease in blood pressure elicited by serotonin is not a direct effect of serotonin on the vasculature, but rather is due to stimulation by serotonin of a non-adrenergic, non-cholinergic vasodilatory pathway, possibly involving a peptide neurotransmitter (Vanhoutte, 1982) or to stimulation of presynaptic 5HT receptors on adrenergic neurons which inhibit norepinephrine release. The more commonly observed vasoconstrictor effect of serotonin results from direct activation of postsynaptic vascular 5HT receptors. On the basis of studies with selective serotonin agonists and antagonists, the postsynaptic vascular 5HT receptor-mediating vasoconstriction has been classified as the $5HT_2$ subtype (Cohen et al., 1981; van Neuten et al., 1981), whereas the presynaptic serotonin receptor that inhibits norepinephrine release is of the $5HT_1$ subtype.

Serotonin also potentiates the vasoconstrictor effect of α-adrenoceptor agonists and angiotensin II. This potentiation can be observed with concentrations of serotonin that have no vasoconstrictor activity (Vanhoutte, 1982; Wenting et al., 1982). This effect, like the direct vasoconstrictor activity of serotonin, is mediated by $5HT_2$ receptors.

Recent studies have shown that serotonin can also interact with receptors on vascular endothelium. Serotonin can dilate dog and pig coronary arteries contracted with a thromboxane agonist (Cocks and Angus, 1983). This dilation is seen only in vessels with intact endothelium and is not sensitive to $5HT_2$ blockade with ketanserin, suggesting that endothelial $5HT_1$ receptors are involved. Endogenous serotonin can also interact with endothelial receptors, since the vasoconstrictor response of dog coronary rings induced by aggregating platelets (which release serotonin) is significantly potentiated by removal of vascular endothelium (Cohen et al., 1983).

In a perfused coronary artery preparation with intact endothelium serotonin can have opposite effects when administered extraluminally or intraluminally. Extraluminal administration of serotonin, which exposes predominantly vascular smooth muscle to serotonin, produces a contractile response, whereas with intraluminal administration of serotonin, in which the endothelium is preferentially exposed to serotonin, relaxation commonly occurs. In fact, intraluminal administration of serotonin can relax contractions induced by extraluminal serotonin. Relaxation can also be produced in this preparation by endogenous serotonin released from aggregating platelets (Cohen et al., 1983).

It is likely that at least some of these vasodilatory effects of serotonin may result from $5HT_1$ receptor activation. The relaxation induced by serotonin in isolated vascular tissues with intact endothelium can be blocked by methiothepin, a moderately selective $5HT_1$ receptor antagonist, but not by ketanserin, a potent and selective $5HT_2$ antagonist. In anaesthetized rats treated with ketanserin (to block $5HT_2$-mediated pressor activity), the hypotensive activity of a series of serotonin agonists correlated well ($r = 0.92$) with their affinity for $5HT_1$ receptors (Kalkman et al., 1983). This hypotensive effect suggests that $5HT_1$ agonists may offer a unique approach to the treatment of hypertension.

5.2.1 Coronary Circulation

Serotonin receptors, like muscarinic cholinergic receptors, mediate a complex response in the coronary circulation: one response may involve the coronary endothelium. Furthermore, $5HT_1$ and $5HT_2$ receptors coexist in coronary arteries, and it appears that these serotonin receptor subtypes mediate opposing responses.

Serotonin has been shown in vitro to dilate coronary arteries when vascular tone is elevated (Cocks and Angus, 1983). This dilation is seen only in vessels with intact endothelium and is not sensitive to $5HT_2$ receptor antagonists, suggesting that endothelial $5HT_1$ receptors mediate coronary artery vasodilation. Endogenous serotonin can also interact with endothelial $5HT_1$ receptors, since the vasoconstrictor response of coronary arteries induced by aggregating platelets (which release serotonin) is significantly potentiated by removal of vascular endothelium (Cohen et al., 1983).

In a perfused coronary artery preparation with intact endothelium, serotonin can have opposite effects when administered extraluminally (adventitial side) or intraluminally (intimal surface) (Cohen et al., 1983). Extraluminal administration of serotonin, which selectively exposes $5HT_2$ receptors located on coronary artery smooth muscle to serotonin, produces a contractile response, whereas intraluminal administration of serotonin, in which endothelial $5HT_1$ receptors are preferentially exposed, commonly produces relaxation. In fact, intraluminal administration of serotonin can relax contractions induced by extraluminally applied serotonin. Relaxation can also be produced in this preparation by endogenous serotonin released from aggregating platelets intraluminally (Cohen et al., 1983).

5.2.2 Pulmonary Circulation

Serotonin produces a vasoconstrictor response in isolated intrapulmonary arteries and veins (Gruetter et al., 1981). It has been suggested that the pulmonary pressor response to thromboembolism results, at least in part, from serotonin released by aggregating platelets. The pulmonary pressor response to serotonin results directly from an increase in pulmonary vascular resistance.

5.2.3 Cerebral Circulation

Serotonin (5HT) produces an intense vasoconstriction of cerebral blood vessels via activation of serotonergic receptors on vascular smooth muscle cells (Edvinsson et al., 1984). This vasoconstriction appears to be mediated by the $5HT_2$ receptor subtype (Griffith et al., 1982), which is the same receptor subtype that mediates vasoconstriction in the peripheral circulation (Cohen et al., 1983). As in peripheral tissues, activation of $5HT_2$ receptors may amplify the cerebral vasoconstrictor responses to a variety of other endogenous compounds, including norepinephrine and angiotensin II. In isolated cerebral arteries with induced vascular tone, serotonin also produces relaxation via inhibitory serotonergic receptors (Fu and Toda, 1983; Vanhoutte, 1982). Serotonin-induced vasodilation has been shown to be endothelial-dependent and to be mediated by $5HT_1$ receptors in other vascular beds; however, this has not been addressed in studies of cerebral blood vessels.

Serotonin may have both a hormonal and a neurotransmitter role in the cerebral circulation, since evidence for a serotonergic innervation to the cerebrovascular bed has been reported, and serotonin can also be released into the circulation from platelets upon aggregation (Edvinsson et al., 1984). Serotonin may be important in the etiology of migraine and cerebral vasospasm following subarachinoid haemorrhage. This is supported by studies that have shown that serotonin antagonists may provide effective prophylactic therapy in some forms of migraine (Raskin, 1981).

5.2.4 Renal Circulation

Serotonin causes renal vasoconstriction (Collis and Vanhoutte, 1977) and has been reported to increase cAMP levels in glomeruli (Shah et al., 1979). Both histamine and serotonin may be involved in the pathogenesis of immunological glomerular diseases (Dousa et al., 1980).

5.2.5 Splanchnic Circulation

The splanchnic vascular responses to serotonin are variable and depend on dose, route of administration, and species (Ormsbee and Fondacaro, 1985;

Richardson, 1984). Generally, intravenous administration of serotonin produces vasodilation in the stomach, small bowel, and colon and vasoconstriction in the liver and pancreas (Chou and Kvietys, 1981). The problems in assessment of the vascular responses to serotonin are compounded by the fact that serotonin also produces motility responses of visceral smooth muscle which influence local blood flow in the mesenteric circulation (Ormsbee and Fondacaro, 1985). Serotonin is found endogenously throughout most of the gastrointestinal tract. Because of the variability of the responses, it has not been possible to classify serotonin receptors in the splanchnic circulation or to establish a physiological role of serotonin in this vascular bed (Richardson, 1984).

5.3 SEROTONERGIC DRUGS USED IN CARDIOVASCULAR DISORDERS

5.3.1 Serotonin Receptor Antagonists in Hypertension

The significance of peripheral serotonin receptors in hypertension is not clear. It has been proposed that peripheral $5HT_2$ receptors, by virtue of their ability to produce vasoconstriction, may be involved in the regulation of blood pressure. Ketanserin is a relatively selective $5HT_2$ receptor antagonist now being clinically evaluated as an antihypertensive drug. In humans, ketanserin is an effective antihypertensive agent (van der Starre et al., 1983; Wenting et al., 1982), suggesting that peripheral vascular $5HT_2$ receptors may, in fact, play a role in hypertension in at least some patients. This observation is somewhat surprising since the vasculature receives no serotonergic innervation. Peripheral serotonin is formed in the enterochromaffin cells of the gastrointenstinal tract; it escapes, is actively accumulated by platelets, and is released upon aggregation (Vanhoutte, 1982). It has been proposed that higher levels of serotonin could reach vascular $5HT_2$ receptors to mediate vasoconstriction in patients with hypertension if platelet uptake of serotonin were reduced and/or platelet aggregation accelerated (Vanhoutte, 1982). Both of these phenomena have been observed in hypertensive patients raising the possibility, in theory, of a non-neuronal serotonergic tone to the vasclature in certain hypertensive states. This explanation has recently been proposed to account for the antihypertensive activity of ketanserin (Vanhoutte, 1982).

However, this explanation for the antihypertensive activity of ketanserin has recently been challenged (Kalkman et al., 1982). The basis for the argument against an antiserotonergic mechanism for the antihypertensive effects of ketanserin is two-fold: (1) other $5HT_2$ antagonists fail to lower blood pressure (Humphrey et al., 1982), and (2) ketanserin is also an

α_1-adrenoceptor antagonist (Kalkman *et al.*, 1982), and it is well documented that α_1-adrenoceptor antagonists (e.g., prazosin) are effective antihypertensive agents because vascular tone is maintained largely by postsynaptic junctional α_1-adrenoceptors which respond to neuronally liberated norepinephrine. It has been shown that the antihypertensive activity of ketanserin in spontaneously hypertensive rats may be completely accounted for by the α_1-adrenoceptor blocking activity of the compound (Kalkman *et al.*, 1982). Whether the same is true for the antihypertensive effects of ketanserin in humans is still not known and awaits further clinical evaluation.

6 Eicosanoid Receptors

6.1 PROSTACYCLIN (PGI$_2$)

6.1.1 Effects of Prostacyclin in the Cardiovascular System and Vascular Smooth Muscle

Prostacyclin is a potent vasodilator in most mammalian species, including humans (Linet, 1982). Prostacyclin also increases cardiac output, but appears to do so indirectly by decreasing afterload (Kadowitz *et al.*, 1984). Infusion of prostacyclin in humans reduces coronary vascular resistance, increases coronary blood flow, and produces flushing of the skin, suggesting generalized systemic vasodilation (Pitt *et al.*, 1983). The primary site of the vasodilator effects of prostacyclin is at the level of the smaller resistance vessels, and not the larger conduit vessels.

The formation of prostacyclin is blocked by aspirin and other cyclo-oxygenase inhibitors. Since cyclo-oxygenase inhibitors do not elevate blood pressure, it is believed that the basal production of prostacyclin does not contribute to vasodilation under normal physiological conditions. However, in some hypoxic, inflammatory, or other pathological states, a vasodilatory role of prostacyclin is probable.

Prostacyclin has been shown to inhibit vasoconstrictor responses elicited by nerve stimulation and by endogenous pressor hormones such as angiotensin II, epinephrine, and norepinephrine. Prostacyclin appears to antagonize neurogenic vasoconstriction by a postjunctional action on vascular smooth muscle rather than by inhibiting neurotransmitter (norepinephrine) release, since nerve-stimulated responses and responses to exogenously administered norepinephrine are inhibited to a similar extent. Furthermore, the responses to angiotensin II and norepinephrine are inhibited to a similar degree, suggesting that prostacyclin non-specifically and functionally antagonizes hormone-induced vasoconstriction (Kadowitz *et al.*, 1984).

The observation that "prostacyclin-like" substances are released spontaneously into the circulation and that prostacyclin is not inactivated in the lung suggests that prostacyclin may serve as a circulating hormone that could act in certain pathological states to maintain the peripheral vascular bed in a dilated state (Gryglewski et al., 1978). Thus, there is an important difference between prostacyclin and other prostaglandins formed from arachidonic acid. Because prostacyclin is not inactivated by the pulmonary circulation, it is equipotent as a vasodilator when given intra-arterially or intravenously, whereas other prostaglandins such as prostaglandins E_1 and E_2 do not escape pulmonary metabolism and are much less active or inactive when given intravenously. Thus, circulating prostacyclin could produce peripheral vasodilation due to the fact that it escapes pulmonary inactivation and may therefore elicit an effect in the arterial circulation (Kadowitz et al., 1984).

Prostacyclin is a potent activator of adenylate cyclase (Larrue et al., 1984), and this has been proposed to be the mechanism responsible for prostacyclin-induced vasodilation. Prostacyclin-mediated increases in cAMP levels also inhibit phospholipase activity in platelets (Lapetina et al., 1977) and vascular endothelium (Brotherton and Hoak, 1982; Hopkins and Gorman, 1981), possibly indirectly by blocking the action of calcium (Brotherton and Hoak, 1982). Prostacyclin-mediated increases in cAMP can inhibit the basal production of prostacyclin, suggesting that prostacyclin has a negative feedback on its own synthesis (Larrue et al., 1984).

6.1.2 Platelet Aggregation

Prostacyclin is the most potent endogenous inhibitor of platelet aggregation, being 30-fold more potent than prostaglandin E_1 and 1000-fold more potent than adenosine (Moncada and Vane, 1977; Mullane et al., 1979). The antiaggregatory effect of prostacyclin appears to result from elevated platelet cAMP levels (Whittle and Moncada, 1984). Prostacyclin also inhibits platelet adhesion. Basal levels of prostacyclin under normal circumstances are not sufficiently high to have a significant effect. However, local concentrations of prostacyclin may become high enough to inhibit platelet aggregation and thrombus formation under some circumstances. Whether levels of prostacyclin in vivo ever reach sufficient concentrations to inhibit platelet adherence to an injured blood vessel is less certain.

6.1.3 Renal Effects of Prostacyclin

Regulation of the renal circulation is complicated by the interplay between hormonal and neurogenic effects acting on vascular resistance, glomerular filtration rate, and renal blood flow. Involved in this delicate interplay are the renin–angiotensin system, catecholamines, prostaglandins, and the kallikrein–kinin system. Furthermore, the relative contribution of these factors may change in a variety of physiological and pathological states.

Prostacyclin is one of the most abundantly produced renal prostaglandins, primarily from arteriolar and glomerular sites. Renal cortical function, such as renal blood flow and glomerular filtration rate, is modulated by cortical prostacyclin synthesis. Prostacyclin increases renal blood flow and antagonizes the renal pressor actions of angiontensin II and vasopressin (antidiuretic hormone). The natriuretic, kaliuretic, and diuretic actions of prostacyclin appear to be independent of the effects of renal blood flow and glomerular filtration rate, suggesting also a tubular action. Prostacyclin is formed in the renal cortex at sites of renin synthesis and storage, and also may modulate renin release (Rosenkranz et al., 1981).

Prostacyclin formation also contributes to the reduction in renal vascular resistance observed during periods of low sodium intake, reduced cardiac output, hypoxaemic and ischaemic renal states, and hepatic disease (Dunn, 1983). A number of studies suggest that prostacyclin has its greatest effect on renal function when circulating blood volume is reduced, and that by blocking synthesis of prostacyclin, cyclo-oxygenase inhibition may exacerbate diminished renal function to the point of renal insufficiency (Dunn, 1983).

Another important effect of prostacyclin in the kidney is its interaction with vasopressin to increase urinary excretion of sodium and water. It is known that prostacyclin has diuretic and natriuretic effects. Furthermore, it has been shown in a variety of species, including humans, that cyclo-oxygenase inhibitors potentiate the hydro-osmotic effect of vasopressin on the renal tubule (Anderson et al., 1975; Berl et al., 1977; Lum et al., 1977), suggesting that prostacyclin may play a physiological role in the renal tubule (Haylor and Lote, 1980).

It appears that renal function significantly depends upon prostacyclin formation during low circulating volume, sodium depletion, low cardiac output, and several other pathological states. These relatively hypovolemic or hypoperfused renal states reduce oxygen transport and impede renal function. In the light of the enormous metabolic activity needed for normal countercurrent exchange of sodium, prostacyclin release may represent part of an "antihypoxic" response and be critical to maintaining normal renal function.

6.1.4 Systemic and Regional Haemodynamic Effect of Prostacyclin

Intra-arterial administration of prostacyclin produces an immediate decrease in mean arterial blood pressure secondary to a decrease in systemic vascular resistance. Cardiac output is significantly increased by prostacyclin, presumably a direct consequence of the reduction in afterload (Kadowitz *et al.*, 1984). Prostacyclin infusion is associated with increases in blood flow in coronary, renal, mesenteric, and hindquarter vascular beds (Kadowitz *et al.*, 1984). These increases in regional blood flow produced by prostacyclin are secondary to decreases in the respective regional vascular resistances, and are consistent with the *in vitro* observations that prostacyclin produces direct arterial vasodilation in isolated strips prepared from the mesenteric, celiac, and coronary arteries (Kadowitz *et al.*, 1984).

Prostacyclin also produces vasodilation in the pulmonary circulation. Thus, prostacyclin infusion has been reported to reduce lobar arterial and small vein pressures without affecting left atrial pressure in normal animals. However, when pulmonary pressures are elevated, prostacyclin is associated with marked reductions in pulmonary vascular resistance. In fact, prostacyclin is the only product of the arachidonic acid cascade known to produce vasodilation in the pulmonary circulation (Kadowitz *et al.*, 1984). It has been proposed that under resting conditions, the pulmonary vascular bed may be maintained in a dilated state by production of prostacyclin in the lung (Kadowitz *et al.*, 1984).

6.1.5 *Effects of Prostacyclin on Local Blood Flow and Reactive Hyperaemia*

The function of the cardiovascular system over a dynamic range of activities and blood pressures depends to a large extent on the capacity of the peripheral vascular beds to autoregulate blood flow according to metabolic demands. Autoregulation of local blood flow is a complex interaction of central, local, and humoral factors, many of which are still unknown. One example is reactive hyperaemia. Reactive hyperaemia is not generally considered to be a true physiological response, but rather a maximal mobilization of the tissue's defences against hypoxia. Cyclo-oxygenase inhibitors reduce both the maximum and the duration of the vasodilatory response after release of arterial occlusion (Messina *et al.*, 1977), and prostacyclin has been implicated as a possible mediator of this response. Similar results have been observed in humans, where total forearm reactive hyperaemia following 5 minutes of arterial occlusion was reduced 50–60% by indomethacin (Kilbom and Wennmalm, 1976; Nowak and Wennmalm, 1979).

6.1.6 *Relationship of Prostacyclin to Cardiovascular Disease*

a. Ischaemic Heart Disease (Angina). Given the vasodilatory and anti-aggregatory properties of prostacyclin, there has been much interest in the possible relation of certain pathological states to disorders in prostacyclin synthesis and/or release. The role of prostacyclin in ischaemic heart disease, such as angina, coronary artery disease, or myocardial infarction, has been the target of many recent investigations.

Clinical trials with prostacyclin in patients with ischaemic heart disease have been equivocal, showing inconsistent relief of anginal pain despite patients' low basal coronary prostacyclin levels upon admission. Many studies show an improvement in some, but not all, patients with angina when prostacyclin was infused (Linet, 1982). Cyclo-oxygenase inhibitors which block the synthesis of prostacyclin have been shown to constrict coronary vessels and to decrease coronary blood flow in patients with ischaemic heart disease, and to exacerbate the imbalance in the ratio between myocardial oxygen supply and demand. It seems likely, therefore, that in patients with coronary artery disease, the endogenous release of prostacyclin in response to hypoxia may be part of a homeostatic mechanism to maintain adequate coronary perfusion (Friedman et al., 1978a,b).

The inconsistent effects of prostacyclin in patients with angina may be attributed, a least in part, to different patient selection criteria, as well as to differences in the stage of the disease. Furthermore, the release of prostacyclin in response to myocardial ischemic episodes is dependent upon local pO_2 levels, and the transient nature of ischaemic attacks may not be of sufficient duration to reduce oxygen tension below 47 mm Hg, a level that has been shown to stimulate prostacyclin synthesis (Wennmalm, 1982).

b. Myocardial Infarction. A number of animal studies have confirmed that infusion of prostacyclin significantly reduces infarct size and mortality following ligation of the left anterior descending coronary artery. Conversely, inhibitors of prostacyclin synthesis increase the size of experimental infarction zones (Lefer et al., 1978). The limiting effect of prostacyclin on infarct size may be related to its cytoprotective effects in the myocardium rather than to an antiaggregatory or coronary vasodilatory effect (Lefer et al., 1978; Ribeiro et al., 1981).

Prostacyclin infused within 6 h of acute myocardial infarction reduced creatinine phosphokinase release from the heart by 50% compared with that in control patients, suggesting that prostacyclin may also limit infarct size in humans (Henriksson et al., 1985). Thus, although prostacyclin infusion may have variable effects in angina, it appears consistently effective in limiting the size of an acute myocardial infarction in animals and humans (Wennmalm, 1982).

c. Effects on Peripheral Vascular Disease. Disorders in prostacyclin synthesis and/or release may be important in the development of certain peripheral vascular diseases, such as chronic atherosclerotic occlusive disease, Buergers disease, Raynaud's phenomenon, and idiopathic vasculopathy. Clinical studies have shown prostacyclin to be beneficial in distal arteriopathies associated with rest pain and ulceration (Linet, 1982). Advanced peripheral vascular insufficiency responds well to prostacyclin infusion, and virtually all patients report relief of rest pain, and healing of ischaemic ulcerations. In these patients prostacyclin may be directly beneficial by augmenting local perfusion, since increases in blood flow to calf muscle have been observed. Studies in patients suffering from a variety of distal arteriosclerotic disorders have demonstrated similar improvement.

6.2 THROMBOXANE A_2 (TXA$_2$)

Thromboxane A_2, a potent vasoconstrictor and promoter of platelet aggregation, is a prostanoid also derived from arachidonic acid via the cyclooxygenase pathway. Thromboxane A_2 is synthesized and released by activated platelets. However, other cells and tissues have the capacity to produce thromboxane A_2; it has been found in polymorphonuclear leukocytes, macrophages, fibroblasts, spleen, iris, conjunctiva, lung, umbilical artery, pulmonary artery, and kidney (Whittle and Moncada, 1984). Thromboxane A_2 may have adverse effects in patients with coronary artery disease because it strongly constricts the systemic vasculature and coronary artery, and because it promotes platelet aggregation, all of which will exacerbate the existing imbalance between myocardial oxygen supply and demand. The pathophysiological role of thromboxane A_2 in the cardiovascular system remains undefined. Increased thromboxane A_2 release has been seen in coronary artery vasospasm and pacing-induced angina (Lewy *et al.*, 1980a,b). Recently, thromboxane A_2 (inferred by detection of its stable metabolite, thromboxane B_2), has been found in peripheral venous samples taken from patients with evolving acute myocardial infarction. Thromboxane A_2 has been shown to promote the synthesis of prostacyclin in vascular smooth muscle.

6.2.1 Platelet Aggregation

Platelet aggregation is a multifactorial phenomenon that can be initiated by many humoral stimuli, including ADP, thrombin, epinephrine, arachidonic acid, and thromboxane A_2. One common denominator of these proaggregatory agents is their ability to decrease platelet levels of cAMP (Whittle and Moncada, 1984). Since the decrease in platelet cAMP can be abolished with thromboxane synthase inhibitors, it may be the formation of thromboxane A_2 by these agents that leads to the decrease in cAMP and subsequently to the induction of platelet aggregation. However, the concept that a decrease in cAMP is a significant factor in causing platelet aggregation has recently been questioned since a number of compounds that inhibit platelet adenylate cyclase do not promote platelet aggregation (Gerrard, 1985).

Thromboxane A_2 plays an important and fundamental role in platelet function (Gerrard, 1985). Thromboxane A_2 stimulates platelet granule centralization. The sequence of events appears to depend upon calcium flux initiating phosphorylation of myosin light chain. The mechanism of thromboxane A_2-induced stimulation of calcium flux, whether direct or indirect (via phosphoinositide breakdown), is uncertain. Furthermore, thromboxane A_2 stimulates granule labilization, one of the essential steps in granule secretion. The biochemical sequence appears to require phosphorylation of critical intracellular proteins. The mechanism of thromboxane A_2-induced phosphorylation, whether due to direct activation of protein kinase C or indirectly via phosphoinositide breakdown and diglyceride production, is also uncertain (Gerrard, 1985). The sequence of events involved in the thromboxane A_2-mediated granule centralization and labilization leading to secretion is summarized in Fig. 3.

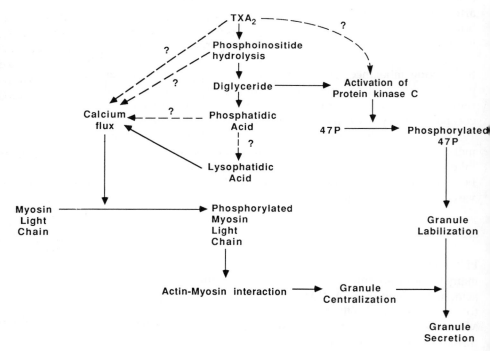

FIG. 3. Schematic representation of the pathways leading from TXA_2 receptor activation to platelet granule secretion.

Platelet aggregation induced by arachidonic acid, prostaglandins H_2 and G_2, and collagen is accompanied by the further formation of thromboxane A_2 (Hamberg and Samuelsson, 1974; Parise et al., 1984). Selective thromboxane receptor antagonists inhibit platelet aggregation induced by arachidonate, prostaglandin endoperoxides, and collagen, suggesting that thromboxane A_2 generation may be a final common pathway leading to platelet aggregation for these substances (Humphrey and Lumley, 1984; Thomas et al., 1984; Whittle and Moncada, 1984). The inhibition of arachidonate-induced platelet aggregation by thromboxane synthase inhibitors could also result from diversion of prostaglandin endoperoxides to prostaglandin D_2, the latter being an inhibitor of platelet aggregation. However, since thromboxane synthase inhibitors do not block platelet aggregation induced by prostaglandin endoperoxides (i.e., prostaglandins G_2 and H_2), it is concluded that these compounds may also act directly on the same receptor as thromboxane A_2.

6.2.2 Coronary Circulation

Thromboxane A_2 is a potent coronary vasoconstrictor (Coleman et al., 1981; Nicolaou et al., 1979; Toda, 1984). The proaggregatory and vasoconstrictor properties of thromboxane A_2 have been implicated in the etiology of several cardiovascular pathologies, such as myocardial ischaemia (Chierchia, 1982; Hoshida et al., 1983), variant angina, coronary vasospasm, myocardial infarction (Hoshida et al., 1983; Kuzuya et al., 1983; Spann, 1983), and sudden death syndrome (Lefer et al., 1981b).

6.2.3 Renal Effects of Thromboxane A_2

Thromboxane A_2 release in the kidneys of young hypertensive rats is relatively high compared with the modest release observed in older hypertensive rats. This finding is consistent with the observation that increased thromboxane A_2 production is seen in isolated glomeruli from hypertensive rats, and suggests further that a primary change resulting in increased renal glomerular thromboxane A_2 synthesis may be a preliminary step leading to increased renal vascular resistance and subsequently to the development of hypertension (Konieczkowski et al., 1982).

6.2.4 Role of Thromboxane A_2 in Cardiovascular Disorders

a. Ischaemic Heart Disease. One minute after coronary artery occlusion in animals, levels of thromboxane A_2 in the great cardiac vein effluent are elevated. This suggests that thromboxane A_2 has a role in acute myocardial infarction. The known vasoconstrictive, platelet aggregatory, and cytolytic actions of thromboxane A_2 may all contribute to myocardial damage following acute infarction (Lefer et al., 1981a,b). Following acute myocardial infarction there is generalized coronary vasoconstriction (Hellstrom, 1971) that may result partly from thromboxane A_2 released into the coronary circulation following platelet aggregation. Coronary venous blood obtained after experimental coronary occlusion caused strips of rabbit aorta and of coronary artery to contract, suggesting that it contained a vasoconstrictive substance (Tanabe et al., 1982). Pretreatment of these animals with a cyclo-oxygenase inhibitor to block thromboxane A_2 synthesis abolishes the constrictive effect of the coronary effluent. Furthermore, after experimental myocardial infarction, administration of a specific thromboxane synthetase inhibitor decreases infarct size (Schror et al., 1980). Conversely, administration of a synthetic thromboxane A_2 mimetic will increase experimental infarct size (Smith et al., 1981).

Several clinical studies have reported increased levels of circulating thromboxane B_2, a stable metabolite and therefore biochemical marker of thromboxane A_2, in patients with angina (Ito et al., 1983; Kuzuya et al., 1983; Yui et al., 1983) or coronary artery vasospasm (Chierchia, 1982; Ohmori et al., 1983). This confirms that platelet aggregation and arachidonic acid metabolism are increased in patients with ischaemic heart disease, and has led to speculation that thromboxane A_2 may have a causative role in this disease. Increased platelet aggregation and thromboxane A_2 release in the coronary circulation during ischaemic attacks has also been noted in several studies. Nonetheless, the importance of thromboxane A_2 in angina remains controversial. Although increased thromboxane B_2 has been demonstrated in pacing-induced angina, no beneficial effect of cyclo-oxygenase inhibitors has been demonstrated, suggesting that thromboxane A_2 may not be the principal causative agent involved. However, aspirin therapy may be beneficial in unstable angina, highly suggestive of a role of thromboxane A_2 in this pathology. Interestingly, the clinical efficacy of calcium channel-blocking agents in coronary artery vasospasm may be related to their ability to block platelet aggregation, and thus, prevent the release of thromboxane A_2 into the coronary circulation (Dahl and Uotila, 1984), thereby eliminating thromboxane A_2-induced coronary vasoconstriction.

Although clinical studies indicate that thromboxane A_2 levels are elevated in patients with ischaemic heart disease, additional factors must also be considered. The balance between prostacyclin and thromboxane A_2 in these cardiovascular conditions appears to be a critical factor regulating coronary perfusion and myocardial dynamics. Higher ratios of prostacyclin:thromboxane A_2 protect the myocardium and increase coronary blood flow, whereas lower ratios worsen ischaemic heart disease by decreasing coronary blood flow and unfavourably altering the ratio between myocardial oxygen supply and demand.

b. *Endotoxin Shock.* The role of thromboxane A_2 in endotoxic shock has been documented in animals. Thromboxane A_2 has been implicated as a causative agent of cardiac and respiratory dysfunction during endotoxin shock. Thromboxane A_2 levels are elevated within 30 min of endotoxin challenge in animals, and this is presumed to be responsible for the observed pulmonary hypertension and thrombocytopenia. The increase in pulmonary vascular resistance and hypoxia observed in experimental endotoxic shock appears to be a direct consequence of the pulmonary vasoconstrictor effects of thromboxane A_2, as well as from microemboli resulting from the aggregation of platelets in the pulmonary circulation, the latter also possibly induced by thromboxane A_2. Studies with either thromboxane synthetase inhibitors (Cook *et al.*, 1980) or thromboxane receptor antagonists (Ball and Parratt, 1984) have shown markedly increased survival rates in animals, but only when administered before or with endotoxin. The mortality rate resulting from endotoxin challenge in animals is not significantly reduced when the thromboxane antagonist/synthetase inhibitor follows the endotoxin challenge, indicating that thromboxane A_2 formation may be a causative factor in the early cascade of events leading to the haemodynamic sequelae of endotoxic shock (Cook *et al.*, 1980).

The haemodynamic effects mediated by thromboxane A_2 in septic shock have been investigated in detail. Thromboxane A_2 has been implicated as a mediator of pulmonary vasoconstriction during endotoxin shock (Slotman *et al.*, 1984). High levels of thromboxane A_2 in sepsis correlate with significantly elevated pulmonary artery pressure, pulmonary capillary wedge pressure, and lung lymph flow, and significantly decreased cardiac output. A significant increase in intrapulmonary shunting accompanies the haemodynamic changes induced by thromboxane A_2. Inhibition of thromboxane A_2 synthesis in septic shock with indomethacin, ibuprofen, or imidazole effectively attenuates the pulmonary vasoconstrictor response to endotoxin.

A strong correlation has been noted between increased plasma thromboxane A_2 levels and decreased cardiac output, decreased stroke volume and decreased left ventricular stroke work (Slotman *et al.*, 1984). Thromboxane A_2-induced elevations in pulmonary vascular resistance preceded late decreases in mean arterial pressure. These interactions support the concept that, in sepsis, increased pulmonary vascular resistance limits the return of blood to the left side of the heart, with subsequent decrements in stroke volume, left ventricular stroke work and cardiac output, followed by a late decline in mean arterial pressure (Slotman *et al.*, 1984). Elevated plasma concentrations of thromboxane A_2 appear to precede impaired cardiopulmonary function, a correlation which suggests that thromboxane A_2 may be involved in the detrimental haemodynamic effects of early septicaemia (Slotman *et al.*, 1984). Thromboxane A_2 mediation of unstable haemodynamics may occur indirectly through increased pulmonary vascular resistance and/or direct myocardial depression elicited by thromboxane A_2 (Friedman *et al.*, 1978b).

6.3 LEUKOTRIENES

Only recently have leukotrienes been identified and their structures elucidated. The major components of slow-reacting substance of anaphylaxis are leukotrienes C_4, D_4, and E_4: leukotriene C_4 being the major component (Hammarstrom, 1983; Samuelsson *et al.*, 1980).

The leukotrienes are released in response to a variety of immunological and non-immunological stimuli, and have been demonstrated to be involved in contraction of bronchial smooth muscle, stimulation of vascular permeability, attraction and activation of leukocytes, and altering myocardial function. The leukotrienes are enzymatic derivatives of arachidonic acid formed via the lipoxygenase enzyme pathway and are synthesized in a variety of tissues and cell types, such as leukocytes, mastocytoma cells, macrophages, lung, kidney and coronary vasculature (Jim *et al.*, 1982; Piper, 1984; Winokur and Morrison, 1981).

Not surprisingly, the synthesis and actions of the leukotrienes, prostacyclin, and thromboxane A_2 may show a direct interplay. The inhibitory effects that hydroperoxy fatty acids derived from the lipoxygenase pathway have on prostacyclin synthetase are well documented (Ham *et al.*, 1979; Moncada *et al.*, 1976; Salmon *et al.*, 1978; Turk *et al.*, 1980). In addition, the production of lipoxygenase products by endothelial cells may be a natural feedback inhibitor of prostacyclin synthesis (Greenwald *et al.*, 1979). Both leukotrienes C_4 and D_4 increase thromboxane A_2 generation, as has been shown by the leukotriene-mediated release of thromboxane A_2 from the guinea pig lung parenchyma. This effect may be due to activation of phospholipase A_2 by certain metabolites of the lipoxygenase pathway (Piper and Samhoun, 1982).

6.3.1 Coronary Circulation

The leukotrienes C_4, D_4, and E_4 are potent mediators of coronary vasoconstriction and produce negative inotropic effects in a variety of species

(Letts and Piper, 1982; Michelassi *et al.*, 1982). Although the leukotriene-mediated negative inotropic response has been repeatedly demonstrated, it has not been conclusively established whether it results from a direct depressant effect of the leukotriene on the myocardium or rather from leukotriene-induced coronary artery vasoconstriction.

Coronary artery vasoconstriction induced by leukotriene C_4 is slower acting than that induced by leukotriene D_4, but is much stronger. Cyclo-oxygenase inhibitors can reduce leukotriene C_4-induced vasoconstriction by nearly 50%, but do not affect leukotriene D_4, indicating that leukotriene C_4-induced coronary artery vasoconstriction may depend on the release of cyclo-oxygenase products, possibly thromboxane A_2. These observations are consistent with previous reports that thromboxane A_2 is released from isolated guinea-pig hearts by products of the lipoxygenase pathway (Allan and Levi, 1981).

Several studies have suggested that leukotrienes C_4 and D_4 may have direct depressant effects on the myocardium, independent of their effects on coronary blood flow. Leukotrienes C_4 and D_4 decrease left ventricular systolic pressure and left ventricular contractility when perfused into guinea-pig hearts (Terashita *et al.*, 1981). Direct depressant effects of leukotrienes C_4, D_4, and E_4 have been demonstrated in the isolated human pectinate muscle and the right ventricular papillary muscle of the guinea-pig (Burke *et al.*, 1982). In isolated working guinea-pig hearts, leukotriene-induced decreases in contractility were found to be largely independent of the changes in coronary flow, and it has been further demonstrated that doses of angiotensin II producing coronary artery vasoconstriction equal to that seen with the leukotrienes have a smaller negative inotropic effect (Burke *et al.*, 1982). This suggests that the leukotrienes have a direct negative inotropic effect above and beyond that which may be attributed to compromised coronary blood flow.

Leukotriene D_4 has been shown to impair regional left ventricular systolic shortening independently of the reduction in coronary blood flow. Cyclo-oxygenase inhibitors do not antagonize the coronary artery vasoconstriction induced by leukotriene D_4, indicating that thromboxane A_2 is not produced. These results indicate that leukotriene D_4 may have a negative inotropic effect on the myocardium, independent of coronary artery vasoconstrictive effects and of the release of cyclo-oxygenase products (Michelassi *et al.*, 1982).

It appears that at least part of the leukotriene C_4-mediated effect on myocardial contractility and the coronary vasculature may be due to the release of thromboxane A_2 into the coronary circulation. Recently it has been demonstrated that a selective thromboxane receptor end-organ antagonist inhibits the leukotriene C_4-induced decrease in coronary blood flow (Burke *et al.*, 1984). Interestingly, the same thromboxane receptor antagonist was relatively more potent in antagonizing the negative inotropic effect of leukotriene C_4 than in antagonizing the leukotriene C_4-induced decrease in coronary blood flow, again suggesting that leukotrienes produce a negative inotropic effect that is independent of coronary artery vasoconstriction (Burke et al., 1984). It has been shown that the negative inotropic effect of leukotrienes results from a reduction in calcium influx through the sarcolemmal membrane. This calcium-blocking effect of the leukotrienes is inhibited by selective leukotriene receptor antagonists, suggesting the involvement of specific leukotriene receptors located in the myocardium (Hattori and Levi, 1984).

The dissociation of coronary blood flow from negative inotropy in the presence of a thromboxane receptor antagonist suggests that thromboxane A_2 may partially mediate the negative inotropic effects of leukotriene C_4. However, other possible explanations have been offered for this observed dissociation in the effects of leukotrienes on coronary artery blood flow and inotropy, including the existence of subpopulations of leukotriene C_4 receptors in the coronary vasculature and cardiac muscle (Burke et al., 1984).

6.3.2 Systemic Haemodynamic Effects of Leukotrienes

The systemic effects of leukotrienes on blood pressure vary with species and routes of administration. When leukotrienes C_4 and D_4 are administered intravenously to the guinea-pig, there is an initial hypertensive response followed by a long-lasting hypotensive response (Drazen et al., 1980; Piper et al., 1981). When the leukotrienes are given intra-arterially, the hypertensive phase is less marked and the hypotension is more prolonged. Cyclooxygenase metabolites may be involved in this leukotriene-mediated response, since inhibitors of the cyclo-oxygenase pathway have been shown to antagonize the hypertensive phase and shorten the duration of the hypotensive phase.

Injection of leukotriene C_4 into the right atrium of monkeys produces an acute rise in mean arterial pressure, pulmonary artery pressure, and right and left atrial pressures (Smedegard et al., 1982). This initial pressor response results from an increase in both pulmonary and systemic vascular resistance, consistent with the known vasoconstrictive effects of leukotriene C_4. Following the acute pressor response there is a marked decrease in cardiac output and reductions in pulmonary artery pressure and right and left atrial pressures occur. This secondary hypotensive response is not the result of peripheral arterial vasodilation, since total peripheral vascular resistance actually increases further. It appears, therefore, that the sustained hypotensive response produced by leukotriene C_4 results primarily from a reduction in cardiac output, possibly from altered cardiac dynamics secondary to coronary vasoconstriction (Letts and Piper, 1982), or from a direct negative inotropic effect of leukotriene C_4 (Hattori and Levi, 1984). Furthermore, the leukotriene C_4-induced pulmonary artery vasoconstriction that leads to increased pulmonary vascular resistance may limit left ventricular filling and thereby also contribute to the observed reduction in cardiac output. Additionally, reduced plasma volume resulting from leukotriene C_4-induced increases in vascular permeability may also be a contributing factor and would also account for the haemoconcentration (rise in haematocrit) observed after leukotriene C_4 administration (Smedegard *et al.*, 1982). an identical haemodynamic profile for leukotriene C_4 and D_4 has also been reported in rats following intravenous administration (Pfeffer *et al.*, 1983).

6.3.3 Involvement of Leukotrienes in Cardiovascular Disease

Elevated leukotriene levels have been detected in sputum or lung lavage specimens from patients with asthma (Dahlen *et al.*, 1983), cystic fibrosis (Cromwell *et al.*, 1981), and neonatal hypoxaemia with pulmonary hypertension (Stenmark *et al.*, 1983). In patients with adult respiratory distress syndrome (ARDS), leukotriene D_4 levels and sometimes leukotriene C_4 levels of lung oedema fluid are significantly elevated (Matthay *et al.*, 1984). Furthermore, the concentration of leukotriene D_4 correlates highly with the ratio of protein concentration in the oedema fluid, suggesting that leukotriene D_4 might contribute to a fundamental abnormality in transcapillary permeability (Goetzel *et al.*, 1984).

The vasoconstriction produced by leukotrienes C_4 and D_4 in the coronary circulation of various species has led to speculation concerning their involvement in pathophysiological conditions such as myocardial ischaemia, angina, and coronary artery vasospasm. A lipoxygenase system exists in porcine coronary and pulmonary arteries, and these blood vessels can synthesize a leukotriene-like substance, indicating that some species can generate leukotrienes locally in the coronary circulation (Piper *et al.*, 1983).

7 Angiotensin II Receptors

7.1 RENIN–ANGIOTENSIN SYSTEM

In the kidney and adrenal gland there is a closed loop feedback system that regulates electrolyte balance and is critical to the regulation of blood pressure. It is currently undergoing intensive study as a target of antihypertensive drug action.

The enzyme renin is released into the blood from the juxtaglomerular apparatus in the kidney. Renin in plasma enzymatically converts angiotensinogen into angiotensin I, which is relatively inert. However, angiotensin I is a substrate for angiotensin-converting enzyme, which generates angiotensin II. Angiotensin II is a potent vasoconstrictor that acts by stimulating postsynaptic vascular angiotensin II receptors to elevate blood pressure by producing systemic arterial vasoconstriction. Another mechanism was recently discovered that may contribute to the elevation in blood pressure elicited by angiotensin II and involves an effect of angiotensin II on presynaptic angiotensin II receptors associated with sympathetic neurons to facilitate norepinephrine release. The elevated synaptic levels of norepinephrine resulting from the presynaptic facilitory effect of angiotensin II will stimulate postsynaptic α_1-adrenoceptors to cause systemic vasoconstriction. In addition, angiotensin II will stimulate aldosterone release from the adrenal cortex which, in turn, causes tubular sodium and water retention, further elevating blood pressure. Elevated blood pressure and increased sodium normally inhibit further renin release to complete the closed loop (long loop) system. In addition, angiotensin II has been shown to directly inhibit renin release (short loop reflex). Clearly, the inability of the kidney to regulate renin release because of damage or an imbalance in the delicate reflex mechanism, can result in the elevation of blood pressure with a concomitant electrolyte imbalance which may produce additional kidney damage, exacerbating the condition and leading to an even greater elevation in blood pressure and further electrolyte imbalance.

7.1.1 Renal Circulation

All of the components of the renin–angiotensin system are present in the region of the juxtaglomerular apparatus (Navar and Rosivall, 1984), which has strengthened the view that locally formed angiotensin II participates in the control of renal vascular resistance, renal blood flow, and glomerular filtration rate.

Infusion of angiotensin II in a number of species elicits a dose-dependent decrease in renal blood flow with smaller and more variable effects on glomerular filtration rate (Navar and Rosivall, 1984). Since filtration fraction increases, it has been proposed that angiotensin II preferentially increases efferent arteriolar resistance (Hall et al., 1977). This notion is supported by in vitro studies in which isolated rabbit afferent arterioles fail to respond to angiotensin II, whereas efferent arterioles are highly sensitive to the vasoconstrictive effect of angiotensin II (Edwards, 1983).

Some studies have shown that under certain conditions, angiotensin II may also increase preglomerular resistance (Navar and Rosivall, 1984). For example, when angiotensin II is infused during inhibition of prostaglandin synthesis, the vasoconstrictive effects of angiotensin II, especially on pre-glomerular resistance vessels, are more pronounced (Bayliss and Brenner, 1978). Therefore, the alteration in renal haemodynamics observed with angiotensin II may depend partly on the status of other intrarenal hormonal systems (Navar and Rosivall, 1984).

Specific angiotensin II receptors have also been found in glomeruli (Skorecki et al., 1983). Mesangial cells, but not glomerular epithelial cells, display a contractile response to angiotensin II (Kreisberg, 1983). Thus, angiotensin II, by modulating mesangial cell contractility, may regulate blood flow along the glomerular capillary and/or the surface area available for filtration (Kreisberg, 1983). This mechanism may account for the decrease in the glomerular ultrafiltration coefficient observed with angio-tensin II (Myers et al., 1975).

Although the exact role of the renin–angiotensin system in regulating renal haemodynamics is uncertain, current evidence suggests that angio-tensin II may maintain glomerular filtration rate during periods of low renal perfusion pressure (Hall et al., 1977). Thus, when renal perfusion pressure is reduced to low levels in dogs, autoregulation of renal blood flow and glomerular filtration rate is well maintained (Hall et al., 1977). However, when renin is depleted or when angiotensin-converting enzyme is inhibited by captopril, regulation of renal blood flow persists, but glomerular filtration rate falls (Hall et al., 1977). Similar observations have been made in humans with renal arterial stenosis, a condition in which the renin–angiotensin system is activated. In these patients, captopril causes a marked decrease in glomerular filtration rate (Blythe, 1983), supporting the view that angioten-sin II, by increasing efferent arteriolar resistance, helps to maintain glomeru-lar capillary pressure, and hence filtration rate, when renal perfusion is compromised (Hall et al., 1977).

7.1.2 Cerebral Circulation

Both angiotensin I and II have been shown to produce concentration-related contraction of isolated cerebral arteries by stimulating angiotensin II recep-tors. Angiotensin I is converted to angiotensin II via angiotensin-converting enzyme, which is localized on the luminal surface of vascular endothelial cells (Whalley et al., 1983). Results from recent studies with captopril suggest that angiotensin II has a physiological role in the autoregulation of cerebral blood flow. Chronic treatment with this angiotensin-converting enzyme inhibitor produces cerebral vasodilation and a subsequent increase in cerebral blood flow in rats. In addition, intravenous infusion of captopril can decrease the pressure range over which cerebral blood flow can be autoregulated (Barry *et al.*, 1984; Koike *et al.*, 1980).

7.2 ANGIOTENSIN-CONVERTING ENZYME INHIBITORS

7.2.1 Hypertension

Angiotensin-converting enzyme converts angiotensin I to angiotensin II, and the latter is responsible directly for vasoconstriction and indirectly, through aldosterone release, for sodium and water retention. It is now known that angiotensin-converting enzyme is not restricted to plasma or lung, but may be found in many organs of the body, including the vasculature (Rubin and Antonaccio, 1980). It has recently been established that inhibiting angiotensin-converting enzyme and subsequently decreasing angiotensin II formation is an effective method of lowering blood pressure in animals and humans. Captopril is a potent competitive inhibitor of angiotensin-converting enzyme and has recently been introduced clinically as an antihypertensive agent.

While originally thought to be useful only in those hypertensive patients with high plasma renin activities, captopril has been shown to be effective in most forms of hypertension (except primary aldosteronism) characterized by either high or normal renin activities. However, greater reductions in blood pressure by captopril have been reported in patients with high plasma renin activity (Atlas *et al.*, 1978). Administration of captopril to humans increases plasma renin activity by abolishing the negative feedback effect elicited by angiotensin II (Case *et al.*, 1978). As a direct consequence of inhibiting antiotensin-converting enzyme, captopril increases circulating angiotensin I and decreases angiotensin II. Since angiotensin II levels are lowered after captopril administration, aldosterone levels likewise fall (Atlas *et al.*, 1979).

The effectiveness of captopril in patients with normal plasma renin activities has led to the proposal that the renin–angiotensin system may be a contributing factor to most forms of hypertension (Rubin and Antonaccio, 1980). For this reason, it is clear that measurements of plasma renin activity are not necessary to predict the likelihood of a response to captopril. Still, the effectiveness of captopril in patients with normal renin activities has been an enigma. It is now known that the arterial wall of animals and humans contains all of the factors necessary to generate angiotensin II locally (Swales, 1979). As indicated earlier, the vasculature also contains angiotensin-converting enzyme, which is capable of converting angiotensin I into angiotensin II, the latter possibly responsible for local vasoconstriction leading to elevated blood pressure. It is possible that the antihypertensive efficacy of captopril in patients and animals with normal plasma renin activity may result from inhibition of angiotensin-converting enzyme, and subsequent blockade of angiotensin II formation, in the vasculature (Rubin and Antonaccio, 1980).

7.2.2 Congestive Heart Failure

Although originally developed for hypertension, the angiotensin-converting enzyme inhibitor, captopril, has proven to be a highly effective agent in the management of congestive heart failure. The primary effect of angiotensin-converting enzyme inhibitors in low output cardiac failure is derived principally from a decrease in total peripheral vascular resistance (afterload). Secondary to the reduction in afterload is a marked increase in cardiac output due primarily to an augmentation in stroke volume, since heart rate is not markedly affected. As expected, stroke-work index increases.

Angiotensin-converting enzyme inhibitors also produce vasodilation on the venous side, and this, combined with improved left ventricular ejection, causes a reduction in left ventricular filling pressure (preload). Thus, in patients with congestive heart failure, angiotensin-converting enzyme inhibitors produce a significant reduction in right atrial pressure, pulmonary artery pressure, and left ventricular end-diastolic pressure.

7.3 ANGIOTENSIN II RECEPTOR ANTAGONISTS

In view of the clinical usefulness of angiotensin-converting enzyme inhibitors, it would be expected that angiotensin II receptor antagonists may represent a novel approach to the treatment of hypertension and congestive heart failure. The angiotensin-converting enzyme inhibitors will inhibit many exopeptidases that cleave dipeptidyl residues from the carboxyl terminal end of peptides, and thus they possess many activities that may be undesirable. Thus, angiotensin II receptor antagonists should provide a more precise inhibition of the effects resulting from activation of the renin–angiotensin system.

All the active peptide angiotensin II antagonists are the result of modification of either the position four (tyrosine) or position eight (phenylalanine) side chains in angiotensin II. Many of these analogues have affinities that are equal to or greater than that of angiotensin II. The first such antagonist to be tested in humans was saralasin ([Sar^1,Ala^8]-angiotensin II) (Pals *et al.*,

1979). Other analogues with greater affinity for the angiotensin II receptor have been studied and found to have pharmacological profiles in humans similar to that of saralasin (Hota *et al.*, 1978; Sneddon, 1981). To date saralasin has only been studied in man by short-term parenteral use. The precise nature of the response to saralasin depends upon salt and renin levels. Following an initial pressor response (resulting from partial agonist activity), saralasin lowers blood pressure in patients with high plasma renin activity, but has little effect in patients with low or normal renin activity (Case *et al.*, 1976). As a result of the peptide nature of saralasin, it is not orally active and the half-life of the hypotensive activity is <10 min (Castillion and Fulton, 1979). Animal experiments suggest that chronic treatment would be more effective than acute administration (Streeton and Anderson, 1984). Furthermore, it has been postulated that removal of the partial agonist activity of saralasin would lead to a blood pressure decrease in patients with normal renin activity (Case *et al.*, 1976), who comprise approximately 55% of the hypertensive population (Laragh, 1980).

Thus, it would appear that a potent non-peptide, orally active angiotensin II receptor antagonist with no intrinsic activity would be useful in the treatment of hypertension. Furthermore, such a compound may also be effective in the treatment of congestive heart failure, possibly leading to a reduction in cardiovascular mortality, in a manner similar to that of the angiotensin-converting enzyme inhibitors (CONSENSUS Trial Study Group, 1987).

8 Purinergic Receptors

8.1 PURINES AND NEUROTRANSMISSION

ATP has been proposed to be the principal neurotransmitter in the non-adrenergic, non-cholinergic (NANC) intrinsic neurones supplying the smooth muscle of the gastrointestinal tract, urinary bladder and rabbit portal vein (Burnstock, 1972). In support of this role of ATP as a NANC neurotransmitter, it has been demonstrated that stimulation of NANC nerves in the taenia coli produces a release of ATP and smooth muscle contraction, both of which are Ca^{2+} dependent (Burnstock *et al.*, 1978). Furthermore, desensitization of the responses to ATP with α,β-methylene ATP also abolishes NANC transmission in the bladder (Kasokov and Burnstock, 1983).

In addition to its role as the primary NANC neurotransmitter in some tissues, ATP is also believed to be a co-transmitter, released and physio-logically active, at several sympathetic and parasympathetic neuroeffector junctions (Burnstock, 1982, 1983). For example, in the rat tail artery the slow depolarization produced by sympathetic nerve stimulation is blocked by the α-adrenoceptor antagonist, phentolamine, whereas the fast depolarizations are abolished by desensitization of the ATP receptors with α,β-methylene ATP (Burnstock *et al.*, 1984). Prejunctional purinergic receptors, activation of which inhibits neurotransmitter release, have also been identified on postganglionic sympathetic and parasympathetic neurones supplying both cardiovascular and non-cardiovascular effector organs (De Mey *et al.*, 1979; Moody and Burnstock, 1982). The norepinephrine and ATP co-released from sympathetic nerves have the potential for a significant degree of interaction in modulating the response via both pre- and post-junctional mechanisms (Burnstock, 1985). Thus, modulation of the metabolism or receptor sites or mechanisms of action of ATP can have profound effects on autonomic neuroeffector transmission.

8.2 PURINERGIC RECEPTOR SUBCLASSIFICATION

In 1978, Burnstock proposed the existence of two distinct types of purinergic receptor. It was proposed that P_1 receptors are more sensitive to adenosine and AMP than to ADP and ATP, and that methylxanthines such as caffeine, theophylline and isobutylmethylxanthine are competitive antagonists at this receptor at lower concentrations than that required for the inhibition of phosphodiesterase. Furthermore, activation of the P_1 receptor acts via an adenylate cyclase system. On the other hand, P_2 receptors are more sensitive to ADP and ATP than to AMP and adenosine, are not antagonized by methylxanthines and do not operate via an adenylate cyclase system, but may stimulate prostaglandin production. However, it was recognized that some actions of ATP and ADP may be mediated via P_1 receptors as a result of their enzymatic breakdown to AMP and adenosine.

In addition to the P_1- and P_2-receptors which are located on the cell surface, an intracellular P-site at which adenosine, 2-chloroadenosine and certain ribose modified analogues, e.g. 9-β-D-xylofuranosyladenosine, are agonists has also been identified (Londos and Wolf, 1977). The 5'- and N^6-substituted analogues of adenosine which are active at P_1 receptors are not agonists at the intracellular P-site (Daly, 1982). In addition, the P-site is insensitive to methylxanthines, but purine transport inhibitors can reduce the activity of P-site agonists by limiting access of the agonist to the intracellular site (Brown and Collis, 1982). Activation of the P-site produces an inhibition of adenylate cyclase (Londos and Wolff, 1977).

P_1-receptors have subsequently been divided into two types, A_1- and A_2-, on the basis of their effects on adenylate cyclase and by ligand binding

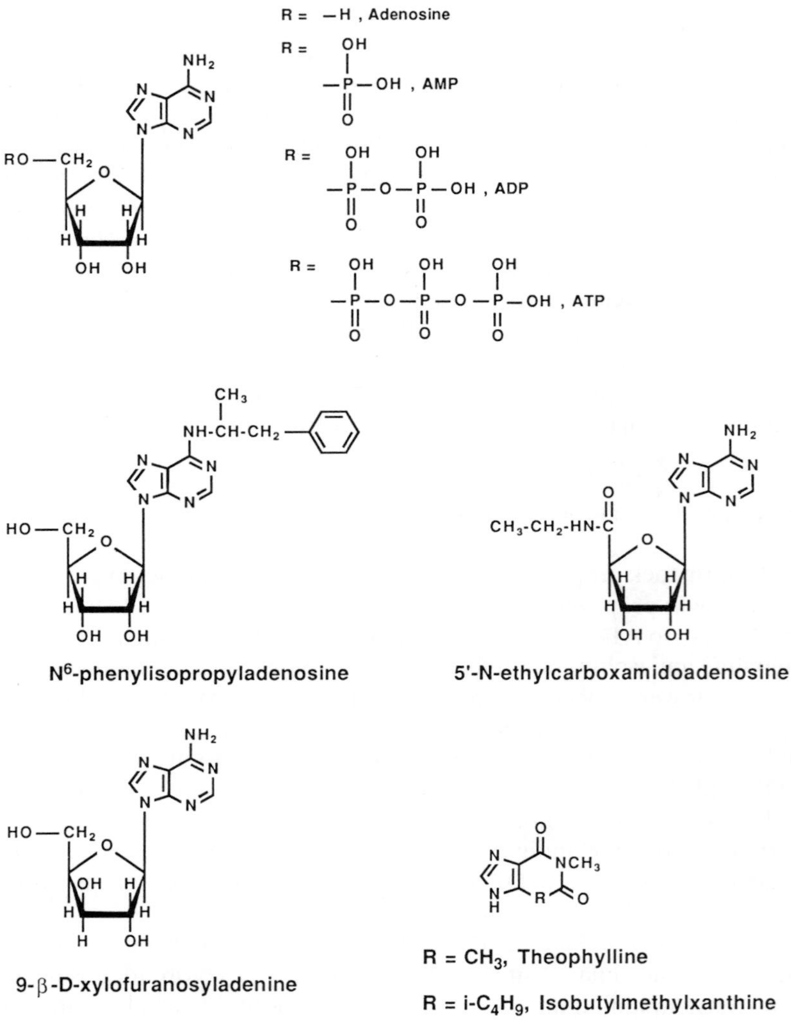

R = —H , Adenosine

R = $-\overset{\overset{\displaystyle OH}{|}}{\underset{\underset{\displaystyle O}{||}}{P}}-OH$, AMP

R = $-\overset{\overset{\displaystyle OH}{|}}{\underset{\underset{\displaystyle O}{||}}{P}}-O-\overset{\overset{\displaystyle OH}{|}}{\underset{\underset{\displaystyle O}{||}}{P}}-OH$, ADP

R = $-\overset{\overset{\displaystyle OH}{|}}{\underset{\underset{\displaystyle O}{||}}{P}}-O-\overset{\overset{\displaystyle OH}{|}}{\underset{\underset{\displaystyle O}{||}}{P}}-O-\overset{\overset{\displaystyle OH}{|}}{\underset{\underset{\displaystyle O}{||}}{P}}-OH$, ATP

N⁶-phenylisopropyladenosine

5'-N-ethylcarboxamidoadenosine

9-β-D-xylofuranosyladenine

R = CH₃, Theophylline

R = i-C₄H₉, Isobutylmethylxanthine

FIG. 4. Structures of selected agents with activity at purinergic receptors.

studies (Londos and Wolff, 1977; van Calker *et al.*, 1979). The A_1-receptor has a high affinity for adenosine and mediates an inhibition of adenylate cyclase, whereas the A_2-receptor has a lower affinity for adenosine and mediates a stimulation of adenylate cyclase. Although both P_1-receptor subtypes are antagonized by methylxanthines, certain adenosine analogues have a differential potency at the A_1- and A_2-receptors (Bruns *et al.*, 1980). For example, 5'-substituted adenosine analogues, e.g. 5'-N-ethylcarboxamidoadenosine, are about 50-fold more potent than N^6-substituted analogues, e.g. N^6-phenylisopropyladenosine, at the A_2-receptors, but there is little difference in potency between these classes of compounds at A_1-receptors (Bruns *et al.*, 1980). The A_1-receptor shows stereoselectivity with $R(-)N^6$-phenylisopropyladenosine being 50–100 times more potent than the $S(+)$-isomer, but the isomeric ratio at the A_2-receptor is only 5 (Bruns *et al.*, 1980). The structure of several of these agents acting on purinergic receptors is shown in Fig. 4.

More recently, it has been proposed that there may be more than one type of P_2-receptor. The P_2-receptor that mediates endothelium-dependent relaxation of the pig aorta appears to have structural requirements for agonists that are different in certain respects from those required by the P_2-receptors on the smooth muscle that mediate vasoconstriction (Burnstock and Kennedy, 1985). This subclassification of P_2-receptors has since been confirmed in canine vascular smooth muscle and endothelium with the receptor on the smooth muscle being termed P_{2x} and that on the endothelium being termed P_{2y} (Houston *et al.*, 1987).

8.3 PURINERGIC RECEPTORS IN THE CARDIOVASCULAR SYSTEM

8.3.1 Coronary Circulation

The coronary circulation contains purinergic receptors that mediate coronary artery vasodilation in response to purine nucleotides. Vasodilation produced by adenosine triphosphate (ATP) and adenosine in the coronary circulation has been studied extensively, largely because of the possible implications in coronary occlusion and the potential relevance to the treatment of angina (Berne, 1975; Burnstock, 1980). Smaller coronary vessels are more sensitive to adenosine than are larger vessels (Schnaar and Sparks, 1972).

ATP and adenosine diphosphate (ADP) are the most potent of the adenyl compounds that relax coronary vessels; adenosine monophosphate (AMP) and adenosine are from one-quarter to one-third as potent as ATP. Adenine, hyoxanthine, guanine, cytosine, and uracil are either inactive or of low potency. Uridine nucleotides may dilate (UTP, UDP) or constrict (UMP) coronary resistance vessels (Burnstock, 1980).

Stimulation of purinergic receptors may result in the influx Ca^{2+} (Herlihy *et al.*, 1976), possibly via elevation of intracellular cAMP after stimulation of adenylate cyclase (Herlihy *et al.*, 1976; Kukovetz *et al.*, 1978). As in cardiac muscle, the vasodilatory action of adenosine on coronary arteries is blocked by theophylline, aminophylline, and caffeine (Herlihy *et al.*, 1976), which is consistent with activation of the A_2 subtype of P_1-purinergic receptors (Herlihy *et al.*, 1976).

8.3.2 Cerebral Circulation

Adenosine may be an important metabolic factor in the autoregulation of cerebral blood flow, since increased cerebral adenosine levels are found during conditions such as ischaemia, hypotension, and hypoxia (Berne *et al.*, 1981). Adenosine dilates cerebral arteries both *in vitro* and *in situ*, with smaller pial vessels being more reactive than larger vessels. Furthermore, *in vivo* studies have demonstrated that adenosine can also increase cerebral blood flow (Winn *et al.*, 1981). The vasodilatory effects of adenosine and related nucleotides are mediated via P_1-purinergic receptors. In addition to its relaxant effects on precontracted vessels, ATP has been shown to constrict some cerebral vessels; this effect is mediated via P_2-purinergic receptors (Muramatsu *et al.*, 1984).

8.3.3 Splanchnic Circulation

In the canine intestinal circulation adenosine induces a dose-dependent vasodilation and an increase in oxygen consumption (Walus *et al.*, 1981). The adenosine antagonist, theophylline, attenuates this response. An adenosine analogue, 2-chloroadenosine, is six-fold more potent than the parent compound in enhancing intestinal blood flow, and this effect is also antagonized by theophylline (Walus *et al.*, 1981). Thus, adenosine and 2-chloroadenosine produce mesenteric vasodilation by acting at P_1-puriner-gic receptors in the intestinal vasculature (Walus *et al.*, 1981).

8.3.4 Myocardium

Purines produce negative inotropic and chronotropic effects in mammalian myocardium (Burnstock, 1980). In most species, ATP is approximately equipotent with adenosine as a myocardial depressant (Green and Stoner, 1950). However, in the guinea-pig atrium adenosine is more potent than ATP (Collis and Pettinger, 1982) suggesting that the purinergic receptor is of the P_1-subtype. Moreover, 2-chloroadenosine, a potent P_1-receptor agonist, is a more potent negative inotropic agent than adenosine

(Burnstock, 1978) and the negative inotropic responses produced by both adenosine and ATP are competitively antagonized by methylxanthines (Collis and Pettinger, 1982). Thus, the purinergic receptor in the myocardium is a P_1-receptor. L-N^6-phenylisopropyladenosine is greater than 100-fold more potent than the D-isomer in guinea-pig atrium and 5'-substituted adenosine analogues are approximately equipotent with N^6-substituted analogues (Collis, 1983). Moreover, ADP-ribosylation of the inhibitory G_i regulatory protein associated with adenylate cyclase abolishes the negative inotropic response to adenosine (Bohm et al., 1986). Taken together, these data show that the subtype of purinergic receptor in the myocardium is the A_1-subtype of the P_1-receptor.

8.3.5 Endothelium

ATP can produce a potent vasodilation that is dependent upon the integrity of the endothelium (De Mey and Vanhoutte, 1981a,b; Kennedy et al., 1985; Vanhoutte and Rimele, 1983). Although AMP and adenosine cause vasodilation mainly by acting directly on vascular smooth muscle, removal of the endothelium does attenuate the vasodilator response to adenosine in pig aorta (Gordon and Martin, 1983) and rat aorta and femoral artery (Konishi and Su, 1983). However, ATP and ADP are 120-fold more potent than AMP and adenosine at producing ^{86}Rb efflux from preloaded pig aortic endothelial cells (Gordon and Martin, 1983), indicating the P_2-nature of the response. As indicated above, the P_2-receptor on the endothelium may be different from that on the vascular smooth muscle (Burnstock and Kennedy, 1985).

8.3.6 Prejunctional Purinergic Receptors

ATP and adenosine produce an inhibition of norepinephrine release at the vascular neuroeffector junction, with both agents having approximately the same potency (De Mey et al., 1979). In addition, the neuroinhibitory response to both ATP and adenosine is antagonized by the P_1-receptor antagonist, theophylline (De Mey et al., 1979). Thus, the prejunctional inhibitory purinergic receptor located on sympathetic postganglionic neurones innervating the vasculature is of the P_1-subtype. In this case it is likely that ATP is rapidly metabolized to adenosine before acting on the P_1-receptors. Thus, at neuroeffector junctions at which ATP and norepinephrine are co-released, there may be a complex interaction of both transmitters with pre- and postjunctional receptors, all of which may be differentially modulated.

9 Vasopressin Receptors

9.1 VASOPRESSIN AND CARDIOVASCULAR REGULATION

9.1.1 Vasoconstrictor Actions of Vasopressin

It was originally believed that only high concentrations of vasopressin in excess of those found physiologically were capable of producing vaso-constriction. However, concentrations of vasopressin in the range commonly found in plasma (0.3 to 30 pg/ml) produced by slow infusion of vasopressin have been shown to produce vasoconstriction in conscious dogs leading to an increase in total peripheral resistance and a reduction in cardiac output (Montani et al., 1980). The vasoconstrictor activity of vaso-pressin is even more pronounced when autonomic reflexes are abolished (Cowley et al., 1983). Moreover, in humans suffering from Shy-Drager's syndrome, in which there is primary autonomic insufficiency, mean arterial pressure is elevated by infusion of arginine vasopressin sufficient to raise plasma levels from 5 to 20 pg/ml (Mohring et al., 1980). However, under conditions where baroreflexes are operating normally, such pressor responses may be masked. Further evidence for a physiological role of the vasoconstrictor activity of vasopressin comes from the observation that blockade of vascular vasopressin receptors with DDAVP produces a significant reduction in diastolic blood pressure in normal human volunteers (Derkx et al., 1983).

In addition to its direct vasoconstrictor activity, very low concentrations of vasopressin can potentiate the response to other vasoconstrictors, e.g. norepinephrine (Bartelstone and Nasmyth, 1965). This potentiation appears to be more pronounced in tissues from hypertensive animals and is such that a combination of subthreshold concentrations of vasopressin and norepin-ephrine can produce a significant vasoconstriction (Sueta et al., 1983). Thus, physiologically relevant concentrations of vasopressin can produce vaso-constriction directly and can potentiate the vasoconstriction produced by other vasoactive agents.

The vasoconstrictor response produced by vasopressin is associated with an increased production of inositol 1,3,4-trisphosphate and 1,2-diacylglycerol as a consequence of the receptor-mediated stimulation of phospholipase C-mediated breakdown of phosphatidyl inositol bisphos-phate (Aiyar et al., 1986). Furthermore, this increased phospholipid tur-nover is believed to be responsible for the mobilization of Ca^{2+} produced by vasopressin (Aiyar et al., 1986).

Vasopressin is also capable of producing vasodilation under certain conditions. Schwartz et al. (1985) have shown that in dogs treated with the

V_1-receptor antagonist, $d(CH_2)_5Tyr(Me)AVP$, exogenous administration of vasopressin produces a decrease in total peripheral resistance with an increase in cardiac output. These authors speculated on the existence of vasodilator vasopressin receptors in the peripheral vasculature, possibly of the V_2-subtype, although the effect of V_2-receptor blockade was not studied (see below for discussion of vasopressin receptor subtypes). *In vitro* studies have shown that low concentrations of vasopressin produce endothelium-dependent relaxation in the canine isolated basilar artery and circumflex coronary artery via the release of the endothelium-derived relaxing factor (EDRF) (Katusic *et al.*, 1984). However, vasopressin only produces contraction in the isolated femoral artery which is not affected by the removal of endothelium, suggesting that vasopressin-induced release of EDRF is vessel dependent (Katusic *et al.*, 1984). The endothelium-dependent vasodilation produced by vasopressin is blocked by the V_1-receptor antagonist, $d(CH_2)_5Tyr(Me)AVP$, demonstrating that the release of EDRF by vasopressin is mediated via V_1-receptors (Katusic *et al.*, 1984).

a. Vasopressin Analogues as Selective Vascular Vasopressin Receptor Agonists and Antagonists. Substitution of the amino acids of vasopressin at the 2-, 3- and 8-positions (tyrosine, phenylalanine and arginine) with phenylalanine, isoleucine and ornithine, respectively, produces only small reductions in vasopressor potency but produces a significant reduction in antidiuretic activity, leading to agonists with selectivity for the vascular vasopressin receptor (Manning and Sawyer, 1985). Thus, the receptors mediating the vasoconstrictor and antidiuretic activities of vasopressin can be differentiated and have been termed V_1- and V_2-, respectively (Michell *et al.*, 1979). Several analogues of vasopressin have been synthesized and been found to possess potent and selective antagonist activity at the vascular V_1-receptor. For example, $d(CH_2)_5DAVP$ and $d(CH_2)_5Tyr(Me)AVP$ are potent antagonists of the vasoconstrictor response to vasopressin, but are in fact weak antidiuretic V_2-receptor agonists (Manning and Sawyer, 1985).

9.1.2 Antidiuretic Actions of Vasopressin

Vasopressin is a potent antidiuretic which stimulates the reabsorption of free water in the renal collecting duct. Body fluid volume is maintained, at least in part, by physiological changes in vasopressin secretion from the posterior pituitary in response to changes in plasma osmolality via a negative feedback servo-control mechanism. In the syndrome of inappropriate secretion of antidiuretic hormone (SIADH), which can occur as the result of a wide variety of disorders (Zerbe *et al.*, 1980), plasma vasopressin levels are elevated leading to disorders of body fluid volume balance. Thus, vaso-pressin also exerts an indirect control over cardiovascular function by producing changes in cardiac output as a result of its effect on water excretion and hence body fluid and plasma volumes. Vasopressin is believed to increase the water permeability of the renal collecting duct via an interaction with V_2-receptors on the basolateral membrane of the epithelial cells (Bockaert *et al.*, 1973). Activation of these V_2-receptors increases adenylate cyclase activity, leading to an increase in intracellular levels of cAMP (Bockaert *et al.*, 1973) which in turn increases the water permeability of the apical membrane (Grantham and Burg, 1966), thus allowing water to move from the lumen of the collecting duct into the renal interstitium and subsequently into the circulation down an osmotic gradient.

a. Vasopressin Analogues as Selective Agonists and Antagonists of Renal Vasopressin Receptors. Several analogues of vasopressin have been developed which show remarkable agonist selectivity for the renal V_2-recep-tor. For example, dDAVP is approximately 3000-fold more potent as an agonist at V_2- *vis-à-vis* V_1-receptors and dVDAVP is a potent V_2-receptor agonist with V_1-receptor antagonist activity (Manning and Sawyer, 1985). In contrast to the V_1-receptors, there are no antagonists with marked selectivity for the V_2-receptor, although some compounds, e.g. $d(CH_2)_5[D-Ile^2,Ile^4]AVP$ and $d(CH_2)[D-Ile^2,Ala^4]AVP$, exhibit nearly a 40-fold selec-tivity for the V_2-receptor (Manning and Sawyer, 1985).

9.1.3 Modulation of Autonomic Reflexes

There is now much evidence to show that vasopressin can modulate the autonomic reflex control of the cardiovascular system via an action on the CNS. The enhancement of vasopressor responses to vasopressin in humans with Shy-Drager's syndrome and in dogs with abolition of autonomic reflexes or CNS ablation suggest a central enhancement of baroreflexes by vasopressin (Cowley *et al.*, 1983). Injection of vasopressin into the fourth cerebral ventricle produces a large bradycardia, whereas the same doses given into the lateral ventricles produce a much smaller effect (Varma *et al.*, 1969). However, it would appear that this effect is not due to direct activation of vagal outflow but rather is the result of an effect on the baroreflex pathway since sino-aortic denervation, which leaves the vagal efferent pathway intact but abolishes baroreflexes, has been shown to prevent vasopressin-induced bradycardia (Montani *et al.*, 1980). Further-more, vasopressin has been shown to enhance the baroreceptor reflex gain when carotid sinus pressure is below, but not above, its normal operating set

However, the precise site of action of vasopressin within the baroreflex loop is unknown, although it would appear that regions in the lower brain stem are involved (Cowley *et al.*, 1983). It is not known whether the arginine vasopressin-containing neurones that have been shown to project from the suprachiasmatic nucleus in the anterior hypothalamus to the nucleus tractus solitarus (Sofroniew and Weindl, 1978) have any role in the reflex control of the cardiovascular system.

9.2 PERIPHERAL VASOPRESSIN RECEPTORS

9.2.1 Coronary Circulation

Vasopressin is a potent direct coronary artery vasoconstrictor that acts on V_1 (vascular) vasopressin receptors. It has been demonstrated in the coronary circulation that exogenously administered vasopressin decreases coronary blood flow by increasing in coronary vascular resistance (Heyndrickx *et al.*, 1976). Additionally, endogenous release of vasopressin has been shown to promote an increase in coronary vascular resistance (Schmid *et al.*, 1974).

Vasopressin-induced increases in coronary resistance and the resulting reductions in coronary blood flow in humans have been implicated as causative factors in specific pathological states, such as myocardial ischaemic injury, myocardial infarction (Mills *et al.*, 1949), anginal pain (Slotnik and Teigland, 1951), ventricular arrhythmias, and sudden death (Mills *et al.*, 1949).

9.2.2 Cerebral Circulation

Recent studies have demonstrated that vasopressin exerts a powerful vaso-constrictor action on isolated human cerebral arteries by directly stimulating specific receptor sites for this neuropeptide (Lluch *et al.*, 1984). In certain pathological conditions in which vasopressin is released in large amounts, such as subarachinoid haemorrhage and hypertension, it is conceivable that vasopressin concentrations may occur sufficient to compromise cerebral blood flow.

9.3 CARDIOVASCULAR EFFECTS OF VASOPRESSIN ANTAGONISTS

9.3.1 Hypertension

Vasopressin may play a role in the maintenance of normal blood pressure (see above). It is also possible that vasopressin may be important in the control of blood pressure in hypertension. Plasma levels of vasopressin are elevated in experimental (Mohring *et al.*, 1979) and human hypertension (Preibisz *et al.*, 1983). However, it has been suggested that the elevated levels of vasopressin play no role in determining blood pressure in human malignant hypertension (Padfield *et al.*, 1981) or in stroke-prone spontaneously hypertensive rats (SHRSP) (Rascher *et al.*, 1981). On the other hand, studies on the effect of interfering with vasopressin function strongly suggest that vasopressin does indeed play a role in hypertension. In a study in rats, Mohring *et al.* (1979) found that antiserum to arginine vasopressin produced a large fall in blood pressure in conscious SHRSP in relation to their elevated plasma vasopressin levels, but produced only a small reduction in blood pressure in normotensive rats. Furthermore, Gavras *et al.* (1984) showed that the V_1-receptor antagonist, $d(CH_2)_5Tyr(Me)AVP$, lowered blood pressure in hypertensive patients with end-stage renal disease. These data strongly suggest that elevated plasma vasopressin levels contribute to the maintenance of blood pressure in hypertension and that this effect is mediated, at least in part, by V_1-receptors. In addition, it would appear that V_1-receptor antagonists may be useful in the treatment of hypertension. At the present time it is unknown whether activation of renal V_2-receptors which increase body fluid volume plays any role in the pathogenesis of hypertension. The potential use of V_2-receptor antagonists in hypertension is unknown.

9.3.2 Congestive Heart Failure

There is evidence to suggest that in some patients suffering from congestive heart failure plasma vasopression levels are elevated. However, it would appear that there is considerable variation in the levels of vasopressin within this group of patients. Preibisz *et al.* (1983) found that although total plasma vasopressin levels were not elevated in New York functional class III or IV heart failure patients, levels of free vasopressin in plasma not containing platelets was significantly, although not greatly, elevated; the levels of vasopressin associated with the platelets was significantly lower in these patients. Thus, free vasopressin levels (that which is available for interaction with the receptor) are probably elevated in congestive heart failure, but perhaps not to the level where they can play a major role in the etiology of the disease. This has been confirmed by Nicod *et al.* (1985), who studied the plasma vasopression levels and the effect of V_1-receptor blockade with $d(CH_2)_5Tyr(Me)AVP$ on haemodynamics in congestive heart failure. This group found that total plasma vasopressin levels were elevated in most patients, in accord with the study of Preibisz *et al.* (1983), and that V_1-receptor blockade had no effect on the abnormal haemodynamics characteristic of congestive heart failure. However, in one patient with very severe failure associated with a very low cardiac index and markedly elevated pulmonary and systemic resistances, plasma vasopressin was abnormally high (55 pg/ml). In this patient the V_1-receptor antagonist produced a marked improvement in systemic and pulmonary haemodynamics and a large increase in cardiac index (Nicod et al., 1985). It would appear, therefore, that vasopressin acting on V_1-receptors does not play a significant role in the etiology of congestive heart failure except in a few cases of very severe failure. Thus, the use of V_1-receptor antagonists in the therapy of congestive heart failure would appear to be limited.

The fluid retention, and hence reduced plasma osmolality, and hyponatremia observed in congestive heart failure does appear to be associated with elevations, albeit small, in plasma vasopressin levels (Szatalowicz et al., 1981). It is possible, therefore, that blockade of renal V_2-receptors may be beneficial in states of hyponatremia associated with heart failure. In this respect, non-selective V_1/V_2-receptor antagonists, e.g. SK&F 101926, may be more beneficial than selective V_2-receptor antagonists (of which there are very few good examples), since any benefit resulting from the additional V_1-receptor blockade in very sick patients may markedly improve the beneficial effects that result from a decrease in body fluid volume and a reduction in the degree of hyponatremia resulting from V_2-receptor blockade.

10 Concluding Remarks

Over the last few years there have been great advances in our knowledge of the pharmacology, biochemistry and molecular biology of receptors. Receptor research has progressed from the random testing of compounds for their ability to act either as an agonist or as an antagonist at a particular receptor or group of receptors to a multitude of approaches starting from the rational design of novel ligands based on quantitative structure–activity relationships to the cloning of the gene for the receptor leading to the determination of the primary amino acid sequence of the receptor protein. Using a variety of mathematical and physicochemical techniques it is now possible to estimate the overall shape and surface charge density of a molecule. Therefore, the rational approach to drug design now includes determining the receptor activity of a series of compounds and looking for a surface of the molecules that is important for receptor activity and then manipulating this surface in order to produce the optimal molecular surface for interaction with the receptor. At the present time, however, this knowledge can only be used to design more potent and specific compounds and to make general predictions about some of the physicochemical properties of the surface of the receptor with which the ligand interacts. With the increasing sophistication of molecular biology it is now possible to determine the primary amino acid structure and some of the important amino acids that are located at the ligand recognition site. In the future it is likely that the combination of receptor chemistry and ligand chemistry will give rise to a full picture of the receptor site on the protein and an insight into how an agonist actually activates the receptor to give rise to the primary biological response, i.e. a change in membrane channel activity or a change in membrane-associated enzyme activity.

Cardiovascular diseases are often accompanied by changes in receptor function or in the concentration of neurohumoral substances which may either underly or exacerbate the disease. This chapter has amply demonstrated that our knowledge of the role of a wide variety of receptors in many cardiovascular diseases is rapidly increasing. Combined with the newer improved methods by which to design ligands to interact with receptors, this knowledge should give rise to more specific agents with which to treat cardiovascular diseases.

References

Aiyar, N., Nambi, P., Stassen, F., and Crooke, S. T. (1986). *Life Sci.* **39**, 37–45

Alabaster, V. A., Keir, R. F., and Peters, C. J. (1985). *Naunyn-Schmiedeberg's Arch. Pharmacol.* **330**, 33–36.

Alkhadhi, K. A., Sabouni, M. H., and Lokhandwala, M. F. (1984). *Fed. Proc.* **43**, 1094.

Allan, G., and Levi, R. (1981). *J. Pharmacol. Exp. Ther.* **217**, 157–161.

Amann, F. W., Bolli, P., Kiowski, W., and Buhler, F. R. (1981). *Hypertension* **3** (Suppl. 1), I-119–123.

Amenta, F., Cavallotti, C., DeRossi, M., and Mione, M. C. (1984). *Eur. J. Pharmacol.* **97**, 105–109.

Anderson, R. J., Berl, T., McDonald, K. W., and Schrier, R. W. (1975). *J. Clin. Invest.* **56**, 420–426.

Angus, J. A., Cocks, T. M., and Satoh, K. (1986). *Fed. Proc.* **45**, 2355–2359.

Appleton, C., Martin, G. V., Algeo, S., Olajos, M., and Goldman, S. (1984). *Circulation* **70** (Suppl. II), 232.

Ariëns, E. J. (1981). *Trends Pharmacol. Sci.* **2**, 170–172.

Ariëns, E. J., and van Rossum, J. M. (1957). *Arch. Int. Pharmacodyn. Ther.* **110**, 275–299.

Arnold, S. B., Williams, R. L., Ports, T. A., Benet, L. Z., Parmley, W. W., and Chatterjee, K. (1979). *Ann. Intern. Med.* **91**, 345–349.

Atlas, S. A., Case, D. B., Sealey, J. E., Sullivan, P. M., and Laragh, J. H. (1978). *Circulation* **58** (Suppl. II), 143.

Atlas, S. A., Case, D. B., Sealey, J. E., Laragh, J. H., and McKinstry, D. N. (1979). *Hypertension* **1**, 274–280.

Auch-Schwelk, W., Starke, K., and Steppler, A. (1983). *Br. J. Pharmacol.* **78**, 543–551.

Awad, R., Payne, R., and Deth, R. C. (1983). *J. Pharmacol. Exp. Ther.* **227**, 60–67.

Awan, N. A., Miller, R. R., Maxwell, K. S., and Mason, D. J. (1977). *Clin. Pharmacol. Ther.* **22**, 79–84.

Awan, N. A., Miller, R. R., Miller, M. P., Vera, Z., Spect. K., and Mason, D. T. (1978). *Am. J. Med.* **65**, 146–154.

Ball, H. A., and Parratt, J. R. (1984). *Br. J. Pharmacol.* **83**, 379P.

Barajas, L., and Wang, P. (1979). *Anat. Res.* **195**, 525–534.

Barajas, L., Powers, K. and Wang, P. (1984). *Am. J. Physiol.* **247**, F50–F60.

Barrett, R. J., and Lokhandwala, M. F. (1982). *Fed. Proc.* **41**, 1587.

Barry, D. I., Paulson, O. B., Jarden, J. O., Juhler, M., Graham, D. I., and Strandgaard, S. (1984). *Am. J. Med.* **76**, 79–85.

Bartelstone, H. J., and Nasmyth, P. A. (1965). *Am. J. Physiol.* **208**, 754–762.

Bayliss, C., and Brenner, B. M. (1978). *Circ. Res.* **43**, 889–898.

Beckeringh, J. J., Thoolen, M. J. M. C., de Jonge, A., Wilffert, B., Timmermans, P. B. M. W. M., and van Zwieten, P. A. (1984). *J. Pharmacol. Exp. Ther.* **229**, 515–521.

Benfey, B. G., and Varma, D. R. (1962). *Int. J. Neuropharmacol.* **1**, 9–12.

Bentley, S. M., Drew, G. M., and Whiting, S. B. (1977). *Br. J. Pharmacol.* **61**, 116P–117P.

Berl, T., Raz, A., Wald, H., Horowitz, J., and Czackes, W. (1977). *Am. J. Physiol.* **232**, F529–F537.

Berne, R. M. (1958). *Circ. Res.* **6**, 644–655.

Berne, R. M. (1975). *In* "The Peripheral Circulation" (R. Zelis, ed.), pp. 117–129. Grune and Stratten Inc., New York.

Berne, R. M., Winn, H. R., and Rubio, R. (1981). *Prog. Cardiovasc. Diseases* **24**, 243–260.

Bertel, O., Burkart, R., and Buhler, F. R. (1981). *Am. Heart J.* **101**, 529–533.

Besse, J. C., and Furchgott, R. F. (1976). *J. Pharmacol. Exp. Ther.* **197**, 66–78.

Bevan, J. A. (1979). *Science* **204**, 635–637.

Bevan, J. A., Bevan, R. D., and Laher, I. (1985). *Clin. Sci.* **68** (Suppl. 10), 83s–85s.

Bhatnagar, R. K., Arneric, S. P., Cannon, J. G., Flynn, J., and Long, J. P. (1982). *Pharmacol. Biochem. Behav.* **17** (Suppl.), 11–19.

Blumberg, A. L., Hieble, J. P., McCafferty, J., Hahn, R. A., and Smith, J. (1982). *Fed. Proc.* **41**, 1345.

Blumberg, A. L., Wislon, J. W. and Hieble, J. P. (1985) *J. Cardiovasc. Pharmacol.* **7**, 723–732.

Blythe, W. B. (1983). *New Engl. J. Med.* **308**, 390–391.

Bockaert, J., Roy, C., Rajerison, R., and Jard, S. (1973). *J. Biol. Chem.* **248**, 5922–5931.

Bohm, M., Bruckner, R., Neumann, J., Schmitz, W., Scholz, H., and Starbatty, J. (1986). *Naunyn-Schmiedeberg's Arch. Pharmacol.* **332**, 403–405.

Bolli, P., Erne, P., Kiowski, W., Ji, B. H., Amann, F. W., and Buhler, F. R. (1983). *J. Hypertension* **1** (Suppl. 2), 257–259.

Bolli, P., Erne, P., Ji, B. H., Block, L. H., Kiowski, W., and Buhler, F. R. (1984). *J. Hypertension* **2** (Suppl. 3), 115–118.

Bousquet, P., and Guertzenstein, P. G. (1973). *Br. J. Pharmacol.* **49**, 573–579.

Breckenridge, A. (1982). *Br. Med. J.* **284**, 765–766.

Bristow, M. R. (1984). *New Engl. J. Med.* **311**, 850–851.

Broadley, K. J. (1970). *Br. J. Pharmacol.* **40**, 617–629.

Broadley, K. J. (1982). *J. Auton. Pharmacol.* **2**, 119–145.

Brodde, O. E. (1982). *Life Sci.* **31**, 289–306.

Brodde, O. E., Motomura, S., Endoh, M., and Schumann, H. J. (1978). *J. Mol. Cell. Cardiol.* **10**, 207–219.

Brotherton, A. F. A., and Hoak, J. C. (1982). *Proc. Natl. Acad. Sci. USA* **79**, 495–499.

Brown, C. M., and Collis, M. G. (1982). *Br. J. Pharmacol.* **76**, 381–387.

Brown, M. J. (1985). *In* "Proceedings of the 5th Vascular Neuroeffector Symposium" (J. A. Bevan, T. Godfraind, R. A. Maxwell, J. C. Stoclet and M. Worcel, eds), pp. 251–258. Elsevier, Amsterdam, New York and Oxford.

Brown, M. J., and Macquin, I. (1981). *Lancet* **ii**, 1079–1081.

Brown, M. J., Brown, D. C., and Murphy, M. B. (1983). *New. Engl. J. Med.* **309**, 1414–1419.

Brown, M. J., Struthers, A. D., Di Silvio, L., Yeo, T., Ghatei, M., and Burrin, J. M. (1985). *Clin. Sci.* **68** (Suppl. 10), 137s–139s.

Bruns, R. F., Daly, J. W., and Snyder, S. H. (1980). *Proc. Natl. Acad. Sci. USA* **77**, 5547–5551.

Buhler, F. R., Laragh, J. H., Baer, J. H., Vaughn, E. D., and Brunner, H. R. (1972). *New Engl. J. Med.* **287**, 1209–1214.

Burke, J. A., Levi, R., Guo, Z.-G., and Corey, E. J. (1982). *J. Pharmacol. Exp. Ther.* **221**, 235–241.

Burke, J. A., Levi, R., and Gleason, J. G. (1984). *J. Cardiovasc. Pharmacol.* **6**, 122–125.

Burnstock, G. (1972). *Pharmacol. Rev.* **24**, 509–581.

Burnstock, G. (1978). *In* "Cell Membrane Receptors for Drugs and Hormones: A Multidisciplinary Approach" (L. Bolis and R. W. Straub, eds), pp. 107–118. Raven Press, New York.

Burnstock, G. (1980). *Circ. Res.* **46**, I-175–182.

Burnstock, G. (1982). *In* "Co-transmission" (A. C. Cuello, ed.), pp. 151–163. Macmillan Press, London.

Burnstock, G. (1983). *In* "Dale's Principle and Communication Between Neurones" (N. N. Osborne, ed.), pp. 7–35. Pergamon Press, Oxford.

Burnstock, G. (1985). *In* "Adenosine: Receptors and Modulation of Cell Function" (V. Skefanovich, K. Rodolphi and P. Schubert, eds), pp. 3–14. IRL Press Ltd., Oxford.

Burnstock, G., and Kennedy, C. (1985). *Gen. Pharmacol.* **16**, 433–440.

Burnstock, G., Cocks, T., Kasakov, L., and Wong, H. (1978). *Eur. J. Pharmacol.* **49**, 145–149.

Burnstock, G., Griffith, S. G., and Sneddon, P. (1984). *J. Cardiovasc. Pharmacol.* **6**, S334–S353.

Calvette, J. A., Hayes, R. J., Oates, N. S., Sever, P. S., and Thom. S. (1984). *Br. J. Pharmacol.* **83**, 364P.

Cambridge, D., and Davey, M. J. (1980). *Br. J. Pharmacol.* **69**, 345P–346P.

Campbell, B. C., Elliot, H. L., Hamilton, C. A., and Reid, J. L. (1980). *Eur. J. Clin. Pharmacol.* **18**, 449–454.

Carey, R. M., Townsend, L. H., Rose, C. E., Kaiser, D. C., Lindsay, C. C., and Ragsdale, N. V. (1983). *Clin. Res.* **31**, 487A.

Case, D. B., Wallace, J. M., Keim, H. J., Sealey, J. E., and Laragh, J. M. (1976). *Am. J. Med.* **60**, 825–836.

Case, D. B., Atlas, S. A., Laragh, J. H., Sealey, J. E., Sullivan, P. A., and McKinstry, D. N. (1978). *Prog. Cardiovasc. Dis.* **21**, 195–206.

Castillion, A. W., and Fulton, R. W. (1979). *Kidney Int.* **15**, 59–519.

Cavero, I., Massingham, R., and Lefevre-Borg, F. (1982). *Life Sci.* **31**, 1059–1064.

Cavero, I., Shepperson, N., Lefevre-Borg, F., and Langer, S. Z. (1983). *Circ. Res.* (Suppl. 1), 69–76.

Chabardes, D., Montegut, M., Imbert-Teboul, M., and Morel, F. (1984). *Mol. Cellular Endocrinol.* **37**, 263–275.

Chierchia, S. (1982). *Acta Med. Scand.* (Suppl.) **660**, 49–56.

Chiu, A. T., McCall, D. E., Thoolen, M. J. M. C., and Timmermans, P. B. M. W. M. (1986). *J. Pharmacol. Exp. Ther.* **238**, 224–231.

Chou, C. C., and Kvietys, P. R. (1981). *In* "Measurements of Blood Flow: Application to the

Splanchnic Circulation" (D. N. Granger and G. B. Buckley, eds), Ch. 27, pp. 447–509. Williams and Wilkins, Baltimore.

Clifton, C. G., O'Neill, W. M., and Wallin, J. D. (1981). *Curr. Ther. Res.* **30**, 397–404.

Cocks, T. M., and Angus, J. A. (1983). *Nature* **305**, 626–630.

Cohen, M. L., Fuller, R. W., and Wiley, K. S. (1981). *J. Pharmacol. Exp. Ther.* **218**, 421–425.

Cohen, R. A., Shepherd, J. T., and Vanhoutte, P. M. (1983). *Science* **221**, 273–274.

Cohen, R. A., Shepherd, J. T., and Vanhoutte, P. M. (1984). *Fed. Proc.* **43**, 2862–2866.

Cohn, J. N., Levine, T. B., Olivari, M. T., Garberg, V., Lura, D., Francis, G. S., Simon, A. B., and Rector, T. (1984). *New Engl. J. Med.* **311**, 819–823.

Coleman, R. A., Humphrey, P. P. A., Kennedy, I., Levy, G. P., and Lumley, P. (1981). *Br. J. Pharmacol.* **73**, 773–778.

Collis, M. G. (1983). *Br. J. Pharmacol.* **78**, 207–212.

Collis, M. G., and Pettinger, S. J. (1982). *Eur. J. Pharmacol.* **81**, 521–529.

Collis, M. G., and Vanhoutte, P. M. (1977). *Circ. Res.* **41**, 759–767.

Connor, H. E., Drew, G. M., and Finch, L. (1982). *J. Pharm. Pharmacol.* **34**, 22–26.

CONSENSUS Trial Study Group (1987). *New Engl. J. Med.* **316**, 1429–1435.

Constantine, J. W., Gunnell, D., and Weeks, R. A. (1980). *Eur. J. Pharmacol.* **66**, 281–286.

Constantine, J. W., Level, W., and Archer, R. (1982). *Eur. J. Pharmacol.* **85**, 325–329.

Conway, E. L., Louis, W. J., and Jarrott, B. (1979). *Neuropharmacol.* **18**, 279–286.

Cook, J. A., Wise, W. C., and Halushka, P. V. (1980). *J. Clin. Invest.* **65**, 227–230.

Cooke, J. H., Johns, E. J., MacLeod, J. H., and Singer, B. (1972). *J. Physiol.* **226**, 15–36.

Cowley, A. W. Jr., Quillen, E. W. Jr., and Skelton, M. M. (1983). *Fed. Proc.* **42**, 3170–3176.

Cromwell, O., Walport, M. J., Morris, H., Taylor, G. W., Hodson, M. E., Batten, J., and Kay, A. B. (1981). *Lancet* **ii**, 164–165.

Cutter, W. E., Bier, D. M., Shah, S. D., and Cryer, P. E. (1980). *J. Clin. Invest.* **66**, 94–101.

Dahl, M., and Uotila, P. (1984). *Prostaglandins Leukotrienes and Medicine* **13**, 217–218.

Dahlen, S., Hansson, G., Hedqvist, P., Bjork, T., Granstrom, E., and Dahlen, B. (1983). *Proc. Natl. Acad. Sci.* **80**, 1712–1716.

Daly, J. W. (1982). *J. Med. Chem.* **25**, 197–207.

Davey, M. J. (1980). *J. Cardiovasc. Pharmacol.* **2** (Suppl. 3), S287–S301.

Davis, D. S., Wing, L. M. H., Reid, J. L., Neill, E., Tippett, P., and Dollery, C. T. (1977). *Clin. Pharmacol. Ther.* **21**, 593–600.

Dawes, P. M., and Vizi, E. S. (1973). *Br. J. Pharmacol.* **48**, 225–232.

Day, M. D., and Roach, A. G. (1974). *Br. J. Pharmacol.* **51**, 325–333.

Day, M. D., and Roach, A. G. (1976). *Br. J. Pharmacol.* **58**, 505–515.

De Mey, J., Burnstock, G., and Vanhoutte, P. M. (1979). *Eur. J. Pharmacol.* **55**, 401–405.

De Mey, J., and Vanhoutte, P. M. (1981a). *Circ. Res.* **48**, 875–884.

De Mey, J. G., and Vanhoutte, P. M. (1981b). *J. Physiol.* **316**, 346–355.

de Jonge, A., Timmermans, P. B. M. W. M., and van Zwieten, P. A. (1981). *Naunyn-Schmiedeberg's Arch Pharmacol.* **317**, 8–12.

de Jonge, A., van den Berg, G., Qian, J. Q., Wilffert, B., Thoolen, M. J. M. C., and Timmermans, P. B. M. W. M. (1986). *J. Pharmacol. Exp. Ther.* **236**, 500–504.

Derkx, F. H., Man in't Veld, A. J., Jones, R., Reid, J. L., and Schealkamp, M. A. D. H. (1983). *J. Hypertension* **1** (Suppl. 2), 58–61.

DiBona, G. F. (1982). *Rev. Physiol. Biochem. Pharmacol.* **94**, 75–181.

Docherty, J. R. (1983a). *Br. J. Pharmacol.* **78**, 655–657.

Docherty, J. R. (1983b). *Br. J. Pharmacol.* **80**, 510P.

Docherty, J. R., and Hyland, L. (1984). *Br. J. Pharmacol.* **83**, 362P.

Docherty, J. R., and Hyland, L. (1985). *Br. J. Pharmacol.* **86**, 335–339.

Docherty, J. R., MacDonald, A., and McGrath, J. C. (1979). *Br. J. Pharmacol.* **67**, 421P–422P.

Dollery, C. T., and Reid, J. L. (1973). *Br. J. Pharmacol.* **47**, 206–216.

Dorward, P. K., and Korner, P. I. (1978). *Eur. J. Pharmacol.* **52**, 61–71.

Dousa, T. P., Shah, S. V., and Abboud, H. E. (1980). *Adv. Cyclic Nuc. Res.* **12**, 285–299.

Doxey, J. C., and Roach, A. G. (1980). *J. Auton. Pharmacol.* **1**, 73–99.

Drazen, J. M., Austen, K. F., Lewis, D. A., Clark, D. A., Goto, G., Marfat, A., and Corey, E. J. (1980). *Proc. Natl. Acad. Sci.* **77**, 4354–4358.

Drew, G. M. (1976). *Eur. J. Pharmacol.* **36**, 313–320.

Drew, G. M. (1978). *Br. J. Pharmacol.* **64**, 293–300.

Drew, G. M., and Whiting, S. B. (1979). *Br. J. Pharmacol.* **67**, 207–215.

Duckles, S. P. (1980). *Br. J. Pharmacol.* **69**, 193–199.

Duckles, S. P., Bevan, R. D., and Bevan, J. A. (1976). *Stroke* **7**, 174–178.

Dunn, M. J. (1983). *In* "Contemporary Nephrology" (S. Klahr and S. G. Massry, eds), Vol. 2, pp. 145–193. Plenum, New York.

Edvinsson, L., Hardebo, J. E., McCulloch, J., and Owman, C. (1978). *Acta Physiol. Scand.* **104**, 349–359.

Edvinsson, L., Emson, P., McCulloch, J., Takemoko, K., and Uddman, R. (1983). *Neurosci. Lett.* **43**, 79–84.

Edvinsson, L., Birath, E., Uddman, R., Lee, J. F., Duverger, D., MacKenzie, E. T., and Scatton, B. (1984). *Acta Physiol. Scand.* **121**, 291–299.

Edwards, R. M. (1983). *Am. J. Physiol.* **244**, F526–F534.

Edwards, R. M. (1985). *Am. J. Physiol.* **248**, F183–F189.

Egleme, C., Godfraind, T., and Miller, R. C. (1984). *Br. J. Pharmacol.* **81**, 16–18.

Elliott, H. L., and Reid, J. L. (1983). *Clin. Sci.* **65**, 237–241.

Elsner, D., Saeed, M., Sommer, O., Holtz, J., and Bassenge, E. (1984). *Hypertension* **6**, 915–925.

Engberg, G., Elam, M., and Svensson, T. H. (1982). *Life Sci.* **30**, 235–243.

Farsang, C., Varga, K., Vajda, L., Alfoldi, S., and Kaposci, J. (1984). *Clin. Pharmacol. Ther.* **36**, 588–594.

Feigl, E. O. (1967). *Circ. Res.* **20**, 262–270.

Feigl, E. O. (1975). *Circ. Res.* **37**, 88–95.

Felder, R. A., Blecher, M., Calcagno, P. L., and Jose, P. A. (1984a). *Am. J. Physiol.* **247**, F499–F505.

Felder, R. A., Blecher, M., Eisner, G. M., and Jose, P. A. (1984b). *Am. J. Physiol.* **246**, F557–F568.

Fennell, W. H., Taylor, A. A., Young, J. B., Brandon, T. A., Ginos, J. Z., Goldberg, L. I., and Mitchell, J. R. (1983). *Circulation* **67**, 829–836.

Flavahan, N. A., and Vanhoutte, P. M. (1986a). *J. Pharmacol. Exp. Ther.* **238**, 131–138.

Flavahan, N. A., and Vanhoutte, P. M. (1986b). *J. Pharmacol. Exp. Ther.* **238**, 139–147.

Flavahan, N. A., Rimele, T. J., Cooke, J. P., and Vanhoutte, P. M. (1984). *J. Pharmacol. Exp. Ther.* **230**, 699–705.

Forster, C., Drew, G. M., Hilditch, A., and Whalley, E. T. (1983). *Eur. J. Pharmacol.* **87**, 227–235.

Fowler, P. J., Grous, M., Price, W., and Matthews, W. D. (1984). *J. Pharmacol. Exp. Ther.* **229**, 712–718.

Friedman, P. L., Brown, E. J. Jr., Gunther, S., Alexander, R. W., Barry, W. H., Mudge, G. H., and Grossman, W. (1978a). *New Engl. J. Med.* **305**, 1171–1175.

Friedman, L. W., Fitzpatrick, T. M., Bloom, M. F., Ramwell, P. W., Rose, J. C., and Kok, P. A. (1978b). *Circ. Res.* **44**, 748–751.

Frisk-Holmberg, M., Paalzow, L., and Wibell, L. (1984). *Eur. J. Clin. Pharmacol.* **26**, 309–313.

Fu, L. H. W., and Toda, N. (1983). *Jap. J. Pharmacol.* **33**, 473–482.

Furchgott, R. F. (1983). *Circ. Res.* **53**, 557–573.

Furchgott, R. F., and Zawadzki, J. V. (1980). *Nature* **288**, 373–376, 1980.

Furster, C., and Whalley, E. T. (1981). *Br. J. Pharmacol.* **74**, 944.

Gaal, G., Kattus, A. A., Kolin, A., and Ross, G. (1967). *Br. J. Pharmacol.* **26**, 713–722.

Gavras, J., Ribeiro, A. B., Kohlman, O., Saragoca, M., Mulinari, R. A., Ramos, O., and Gavras, I. (1984). *Hypertension* **6** (Suppl. 1), 156–160.

Gellai, M., and Ruffolo, R. R. Jr. (1987). *J. Pharmacol. Exp. Ther.* **240**, 723–728.

Gerold, M., and Haeusler, G. (1983). *Naunyn-Schmiedeberg's Arch. Pharmacol.* **322**, 29–33.

Gerrard, J. M. (1985). *In* "Prostaglandins and Leukotrienes: Blood and Vascular Cell Function", pp. 77–106. Marcel Dekker, New York.

Giles, T. D., Thomas, M. G., Sander, G. E., and Quiroz, A. C. (1985). *J. Cardiovasc. Pharmacol.* **7**, (Suppl. 8), S51–S55.

Gillis, R. A., Gatti, P. J., and Quest, J. A. (1985). *J. Cardiovasc. Pharmacol.* **7** (Suppl. 8), S38–S44.

Glomstein, A., Kauge, A., Oye, I., and Sinclair, D. (1967). *Acta Physiol. Scand.* **69**, 102–110.

Glusa, E., and Markwardt, F. (1983). *Naunyn-Schmiedeberg's Arch Pharmacol.* **323**, 101–105.

Goetzel, E. J., Payan, D. G., and Goldman, D. W. (1984). *J. Clin. Immun.* **4**, 79–84.

Goldberg, L. I., Sonneville, P. F., and McNay, J. L. (1968). *J. Pharmacol. Exp. Ther.* **163**, 188–197.

Goldberg, L. I., Hsieh, Y. Y., and Resnekov, L. (1977). *Prog. Cardiovasc. Dis.* **19**, 327–340.

Goldberg, L. I., Volkman, P. H., and Kohli, J. D. (1978). *Ann. Rev. Pharmacol. Toxicol.* **18**, 57–79.

Goldberg, M. R., and Robertson, D. (1984). *Hypertension* **6**, 551–556.

Goldstein, J. A. (1983). *Biol. Psychiatry* **18**, 1339–1340.

Gordon, J. L., and Martin, W. (1983). *Br. J. Pharmacol.* **79**, 531–541.

Göthert, M., Schlicker, E., Hentrich, F., Rohm, N., and Zerkowski, H.-R. (1984). *Eur. J. Pharm.* **102**, 261–267.

Govier, W. C. (1967). *Life Sci.* **6**, 1361–1365.

Granger, D. N., Richardson, P. D. I., Kvietys, P. R., and Mortillaro, N. A. (1980). *Gastroenterology* **78**, 837–863.

Grantham, J. J., and Burg, M. B. (1966). *Am. J. Physiol.* **211**, 255–259.

Green, H. N., and Stoner, H. B. (1950). "Biological Actions of the Adenine Nucleotides". Lewis, London.

Green, M. G., and Pettinger, S. J. (1982). *Eur. J. Pharmacol.* **81**, 521–529.

Greengard, P., and Kebabian J. W. (1974). *Fed. Proc.* **33**, 1059–1067.

Greenwald, J. E., Bianchine, J. R., and Wong, L. K. (1979). *Nature* **281**, 588–589.

Greenway, C. V., and Innes, I. R. (1981). *J. Cardiovasc. Pharmacol.* **3**, 1321–1331.

Grega, G. J., Barrett, R. J., Adamski, S. W., and Lokhandwala, M. F. (1984). *J. Pharmacol. Exp. Ther.* **229**, 756–762.

Griffith, S. G., Lincoln, J., and Burnstock, G. (1982). *Brain Res.* **247**, 388–392.

Gross, G. J., and Feigl, E. O. (1975). *Am. J. Physiol.* **228**, 1909–1913.

Gross, G. J., and Urquilla, P. R. (1982). *In* "Modern Pharmacology" (C. R. Craig and R. E. Stitzel, eds), pp. 283–294. Little, Brown and Co., Boston.

Gruetter, C. A., Ignaro, L. J., Hyman, A. L., and Kadowitz, P. J. (1981). *Can. J. Pharmacol.* **59**, 157–162.

Gryglewski, R. J., Korbut, R., Ogetkiewicz, A., Splawinski, J., Wojtaszek, B., and Swies, J. (1978). *Naunyn-Schmiedeberg's Arch. Pharmacol.* **304**, 45–50.

Gunnar Wallin, B., and Frisk-Holmberg, M. (1981). *Hypertension* **3**, 340–346.

Haeusler, G. (1974). *Naunyn-Schmiedeberg's Arch. Pharmacol.* **286**, 97–111.

Hall, J. E., Guyton, A. C., Jackson, T. E., Coleman, T. G., Lohmeier, T. E., and Trippodo, N. C. (1977). *Am. J. Physiol.* **233**, F366–F372.

Ham, E. A., Egan, R. W., Soderman, D. D., Gale, P. H., and Keuhl, F. A. (1979). *J. Biol. Chem.* **254**, 2191–2194.

Hamberg, M., and Samuelsson, B. (1974). *Proc. Natl. Acad. Sci.* **71**, 3400–3404.

Hamed, A. T., Jandhyala, B. S., Ginos, J. Z., and Lokhandwala, M. F. (1981). *Eur. J. Pharmacol.* **74**, 83.

Hamilton, C. A., and Reid, J. L. (1982). *Cardiovasc. Res.* **16**, 11–15.

Hamilton, C. A., Reid, J. L., and Sumner, D. J. (1983). *J. Cardiovasc. Pharmacol.* **5**, 868–873.

Hamilton, F. M., and Feigl, E. (1976). *Am. J. Physiol.* **230**, 1569–1576.

Hammarstrom, S. (1983). *Ann. Rev. Biochem.* **52**, 355–377.

Hannah, J. A. M., Hamilton, C. A., and Reid, J. L. (1983). *Naunyn-Schmiedeberg's Arch. Pharmacol.* **322**, 221–227.

Hansson, L. (1983). *Br. J. Clin. Pharmacol.* **15**, 485S–489S.

Hansson, L., Hunyor, S. N., Julius, S., and Hoobler, S. W. (1973). *Am. Heart J.* **85**, 605–610.

Harvey, J. N., Worth, D. P., Brown, J. R., and Lee, M. R. (1986). *Br. J. Clin. Pharmacol.* **21**, 53–62.

Hashimoto, K., Shigel, T., Imai, S., Saito, Yo., Yago, N., Uei, I., and Clark, R. E. (1960). *Am. J. Physiol.* **198**, 965–970.

Hattori, Y., and Levi, R. (1984). *J. Pharmacol. Exp. Ther.* **230**, 646–651.

Haylor, J., and Lote, C. J. (1980). *J. Physiol.* **298**, 371–381.

Hellstrom, H. R. (1971). *Cardiovasc. Res.* **5**, 371–375.

Henriksson, P., Edhag, O., and Wennmalm, A. (1985). *In* "Prostacyclin, Clinical Trials" (R. Gryglewski, ed.), pp. 31–42. Raven Press, New York.

Herlihy, J. T., Bockman, E. L., Berne, R. M., and Rubio, R. (1976). *Am. J. Physiol.* **230**, 1239–1243.

Hesse, I. F. A., and Johns, E. J. (1984). *J. Autonom. Pharmacol.* **4**, 145–152.

Heusch, G., and Deussen, A. (1983). *Circ. Res.* **53**, 8–15.

Heusch, G., Deussen, A., Schipke, J., and Thamer, V. (1984). *J. Cardiovasc. Pharmacol.* **6**, 961–968.

Heyndrickx, G. R., Boettcher, D. H., and Vatner, S. F. (1976). *Am. J. Physiol.* **231**, 1579–1587.

Hicks, P. E., and Waldron, C. (1982). *Br. J. Pharmacol.* **75**, 152P.

Hieble, J. P., and Pendleton, R. G. (1979). *Naunyn-Schmiedeberg's Arch. Pharmacol.* **309**, 217–224.

Hieble, J. P., and Woodward, D. F. (1984). *Naunyn-Schmiedeberg's Arch. Pharmacol.* **328**, 44–50.

Hieble, J. P., Roesler, J. M., Fowler, P. J., Matthews, W. D., and DeMarinis, R. M. (1985). *In* "Proceedings of the 5th Vascular Neuroeffector Symposium" (J. A. Bevan, T. Godfraind, R. A. Maxwell, J. C. Stoclet and M. Worcel, eds), pp. 159–164. Elsevier, Amsterdam, New York and Oxford.

Hieble, J. P., DeMarinis, R. M., Matthews, W. D., and Fowler, P. J. (1986). *J. Pharm. Exp. Ther.* **236**, 90–96.

Hiley, C. R., and Thomas, G. R. (1987). *Br. J. Pharmacol.* **90**, 61–70.

Hoffman, B. B., and Lefkowitz, R. J. (1980). *Ann. Rev. Pharmacol. Toxicol.* **20**, 581–608.

Holtz, J., Saeed, M., Sommer, O., and Bassenge, E. (1982). *Eur. J. Pharmacol.* **82**, 199–202.

Hopkins, N. K., and Gorman, R. R. (1981). *J. Clin. Invest.* **67**, 540–546.

Horn, P. T., Kohli, J. D., and Goldberg, L. I. (1981). *Fed. Proc.* **40**, 291.

Horn, P. T., Kohli, J. D., Listinsky, J. J., and Goldberg, L. I. (1982). *Naunyn-Schmiedeberg's Arch. Pharmacol.* **318**, 166–172.

Hoshida, S., Ohmori, M., Kuzuya, T., Tada, M., Tanaka, T., Fukui, S., and Minamino, T. (1983). *Jap. Circ. J.* **47**, 1026.

Houston, D. A., Burnstock, G., and Vanhoutte, P. M. (1987). *J. Pharmacol. Exp. Ther.* **241**, 501–506.

Hota, T., Oginara, T., Mikami, M., Nakamura, M., Maruyama, A., Mandai, T., and Kumanara, Y. (1978). *Life Sci.* **22**, 1955–1962.

Humphrey, P. P. A., and Lumley, P. (1984). *Br. J. Pharmacol.* **83**, 378.

Humphrey, P. P. A., Feniuk, W., and Watts, A. D. (1982). *J. Pharm. Pharmacol.* **34**, 541.

Hyman, A. L., Nandiwada, P., Knight, D. S., and Kadowitz, P. J. (1981). *Circ. Res.* **48**, 407–415.

Hyman, A. L., and Kadowitz, P. J. (1985). *Am. J. Physiol.* **249**, H891–H898.

Hyman, A. L., Lippton, H. L., and Kadowitz, P. J. (1985). *J. Cardiovasc. Pharmacol.* **7**, S80–S95.

Immink, W. F. G. A., Beijer, H. J. M., and Charbon, G. A. (1976). *Pfluegers Arch.* **365**, 107–118,

Insel, P. A., and Snavely, M. D. (1981). *Ann. Rev. Physiol.* **43**, 625.

Ito, T., and Chiba, S. (1985). *J. Pharmacol. Exp. Ther.* **234**, 698–702.

Ito, T., Sikano, M., Chen, L. S., Hitoshi, K., Kazumasa, I., Okumura, K., Ban, M., Ogawa, K., and Satake, T. (1983). *Jap. Circ. J.* **47**, 896.

Iversen, L. L. (1977). *J. Neurochem.* **29**, 5–12.

Jain, A. K., Hiremath, A., Michael, R., Ryan, J. R., and McMahon, F. G. (1985). *Clin. Pharmacol. Ther.* **37**, 271–276.

Jarrott, B., Summers, R. J., Culvenor, A. J., and Louis, W. J. (1980). *Cir. Res.* **46** (Suppl. I), I-15–20.

Jarrott, B., Lewis, S., Conway, E. L., Summers, R., and Louis, W. J. (1984). *Clin. Exp. Hyperten.* **A6**, 387–400.

Jauernig, R. A., Moulds, R. F. W., and Shaw, J. (1978). *Arch. Int. Pharmacodyn.* **231**, 81–89.

Jewitt, D., Mitchell, A., Birkhead, J., and Dollery, C. (1974). *Lancet* **ii**, 363–367.

Jie, K., van Brummelen, P., Vermey, P., Timmermans, P. B. M. W. M., and van Zwieten, P. A. (1986). *J. Cardiovasc. Pharmacol.* **8**, 190–196.

Jim, K., Hassid, A., Sun, F., and Dunn, M. J. (1982). *J. Biol. Chem.* **257**, 10294–10299.

Jim, K. F., and Matthews, W. D. (1985). *J. Pharmacol. Exp. Ther.* **234**, 161–165.

Kadowitz, P. J., Lippton, H. L., McNamara, D. B., Wolin, M. S., and Hyman, A. L. (1984). *In* "Cardiovascular Pharmacology" (M. Antonaccio, ed.), pp. 453–474. Raven Press, New York.

Kalkman, H. O., Boddeke, W. G. M., Doods, H. N., Timmermans, P. B. M. W. M., and van Zwieten, P. A. (1983). *Eur. J. Pharmacol.* **91**, 155–156.

Kalkman, H. O., Thoolen, M. J. M. C., Timmermans, P. B. M. W. M., and Van Zwieten, P. A. (1984). *J. Pharm. Pharmacol.* **36**, 265–268.

Kalkman, H. O., Timmermans, P. B. M. W. M., and Van Zwieten, P. A. (1982). *J. Pharmacol. Exp. Ther.* **222**, 227–231.

Kaneda, Y., and Bello-Reuss, E. (1983). *Mineral Electrolyte Metab.* **9**, 147–150.

Kasokov, L., and Burnstock, G. (1983). *Eur. J. Pharmacol.* **86**, 291–294.

Katusic, S. Z., Shepherd, J. T., and Vanhoutte, P. M. (1984). *Circ. Res.* **55**, 575–579.

Kebabian, J. W., and Greengard, P. (1971). *Science* **174**, 1346–1349.

Keeton, T. K., and Campbell, W. B. (1980). *Pharmacol. Rev.* **32**, 81–227.

Kennedy, C., Delbro, D., and Burnstock, G. (1985). *Eur. J. Pharmacol.* **107**, 161–168.

Kho, T. L., Schalekamp, M. A. D. H., Zaal, G. A., Wester, A., and Birkenhager, W. H. (1975). *Arch. Int. Pharmacodyn.* **217**, 162–169.

Kilbom, A., and Wennmalm, A. (1976). *J. Physiol.* **257**, 109–121.

Kinter, L. B., Mann, W. A., and Naselsky, D. (1985). *Fed. Proc.* **44**(4), 1014.

Kobayashi, H., Maoret, M., Ferrante, M., Spano, P., and Trabucchi, M. (1981). *Brain Res.* **220**, 194–198.

Kobinger, W. (1978). *Rev. Physiol. Biochem. Pharmacol.* **81**, 39–100.

Kobinger, W., and Pichler, L. (1976). *Eur. J. Pharmacol.* **40**, 311–320.

Kobinger, W., and Pichler, L. (1981). *Eur. J. Pharmacol.* **76**, 101–105.

Kobinger, W., and Pichler, L. (1982). *Eur. J. Pharmacol.* **82**, 203–206.

Kobinger, W., Lillie, C., and Pichler, L. (1980). *Circ. Res.* **46**, I-21–25.

Koike, H., Ito, K., Miyamoto, M., and Nishino, H. (1980). *Hypertension* **2**, 299–303.

Konieczkowski, M., Dunn, M. J., and Hassid, A. (1982). *Fed. Proc.* **41**, 1543.

Konishi, M., and Su, C. (1983). *Hypertension* **5**, 881–886.

Kopia, G. A., Kopaciewicz, L. J., and Ruffolo, R. R. Jr. (1986). *J. Pharmacol. Exp. Ther.* **239**, 641–647.

Korner, P. I. (1976). *In* "Regulation of Blood Pressure by the Central Nervous System" (G. Onesti, M. Fernandes and K. E. Kim, eds), pp. 412. Grune and Stratton, New York.

Korner, P. I., and Angus, J. A. (1981). *Pharmacol. Ther.* **13**, 321–356.

Kreisberg, J. I. (1983). *Fed. Proc.* **42**, 3053.

Krothapalli, R. K., Duffy, B., Senekjian, H., and Suki, W. (1983). *J. Clin. Invest.* **72**, 287–294.

Kukovetz, W. R., Poch, G., Holzmann, S., Wurm, A., and Rinner, I. (1978). *Adv. Cyclic Nucleotide Res.* **9**, 397–409.

Kuzuya, T., Tada, M., Hoshida, S., Ohmori, M., Matsuda, H., Inoue, M., Abe, H., and Minamino, T. (1983). *Circulation* **68**, 111–398.

Langer, S. Z. (1977). *Br. J. Pharmacol.* **60**, 481–497.

Langer, S. Z., and Hicks, P. E. (1984). *J. Cardiovasc. Pharmacol.* **6** (Suppl. 4), S547–S558.

Langer, S. Z., and Shepperson, N. B. (1981). *Br. J. Pharmacol.* **74**, 942.

Langer, S. Z., and Shepperson, N. B. (1982a). *J. Cardiovasc. Pharmacol.* **4**, S8–S13.

Langer, S. Z., and Shepperson, N. B. (1982b). *Trends Pharmacol. Sci.* **3**, 440–444.

Langer, S. Z., Shepperson, N. B., and Massingham, R. (1981). *Hypertension* **3** (Suppl. 1), I-112–I-118.

Langer, S. Z., Duval, N., and Massingham, R. (1985). *J. Cardiovasc. Pharmacol.* **6** (Suppl. 4), S547–S558.

Lapetina, E. G. (1982). *Trends Pharmacol. Sci.* **3**, 115.

Lapetina, E. G., Schmitges, C. J., Chandrabose, K., and Cuatrecasas, P. (1977). *Biochem. Biophys. Res. Commun.* **76**, 828–835.

Laragh, J. H. (1980). *In* "Captopril and Hypertension" (D. B. Case, E. H. Sonnenblick and J. H. Laragh, eds), pp. 173–184. Plenum Medical Books Co., New York.

Larrue, J., Dorian, B., Daret, D., Demond-Henri, J., and Bricaud, H. (1984). *In* "Advances in Cyclic Nucleotide Research" (P. Greengard, ed.), Vol. 17, pp. 585–593. Raven Press, New York.

Lebet, B., and Tosaka, T. (1970). *Proc. Natl. Acad. Sci.* **67**, 667–673.

Lefer, A. M., Ogletree, M. L., Smith, J. B., Silver, M. J., Nicolaou, K. C., Barnette, W. E., and Gasic, G. P. (1978). *Science* **200**, 52–54.

Lefer, A. M., Okamatsu, S., Smith, E. F., and Smith, J. B. (1981a). *Thrombosis Res.* **23**, 265–273.

Lefer, A. M., Smith, J. B., and Nicolaou, K. C. (1981b). *In* "Cardiovascular Physiology: Microcirculation and capillary exchange. Advances in Physiological Science 7" (J. Hamar and L. Szabo, eds), pp. 91–98. Pergamon Press, London.

Leier, C. V., and Unverferth, D. V. (1983). *Ann. Intern. Med.* **99**, 490–496.

Letts, L. G., and Piper, P. J. (1982). *Br. J. Pharmacol.* **76**, 169–176.

Levine, T. B., Francis, G. S., and Goldsmith, S. R. (1982). *Am. J. Cardiol.* **49**, 1659–1666.

Levitt, B., and Hieble, J. P. (1985). *Fed. Proc.* **44**, 1465.

Lewis, P. J., and Haeusler, G. (1975). *Nature* **256**, 440.

Lewis, S. J., Fennessy, M. R., and Taylor, D. A. (1981). *Clin. Exp. Pharmacol. Physiol.* **8**, 489–495.

Lewy, R. I., Wiener, L., Smith, J. B., Walensky, P., Silver, M. J., and Saia, J. (1980a). *Clin. Cardiol.* **2**, 404–406.

Lewy, R. I., Wiener, L., Walinsky, P., Lefer, A. M., Silver, M. J., and Smith, J. B. (1980b). *Circulation* **61**, 1165–1171.

Liang, C. S., and Hood, W. B. (1979). *J. Pharmacol. Exp. Ther.* **211**, 698–705.

Linet, O. I. (1982). *Postgraduate Medicine* **72**, 105–120.

Lioy, F. (1967). *Am. J. Physiol.* **213**, 487–491, 1967.

Lluch, S., Conde, M. V., Diéguez, G., De Pablo, A. L. L., Gonzalez, M. C., Estrada, C., and Gomez, B. (1984). *J. Pharmacol. Exp. Ther.* **228**, 749–755.

Lokhandwala, M. F., and Barrett, R. J. (1982). *J. Auton. Pharmacol.* **3**, 189–215.

Lokhandwala, M. F., Watkins, H., and Alkhadhi, K. A. (1984). *Fed. Proc.* **43**, 1094.

Londos, C., and Wolff, J. (1977). *Proc. Natl. Acad. Sci.* **74**, 5482–5486.

Lopez, L. M., and Mehta, J. L. (1984). *Am. J. Cardiol.* **53**, 787–790.

Lowenthal, D. T. (1980). *J. Cardiovasc. Pharmacol.* **2**, S29–S37.

Lum, G. M., Aisenbrey, G. A., Dunn, M. J., Berl, T., and McDonald, K. M. (1977). *J. Clin. Invest.* **59**, 8–13.

Madjar, H., Docherty, J. R., and Starke, K. (1980). *J. Cardiovasc. Pharmacol.* **2**, 619–627.

Magnoni, M. S., Kobayashi, H., Cazzaniga, F., Izumi, F., Spano, P. F., and Trabucchi, M. (1983). *Circulation* **67**, 610–613.

Majewski, H., Rand, M. J., and Tung, L. H. (1981). *Br. J. Pharmacol.* **73**, 669–679.

Majewski, H., Hedler, L., and Starke, K. (1982a). *Naunyn-Schmiedeberg's Arch. Pharmacol.* **321**, 20–27.

Majewski, H., Tung, L. H., and Rand, M. J. (1982b). *J. Cardiovasc. Pharmacol.* **4**, 99–106.

Malindzak, G. S., Kosinski, E. J., Green, H. D., and Yarborough, G. W. (1978). *J. Pharmacol. Exp. Ther.* **206**, 248–258.

Malta, E., McPherson, G. A., and Raper, C. (1979). *Br. J. Pharmacol.* **65**, 249–256.

Malta, E., Schini, V., and Miller, R. C. (1986). *J. Pharm. Pharmacol.* **38**, 209–213.

Manning, M., and Sawyer, W. H. (1985). *In* "Vasopressin" (R. W. Schrier, ed.), pp. 131–144. Raven Press, New York.

Martin, W., Furchgott, R. F., Villani, G. M., and Jothianandan, D. (1986). *J. Pharmacol. Exp. Ther.* **237**, 529–538.

Matsuda, H., Kuon, E., Holtz, J., and Brusse, R. (1985). *J. Cardiovasc. Pharmacol.* **7**, 680–688.

Matthay, M. A., Eschenbacher, W. C., and Goetzel, E. J. (1984). *Clin. Res.* **32**, 529A.

Matthews, W. D., Jim, K. F., Hieble, J. P., and DeMarinis, R. M. (1984a). *Fed. Proc.* **43**, 2923–2928.

Matthews, W. D., McCafferty, G. P., and Grous, M. (1984b). *J. Pharmacol. Exp. Ther.* **231**, 355–360.

McAdams, R. P., and Waterfall, J. F. (1984). *Br. J. Pharmacol.* **83**, 412.

McCalden, T. A. (1981). *J. Auton. Pharmacol.* **1**, 421–431.

McCannel, K. L., McNay, J. L., Meyer, M. D., and Goldberg, L. I. (1966). *New Engl. J. Med.* **275**, 1389–1398.

McGrath, J. C. (1982). *Biochem. Pharmacol.* **31**, 467–484.

McGrath, J. C., Flavahan, N. A., and McKean, C. E. (1982). *J. Cardiovasc. Pharmacol.* **4**(Suppl. 1), S101–S107.

McPherson, G. A., and Summers, R. J. (1981). *J. Pharm. Pharmacol.* **33**, 189–191.

Medgett, I. C., Hicks, P. E., and Langer, S. Z. (1984). *J. Pharmacol. Exp. Ther.* **231**, 159–165.

Meier, M., Orwin, J., Rogg, H., and Brunner, H. (1980). *In* "Pharmacology of Antihypertensive Drugs" (A. Scriabine, ed.), pp. 179–194. Raven Press, New York.

Messina, E. J., Weiner, R., and Kaley, G. (1977). *Am. J. Physiol.* **232**, H571–H575.

Michelassi, F., Castorena, G., Hill, R. D., Phil, D., Lowenstein, E., Watkins, D., Petkau, A. J., and Zapol, W. M. (1982). *Surgery* **93**, 267–275.

Michell, R. H. (1979). *Trends Biochem. Sci.* **4**, 128–131.

Michell, R. H., Kirk, C. J., and Billah, M. M. (1979). *Biochem. Soc. Trans.* **7**, 861–865.

Mills, M. D., Burchell, H. B., Parker, R. L., and Kirklin, B. R. (1949). *Staff Meeting of the Mayo Clinic.* **24**, 254–258.

Mohring, J., Kintz, J., and Schoun, J. (1979). *J. Cardiovasc. Pharmacol.* **1**, 593–608.

Mohring, J., Glanger, K., Maciel, J. A. Jr., Dusing, R., Kramer, J. H., Arbogast, R., and Koch-Weser, J. (1980). *J. Cardiovasc. Pharmacol.* **2**, 367–376.

Montani, J. P., Liard, J. F., Schoun, J., and Mohring, J. (1980). *Circ. Res.* **47**, 346–355.

Moncada, S., and Vane, J. R. (1977). *In* "Biochemical Aspects of Prostaglandins and Thromboxanes" (N. Kharasch and J. Fried, eds), pp. 155–177. Academic Press, New York.

Moncada, S., Gryglewski, R. J., Bunting, S., and Vane, J. R. (1976). *Prostaglandins* **12**, 715–737.

Montastruc, J.-L., and Montastruc, P. (1980). *Eur. J. Pharmacol.* **63**, 103–116.

Moody, C. J., and Burnstock, G. (1982). *Eur. J. Pharmacol.* **77**, 1–9.

Mullane, K. M., Dusting, G. J., Salmon, J. A., Moncada, S., and Vane, J. R. (1979). *Eur. J. Pharmacol.* **54**, 217–228.

Muller-Schweinitzer, E. (1984). *Naunyn-Schmiedeberg's Arch. Pharmacol.* **327**, 299–303.

Muramatsu, I., Sakakibara, Y., Hong, S. C., and Fujiwara, M. (1984). *Pharmacology* **28**, 27–33.

Murthy, V. V., Gilbert, J. C., Goldberg, L. I., and Kuo, J. F. (1973). *J. Pharm. Pharmacol.* **28**, 567.

Myers, B. D., Deen, W. M., and Brenner, B. M. (1975). *Circ. Res.* **37**, 101–110.

Navar, L. G., and Rosivall, L. (1984). *Kidney Int.* **25**, 857–868.

Nicod, P., Waeber, B. Bussien, J.-P., Goy, J. J., Turini, G., Nussberger, J., Hofbauer, K. G., and Brunner, H. R. (1985). *Am. J. Cardiol.* **55**, 1043–1047.

Nicolaou, K. C., Magolda, R. L., Smith, J. B., Aharony, D., Smith, E. F., and Lefer, A. M. (1979). *Proc. Natl. Acad. Sci.* **76**, 2566–2570.

Nichols, A. J. (1985). Ph.D. Thesis, University of Cambridge.

Nichols, A. J., and Hiley, C. R. (1985). *J. Pharm. Pharmacol.* **37**, 110–115.

Nichols, A. J., and Ruffolo, R. R. Jr. (1986). *Eur. J. Pharmacol.* **126**, 297–301.

Nowak, J., and Wennmalm, A. (1979). *Acta Physiol. Scand.* **106**, 365–369.

Ogasawara, B., Ogawa, K., Hayashi, H., and Sassa, H. (1981). *Clin. Pharmacol. Ther.* **29**, 464–471.

Ohlstein, E. H., Shebuski, R. J., and Ruffolo, R. R. Jr. (1986). *The Pharmacologist* **28**, 141.

Ohmori, M., Tada, M., Kuzuya, T., Yamagishi, H., Matsuda, H., Inoue, M., Abe, H., and Kodama, K. (1983). *Circulation* **68**, III–22.

Olsen, U. B. (1976). *Eur. J. Pharmacol.* **36**, 95–101.

Onesti, G., Schwartz, A. B., and Kim, K. E. (1971). *Circ. Res.* **28** (Suppl. 2), 53–69.

Oriowo, M. A., Bevan, R. D., and Bevan, J. A. (1985). *Fed. Proc.* **44**, 883.

Ormsbee, H. S., III, and Fondacaro, J. D. (1985). *Proc. Soc. Exp. Biol. Med.* **178**, 333–338.

Osborn, J. L., DiBona, G. F., and Thames, M. D. (1981). *J. Pharmacol. Exp. Ther.* **216**, 265–269.

Osborn, J. L., DiBona, G. F., and Thames, M. D. (1982). *Am. J. Physiol.* **242**, F620–F626.

Osborn, J. L., Holdaas, H., Thames, M. D., and DiBona, G. F. (1983). *Circ. Res.* **53**, 298–305.

Osnes, J.-B. (1976). *Acta Pharmac. Tox.* **398**, 232–240.

Oswald, H., and Greven, J. (1981). *In* "Handbook of Experimental Pharmacology" (L. Szekeres, ed.), Vol. 54, pp. 241–288. Springer Verlag, Berlin.

Owen, M. P., and Bevan, J. A. (1985). *Fed. Proc.* **44**, 1733.

Padfield, P. L., Brown, J. J., Lever, A. F., Morton, J. J., and Robertson, J. I. S. (1981). *New Engl. J. Med.* **304**, 1067–1070.

Pals, D. T., Denning, G. S., and Keenan, R. E. (1979). *Kidney Int.* **15**, 57–511.

Parise, L. V., Venton, D. L., and Le Breton, G. C. (1984). *J. Pharmacol. Exp. Ther.* **228**, 240–244.

Parratt, J. R. (1969). *Cardiovas. Res.* **3**, 306–314.

Patel, P., Bose, D., and Greenway, C. (1981). *J. Cardiovasc. Pharmacol.* **3**, 1050–1059.

Paton, W. D. M., and Vizi, E. S. (1969). *Br. J. Pharmacol.* **35**, 10–28.

Pawlik, W. W., Shepherd, A. P., Mailman, D., and Jacobsen, E. D. (1976). *Adv. Exp. Med. Biol.* **75**, 511–516.

Pettinger, W. A. (1987). *Hypertension* **9**, 3–6.

Pfeffer, M. A., Pfeffer, J. M., Lewis, R. A., Braunwald, E., Corey, E. J., and Austen, K. F. (1983). *Am. J. Physiol.* **244**, H628–H633.

Piper, P. J. (1984). *Physiol. Rev.* **64**, 744–761.

Piper, P. J., and Samhoun, M. N. (1982). *Br. J. Pharmacol.* **77**, 267–275.

Piper, P. J., Samhoun, M. N., Tippins, J. R., Williams, T. J., Palmer, M. A., and Peck, M. J. (1981). *In* "SRS-A and leukotrienes" (P. J. Piper, ed.), pp. 81–99. John Wiley, New York.

Piper, P. J., Letts, L. G., and Galton, S. A. (1983). *Prostaglandins* **25**, 591–599.

Pitt, B., Elliot, E. C., and Gregg, D. E. (1967). *Circ. Res.* **21**, 75–84.

Pitt, B., Shea, M. J., Romson, J. L., and Lucchesi, B. A. (1983). *Ann. Rev. Intern. Med.* **99**, 83–92.

Planitz, V. (1984). *Eur. J. Clin. Pharmacol.* **27**, 147–152.

Powis, D. A., and Baker, P. F. (1986). *Mol. Pharmacol.* **29**, 134–141.

Preibisz, J. J., Sealey, J. E., Laragh, J. H., Cody, R. J., and Weksler, B. B. (1983). *Hypertension* **5** (Suppl. 1), 129–138.

Proctor, E. (1968). *J. Pharm. Pharmacol.* **20**, 36–40.

Purdy, R. E., and Stupecky, G. L. (1984). *J. Pharmacol. Exp. Ther.* **229**, 459–468.

Raab, W., and Gigee, W. (1953). *Naunyn-Schmiedeberg's Arch. Pharmacol.* **219**, 248–262.

Raisman, R., Brile, M., and Langer, S. Z. (1979). *Naunyn-Schmiedeberg's Arch. Pharmacol.* **307**, 223–226.

Rajfer, S. I., Anton, A. H., Rossen, J. D., and Goldberg, L. I. (1984). *New Engl. J. Med.* **310**, 1352–1362.

Rascher, W., Weidman, E., and Gross, F. (1981). *Clin. Sci.* **61**, 295–298.

Raskin, N. H. (1981). *Ann. Rev. Pharmacol. Toxicol.* **21**, 463–478.

Reese, J. B., and Matthews, W. D. (1986). *The Pharmacologist* **28**, 161.

Reid, I. A., Nolan, P. L., Wolf, J. A., and Keil, L. C. (1979). *Endocrinology* **104**, 1403–1406.

Reid, J. L. (1985). *J. Cardiovasc. Pharmacol.* **7** (Suppl. 8), S45–S50.

Reid, J. L., Dargie, H. J., Davies, D. S., Wing, L. M. H., Hamilton, C. A., and Dollery, C. T. (1977). *Lancet* **i**, 1171–1174.

Reid, J. L. Hamilton, C. A., and Hannah, J. A. M. (1983a). *Chest* **83**, 302–304.

Reid, J. L., Rubin, P. C., and Howden, C. W. (1983b). *Br. J. Clin. Pharmacol.* **15** (Suppl. 4), 463–469.

Reis, D. J. (1984). *Circulation* **70**, III-31–45.

Ribeiro, L. G. T., Brandon, T. A., Hopkins, D. G., Redutu, L. A., Taylor, A. A., and Miller, R. R. (1981). *Am. J. Cardiol.* **47**, 835–840.

Richardson, P. D. I., and Withrington, P. G. (1978). *Eur. J. Pharmacol.* **48**, 337–349.

Richardson, P. D. I. (1984). *In* "Physiology of the Intestinal Circulation" (A. P. Shepherd and D. N. Granger, eds), Ch. 32, pp. 393–402. Raven Press, New York.

Roesler, J. M., Hieble, J. P., McCafferty, J. P., DeMarinis, R. M., and Matthews, W. D. (1986). *J. Pharmacol. Exp. Ther.* **236**, 1–7.

Roman, R. J., Cowley, A. W. Jr., and Lecherie, C. (1979). *J. Pharmacol. Exp. Ther.* **221**, 385–393.

Rosendorff, C., Mitchell, G., Scriven, D. R., and Shapiro, C. (1976). *Circ. Res.* **38**, 140–145.

Rosenkranz, B., Wilson, T. W., Seyberth, H., and Frolich, J. C. (1981). Proc. 8th Int. Congr. Nephrol., Athens, pp. 1045–1052.

Rubin, B., and Antonaccio, M. J. (1980). *In* "The Pharmacology of Antihypertensive Drugs" (A. Scriabine, ed.), pp. 21–42. Raven Press, New York.

Rubin, S. A., Chatterjee, K., Gelberg, H. J., Ports, T. A., Brundage, B. H., and Parmley, W. W. (1979). *Am. J. Cardiol.* **43**, 810–815.

Ruffolo, R. R. Jr. (1982). *J. Auton. Pharmacol.* **2**, 277–294.

Ruffolo, R. R. Jr. (1984a). Monographs in Neural Science, Vol. 10, pp. 224–253. Karger, Basel.

Ruffolo, R. R. Jr. (1984b). *Fed. Proc.* **43**, 2910–2916.

Ruffolo, R. R. Jr. (1984c). *Trends Pharmacol. Sci.* **5**, 160–164.

Ruffolo, R. R. Jr. (1985a). *Clin. Sci.* **68** (Suppl. 10), 9s–14s.

Ruffolo, R. R. Jr. (1985b). *Pharmacol. Biochem. Behav.* **22**, 827–833.

Ruffolo, R. R. Jr. (1986). *Fed. Proc.* **45**, 2341–2346.

Ruffolo, R. R. Jr., and Morgan, E. L. (1984). *J. Pharmacol. Exp. Ther.* **229**, 364.

Ruffolo, R. R. Jr., and Waddell, J. E. (1982). *J. Pharmacol. Exp. Ther.* **222**, 29–36.

Ruffolo, R. R. Jr., and Yaden, E. L. (1984). *J. Cardiovasc. Pharmacol.* **6**, 1011–1019.

Ruffolo, R. R. Jr., and Zeid, R. L. (1985). *J. Pharmacol. Exp. Ther.* **235**, 636–643.

Ruffolo, R. R. Jr., Rosing, E. L., and Waddell, J. E. (1979a). *J. Pharmacol. Exp. Ther.* **209**, 429–436.

Ruffolo, R. R., Rosing, E. L., and Waddell, J. E. (1979b). *J. Pharmacol. Exp. Ther.* **211**, 733–738.

Ruffolo, R. R., Anderson, K. S., and Miller, D. D. (1982a). *Mol. Pharmacol.* **21**, 259–265.

Ruffolo, R. R., Yaden, E. L., and Waddell, J. E. (1982b). *J. Pharmacol. Exp. Ther.* **222**, 645–651.

Ruffolo, R. R., Yaden, E. L., Waddell, J. E., and Ward, J. S. (1982c). *Pharmacology* **25**, 187–201.

Ruffolo, R. R., Yaden, E. L., and Ward, J. S. (1982d). *Eur. J. Pharmacol.* **81**, 367–375.

Ruffolo, R. R. Jr., Banning, J. W., Patil, P. N., Hamada, A., and Miller, D. D. (1983). *J. Auton. Pharmacol.* **3**, 185–193.

Ruffolo, R. R. Jr., Morgan, E. L., and Messick, K. (1984). *J. Pharmacol. Exp. Ther.* **230**, 587–594.

Sabouni, M. H., and Lokhandwala, M. F. (1984). *Fed. Proc.* **43**, 1094.

Sakakibara, Y., Fujiwara, M., and Muramatsu, I. (1982). *Naunyn-Schmiedeberg's Arch. Pharmacol.* **319**, 1–7.

Salmon, J. A., Smith, D. R., Flower, R. J., Moncada, S., and Vane, J. R. (1978). *Biochem. Biophys. Acta.* **523**, 250–262.

Samuelsson, B., Hammarstrom, S., Murphy, R. C., and Borgeat, P. (1980). *Allergy* **35**, 375–381.

Sanchez, A., and Pettinger, W. A. (1981). *Life Sci.* **29**, 2795–2802.

Sastre, A., Griendling, K. K., Rusher, M. M., and Milnor, W. R. (1984). *J. Pharmacol. Exp. Ther.* **229**, 887–896.

Sawyer, R., Warnock, P., and Docherty, J. R. (1985). *J. Cardiovasc. Pharmacol.* **7**, 809–812.

Schmid, P. G., Abboud, F. M., Wendling, M. G., Ramberg, E. S., Mark, A. L., Heiskad, D. D., and Eckstein, J. W. (1974). *Am. J. Physiol.* **227**, 998–1004.

Schmitt, H. (1971). *Acta Pharmacol.* **24**, 93–131.

Schmitt, H., and Schmitt, H. (1969). *Eur. J. Pharmacol.* **6**, 8–12.

Schmitz, J. M., Graham, K. M., Saglowsky, A., and Pettinger, W. A. (1981). *J. Pharmacol. Exp. Ther.* **219**, 400–406.

Schnaar, R. L., and Sparks, H. V. (1972). *Am. J. Physiol.* **223**, 223–228.

Scholtysik, G. (1980). *Br. J. Clin. Pharmacol.* **10**, 21S–24S.

Scholtysik, G., Lauener, H., Eichenberger, E., Burki, H., Salzmann, R., Muller-Schweinitzer, E., and Waite, R. (1975). *Arzneimittel Forsch.* **25**, 1483–1491.

Schror, K., Smith, E. F., Bickerton, M., Smith, J. B., Nicolaou, K. C., Magolda, R., and Lefer, A. M. (1980). *Am. J. Physiol.* **238**, H87–H92.

Schultz, H. S., Chertien, S. D., Brewer, D. D., Eltorai, M. T., and Weber, M. A. (1981). *J. Clin. Pharmacol.* **21**, 65–71.

Schumann, H. J., and Brodde, O.-E. (1979). *Arch. Pharmacol.* **308**, 191–198.

Schumann, H. J., and Endoh, M. (1976). *Eur. J. Pharmacol.* **36**, 413–421.

Schumann, H. J., Endoh, M., and Brodde, O.-E. (1975). *Arch. Pharmacol.* **289**, 291–302.

Schwartz, J., Liard, J. F., Ott, C., and Cowley, A. W. (1985). *Am. J. Physiol.* **249**, H1001–H1008.

Segstro, R., and Greenway, C. (1986). *J. Pharmacol. Exp. Ther.* **236**, 224–229.

Sercombe, R., Aubineau, P., Edvinsson, L., Mamo, H., Owman, C. H. and Seylaz, J. (1977). *Pflüger's Arch.* **368**, 241–244.

Shah, S. V., Northrup, T. E., Hui, Y. S. F., and Dousa, T. P. (1979). *Kidney Int.* **15**, 463–472.

Shebuski, R. J., Fujita, T., and Ruffolo, R. R. Jr. (1986). *J. Pharmacol. Exp. Ther.* **238**, 217–223.

Shebuski, R. J., Ohlstein, E. H., Smith, J. M. Jr., and Ruffolo, R. R. Jr. (1987). *J. Pharmacol. Exp. Ther.* **242**, 158–165.

Shepperson, N. B., Duval, N., and Langer, S. Z. (1982). *Eur. J. Pharmacol.* **81**, 627–635.

Shoji, T., Tsuru, H., and Shigei, T. (1983). *Naunyn-Schmiedeberg's Arch. Pharmacol.* **324**, 246–255.

Sioufi, A., Pommier, F., Mangoni, P., Gauron, S., and Metayer, J. P. (1981). *J. Chromatogr.* **222**, 429–435.

Skarby, T. (1984). *Acta Physiol. Scand.* **122**, 165–174.

Skarby, T. V. C., Anderson, K. E., and Edvinsson, L. (1983). *Acta. Physiol. Scand.* **117**, 63–73.

Skorecki, K. L., Ballermann, B. J., Rennke, H. G., and Brenner, B. M. (1983). *Fed. Proc.* **42**, 3064–3070.

Slotman, G. J., Quinn, J. V., Burchard, K. W., and Gann, D. S. (1984). *J. Trauma* **24**, 803–810.

Slotnik, I. L., and Teigland, J. D. (1951). *J. Am. Med. Assoc.* **146**, 1126–1129.

Smedegard, G., Hedqvist, P., Dahlen, S.-E., Revenas, B., Hammarstrom, S., and Samuelsson, B. (1982). *Nature, London* **295**, 327–329.

Smith, E. F., Lefer, A. M., Aharony, D., Smith, J. B., Magolda, R. L., Claremon, D., and Nicolaou, K. C. (1981). *Prostaglandins* **21**, 443–456.

Smyth, D. D., Umemura, S., and Pettinger, W. A. (1984). *Am. J. Physiol.* **247**, F680–F685.

Smyth, D. D., Umemura, S., and Pettinger, W. A. (1985a). *Am. J. Physiol.* **248**, F767–F772.

Smyth, D. D., Umemura, S., and Pettinger, W. A. (1985b). *Circ. Res.* **57**, 304–311.

Sneddon, J. M. (1981). *Drugs of the Future* **6**, 159–161.

Sofroniew, M. W., and Weindl, A. (1978). *Am. J. Anat.* **153**, 391–430.

Sonnenblick, E. H., Frishman, W. H., and LeJemtel, T. H. (1979). *New Engl. J. Med.* **300**, 17–22.

Spann, J. F. (1983). *Am. J. Med.* **74**, 877–886.

Srimal, R. C., Gulati, K., and Dhawan, B. N. (1977). *Can. J. Physiol. Pharmacol.* **55**, 1007–1014.

Stanaszek, W. F., Kellerman, D., Brogden, R. N., and Romankiewicz, J. A. (1983). *Drugs* **25**, 339–384.

Starke, K. (1981). *Rev. Physiol. Biochem. Pharmacol.* **88**, 199–236.

Starke, K., Montel, H., and Schumann, H. J. (1971a). *Naunyn-Schmiedeberg's Arch. Pharmacol.* **270**, 210–214.

Starke, K., Montel, H., and Wagner, J. (1971b). *Naunyn-Schmiedeberg's Arch. Pharmacol.* **271**, 181–192.

Stenmark, K. R., James, S. L., Voelkel, N. F., Toews, W. H., Reeves, J. R., and Murphy, R. (1983). *New Engl. J. Med.* **309**, 77–80.

Stephenson, J. A., and Summers, R. J. (1985). *Eur. J. Pharmacol.* **116**, 271–278.

Stevens, M. J., and Moulds, R. F. W. (1982). *Cardiovasc. Pharmacol.* **4**, (Suppl. 1), S129–S133.

Stokes, G. S., and Marwood, J. F. (1984). *Meth. Find. Exp. Clin. Pharmacol.* **6**, 197–204.

Story, D. F., McCulloch, M. W., Rand, M. J., and Stanford-Starr, C. A. (1981). *Nature* **293**, 62–65.

Story, D. F., Standford-Starr, C. A., and Rand, M. J. (1985). *Clin. Sci.* **68** (Suppl. 10), 111s–115s.

Stote, R. M., Dubb, J. W., Familiar, R. G., Erb, B. B., and Alexander, F. (1983). *Clin. Pharmacol. Ther.* **34**, 309–315.

Strandhoy, J. W., Morris, M., and Buckalew, V. M. Jr. (1982). *J. Pharmacol. Exp. Ther.* **221**, 347–352.

Streeton, D. H. P., and Anderson, G. H. (1984). *In* "Handbook of Hypertension" (A. E. Doyle, ed.), Vol. 5, pp. 246–271. Elsevier, Amsterdam.

Sueta, C. A., Hutchins, P. M., and Dusseau, J. W. (1983). *Hypertension* **5**, 321–327.

Sullivan, A. T., and Drew, G. M. (1980). *Naunyn-Schmiedeberg's Arch Pharmacol.* **314**, 249–258.

Sulpizio, A. C., and Hieble, J. P. (1985). *The Pharmacologist* **27**, 205.

Sulpizio, A. C., and Hieble, J. P. (1987). *Eur. J. Pharmacol.* **135**, 107–110.

Summers, R. J. (1984). *Fed. Proc.* **43**, 2917–2922.

Summers, R. J., and McPherson, G. A. (1982). *Trends Pharmacol. Sci.* **3**, 291–294.

Swales, J. D. (1979). *Clin. Sci.* **56**, 293–298.

Szatalowicz, V. L., Arnold, P. E., Chaimovitz, C., Bichet, D., Berl, T., and Schrier, R. W. (1981). *New Engl. J. Med.* **305**, 263–266.

Tanabe, M., Terashita, Z.-I., Fijiwara, S., Shimamoto, N., Goto, N., Nishikawa, K., and Hiraka, M. (1982). *Cardiovasc. Res.* **16**, 99–106.

Taylor, A. A., Fennell, W. A., Ruud, C. O., Pool, J. L., Nelson, E. B., Ginos, J. Z., and Mitchell, J. R. (1984). *Hypertension* **6** (Suppl. 1), I-40–45.

Terashita, Z.-I., Fukui, H., Hirata, M., Terao, S., Ohkawa, S., Nishikawa, K., and Kikuchi, S. (1981). *Eur. J. Pharmacol.* **73**, 357–361.

Thomas, J. A., and Marks, B. H. (1978). *Am. J. Cardiol.* **41**, 233–243.

Thomas, M., Lumley, P., and Hornby, E. J. (1984). *Br. J. Clin. Pharmacol.* **19**, 123P.

Thoolen, J. M. C., Timmermans, P. B. M. W. M., and van Zweiten, P. A. (1983). *Br. J. Clin. Pharmacol.* **15**, 491S–505S.

Timmermans, P. B. M. W. M., and Thoolen, M. J. M. C. (1987). *In* "The α_1-Adrenergic Receptors" (R. R. Ruffolo, Jr., ed.), in press. Humana Press, Clifton, New Jersey.

Timmermans, P. B. M. W. M., and van Zwieten, P. A. (1978). *Arzneimittel-Forsch.* **28**, 1676–1681.

Timmermans, P. B. M. W. M., and van Zwieten, P. A. (1982). *J. Med. Chem.* **25**, 1390–1401.

Timmermans, P. B. M. W. M., Brands, A., and van Zwieten, P. A. (1977). *Naunyn-Schmiedeberg's Arch. Pharmacol.* **300**, 217–226.

Timmermans, P. B. M. W. M., Kwa, H. Y., and van Zwieten, P. A. (1979). *Naunyn-Schmiedeberg's Arch. Pharmacol.* **310**, 189–193.

Timmermans, P. B. M. W. M., Hoefke, W., Stahle, H., and van Zwieten, P. A. (1980). *Prog. Pharmacol.* **3**, 1–104.

Timmermans, P. B. M. W. M., de Jonge, A., van Meel, J. C. A., Slothorst-Grisdijk, F. P., Lam, E., and van Zwieten, P. A. (1981). *J. Med. Chem.* **24**, 502–507.

Timmermans, P. B. M. W. M., de Jonge, A., van Meel, J. C. A., Mathy, M. J., and van Zwieten, P. A. (1983). *J. Cardiovasc. Pharmacol.* **5**, 1–11.

Toda, N. (1983). *J. Pharmacol. Exp. Ther.* **226**, 861–868.

Toda, N. (1984). *Br. J. Pharmacol.* **83**, 399.

Tung, L. H., Rand, M. J., and Majewski, H. (1981). *Clin. Sci.* **61**, 191s–193s.

Turk, J., Wyche, A., and Needleman, P. (1980). *Biochem. Biophys. Res. Commun.* **95**, 1628–1634.

Uchida, W., Kimura, T., and Satoh, S. (1984). *Eur. J. Pharmacol.* **103**, 51–56.

Ueda, S., Yano, S., and Sakanashi, M. (1982). *J. Cardiovasc. Pharmacol.* **4**, 76–81.

Umemura, S., Marver, D., Smyth, D. M., and Pettinger, W. A. (1985). *Am. J. Physiol.* **249**, F28–F33.

Usui, H., Fujiwara, M., Tsukahara, T., Taniguchi, T., and Kurahashi, K. (1985). *J. Cardiovasc. Pharmacol.* **7** (Suppl. 3), S47–S52.

van Breeman, C., Hwang, O., and Cauvin, C. (1982). In "International Symposium on Calcium Modulators" (T. Godfraind, ed.), pp. 93–116. Elsevier/North Holland, Amsterdam.

van Calker, D., Muller, H., and Hamprecht, B. (1979). *J. Neurochem.* **33**, 999–1005.

van der Starre, P. J. A., Scheijgrond, H. W., Reneman, R. S., and Kolling, J. B. (1983). *Anesth. Analg.* **62**, 63–69.

van Meel, J. C. A., Timmermans, P. B. M. W. M., and van Zwieten, P. A. (1983). *J. Cardiovasc. Pharmacol.* **5**, 580–585.

van Meel, J. C. A., de Jonge, A., Kalkman, H. O., Wilffert, B., Timmermans, P. B. M. W. M., and van Zwieten, P. A. (1981a). *Eur. J. Pharmacol.* **69**, 205–208.

van Meel, J. C. A., de Jonge, A., Kalkman, H. O., Wilffert, B., Timmermans, P. B. M. W. M., and van Zwieten, P. A. (1981b). *Naunyn-Schmiedeberg's Arch. Pharmacol.* **316**, 288–293.

van Meel, J. C. A., de Jonge, A., Timmermans, P. B. M. W. M., and van Zwieten, P. A. (1981c). *J. Pharmacol. Exp. Ther.* **219**, 760–767.

van Meel, J. C. A., de Zoeten, K., Timmermans, P. B. M. W. M., and van Zwieten, P. A. (1982). *J. Auton. Pharmacol.* **2**, 13–20.

van Neuten, J. M., Janssen, P. A. J., van Beek, J., Xhonneaux, R., Verbeuren, T. J., and Vanhoutte, P. M. (1981). *J. Pharmacol. Exp. Ther.* **218**, 217–230.

van Zwieten, P. A. (1980). *Br. J. Clin. Pharmacol.* **10**, 13S–20S.

van Zwieten, P. A., Thoolen, M. J. M. C., and Timmermans, P. B. M. W. M. (1983). *Br. J. Clin. Pharmacol.* **15**, 455S–462S.

Vanhoutte, P. M. (1982). *Trends Pharmacol. Sci.* **3**, 370–373.

Vanhoutte, P. M., and Rimele, T. J. (1983). *J. Physiol. (Paris)* **78**, 681–686.

Varma, S., Bhuwaneshwar, P. J., and Bhargava, K. P. (1969). *Circ. Res.* **54**, 787–792.

Veda, S., Yuno, S., and Sakanashi, M. (1982). *J. Cardiovasc. Pharmacol.* **4**, 76–81.

Ventura, H. O., Messerli, F. H., Oigmun, W., Dunn, F. G., Kobrin, I., and Frohlich, E. D. (1983). *Circulation* **68** (Suppl. III), 46.

Villalobos-Molina, R., Uc, M., Hong, E., and Garcia-Sainz, J. A. (1982). *J. Pharmacol. Exp. Ther.* **222**, 258–261.

Vizi, E. S., and Knoll, J. (1971). *J. Pharm. Pharmacol.* **23**, 918–925.

Wahl, M., Kuschinsky, W., Bosse, O., and Neiss, A. (1974). *Pflügers Arch.* **348**, 293–303.

Walland, A. (1978). *Eur. J. Pharmacol.* **47**, 211–221.

Walus, K. M., Fondacaro, J. D., and Jacobson, E. D. (1981). *Gastroenterol.* **81**, 327–324.

Warnock, P., Hyland, L., and Docherty, J. R. (1985). *Eur. J. Pharmacol.* **113**, 239–245.

Weber, M. A. (1980). *J. Cardiovasc. Pharmacol.* **2** (Suppl. 1), S73–S89.

Wennmalm, A. (1982). *In* "Prostaglandins and the Cardiovascular System" (J. Oates, ed.), pp. 303–331. Raven Press, New York.

Wenting, G. J., Man in't Veld, A. J., Woittiez, A. J., Boomsma, F., and Schalekamp, M. A. D. H. (1982). *Br. Med. J.* **284**, 537–539.

Whalley, E. T., Fritz, H., and Geiger, R. (1983). *Naunyn-Schmiedeberg's Arch. Pharmacol.* **324**, 296–301.

Whittle, B. J. R., and Moncada, S. (1984). *In* "Cardiovascular Pharmacology" (M. Antonaccio, ed.), pp. 519–534. Raven Press, New York.

Wilffert, B., Timmermans, P. B. M. W. M., and van Zwieten, P. A. (1982). *J. Pharmacol. Exp. Ther.* **221**, 762–768.

Wilkins, K. H., Wintermitz, S. R., Oparil, S., Smith, L. R., and Sustan, H. P. (1981). *Clin. Pharmacol. Ther.* **30**, 752–757.

Willems, J. L. (1973). *Naunyn-Schmiedeberg's Arch. Pharmacol.* **279**, 115–126.

Williams, D. O., and Most, A. S. (1981). *Circulation* **63**, 11–16.

Winn, H. R., Rubio, R., Curnish, R. R., and Berne, R. M. (1981). *J. Cerebral Blood Flow Metabol.* **1** (Suppl. 1), S401.

Winokur, T. S., and Morrison, A. R. (1981). *Biol. Chem.* **256**, 10 221–10 223.

Winquist, R. J., Webb, R. C., and Bohr, D. E. (1982). *Circ. Res.* **51**, 769–776.

Yamaguchi, I., and Kopin, I. J. (1980). *J. Pharmacol. Exp. Ther.* **214**, 275–281.

Yeh, B. K., McKay, J. L., and Goldberg, L. I. (1969). *J. Pharmacol. Exp. Ther.* **168**, 303–309.

Yui, Y., Hattori, R., Takatsu, Y., Kadota, K., Kambara, H., Nakajima, H., Murakami, M., and Kawai, C. (1983). *Circulation* **68**, III–397.

Zandberg, P., Timmermans, P. B. M. W. M., and van Zwieten, P. A. (1984). *J. Cardiovasc. Pharmacol.* **6**, 256–262.

Zerbe, R., Stropes, L., and Robertson, G. (1980). *Ann. Rev. Med.* **31**, 315–327.

The Pharmacology and Therapeutic Potential of Serotonin Receptor Agonists and Antagonists

RAY W. FULLER

Lilly Research Laboratories, Eli Lilly and Company, Lilly Corporate Center, Indianapolis, Indiana, USA

ADVANCES IN DRUG RESEARCH, VOL. 17
ISBN 0-12-013317-2

1 Introduction

Serotonin (5-hydroxytryptamine, 5HT) is synthesized from the amino acid tryptophan via a specific hydroxylase that forms the intermediate, 5-hydroxytryptophan, which is then decarboxylated to serotonin. Serotonin is metabolized primarily by monoamine oxidase type A, forming 5-hydroxy-indoleacetic acid. The occurrence of serotonin in and release of serotonin from neurons will be the focus and the reference point in this article; however serotonin is also formed by non-neuronal cells such as the entero-chromaffin cells in the gut, and is stored and released by cells such as blood platelets, which take up serotonin but do not synthesize it. There are serotonin receptors at many locations in peripheral tissues that apparently do not receive serotonergic innervation. In most cases, the physiological roles of these receptors are poorly understood.

In a recent review, Azmitia and Gannon (1986) made the point that serotonin-producing neurons in the mammalian brain comprise a very expansive neuronal circuitry. Although a small percentage of brain neurons are serotonin neurons, these serotonin neurons innervate many different areas in the brain. Because of this extensive innervation by serotonin neurons, they appear to be involved in numerous functions of the brain. Serotonin can also influence many peripheral tissues. Drugs that alter serotonergic function therefore have the potential of altering several physio-logical processes and of having therapeutic effects in several pathological conditions.

2 Sites of Intervention in Serotonergic Neuron Function

A schematic representation of the events that occur at a serotonergic synapse is shown in Fig. 1. Serotonin is formed within the nerve terminal, is held in storage granules or vesicles, and is released at nerve impulse into the synaptic cleft. There it acts on receptors on the postsynaptic neuron to complete the process of neurotransmission across this synapse. The seroto-nin in the synaptic cleft is inactivated primarily by being transported back into the nerve terminal through the action of specific membrane carriers or uptake pumps on the nerve membrane. Once inside the serotonin neuron, serotonin is already inactive insofar as the synaptic receptors are concerned, and may either be re-used in storage granules or degraded metabolically by monoamine oxidase. In addition to the postsynaptic receptors, presynaptic autoreceptors also appear to exist on the serotonin nerve terminal itself. Activation of these receptors leads to a diminution in the synthesis and

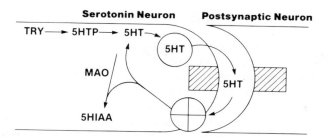

FIG. 1. Representation of a serotonergic synapse to illustrate possible sites of drug action. Drugs can act directly on the postsynaptic receptor by mimicking or blocking the action of serotonin. Drugs can increase the amount of serotonin acting on the postsynaptic receptor by increasing intraneuronal stores of serotonin so that more is released, by releasing serotonin directly, or by inhibiting serotonin reuptake. Drugs can decrease the amount of serotonin acting on the postsynaptic receptor by depleting intraneuronal stores of serotonin or by activating the autoreceptor to turn down serotonin release.

release of serotonin. The autoreceptor apparently has the physiological role of sensing the concentration of serotonin in the synaptic cleft and modulating the further release and synthesis of serotonin accordingly. Drug intervention in this overall process is possible at several sites, as discussed below.

2.1 ENHANCEMENT OF FUNCTION

Drugs may enhance serotonergic transmission by mimicking the action of serotonin at the postsynaptic receptor. Direct agonists that stimulate the serotonin receptor would enhance serotonergic function independently of the functional state of the presynaptic neuron. Indirect agonists increase the amount of serotonin acting on the postsynaptic receptor. Serotonin uptake inhibitors block the re-uptake of serotonin, thereby prolonging the action of serotonin that has been released into the synaptic cleft on the postsynaptic receptors. Serotonin-releasing drugs release serotonin from intraneuronal storage granules into the synaptic cleft, where it activates receptors. The serotonin precursors, tryptophan and 5-hydroxytryptophan, can increase the amount of serotonin formed and released into the synaptic cleft. 5-Hydroxytryptophan appears to be more effective than tryptophan in this regard. Monoamine oxidase inhibitors, by blocking serotonin degradation, increase the amount of serotonin in the storage granules that is available for release. Drugs that act in these various ways to enhance serotonergic neurotransmission do so with various degrees of specificity.

2.2 DEPRESSION OF FUNCTION

Drugs can decrease serotonergic function by decreasing the amount of serotonin that is released into the synaptic cleft or by blocking the action of serotonin on the postsynaptic receptor. Direct-acting serotonin antagonists have been particularly useful as pharmacological tools. Inhibitors of serotonin biosynthesis, such as p-chlorophenylalanine (Koe and Weissman, 1966), deplete serotonin stores and decrease the amount of serotonin that is released physiologically. Agents like reserpine, tetrabenazine and Ro 4-1284 deplete granular stores of serotonin, but these agents are not specific; they also deplete catecholamines, for example. p-Chloroamphetamine and fenfluramine deplete serotonin stores more specifically. Serotonin neurotoxins impair serotonergic function by destruction of the serotonergic terminals. 5,6- and 5,7-Dihydroxytryptamines have been most commonly used as serotonin neurotoxins, but high doses of p-chloroamphetamine or fenfluramine can also act in this way (Jacoby and Lytle, 1978).

3 Serotonin Receptor Heterogeneity

Serotonin receptors occur in the brain and in various peripheral tissues, including the gut, the uterus, the.heart, and blood vessels. Serotonin receptors occur on various types of cells. For example, in the brain, serotonin receptors are present on neurons and on glial cells (Fillion *et al.*, 1983). Serotonin receptors are also present on some neurons in peripheral tissues (Richardson and Engel, 1986). Serotonin receptors are present on various smooth muscle cells and on blood platelets. Serotonin receptors on neurons may occur either presynaptically or postsynaptically. Presynaptic serotonin receptors present on non-serotonergic nerve terminals may modulate the release of neurotransmitters; serotonin receptors present on serotonergic nerve terminals that modulate the release of serotonin itself are termed autoreceptors.

3.1 EVIDENCE FOR MULTIPLE SEROTONIN RECEPTORS

Gaddum and Picarelli (1957) reported evidence for two separate serotonin receptors present in peripheral smooth muscle preparations studied *in vitro*, the receptors being distinguished on the basis of their pharmacological properties. One receptor was termed the "D" receptor because it was affected by dibenzyline, and the other receptor was termed the "M" receptor because it was affected by morphine. Evidence for heterogeneity of serotonin receptors in brain has been revealed by electrophysiological studies (McCall and Aghajanian, 1979). At least three types of receptors could be differentiated in these electrophysiological studies. One postsynaptic receptor mediated depression of firing by serotonin and was not blocked by the classical serotonin antagonists. A second postsynaptic receptor facilitated excitatory inputs and was blocked by methysergide. A third type of receptor, located presynaptically, mediated serotonin-induced inhibition of serotonergic neurons; this receptor also was not blocked by classical antagonists of peripheral serotonin receptors. In the late 1970s, radioligand-binding techniques became useful in studying and characterizing serotonin receptors in brain membranes. In 1979, Peroutka and Snyder defined two types of brain serotonin receptors based on radioligand binding. The 5HT-1 receptor was labelled with tritiated serotonin. Agonists generally had higher affinity than antagonists for this receptor. There was some evidence for the receptor being linked to adenylate cyclase. The 5HT-2 receptor was labelled in the frontal cortex with tritiated spiperone. This receptor was termed the 5HT-2 receptor. Antagonists had higher affinity for this receptor than did agonists. There was no evidence that the 5HT-2 receptor was coupled to adenylate cyclase; guanine nucleotides did not alter the affinity of agents for this site. Subsequently, it has become recognized that tritiated serotonin binds not to a single site, but to multiple sites which can be differentiated based on their affinity for other agents.

3.2 SUBTYPES OF SEROTONIN RECEPTORS CURRENTLY DEFINED BY RADIOLIGAND BINDING

Five subtypes of serotonin receptors in brain tissue have been clearly defined and characterized based on radioligand binding. There is recent evidence for additional binding sites that do not fit within one of these categories.

3.2.1 5HT-1A Receptors

A portion of the binding of tritiated serotonin to brain membrane receptors was displaceable by low concentrations of spiperone. This binding site, having high affinity for both serotonin and spiperone, was termed the 5HT-1A site (Nelson et al., 1980). Tritiated 8-hydroxy-N,N-dipropyl-2-

aminotetralin (8-OH-DPAT) (see Fig. 4) is generally used as a selective radioligand for this 5HT-1A receptor (Hall *et al.*, 1985), although tritiated LY 165 163 (see Fig. 4) has also been used (Ransom *et al.*, 1986). The 5HT-1A receptor may mediate certain behavioural effects, the hypothermic effect, and antihypertensive effects of some serotonin agonists (Peroutka *et al.*, 1986).

3.2.2 5HT-1B Receptors

That portion of the binding of tritiated serotonin to brain membranes that was not sensitive to displacement by spiperone was termed the 5HT-1B receptor (Nelson *et al.*, 1983). The 5HT-1B receptor has also been labelled with $(-)$-[^{125}I]iodocyanopindolol, with isoprenaline present to block the binding of this radioligand to β-adrenergic receptors (Hoyer *et al.*, 1985a). Some presynaptic autoreceptors on serotonin neurons in rat brain may be 5HT-1B sites (Engel *et al.*, 1986). The 5HT-1B receptor is thought not to exist in human brain (Hoyer *et al.*, 1986).

3.2.3 5HT-1C Receptors

A third subtype of binding site labelled with tritiated serotonin was recognized later (Pazos *et al.*, 1984a). The 5HT-1C sites are mainly concentrated in the choroid plexus, where their activation leads to increased phosphatidylinositol turnover (Conn *et al.*, 1986). These sites may be selectively labelled with tritiated mesulergine (Pazos *et al.*, 1984b) or with N_1-methyl-2-[^{125}I]lysergic acid diethylamide (Yagaloff and Hartig, 1986). The 5HT-1C binding sites in pig brain have been solubilized (Yagaloff and Hartig, 1986).

3.2.4 5HT-1D Receptors

Recently Heuring and Peroutka (1987) reported that a majority of tritiated serotonin binding sites in the bovine caudate did not conform to 5HT-1A, 5HT-1B or 5HT-1C sites, but represented a new subclass of binding sites designated 5HT-1D sites. Agents with high affinity and selectivity for 5HT-1A sites, such as 8-OH-DPAT, ipsapirone and buspirone, had relatively low affinity for these sites. Both RU 24969 and $(-)$-pindolol, which have high affinity for 5HT-1B sites, had low affinity for the newly defined sites. Mianserin and mesulergine had high affinity for 5HT-1C sites but low affinity for the 5HT-1D sites. The 5HT-1D sites were most dense in the basal ganglia but were found in all regions of bovine brain and represented the most common subtype of 5HT-1 binding site in bovine brain.

3.2.5 5HT-2 Receptors

The 5HT-2 receptor was originally defined based on its labelling with tritiated spiperone (Peroutka and Snyder, 1979). Spiperone also is a potent dopamine antagonist and binds to dopamine receptors. More specific radioligands for the 5HT-2 site are tritiated ketanserin (Leysen et al., 1982) or tritiated 7-aminoketanserin (Wouters et al., 1986). In some brain regions, 5HT-2 receptors may be coupled to phosphatidylinositol turnover (Conn and Sanders-Bush, 1985; Kendall and Nahorski, 1985). Activation of 5HT-2 sites may be associated with hallucinogenic activity of some amphetamine-related drugs (Glennon et al., 1984) and with activation of the pituitary–adrenocortical axis in rats (Fuller et al., 1983; Koenig et al., 1985). The 5HT-2 subtype defined by radioligand binding seems to be identical to the "D" receptor of Gaddum and Piccarelli (1957), and the receptors mediating the contractile response to serotonin in most blood vessels are 5HT-2 receptors (Cohen, 1984).

3.3 NOMENCLATURE OF SEROTONIN RECEPTOR SUBTYPES

Up to now, it has not been possible to integrate completely the subtypes of serotonin receptors present in various tissues and studied in different ways, such as by radioligand binding, electrophysiological or pharmacological differentiation. In a recent attempt to provide a broad framework for classification of serotonin receptors, Bradley et al. (1986) proposed that three types of serotonin receptors be defined: a "5HT-1-like" receptor, a 5HT-2 receptor and a 5HT-3 receptor. The 5HT-1-like receptor is associated with prejunctional inhibition of neuronal transmitter release, with smooth muscle relaxation, with contraction of some vascular smooth muscles, and with tachycardia in the cat. The receptor mediating these responses appears to have much in common with the 5HT-1 site defined in the brain by radioligand binding. One impediment to the complete characterization of the 5HT-1-like receptors has been the lack of selective antagonist drugs. The 5HT-2 receptor that mediates gastrointestinal and vascular smooth muscle contraction, platelet aggregation, and neuronal depolarization appears to be identical to the "D" receptor defined by Gaddum and Picarelli (1957).

The 5HT-3 nomenclature was proposed to replace the term "M" receptor used by Gaddum and Picarelli (1957). This receptor mediates the depolarization of peripheral neurons.

A shortcoming of the Bradley *et al.* (1986) paper is its inadequate coverage of 5HT-1 receptor subtypes, due to the bias of the paper toward peripheral receptors for serotonin and against the use of radioligands in characterizing receptors. The authors recommended calling all serotonin receptors which were not 5HT-2 or 5HT-3 receptors "5HT-1-like", but did not define clearly what they considered 5HT-1 sites to be, a prerequisite to calling something "5HT-1-like".

It is important to recognize that binding sites might not be receptors that mediate physiological events, but it is equally important to recognize that radioligand binding offers a direct means of identifying, characterizing, localizing and quantitating receptors. We try to create categories for our own convenience as researchers, but our current attempts at doing that with serotonin receptors probably are primitive and inaccurate, even if they represent an advance over the receptor classification existing at the beginning of this decade. Several years ago, some workers were arguing that the 5HT-2 sites defined by radioligand binding could not be serotonin receptors because of the low affinity of serotonin itself for those sites. Subsequently, some have argued that 5HT-1 binding sites could not be receptors because they would always be fully saturated with neurotransmitter due to its high affinity. Such arguments, which presuppose knowing the concentration of serotonin in the synaptic cleft and fail to account for factors like possible differences in distance of the receptor from the nerve terminal, usually generate more heat than light.

No radioligand binding studies of 5HT-3 receptors in brain tissue have been published. However, central actions of compounds considered to be selective 5HT-3 antagonists have been reported. For instance, 5HT-3 antagonists have been reported to inhibit "anxiety-mediated" behaviour in mice and marmosets (Costall *et al.*, 1987a), hyperactivity induced by bilateral infusion of dopamine into the nucleus accumbens of rats or marmosets (Costall *et al.*, 1987b), and hyperactivity induced by dopamine infused into the amygdala of rats (Costall *et al.*, 1987c). One interpretation is that 5HT-3 receptors do exist in brain and do modulate dopaminergic function and anxiogenic responses. Another possibility is that some agents which are known to be 5HT-3 antagonists also have other, yet uncharacterized, pharmacological interactions that account for the above-mentioned effects.

The research on serotonin must now be directed towards a better understanding of the heterogeneity of its receptors and an integration of information obtained from studies including radioligand binding, electrophysiology, second messenger coupling, whole animal physiology, etc.

4 Direct-acting Serotonin Agonists

4.1 INDOLES

Several indoles closely related in structure to serotonin can mimic the action of serotonin at receptors (Fig. 2). These include especially N-methyl and O-methyl substituted compounds (Haigler and Aghajanian, 1977). Bufotenin (N,N-dimethylserotonin) is an example of such a compound that occurs in nature. N,N-Dimethyl-5-methoxytryptamine is probably the serotonin analogue most widely used as a centrally acting serotonin agonist; the methyl substituents protect it somewhat from metabolic inactivation and permit it to cross the blood–brain barrier. It decreases brain serotonin turnover (Fuxe et al., 1972), elicits the serotonin behavioural syndrome (Grahame-Smith, 1971), increases serum corticosterone (Fuller and Snoddy, 1979) and prolactin (Simonovic and Meltzer, 1983) concentrations, and produces various other effects characteristic of central serotonin receptor activation (Green and Heal, 1985).

RU 24969 (Fig. 2) is a synthetic indole, less closely resembling serotonin in structure than some of the above compounds, that has serotonin agonist activity (Euvrard and Boissier, 1980). It decreases brain serotonin turnover

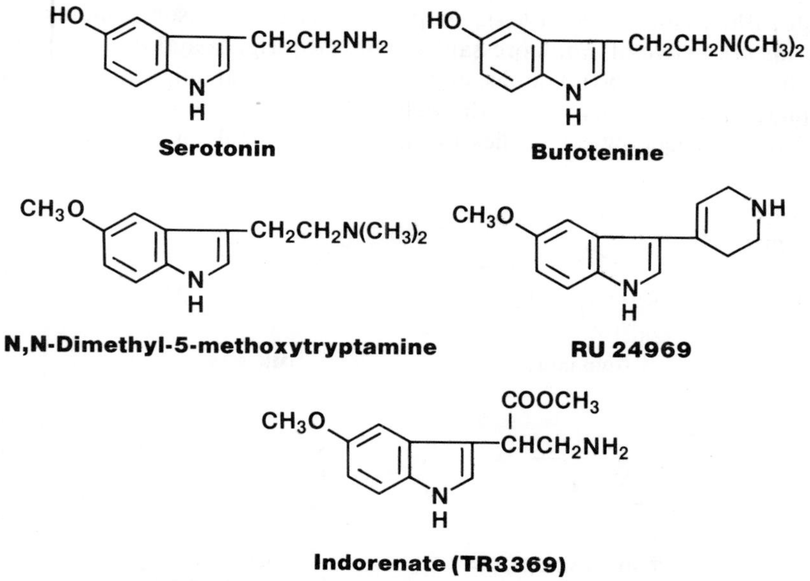

FIG. 2. Indoles that act as agonists at serotonin receptors.

and increases serum concentrations of prolactin and corticosterone in rats (Euvrard and Boissier, 1980). RU 24969 increases locomotor activity in mice and rats but does not cause components of the serotonin behavioural syndrome (head-weaving, head-twitching and reciprocal forepaw treading) seen with other serotonin agonists (Green et al., 1984), apparently because of its selective affinity for 5HT-1 receptors (Green and Heal, 1985). RU 24969 has high affinity for 5HT-1A and 5HT-1B receptor subtypes, but low affinity for 5HT-1C and 5HT-2 receptors (Hoyer et al., 1985b).

Indorenate (TR 3369) (Fig. 2) is another synthetic indole; it has antihypertensive properties, apparently resulting from agonist activity at central serotonin receptors (Hong, 1981). Indorenate has relatively high affinity for 5HT-1A sites (Hoyer et al., 1985b) and, like RU 24969, does not elicit the serotonin behavioural syndrome (Safdy et al., 1982).

Tetrahydro-β-carbolines are indoles, capable of being formed by cyclization of tryptamines and found to occur in mammalian brain, that apparently can act directly as agonists on serotonin receptors (Nielsen et al., 1982).

4.2 PIPERAZINES

Quipazine (Fig. 3), 2-(1-piperazinyl)quinoline, was the first substituted piperazine to be described as a direct-acting serotonin agonist (Hong and Pardo, 1966; Hong et al., 1969). Quipazine was active in some animal test systems predictive of antidepressant activity (Rodriguez and Pardo, 1971), but there appear to be no published data indicating that quipazine has been evaluated as an antidepressant drug clinically. Quipazine has been widely used in pharmacological studies in laboratory animals as a direct-acting

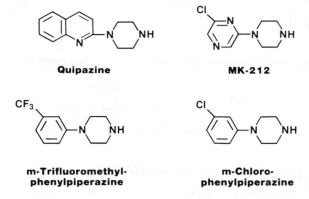

FIG. 3. Arylpiperazines that act as agonists at some serotonin receptors.

serotonin agonist, although there is some evidence that it has other actions as well. For example, its effects on serotonergic systems are not entirely due to activation of postsynaptic receptors. Presynaptic effects of quipazine include inhibition of serotonin uptake (Medon et al., 1973) and inhibition of monoamine oxidase (Fuller et al., 1976; Green et al., 1976). In addition, quipazine has been suggested to have some β-adrenergic agonist activity (Frances et al., 1980). Some investigators have also attributed certain effects of quipazine to direct or indirect stimulation of dopamine receptors in brain (Ponzio et al., 1981; Feigenbaum et al., 1983; Schecter and Concannon, 1982). Nonetheless, the most prominent actions of quipazine seem to result from its serotonin agonist activity. For example, the elevation of serum corticosterone concentration by quipazine in rats is blocked completely by serotonin antagonists such as metergoline, mianserin and LY 53857 at doses that do not block the elevation of serum corticosterone concentration by a dopamine agonist, pergolide (Fuller and Snoddy, 1984). This implies that quipazine at the doses used (2.5–10 mg/kg) has insufficient dopaminergic agonist activity to produce this effect.

There are some serotonin receptors at which quipazine behaves as an antagonist instead of an agonist. For example, quipazine antagonized serotonin-induced depolarization of rabbit superior cervical ganglion neurons and antagonized serotonin-induced contraction of the rat stomach fundus (Lansdown et al., 1980). Quipazine also blocked presynaptic autoreceptors that modulate serotonin release from rat brain slices (Schlicker and Gothert, 1981) or synaptosomes (Martin and Sanders-Bush, 1982). Quipazine is relatively non-selective for serotonin receptor subtypes, the order of affinity for ligand binding sites being 5HT-1C > 5HT-1B > 5HT-2 > 5HT-1A (Hoyer et al., 1985b).

m-Trifluoromethylphenylpiperazine (Fig. 3) was reported to be a direct-acting serotonin agonist based on its affinity for serotonin binding sites in vitro and its ability to decrease brain serotonin turnover in rats in vivo (Fuller et al., 1978). m-Trifluoromethylphenylpiperazine has the advantage over quipazine of acting more purely on serotonin systems as a direct agonist, apparently with no presynaptic actions (inhibition of monoamine oxidase or inhibition of serotonin uptake) at effective doses (Fuller et al., 1981a). m-Trifluoromethylphenylpiperazine produces numerous pharmacological effects apparently as a consequence of the activation of central serotonin receptors, e.g. increases in serum corticosterone and prolactin concentration (Fuller et al., 1981a), stimulation of corticotropin-releasing factor and arginine vasopressin release from the hypothalamus (Hashimoto et al., 1982), and decreased response of squirrel monkeys on food- and shock-presentation schedules (Brady and Barrett, 1985). Quipazine serves as a discriminative stimulus in rats, apparently by activating 5HT-1 receptors (Cunningham and Appel, 1986).

m-Chlorophenylpiperazine (Fig. 3) was patented as an appetite suppressant drug long before its mechanism of action was known (Moser *et al.*, 1966). In 1979, Samanin *et al.* reported that the anorectic effect of *m*-chlorophenylpiperazine was due to its action as a direct serotonin agonist in brain. *m*-Chlorophenylpiperazine, like *m*-trifluoromethylphenylpiperazine, decreases brain serotonin turnover and increases serum corticosterone and prolactin concentrations in rats (Fuller *et al.*, 1981b; Invernizzi *et al.*, 1981; Quattrone *et al.*, 1981). *m*-Chlorophenylpiperazine is a metabolite of the antidepressant drug trazodone (Melzacka *et al.*, 1979), and accounts for some of the pharmacological actions of trazodone given in high doses to laboratory animals (Maj *et al.*, 1979). *m*-Chlorophenylpiperazine has been found in plasma of humans as a metabolite of trazodone (Suckow, 1983), and on this basis *m*-chlorophenylpiperazine itself has been administered to humans (Mueller *et al.*, 1986). *m*-Chlorophenylpiperazine elicits some of the same hormonal responses in humans as it does in rats, e.g. an increase in cortisol and in prolactin, and offers promise as a means of evaluating the functional state of brain serotonin receptors in disease states and after drug treatments by measuring the responses in these serum hormones.

Sills *et al.* (1984) suggested that *m*-chlorophenylpiperazine and *m*-trifluoromethylphenylpiperazine have selective affinity for 5HT-1B receptors. On this basis, some investigators have used these compounds as tools believed to activate 5HT-1B receptors selectively. For example, the neuroendocrine effects of *m*-chlorophenylpiperazine in humans have been attributed to 5HT-1B receptor mediation (Heninger *et al.*, 1985). Other investigators have suggested that 5HT-1B receptors do not exist in human brain (Hoyer *et al.*, 1986). Some effects of these phenylpiperazines in rats may be mediated by 5HT-1B receptor activation (McKenney and Glennon, 1986), but these compounds do not appear to be selective enough for 5HT-1B receptors that all of their effects can be attributed to 5HT-1B activation. Sills *et al.* (1984) suggested that *m*-trifluoromethylphenylpiperazine had as much as 70-fold selectivity toward 5HT-1B versus 5HT-1A sites, but more recent estimates are that this selectivity is only 30-fold (Asarch *et al.*, 1985), four-fold (Hamon *et al.*, 1986) or three-fold (Peroutka, 1986). *m*-Chlorophenylpiperazine has been slightly less selective than *m*-trifluoromethylphenylpiperazine when the two were compared (Sills *et al.*, 1984; Hamon *et al.*, 1986).

MK-212 (Fig. 3) was originally described as a centrally-acting anorectic drug whose mechanism of action apparently involved serotonin (Clineschmidt *et al.*, 1977a,b). Subsequently, MK-212 was shown to produce numerous effects characteristic of serotonin agonists, including head twitches in mice and the serotonin behavioural syndrome in rats (Clineschmidt, 1979). There is electrophysiological evidence that MK-212 discriminates between subsets of serotonergic receptors in the brain; it was equivalent to serotonin in inhibiting raphe cell firing but did not mimic serotonin in inhibiting the firing of cortical neurons (Yarbrough *et al.*, 1984). The ability of MK-212 to serve as a discriminative cue in rats was substituted by fenfluramine and *m*-chlorophenylpiperazine and blocked by serotonin antagonists having affinity for 5HT-1 as well as 5HT-2 receptors (Cunningham *et al.*, 1986). The increase in body temperature elicited by MK-212 in rats was antagonized by selective antagonists of 5HT-2 receptors (Gudelsky *et al.*, 1986).

4.3 8-HYDROXY-DPAT

A compound that is neither an indole nor a piperazine, 8-OH-DPAT (8-hydroxy-N,N-dipropyl-2-aminotetralin, Fig. 4), was reported to be a direct-acting serotonin agonist based on its ability to decrease brain serotonin synthesis and to cause the serotonin behavioural syndrome, even in rats depleted of serotonin (Arvidsson *et al.*, 1981; Hjorth *et al.*, 1982). Unlike other hydroxylated 2-aminotetralins, the compound appeared to lack dopamine agonist activity. The compound altered sexual behaviour in male

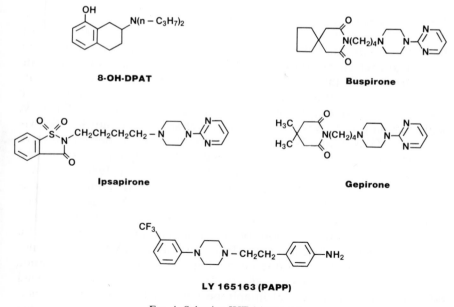

FIG. 4. Selective 5HT-1A agonists.

rats (Ahlenius *et al.*, 1981), enhanced the acoustic startle response in rats (Svensson and Ahlenius, 1983), caused rotational behaviour in rats with unilateral lesions of the dorsal raphe nucleus (Blackburn *et al.*, 1984), and decreased body temperature in mice (Goodwin *et al.*, 1986) and rats (Goodwin and Green, 1985; Hjorth, 1985), effects attributed to activation of central serotonin receptors. The compound also stimulated serotonin-sensitive adenylate cyclase in brain preparations from newborn rats (Hamon *et al.*, 1984). Some evidence has suggested that 8-OH-DPAT is not devoid of dopamine agonist activity (Simonovic *et al.*, 1984).

8-OH-DPAT is much more potent in decreasing serotonin turnover in rat brain when injected subcutaneously than when injected intraperitoneally (unpub. obs.). Perhaps the explanation is that 8-OH-DPAT is susceptible to rapid first-pass metabolism in the liver. In any event, it is important to consider route of administration in comparing various effects of 8-OH-DPAT.

Radioligand binding studies revealed that 8-OH-DPAT had selective affinity for the 5HT-1A subtype of serotonin receptors (Middlemiss and Fozard, 1983). Thus, the effects of the compound are thought to be mediated by activation of 5HT-1A receptors located presynaptically or postsynaptically.

4.4 OTHER SELECTIVE 5HT-1A AGONISTS

In contrast to the limited selectivity of agonists at other receptor subtypes, some highly selective agonists at 5HT-1A receptors are known. In addition to 8-OH-DPAT, the most selective 5HT-1A agonist currently known (Hamon *et al.*, 1986), others include buspirone, gepirone, ipsapirone and LY 165163 (Fig. 4). Buspirone is an anxiolytic drug (Goldberg and Finnerty, 1979) that only recently was found to have high selective affinity for 5HT-1A receptors (Glaser and Traber, 1983; Peroutka, 1985). Several lines of evidence from *in vitro* and *in vivo* studies indicate buspirone is a partial agonist at 5HT-1A receptors (Yocca *et al.*, 1986a; Lucki, 1986; Smith and Peroutka, 1986; Reynolds *et al.*, 1986). Gepirone is a structural analogue of buspirone which also has affinity for 5HT-1A receptors (Yocca *et al.*, 1986b) and produces functional effects such as increases in plasma concentrations of corticosterone in rats like those of buspirone and attributed to 5HT-1A receptor activation (Koenig *et al.*, 1986). Ipsapirone (TVXQ 7821) is also structurally related to buspirone and has high affinity for 5HT-1A receptors (Traber *et al.*, 1984; Hiner *et al.*, 1985). In rats trained to discriminate 8-OH-DPAT, buspirone and ipsapirone completely mimic the discriminative cue effects of 8-OH-DPAT (Cunningham *et al.*, 1985). Gepirone and ipsapirone, like buspirone, appear to be partial agonists at 5HT-1A receptors (Reynolds et al., 1986; Smith and Peroutka, 1986; Yocca et al., 1986a).

A third structural type of compound acting as a selective 5HT-1A agonist is LY 165163 or PAPP, 1-(m-trifluoromethylphenyl)-4-p-aminophenylethyl-piperazine (Asarch et al., 1985). This compound is from a series of m-halophenylpiperazines (Fuller et al., 1978, 1980). It was studied first as a potential precursor to a photoaffinity label for serotonin receptors (Fuller et al., 1986b; Shih et al., 1986). The idea was to convert the amino group to an azido group and thus produce a photolabile compound with high affinity for serotonin receptors. LY 165163 itself was found to have high selectivity for the 5HT-1A subtype of serotonin receptors (Asarch et al., 1985). This was unexpected, since the parent compound, m-trifluoromethylphenylpiperazine, has higher affinity for 5HT-1B sites than for 5HT-1A sites (Hamon et al., 1986). LY 165163 produces functional effects like other 5HT-1A agonists, e.g. decreased brain serotonin turnover and increased serum corticosterone concentration in rats (Fuller et al., 1986b). Tritiated PAPP has been used as a radioligand for labelling 5HT-1A sites (Ransom et al., 1986; Shih et al., 1986).

5 Serotonin Antagonists

Some antagonists have selective affinity for 5HT-1 sites versus 5HT-2 sites in vitro, such as (−)-pindolol and cyanopindolol (Hoyer et al., 1985b) and spiroxatrine (Nelson and Taylor, 1986). However, no selective 5HT-1 antagonists have been reported to be specific and effective 5HT-1 antagonists in a variety of systems in vivo. There are, however, potent and selective antagonists of 5HT-2 and 5HT-3 receptors.

5.1 5HT-2 ANTAGONISTS

Many of the classic serotonin antagonists that have been available for years turn out to be more or less selective for 5HT-2 receptors (Peroutka and Snyder, 1979). That may be explained partly because most test systems used in the discovery and development of those antagonists, e.g. contractile responses in vascular or other smooth muscle tissue, measured responses that happen to be mediated by 5HT-2 receptors. Currently there is an abundance of 5HT-2 antagonists, including methysergide, metergoline, cyproheptadine, danitracen, pizotifen, mianserin, cinanserin, trazodone, benzoctamine and metitepine. Not all are highly selective, some having affinity for other serotonin receptor subtypes or for other types of receptors

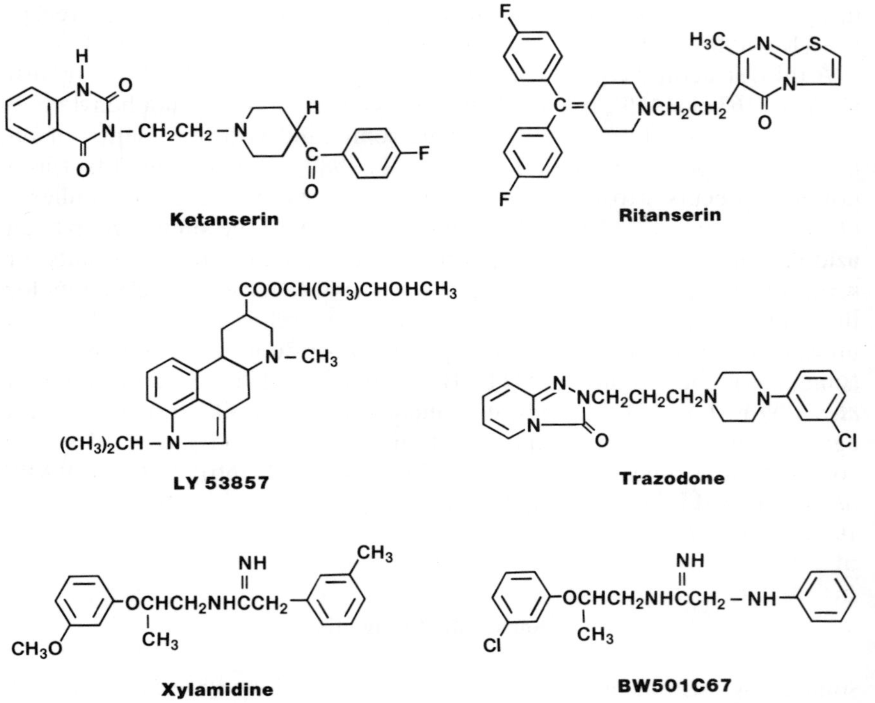

Ketanserin   Ritanserin

LY 53857   Trazodone

Xylamidine   BW501C67

FIG. 5. 5HT-2 antagonists.

such as histamine H1 or α_1-adrenergic receptors (Leysen et al., 1981; Cohen et al., 1983).

Ketanserin (Fig. 5) is a relatively recently described serotonin antagonist that has often been considered to be a selective 5HT-2 antagonist. Ketanserin has selective affinity for 5HT-2 sites in comparison to 5HT-1 sites. However, even in the original description of ketanserin based on radioligand binding (Leysen et al., 1981), it was shown to have affinity for α_1-adrenergic receptors and for H1 histaminergic receptors about one-fifth as high as its affinity for 5HT-2 receptors. It is now clear that some of the functional effects of ketanserin previously attributed to its 5HT-2 block are in fact results of α_1-receptor block. For example, lowering of blood pressure by ketanserin in rats is due to block of α_1-receptors (Fozard, 1982; Kalkman et al., 1982). Ketanserin remains one of the most selective agents for distinguishing 5HT-2 from 5HT-1 receptors, but its affinity for H1 histamine receptors and especially for α_1-adrenergic receptors must be considered in interpreting functional changes that result from ketanserin administration.

The claim that ketanserin does not have "central side effects" (Symoens, 1982) led to the impression that it does not cross the blood–brain barrier (Wenting *et al.*, 1982), but clearly ketanserin does block central 5HT-2 receptors (Niemegeers *et al.*, 1983) and in fact has been used to label central 5HT-2 receptors (Laduron *et al.*, 1982).

Some structural relatives of ketanserin such as ritanserin appear to be more selective for 5HT-2 receptors in regard to α_1- and H1-receptors, although others including altanserin and setoperone still have ketanserin-like affinity for α_1-receptors (Janssen, 1985). Pirenperone is another 5HT-2 antagonist that has relatively high affinity for other neurotransmitter receptors *in vitro* (Kennis *et al.*, 1986) and blocks receptors in addition to 5HT-2 receptors *in vivo* (Pawlowski *et al.*, 1985; Kennis *et al.*, 1986).

LY 53857 (Fig. 5) is from a series of ergoline esters that are potent and selective antagonists of 5HT-2 receptors (Fuller and Snoddy, 1979; Cohen *et al.*, 1983). LY 53857 is a potent antagonist of vascular and brain 5HT-2 receptors but has no significant affinity for α_1-adrenergic receptors and low affinity for α_2-adrenergic receptors (Cohen *et al.*, 1983, 1985a). The compound also does not interact significantly with histamine H1-, β_1- or β_2-adrenergic, muscarinic or angiotensin I receptors (Cohen *et al.*, 1985a).

Two antagonists of 5HT-2 receptors, xylamidine and BW 501C67 (Fig. 5), are noteworthy because they apparently penetrate the blood–brain barrier poorly and can be used to discriminate whether central or peripheral serotonin receptors are involved in functional effects of direct or indirect agonists (Copp *et al.*, 1967; Mawson and Whittington, 1970). These compounds are potent antagonists of several peripheral responses to serotonin, including foot paw oedema in rats following intraplantar injection of serotonin, the pressor response to intravenously injected serotonin in pithed rats and in dogs after block of ganglionic transmission, the bronchoconstrictor response to intravenously injected serotonin in guinea-pigs, the dyspnea induced by a serotonin aerosol in guinea-pigs, and serotonin-induced arterial spasm in baboons (Copp *et al.*, 1967; Mawson and Whittington, 1970; Bouillin *et al.*, 1978; Fozard, 1982). In contrast, xylamidine and BW 501C67 do not antagonize serotonergic effects that are mediated by central serotonin receptors, such as head twitches induced by intraventricular injection of serotonin in mice, behavioural changes induced by intravenous injection of tryptamine in rats, behavioural changes induced by 5-hydroxytryptophan in iproniazid-pretreated rats, serum corticosterone elevation by quipazine in rats, and hyperthermia elicited by MK-212 in rats (Mawson and Whittington, 1970; Copp *et al.*, 1967; Fuller *et al.*, 1986a; Gudelsky *et al.*, 1986).

5.2 5HT-3 ANTAGONISTS

The original naming of the "M" receptor was based on the ability of morphine to antagonize the serotonin receptor mediating depolarization of cholinergic nerves in the guinea-pig ileum (Gaddum and Picarelli, 1957). Morphine is not a specific antagonist of this receptor, now referred to as the 5HT-3 receptor (Bradley *et al.*, 1986). These 5HT-3 receptors are present on postganglionic autonomic neurons in the peripheral sympathetic and parasympathetic nervous systems, on enteric neurons, and on sensory neurons in various tissues (Richardson and Engel, 1986).

Fozard (1984) described MDL 72222 (Fig. 6), a potent and highly selective antagonist at excitatory serotonin receptors on sympathetic fibres in the rabbit heart. The compound antagonized the Bezold–Jarisch reflex in rats *in vivo*, but had little effect on responses mediated by the M receptor on cholinergic nerves of the guinea-pig ileum. Richardson *et al.* (1985) described another compound, ICS 205-930 (Fig. 6), even more potent as an antagonist of M receptors on peripheral neurons. Subsequently, additional compounds, BRL 24924 (Dunbar *et al.*, 1986) and GR 38032F (Brittain *et al.*, 1987), have been described as potent 5HT-3 antagonists (Fig. 6). These 5HT-3 antagonists antagonize emetic effects of anticancer drugs (Miner and Sanger, 1986; Costall *et al.*, 1986a) and may act in the hypothalamus to facilitate gastric emptying in the guinea-pig (Costall *et al.*, 1986b).

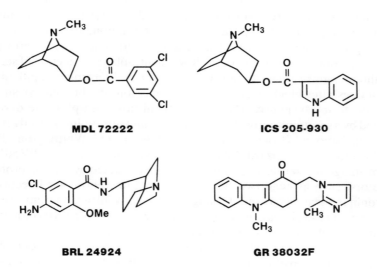

MDL 72222   **ICS 205-930**

BRL 24924   **GR 38032F**

FIG. 6. 5HT-3 antagonists.

6 Therapeutic Uses of Serotonergic Drugs

Potential uses of direct-acting serotonin agonists and antagonists in clinical therapy can be suggested based on current knowledge of disease pathology and functional involvement of serotonin, on effects of these agents in experimental animals, and on clinical experience with drugs that alter serotonergic function. Direct agonists could be expected to mimic the effects of indirect agonists generally, although the specificity of the direct agonist for receptor subtypes may be different from the specificity of serotonin itself, which activates receptors when serotonin uptake inhibitors or serotonin releasers are administered. Thus, some effects of direct agonists may be different from those of indirect agonists.

6.1 PSYCHIATRIC DISORDERS

6.1.1 Mental Depression

Consideration of serotonin involvement in depression and/or in the action of antidepressant drugs stemmed from neurochemical studies in depressed patients and known mechanisms of some antidepressant drugs. Numerous reports of decreased serotonin concentration in brain tissue taken from depressed patients who had died from suicide or other causes have appeared, but not all studies have revealed such differences (see Murphy *et al.*, 1978; Burns and Mendels, 1979). The concentration of 5-hydroxyindoleacetic acid in cerebrospinal fluid of depressed patients has often been reported to be decreased (Murphy *et al.*, 1978; Burns and Mendels, 1979). The decrease may occur specifically in some subtypes of patients (Asberg *et al.*, 1986). Monoamine oxidase inhibitors, effective in treating depression, increase brain concentrations of serotonin along with those of other monoamines. Some uptake-inhibiting antidepressant drugs inhibit the neuronal uptake of serotonin, although the original drugs in this class were relatively unspecific, also inhibiting the neuronal uptake of catecholamines and interacting directly with neuronal receptors such as the muscarinic cholinergic receptor, the histamine H1-receptor, α_1- and α_2-adrenergic receptors, and others. The mechanism of antidepressant action of the latter drugs was difficult to establish because of their lack of specificity.

Within the past decade or so, numerous drugs have emerged that inhibit selectively the neuronal reuptake of serotonin without directly affecting catecholamine neurons or neurotransmitter receptors. Several of these drugs, including fluoxetine, zimelidine, fluvoxamine, citalopram and paroxetine, have shown antidepressant efficacy in humans (Lemberger *et al.*, 1985; Asberg *et al.*, 1986). These latter drugs lack some of the side effects of tricyclic antidepressant drugs that result from block of cholinergic, histaminergic and adrenergic receptors and also lack the direct cardiac effects of the tricyclic drugs. Zimelidine was marketed as an antidepressant drug but had to be withdrawn because of side effects, including rare instances of the Guillain–Barre syndrome (Fagius *et al.*, 1985), which were not thought to be related to serotonin uptake inhibition. Some of the other selective inhibitors of serotonin uptake are being introduced into the marketplace as antidepressant drugs and offer the promise of effective treatment with reduction in side effects compared to most existing drugs.

The efficacy in depression of several structurally unrelated compounds that inhibit serotonin uptake but apparently lack other pharmacological similarities supports the idea that enhancement of central serotonergic function is a mechanism that can lead to alleviation of depressive symptoms. It follows that direct-acting serotonin agonists may also be effective anti-depressant agents, but so far this has not been demonstrated in clinical trials. An expected advantage of direct agonists would be efficacy independent of functionality of serotonin neurons. If the function of a serotonergic system was impaired such that the neurons were not releasing serotonin, then uptake inhibition would be unable to restore function, but a direct agonist acting on the appropriate receptor would be effective. There is little or no evidence of the identity of the serotonin receptor(s) involved in depression or in the action of antidepressant serotonergic drugs. Clinical evaluation of direct-acting serotonin agonists acting on 5HT-1A, 5HT-1B, 5HT-1C, 5HT-2 or other types of serotonin receptors may not only lead to superior, possibly faster acting, antidepressant drugs, but may also reveal more information about the etiology of the disease.

Several antidepressant drugs also are potent 5HT-2 antagonists (Fuxe *et al.*, 1977; Maj, 1981), and the possibility that antagonism of serotonin receptors is a (the) mechanism of their antidepressant action has been considered. Because most of those drugs also are amine uptake inhibitors, alternative possible mechanisms are obvious. Trazodone (Fig. 6) is an antidepressant drug whose major pharmacological action is antagonism of 5HT-2 receptors (Maj, 1981; Fuller *et al.*, 1984). Even with this drug, however, there is uncertainty about serotonin antagonism being its mechanism of antidepressant action, because it is metabolized extensively to *m*-chlorophenylpiperazine, a direct-acting serotonin agonist (Rurak and Melzacka, 1983; Suckow, 1983). The possible role of the metabolite acting to enhance serotonergic function must be considered as a potential explanation for the antidepressant efficacy of trazodone.

Although the more prevalent view has been that depression might be related to deficiency of central serotonergic function and that some antidepressant drugs might act by enhancing serotonergic function, an alternative view that depression might be a hyperfunctional serotonergic state and that serotonin antagonists would be effective treatments has been advanced (Aprison et al., 1982). Adaptive changes (up-regulation or down-regulation) in neurotransmitter receptors can occur after chronic treatment with antidepressant drugs, offering one possibility of reconciling these seemingly opposing views about serotonergic function following treatment with antidepressant drugs.

6.1.2 Anxiety

A possible relationship of brain serotonin to anxiety has long been considered. In the mid-1970s, the idea was suggested that a reduction in serotonergic function might be a mechanism involved in the anxiolytic action of benzodiazepines (Stein et al., 1975; Tye et al., 1977). This particular idea has fallen into disfavour (Panksepp and Cox, 1986) but has not been excluded as a possibility (Thiebot, 1986). Recently, two classes of serotonergic drugs—5HT-1A agonists and 5HT-2 antagonists—have been considered as anxiolytic agents.

Ritanserin is a relatively selective antagonist of 5HT-2 receptors that antagonizes LSD (Colpaert et al., 1985) and produces anxiolytic-like actions in animals (Gardner, 1986). A double-blind study in humans with generalized anxiety disorder has indicated ritanserin to be similar to lorazepam and better than placebo in efficacy, lacking the side effects associated with lorazepam (Ceulemans et al., 1985).

Buspirone is an anxiolytic drug with high affinity for the 5HT-1A subtype of serotonin receptor (Peroutka, 1985; Wander et al., 1986), apparently acting as a partial agonist at 5HT-1A receptors (Smith and Peroutka, 1986). The possibility that 5HT-1A interactions are involved in the anxiolytic efficacy of buspirone has been suggested (Peroutka, 1985). Consistent with that idea are the findings that other 5HT-1A agonists have anxiolytic-like actions in animals, and some have anxiolytic efficacy in humans. Ipsapirone and gepirone are structural analogues of buspirone with affinity for 5HT-1A sites and with anxiolytic actions in both animals and in humans (Traber et al., 1984; Eison et al., 1986; Csanalosi et al., 1987). 8-OH-DPAT is a selective 5HT-1A agonist with anxiolytic actions in some animal models (Engel et al., 1984). Compelling evidence for an involvement of 5HT-1A receptors in the clinical anxiolytic activity of buspirone and related compounds has not been presented. If 5HT-1A receptors are involved, is it activation or antagonism of those receptors that mediates the anxiolytic effect of buspirone? If buspirone is a partial agonist, either action might occur in vivo, depending on the number of receptors in the serotonergic system involved and on the tone of their activation by endogenous serotonin.

Another effect of selective 5HT-1A agonists, namely the increase in food intake, is suggested to occur by reduction of input to postsynaptic serotonin receptors secondary to activation of 5HT-1A autoreceptors that modulate serotonin release (Dourish *et al.*, 1986a). If a similar mechanism were involved in the anxiolytic action of buspirone, namely a reduction in serotonergic transmission, a commonality to the earlier postulate that benzodiazepines reduce anxiety by decreasing serotonergic transmission is suggested. Further consideration of that possibility might be warranted.

6.1.3 Alcoholism

Serotonin uptake inhibitors, serotonin precursors and direct-acting serotonin agonists have been reported to suppress alcohol drinking in rats selected or bred to drink ethanol solutions (Rockman *et al.*, 1982; Murphy *et al.*, 1985; Zabik *et al.*, 1985; Naranjo *et al.*, 1986), even in animals given a choice between an ethanol solution or water. Since many of the social factors involved in alcohol consumption in humans presumably are absent in rats, one should be cautious about extrapolating these findings to a therapeutic use for such drugs in human alcoholism. However, a limited amount of clinical data so far presented suggests that selective inhibitors of serotonin uptake can reduce alcohol intake in human subjects as well (Naranjo *et al.*, 1984, 1987).

6.2 OBESITY AND EATING DISORDERS

There is extensive evidence that brain serotonin neurons participate in the hypothalamic regulation of food intake (Blundell, 1984; Leibowitz and Shor-Posner, 1986). Numerous drugs that increase serotonin receptor activation by direct stimulation of the receptor or by increasing serotonin concentrations in the synaptic cleft decrease food intake in rats. *m*-Chlorophenylpiperazine (Samanin *et al.*, 1979), *m*-trifluoromethylphenylpiperazine (Fuller *et al.*, 1981b), quipazine (Samanin *et al.*, 1977), MK212 (Clineschmidt *et al.*, 1977a,b) and RU 24969 (Dourish *et al.*, 1986b) are examples of direct-acting serotonin agonists that decrease food intake. Serotonin uptake inhibitors decrease food intake in rats (Goudie *et al.*, 1976; Dumont *et al.*, 1981), as do serotonin-releasing drugs including fenfluramine (Rowland and Carlton, 1986) and *p*-chloroamphetamine (Kaergaard Nielsen *et al.*, 1967). Serotonergic drugs decrease stress-induced eating in rats, whereas amphetamine-related drugs do not (Antelman *et al.*, 1981). Serotonergic drugs selectively decrease carbohydrate consumption in rats, whereas amphetamine-related drugs non-selectively decrease total caloric intake (Wurtman and Wurtman, 1979). ($\pm$)-Fenfluramine has been marketed as an antiobesity drug for several years, and now (+)-fenfluramine, the active enantiomer in releasing serotonin, is being introduced into clinical use. Fluoxetine, zimelidine and fluvoxamine are serotonin uptake inhibitors that have caused decreases in body weight rather than increases typically seen with antidepressant drugs in patients being treated for mental depression and have decreased body weight in non-depressed obese patients (Simpson *et al.*, 1981; Smedegaard *et al.*, 1981; Abell *et al.*, 1986).

Recently, a certain class of direct-acting serotonin agonists have been found to increase food intake in rats, instead of decreasing it as most other serotonin agonists do. Those agonists which increase food intake are agonists that selectively activate the 5HT-1A receptor. In freely feeding rats, 8-OH-DPAT increased food intake at lower doses than those causing serotonin-related behavioural changes, although much higher doses decreased food intake in rats deprived of food for 24 h (Dourish *et al.*, 1985a,b). Apparently 8-OH-DPAT increases feeding by acting on autoreceptors on serotonin neurons, reducing serotonergic output (Bendotti and Samanin, 1986; Dourish *et al.*, 1986a), suggesting that feeding in rats was being limited by serotonergic tone. Subsequently, other selective 5HT-1A agonists, e.g. buspirone (Dourish *et al.*, 1986b), ipsapirone (Dourish *et al.*, 1986b) and LY 165163 (Wong and Fuller, 1987), have also been shown to increase food intake in rats.

6.3 ANALGESIA

Several lines of evidence implicate serotonin neurons in the central nervous system in pain and in the action of analgesic drugs. Serotonin neurons project to regions of the central nervous system known to be involved in nociceptive responsiveness (Basbaum and Fields, 1978; Roberts, 1984; Hylden *et al.*, 1986). Serotonin neurons apparently make synaptic input to enkephalin neurons (Glazer and Basbaum, 1984) and vice versa (Parenti *et al.*, 1983). Serotonin and enkephalin-related peptides co-exist in some neurons (Leger *et al.*, 1986). Drugs that enhance serotonergic transmission have antinociceptive activity in many animal tests (Ogren and Berge, 1984; Archer *et al.*, 1985), and drugs that decrease serotonergic transmission enhance nociceptive responses (Messing and Lytle, 1977). Serotonin uptake inhibitors enhance morphine analgesia in animals (Messing *et al.*, 1975; Hynes *et al.*, 1985). Zimelidine, a serotonin uptake inhibitor, has been reported to have clinically useful analgesic activity (Johansson and von Knorring, 1979; Gourlay *et al.*, 1986). Recently ritanserin, a 5HT-2 antagonist, has been reported to have analgesic effects in humans (Sandrini *et al.*, 1986).

6.4 MIGRAINE

Serotonin antagonists have been used for several years in the treatment of migraine (Lance *et al.*, 1970; Speight and Avery, 1972), although the exact mechanism of their action has been unknown. Serotonin receptors exist on cerebral blood vessels, on sensory nerves and in central pain pathways, providing at least three possible sites of action. Three types of serotonin receptors, namely 5HT-1A, 5HT-2 and 5HT-3 receptors, have been implicated in the actions of antimigraine drugs.

The efficacy of antimigraine drugs such as methysergide, ergotamine, dihydroergotamine and danitracen generally has been attributed to their ability to block vascular 5HT-2 receptors (Sulman *et al.*, 1977). However, at least some of these compounds can act as partial agonists and can potentiate serotonin-induced contraction of intracranial blood vessels (Hardebo *et al.*, 1978). Thus the exact involvement of vascular 5HT-2 receptors in the action of antimigraine drugs remains uncertain.

Hiner *et al.* (1986) reported that four antimigraine drugs, methysergide, cyproheptadine (−)-propranolol and pizotifen, all have high affinities for 5HT-1A receptors, and suggested that the 5HT-1A receptor may be a common site involved in the antimigraine action of these agents.

Recently, a 5HT-3 antagonist, MDL 72222, was reported to be efficacious in the treatment of migraine (Loisy *et al.*, 1985). Possibly, the stimulation of 5HT-3 receptors located on sensory neurons on intracranial blood vessels is involved in vascular headaches (Richardson *et al.*, 1986).

6.5 HYPERTENSION

There is some basis for considering that centrally acting serotonin agonists or peripheral serotonin antagonists might be antihypertensive agents. A role of central serotonin neurons in regulating blood pressure has been investigated extensively, but the physiological significance of such regulation is still uncertain (Kuhn *et al.*, 1980; Chalmers *et al.*, 1984). Some centrally acting serotonin agonists do lower blood pressure, perhaps acting via 5HT-1A receptors (Antonaccio and Kerwin, 1981; Martin and Lis, 1985).

Ketanserin has antihypertensive effects in experimental animals and in humans, and these effects had originally been attributed to block of vascular 5HT-2 receptors (De Cree et al., 1981; Wenting et al., 1982). Now it is clear that the lowering of blood pressure by ketanserin in rats is due to its α_1 blocking efficacy (Fozard, 1982; Kalkman et al., 1982). There continues to be uncertainty about the importance of 5HT-2 antagonism versus α_1 antagonism in the antihypertensive effects of ketanserin in humans (Ball et al., 1983; Vanhoutte, 1985) and therefore about the possibility that blockade of vascular 5HT-2 receptors is a mechanism that can be effective in treating hypertension in humans.

6.6 THROMBOSIS AND OTHER VASCULAR DISORDERS

The ability of serotonin to constrict most blood vessels and to amplify the vasoconstrictor responses to other substances, to enhance aggregation of blood platelets, and to be released from platelets upon aggregation and the serotonergic innervation of cerebral blood vessels raise the possibility of involvement of serotonin in various circulatory disorders (Houston and Vanhoutte, 1986; Scatton et al., 1985). Experimental findings in laboratory animals support the potential utility of serotonin antagonists in therapy of thrombosis or other vascular disorders. For instance, 5HT-2 antagonists abolished cyclic flow reductions in stenosed coronary arteries of open-chest dogs (Bush, 1987), a phenomenon believed due to repetitive occlusive platelet thrombus formation and dislodgement and thought to be mediated by serotonin (Ashton et al., 1986). Ketanserin restored peripheral collateral circulation in cats after acute thrombotic obstruction of the aorta (Nevel-steen et al., 1984). Mianserin, another 5HT-2 antagonist, had earlier been reported to improve hindlimb collateral blood flow in cats after aortic occlusion, suggesting that serotonin contributes to the inhibition of collateral blood flow following arterial thrombosis (Schaub et al., 1977).

7 Conclusion

Impressive advances have been made in the identification and development of drugs that increase or decrease serotonergic function by direct actions on serotonin receptors or by altering the amount of serotonin acting on those receptors. Currently such drugs are being used in the therapy of diseases like depression, migraine and obesity, and the promise of broader therapeutic uses is one factor that attracts researchers to the area. Selective inhibitors of serotonin uptake are available. Classes of drugs that are needed include serotonin releasers that act selectively and are not neurotoxic, and direct-acting agonists and antagonists acting specifically on each of the subtypes of serotonin receptors. The latter drugs not only have potential therapeutic applications but will be valuable tools in increasing our understanding of serotonin receptor subtypes and their mediation of the numerous physiological actions of serotonin.

References

Abell, C. A., Farquhar, D. L., Galloway, S. M., Steven, F., Philip, A. E., and Munro, J. F. (1986). *J. Psychosomatic Res.* **30**, 143–146.

Ahlenius, S., Larsson, K., Svensson, L., Hjorth, S., Carlsson, A., Lindberg, P., Wikstrom, H., Sanchez, D., Arvidsson, L.-E., Hacksell, U., and Nilsson, J. L. G. (1981). *Pharmacol. Biochem. Behav.* **15**, 785–792.

Antelman, S. M., Rowland, N., and Kocan, D. (1981). *In* "Anorectic Agents, Mechanisms of Action and Tolerance" (S. Garattini and R. Samanin, eds), pp. 45–62. Raven Press, New York.

Antonaccio, M. J., and Kerwin, L. (1981). *J. Cardiovasc. Pharmacol.* **3**, 1306–1311.

Aprison, M. H., Hingtgen, J. N., and Nagayama, H. (1982). *In* "New Vistas in Depression" (S. Langer, R. Takahashi, T. Segawa and M. Briley, eds), pp. 171–178. Pergamon Press, New York.

Archer, T., Minor, B. G., and Post, C. (1985). *Brain Res.* **333**, 55–61.

Arvidsson, L.-E., Hacksell, U., Nilsson, J. L. G., Hjorth, S., Carlsson, A., Lindberg, P., Sanchez, D., and Wikstrom, H. (1981). *J. Med. Chem.* **24**, 921–923.

Asarch, K. B., Ransom, R. W., and Shih, J. C. (1985). *Life Sci.* **36**, 1265–1273.

Asberg, M., Eriksson, B., Martensson, B., Traskman-Bendz, L., and Wagner, A. (1986). *J. Clin. Psychiat.* **47** (Suppl. 4), 23–35.

Ashton, J. H., Benedict, C. R., Fitzgerald, C., Raheja, S., Taylor, A., Campbell, W. B., Buma, L. M., and Willerson, J. T. (1986). *Circulation* **73**, 572–578.

Azmitia, E. C., and Gannon, P. J. (1986). *In* "Advances in Neurology", Vol. 43: Myoclonus, pp. 407–468. Raven Press, New York.

Ball, S. G., Zabludowski, J. R., and Robertson, J. I. S. (1983). *Br. Med. J.* **287**, 1065.

Basbaum, A. I., and Fields, H. L. (1978). *Ann. Neurol.* **4**, 451–462.

Bendotti, C., and Samanin, R. (1986). *Eur. J. Pharmacol.* **121**, 147–150.

Blackburn, T. P., Kemp, J. D., Martin, D. A., and Cox, B. (1984). *Psychopharmacology* **83**, 163–165.

Blundell, J. E. (1984). *Neuropharmacology* **23**, 1537–1551.

Bouillin, D. J., DuBoulay, G. H., and Rogers, A. T. (1978). *Br. J. Clin. Pharmacol.* **6**, 203–215.

Bradley, P. B., Engel, G., Feniuk, W., Fozard, J. R., Humphrey, P. P. A., Middlemiss, D. N., Mylecharane, E. J., Richardson, B. P., and Saxena, P. R. (1986). *Neuropharmacology* **25**, 563–576.

Brady, L. S., and Barrett, J. E. (1985). *J. Pharmacol. Exp. Ther.* **235**, 436–441.

Brittain, R. T., Butler, A., Coates, I. H., Fortune, D. H., Hagan, R., Hill, J. M., Humber, D. C., Humphrey, P. P. A., Ireland, S. J., Jack, D., Jordan, C. C., Oxford, A., Straughan, D. W., and Tyers, M. B. (1987). *Br. J. Pharmacol.* **90**, 87P.

Burns, D. B., and Mendels, J. (1979). *In* "Current Developments in Psychopharmacology"

(W. B. Essman and L. Valzelli, eds), Vol. 5, pp. 293–359. SP Medical and Scientific Books, New York.

Bush, L. R. (1987). *J. Pharmacol. Exp. Ther.* **240**, 674–682.

Ceulemans, D. L. S., Hoppenbrouwers, M.-L. J. A., Gelders, Y. G., and Reyntjens, A. J. M. (1985). *Pharmacopsychiatry* **18**, 303–305.

Chalmers, J. P., Minson, J. B., and Choy, V. (1984). *Hypertension 6* (Suppl. II), II-16–II-21.

Clineschmidt, B. V. (1979). *Gen. Pharmacol.* **10**, 287–290.

Clineschmidt, B. V., Hanson, H. M., Pflueger, A. B., and McGuffin, J. C. (1977a). *Psychopharmacology* **55**, 27–33.

Clineschmidt, B. V., McGuffin, J. C., and Pflueger, A. B. (1977b). *Eur. J. Pharmacol.* **44**, 65–74.

Clineschmidt, B. V., McGuffin, J. C., Pflueger, A. B., and Totaro, J. A. (1978). *Br. J. Pharmacol.* **62**, 579–589.

Cohen, M. L. (1984). *Drug Dev. Res.* **4**, 301–313.

Cohen, M. L., Fuller, R. W., and Kurz, K. D. (1983). *J. Pharmacol. Exp. Ther.* **227**, 327–332.

Cohen, M. L., Colbert, W., and Wittenauer, L. A. (1985a). *Drug Dev. Res.* **5**, 313–321.

Cohen, M. L., Kurz, K. D., Mason, N. R., Fuller, R. W., Marzoni, G. P., and Garbrecht, W. L. (1985b). *J. Pharmacol. Exp. Ther.* **235**, 319–323.

Colpaert, F. C., Meert, T. F., Niemegeers, C. J. E., and Janssen, P. A. J. (1985). *Psychopharmacology* **86**, 45–54.

Conn, P. J., and Sanders-Bush, E. (1985). *J. Pharmacol. Exp. Ther.* **234**, 195–203.

Conn, P. J., Sanders-Bush, E., Hoffman, B. J., and Hartig, P. R. (1986). *Proc. Natl. Acad. Sci.* **83**, 4086–4088.

Copp, F. C., Green, A. F., Hodson, H. F., Randall, A. W., and Sim, M. F. (1967). *Nature* **214**, 200–201.

Costall, B., Domeney, A. M., Naylor, R. J., and Tattersall, F. D. (1986a). *Neuropharmacology* **25**, 959–961.

Costall, B., Kelly, M. E., Naylor, R. J., Tan, C. C. W., and Tattersall, F. D. (1986b). *Neuropharmacology* **25**, 1293–1296.

Costall, B., Domeney, A. M., Hendrie, C. A., Kelly, M. E., Naylor, R. J., and Tyers, M. B. (1987a). *Br. J. Pharmacol.* **90**, 257P.

Costall, B., Domeney, A. M., Kelly, M. E., Naylor, R. J., and Tyers, M. B. (1987b). *Br. J. Pharmacol.* **90**, 89P.

Costall, B., Domeney, A. M., Naylor, R. J., and Tyers, M. B. (1987c). *Br. J. Pharmacol.* **90**, 243P.

Csanalosi, I., Schweizer, E., Case, W. G., and Rickels, K. (1987). *J. Clin. Psychopharmacol.* **7**, 31–33.

Cunningham, K. A., and Appel, J. B. (1986). *J. Pharmacol. Exp. Ther.* **237**, 369–377.

Cunningham, K. A., Callahan, P. M., and Appel, J. B. (1985). *Soc. Neurosci. Abstr.* **11**, 45.

Cunningham, K. A., Callahan, P. M., and Appel, J. B. (1986). *Psychopharmacology* **90**, 193–197.

De Cree, J., Leempoels, J., De Cock, W., Geukens, H., and Verhaegen, H. (1981). *Angiology* **32**, 137–144.

Dourish, C. T., Hutson, P. H., and Curzon, G. (1985a). *Brain Res. Bull.* **15**, 377–384.

Dourish, C. T., Hutson, P. H., and Curzon, G. (1985b). *Psychopharmacology* **86**, 197–204.

Dourish, C. T., Hutson, P. H., and Curzon, G. (1986a). *Psychopharmacology* **89**, 467–471.

Dourish, C. T., Hutson, P. H., Kennett, G. A., and Curzon, G. (1986b). *Appetite* **7** (Suppl.), 127–140.

Dumont, C., Laurent, J., Grandadam, A., and Boissier, J. R. (1981). *Life Sci.* **28**, 1939–1945.

Dunbar, A. W., McClelland, C. M., and Sanger, G. J. (1986). *Br. J. Pharmacol.* **88**, 319P.

Eison, A. S., Eison, M. S., Stanley, M., and Riblet, L. A. (1986). *Pharmacol. Biochem. Behav.* **24**, 701–707.

Engel, G., Gothert, M., Hoyer, D., Schlicker, E., and Hillenbrand, K. (1986). *Naunyn-Schmiedeberg's Arch. Pharmacol.* **332**, 1–7.

Engel, J. A., Hjorth, S., Svensson, K., Carlsson, A., and Liljequist, S. (1984). *Eur. J. Pharmacol.* **105**, 365–368.

Euvrard, C., and Boissier, J. R. (1980). *Eur. J. Pharmacol.* **63**, 65–72.

Fagius, J., Osterman, P. O., Siden, A., and Wilholm, B.-E. (1985). *Neurol. Neurosurg. Psychiatry* **48**, 65–69.

Feigenbaum, J., Yanai, J., and Klawans, H. L. (1983). *Int. J. Neurosci.* **18**, 205–210.

Fillion, G., Beaudoin, D., Fillion, M.-P., Rousselle, J.-C., Robaut, C., and Netter, Y. (1983). *J. Neural. Trans. Suppl.* **18**, 307–317.

Fozard, J. R. (1982). *J. Cardiovasc. Pharmacol.* **4**, 829–838.

Fozard, J. R. (1984). *Naunyn-Schmiedeberg's Arch. Pharmacol.* **326**, 36–44.

Frances, H., Lecrubier, Y., Puech, A. J., and Simon, P. (1980). *Psychopharmacology* **67**, 307–310.

Fuller, R. W., and Snoddy, H. D. (1979). *Endocrinology* **105**, 923–928.

Fuller, R. W., and Snoddy, H. D. (1984). *The Pharmacologist* **26**, 179.

Fuller, R. W., Snoddy, H. D., Perry, K. W., Roush, B. W., Molloy, B. B., Bymaster, F. P., and Wong, D. T. (1976). *Life Sci.* **18**, 925–934.

Fuller, R. W., Snoddy, H. D., Mason, N. R., and Molloy, B. B. (1978). *Eur. J. Pharmacol.* **52**, 11–16.

Fuller, R. W., Mason, N. R., and Molloy, B. B. (1980). *Biochem. Pharmacol.* **29**, 835–838.

Fuller, R. W., Snoddy, H. D., Mason, N. R., Hemrick-Luecke, S. K., and Clemens, J. A. (1981a). *J. Pharmacol. Exp. Ther.* **218**, 636–641.

Fuller, R. W., Snoddy, H. D., Mason, N. R., and Owen, J. E. (1981b). *Neuropharmacology* **20**, 155–162.

Fuller, R. W., Snoddy, H. D., and Mason, N. R. (1983). *Fed. Proc.* **42**, 459.

Fuller, R. W., Snoddy, H. D., and Cohen, M. L. (1984). *Neuropharmacology* **23**, 539–544.

Fuller, R. W., Kurz, K. D., Mason, N. R., and Cohen, M. L. (1986a). *Eur. J. Pharmacol.* **125**, 71–77.

Fuller, R. W., Snoddy, H. D., and Molloy, B. B. (1986b). *J. Pharmacol. Exp. Ther.* **239**, 454–459.

Fuxe, K., Holmstedt, B., and Jonsson, G. (1972). *Eur. J. Pharmacol.* **19**, 25–34.

Fuxe, K., Ogren, S.-O., Agnati, L., Gustafsson, J. A., and Jonsson, G. (1977). *Neurosci. Lett.* **6**, 339–343.

Gaddum, J. H., and Picarelli, Z. P. (1957). *Br. J. Pharmacol. Chemother.* **12**, 323–328.

Gardner, C. R. (1986). *Pharmacol. Biochem. Behav.* **24**, 1479–1485.

Glaser, T., and Traber, J. (1983). *Eur. J. Pharmacol.* **88**, 137–138.

Glazer, E. J., and Basbaum, A. I. (1984). *Brain Res.* **29**, 386–391.

Glennon, R. A., Titeler, M., and McKenney, J. D. (1984). *Life Sci.* **35**, 2505–2511.

Goldberg, H. L., and Finnerty, R. J. (1979). *Am. J. Psychiatr.* **136**, 1184–1187.

Goodwin, G. M., and Green, A. R. (1985). *Br. J. Pharmacol.* **84**, 743–753.

Goodwin, G. M., De Souza, R. J., and Green, A. R. (1986). *Neuropharmacology* **24**, 1187–1194.

Goudie, A. J., Thornton, E. W., and Wheeler, T. J. (1976). *J. Pharm. Pharmacol.* **28**, 318–320.

Gourlay, G. K., Cherry, D. A., Cousins, M. J., Love, B. L., Graham, J. R., and McLachlan, M. O. (1986). *Pain* **25**, 35–52.

Grahame-Smith, D. G. (1971). *Br. J. Pharmacol.* **43**, 856–864.

Green, A. R., and Heal, D. J. (1985). *In* "Neuropharmacology of Serotonin" (A. R. Green, ed.), pp. 326–365. Oxford University Press, Oxford.

Green, A. R., Youdim, M. B. H., and Grahame-Smith, D. G. (1976). *Neuropharmacology* **15**, 173–179.

Green, A. R., Guy, A. P., and Gardner, C. R. (1984). *Neuropharmacology* **23**, 655–661.

Gudelsky, G. A., Koenig, J. I., and Meltzer, H. Y. (1986). *Neuropharmacology* **25**, 1307–1313.

Haigler, H. J., and Aghajanian, G. K. (1977). *Fed. Proc.* **36**, 2159–2164.

Hall, M. D., El Mestikawy, S., Emerit, M. B., Pichat, L., Hamon, M., and Gozlan, H. (1985). *J. Neurochem.* **44**, 1685–1696.

Hamon, M., Bourgoin, S., Enjalbert, A., Bockaert, J., Hery, F., Turneaux, J. P., and Glowinski, J. (1976). *Naunyn-Schiedeberg's Arch. Pharmacol.* **294**, 99–108.

Hamon, M., Bourgoin, S., Gozlan, H., Hall, M. D., Goetz, C., Artaud, F., and Horn, A. S. (1984). *Eur. J. Pharmacol.* **100**, 263–276.

Hamon, M., Cossery, J.-M., Spampinato, U., and Gozlan, H. (1986). *Trends Pharmacol. Sci.* **7**, 336–338.

Hardebo, J. E., Edvinsson, L., Owman, C., and Svendgaard, N.-A. (1978). *Neurology* **28**, 64–70.

Hashimoto, K., Ohno, N., Murakami, K., Kageyama, J., Aoki, Y., and Takahara, J. (1982). *Endocrinol. Japon* **29**, 383–388.

Heninger, G. R., Charney, D. S., and Price, L. H. (1985). *Abstr. Am. Coll. Neuropsychopharmacol.*, p. 65.

Heuring, R. E., and Peroutka, S. J. (1987). *J. Neurosci.* **7**, 894–903.

Hiner, B. C., Ison, P. J., and Peroutka, S. J. (1985). *Soc. Neurosci. Abstr.* **11**, 135.

Hiner, B. C., Roth, H. L., and Peroutka, S. J. (1986). *Ann. Neurol.* **19**, 511–513.

Hjorth, S. (1985). *J. Neural Trans.* **61**, 131–135.

Hjorth, S., Carlsson, A., Lindberg, P., Sanchez, D., Wikstrom, H., Arvidsson, L.-E., Hacksell, U., and Nilsson, J. L. G. (1982). *J. Neural Trans.* **55**, 169–188.

Hong, E. (1981). *In* "Molecular Basis of Drug Action" (T. P. Singer and R. N. Ondarza, eds), pp. 247–252. Elsevier-North Holland, New York.

Hong, E., and Pardo, E. G. (1966). *J. Pharmacol. Exp. Ther.* **153**, 259–265.

Hong, E., Sancilio, L. F., Vargas, R., and Pardo, E. G. (1969). *Eur. J. Pharmacol.* **6**, 274–280.

Houston, D. S., and Vanhoutte, P. M. (1986). *Drugs* **31**, 149–163.

Hoyer, D., Engel, G., and Kalkman, H. O. (1985a). *Eur. J. Pharmacol.* **118**, 1–12.

Hoyer, D., Engel, G., and Kalkman, H. O. (1985b). *Eur. J. Pharmacol.* **118**, 13–23.

Hoyer, D., Pazos, A., Probst, A., and Palacios, J. M. (1986). *Brain Res.* **376**, 85–96.

Hylden, J. L. K., Hayashi, H., Ruda, M. A., and Dubner, R. (1986). *Brain Res.* **370**, 401–404.

Hynes, M. D., Lochner, M. A., Bemis, K. G., and Hymson, D. L. (1985). *Life Sci.* **36**, 2317–2323.

Invernizzi, R., Cotecchia, S., De Blasi, A., Mennini, T., Pataccini, R., and Samanin, R. (1981). *Neurochem. Int.* **3**, 239–244.

Jacoby, J. H., and Lytle, L. D. (eds) (1978). *Ann. N.Y. Acad. Sci.* **305**, 1–702.

Janssen, P. A. J. (1985). *J. Cardiovasc. Pharmacol.* **7** (Suppl. 7), S2–S11.

Johansson, F., and von Knorring, L. (1979). *Pain* **7**, 69–78.

Kaergaard Nielsen, C., Magnussen, M. P., Kampmann, E., and Frey, H.-H. (1967). *Arch. Int. Pharmacodyn.* **170**, 428–444.

Kalkman, H. O., Timmermans, P. B. M. W. M., and Van Zwieten, P. A. (1982). *J. Pharmacol. Exp. Ther.* **222**, 227–231.

Kendall, D. A., and Nahorski, S. R. (1985). *J. Pharmacol. Exp. Ther.* **233**, 473–479.

Kennis, L. E. J., Vandenberk, J., Boey, J. M., Mertens, J. C., Van Heertum, A. H. M., Janssen, M., and Awouters, F. (1986). *Drug Dev. Res.* **8**, 133–140.

Koe, B. K., and Weissman, A. (1966). *J. Pharmacol. Exp. Ther.* **154**, 499–516.

Koenig, J. I., Gudelsky, G. A., and Meltzer, H. Y. (1985). *Soc. Neurosci. Abstr.* **11**, 359.

Koenig, J. I., Meltzer, H. Y., and Gudelsky, G. A. (1986). *Soc. Neurosci. Abstr.* **12**, 1235.

Kuhn, D. M., Wolf, W. A., and Lovenberg, W. (1980). *Hypertension* **2**, 243–255.

Laduron, P. M., Janssen, P. F. M., and Leysen, J. E. (1982). *Eur. J. Pharmacol.* **81**, 43–48.

Lance, J. W., Anthony, M., and Somerville, B. (1970). *Br. Med. J.* **2**, 327–330.

Lansdown, M. J. R., Nash, H. L., Preston, P. R., Wallis, D. I., and Williams, R. G. (1980). *Br. J. Pharmacol.* **68**, 525–532.

Leger, L., Charnay, Y., Dubois, P. M., and Jouvet, M. (1986). *Brain Res.* **362**, 63–73.

Leibowitz, S. F., and Shor-Posner, G. (1986). *Appetite* **7** (Suppl.), 1–14.

Lemberger, L., Fuller, R. W., and Zerbe, R. L. (1985). *Clin. Neuropharmacol.* **8**, 299–327.

Leysen, J. E., Awouters, F., Kennis, L., Laduron, P. M., Vandenberk, J., and Janssen, P. A. J. (1981). *Life Sci.* **28**, 1015–1022.

Leysen, J. E., Niemegeers, C. J. E., van Nueten, J. M., and Laduron, P. M. (1982). *Mol. Pharmacol.* **21**, 301–314.

Loisy, C., Beorchia, S., Centonze, V., Fozard, J. R., Schechter, P. J., and Tell, G. P. (1985). *Cephalalgia* **5**, 79–82.

Lucki, I. (1986). *Psychopharmacology* **89**, S55.

Maj, J. (1981). *Pharmakopsychiatry* **14**, 35–39.

Maj, J., Palider, W., and Rawlow, A. (1979). *J. Neural Transmission* **44**, 237–248.

Martin, G. E., and Lis, E. V. Jr. (1985). *Arch. Int. Pharmacodyn.* **273**, 251–261.

Martin, L. L., and Sanders-Bush, E. (1982). *Neuropharmacology* **21**, 445–450.

Mawson, C., and Whittington, H. (1970). *Br. J. Pharmacol.* **39**, 223P.

McCall, R. B., and Aghajanian, G. K. (1979). *Brain Res.* **169**, 11–27.

McKenney, J. D., and Glennon, R. A. (1986). *Pharmacol. Biochem. Behav.* **24**, 43–47.

Medon, P. J., Leeling, J. L., and Phillips, B. M. (1973). *Life Sci.* **13**, 685–691.

Melzacka, M., Boksa, J., and Maj, J. (1979). *J. Pharm. Pharmacol.* **31**, 855–856.

Messing, R. B., and Lytle, L. D. (1977). *Pain* **4**, 1–21.

Messing, R. B., Phebus, L., Fisher, L. A., and Lytle, L. D. (1975). *Psychopharmacol. Commun.* **1**, 511–521.

Middlemiss, D. N., and Fozard, J. R. (1983). *Eur. J. Pharmacol.* **90**, 151–153.

Miner, W. D., and Sanger, G. J. (1986). *Br. J., Pharmacol.* **88**, 497–499.

Moser, L. R., Kaiser, J. A., and Hardy, R. A. Jr. (1966). U.S. Patent No. 3,253,989, 31 May.

Mueller, E. A., Murphy, D. L., and Sunderland, T. (1986). *Psychopharmacology* **89**, 388–391.

Murphy, D. L., Campbell, I. C., and Costa, J. L. (1978). *Progr. Neuro-Psychopharmacol.* **2**, 1–31.

Murphy, J. M., Waller, M. B., Gatto, G. J., McBride, W. J., Lumeng, L., and Li, T.-K. (1985). *Alcohol* **2**, 349–352.

Naranjo, C. A., Sellers, E. M., and Lawrin, M. O. (1986). *J. Clin. Psychiatr.* **47** (Supp. 4), 16–22.

Naranjo, C. A., Sellers, E. M., Roach, C. A., Woodley, D. V., Sanchez-Craig, M., and Sykora, K. (1984). *Clin. Pharmacol. Ther.* **35**, 374–381.

Naranjo, C. A., Sellers, E. M., Sullivan, J. T., Woodley, D. V., Kadlec, K., and Sykora, K. (1987). *Clin. Pharmacol. Ther.* **41**, 266–274.

Nelson, D. L., and Taylor, E. W. (1986). *Eur. J. Pharmacol.* **124**, 207–208.

Nelson, D. L., Pedigo, N. W., and Yamamura, H. I. (1980). *In* "Psychopharmacology and Biochemistry of Neurotransmitter Receptors" (H. I. Yamamura, R. W. Olsen and E. Usdin, eds), pp. 325–338. Elsevier, North-Holland, Amsterdam.

Nelson, D. L., Schnellmann, R., and Smitt, M. (1983). *In* "Molecular Pharmacology of Neurotransmitter Receptors" (T. Segawa, H. I. Yamamura and K. Kurijama, eds), pp. 103–114. Raven Press, New York.

Nevelsteen, A., De Clerck, F., Loots, W., and De Gryse, A. (1984). *Arch. Int. Pharmacodyn.* **270**, 268–279.

Nielsen, E. B., White, F. J., Holohean, A. M., Callahan, P. M., and Appel, J. B. (1982). *Life Sci.* **31**, 2433–2439.

Niemegeers, C. J. E., Colpaert, F. C., Leysen, J. E., Awouters, F., and Janssen, P. A. J. (1983). *Drug Dev. Res.* **3**, 123–135.

Panksepp, J., and Cox, J. F. (1986). *Behav. Brain Sci.* **9**, 340–341.

Ogren, S.-O., and Berge, O.-G. (1984). *Neuropharmacology* **23**, 915–924.

Parenti, M., Tirone, F., Olgiati, V. R., and Groppetti, A. (1983). *Brain Res.* **280**, 317–322.

Pawlowski, L., Siwanowicz, J., Bigajska, K., and Przegalinski, E. (1985). *Pol. J. Pharmacol. Pharm.* **37**, 179–186.

Pazos, A., Hoyer, D., and Palacios, J. M. (1984a). *Eur. J. Pharmacol.* **106**, 539–546.

Pazos, A., Hoyer, D., and Palacios, J. M. (1984b). *Eur. J. Pharmacol.* **106**, 531–538.

Peroutka, S. J. (1985). *Biol. Psychiatr.* **20**, 971–979.

Peroutka, S. J. (1986). *J. Neurochem.* **47**, 529–540.

Peroutka, S. J., and Snyder, S. H. (1979). *Mol. Pharmacol.* **16**, 687–689.

Peroutka, S. J., Heuring, R. E., Mauk, M. D., and Kocsis, J. D. (1986). *Psychopharmacol. Bull.* **22**, 813–817.

Ponzio, F., Consolazione, A., Calderini, G., Achilli, G., Rochetti, M., and Algeri, S. (1981). *Life Sci.* **29**, 83–91.

Quattrone, A., Schettini, G., Annunziato, L., and Di Renzo, G. (1981). *Eur. J. Pharmacol.* **76**, 9–13.

Ransom, R. W., Asarch, K. B., and Shih, J. C. (1986). *J. Neurochem.* **46**, 68–75.

Reynolds, L. S., Seymour, P. A., and Heym, J. H. (1986). *J. Soc. Neurosci. Abstr.* **12**, 481.

Richardson, B. P., and Engel, G. (1986). *Trends Neurol. Sci.* **9**, 424–428.

Richardson, B. P., Engel, G., Donatsch, P., and Stadler, P. A. (1985). *Nature* **316**, 126–131.

Richardson, B. P., Donatsch, P., Engel, G., and Giger, R. (1986). *J. Pharmacol.* **17**, 99–100.

Roberts, M. H. T. (1984). *Neuropharmacology* **23**, 1529–1536.

Rockman, G. E., Amit, Z., Brown, Z. W., Bourque, C., and Ogren, S.-O. (1982). *Neuropharmacology* **21**, 341–347.

Rodriguez, R., and Pardo, E. G. (1971). *Psychopharmacologia* **21**, 89–100.

Rowland, N. E., and Carlton, J. (1986). *Progr. Neurobiol.* **27**, 13–62.

Rurak, A., and Melzacka, M. (1983). *Pol. J. Pharmacol. Pharm.* **35**, 241–247.

Safdy, M. E., Kurchacova, E., Schut, R. N., Vidrio, H., and Hong, E. (1982). *J. Med. Chem.* **25**, 723–730.

Samanin, R., Bendotti, C., Miranda, F., and Garattini, S. (1977). *J. Pharm. Pharmacol.* **29**, 53.

Samanin, R., Mennini, T., Ferraris, A., Bendotti, C., Borsini, F., and Garattini, S. (1979). *Naunyn-Schmiedeberg's Arch. Pharmacol.* **308**, 159–163.

Sandrini, G., Alfonsi, E., De Rysky, C., Marini, S., Facchinetti, F., and Nappi, G. (1986). *Eur. J. Pharmacol.* **130**, 311–314.

Scatton, B., Duverger, D., L'Heureux, R., Serrano, A., Fage, D., Nowicki, J.-P., and MacKenzie, E. T. (1985). *Brain Res.* **345**, 219–229.

Schaub, R. G., Meyers, K. M., and Sande, R. D. (1977). *J. Lab. Clin. Med.* **90**, 645–653.

Schecter, M. D., and Concannon, J. T. (1982). *Pharmacol. Biochem. Behav.* **17**, 393–397.

Schlicker, E., and Gothert, M. (1981). *Naunyn-Schmiedeberg's Arch. Pharmacol.* **317**, 204–208.

Shih, J. C., Asarch, K. B., and Ransom, R. (1986). *Psychopharmacol. Bull.* **22**, 818–824.

Sills, M. A., Wolfe, B. B., and Frazer, A. (1984). *J. Pharmacol. Exp. Ther.* **231**, 480–487.

Simonovic, M., and Meltzer, H. Y. (1983). *Brain Res.* **272**, 269–275.

Simonovic, M., Gudelsky, G. A., and Meltzer, H. Y. (1984). *J. Neural Trans.* **59**, 143–149.

Simpson, R. J., Lawton, D. J., Watt, M. H., and Tiplady, B. (1981). *Br. J. Clin. Pharmacol.* **11**, 96–98.

Smedegaard, J., Christiansen, P., and Skrumsager, B. (1981). *Int. J. Obesity* **5**, 377–378.

Smith, L. M., and Peroutka, S. J. (1986). *Pharmacol. Biochem. Behav.* **24**, 1513–1519.

Speight, T. M., and Avery, G. S. (1972). *Drugs* **3**, 159–203.

Stein, L., Wise, C. D., and Belluzzi, J. D. (1975). *In* "Mechanism of Action of Benzo-diazepines" (E. Costa and P. Greengard, eds), pp. 29–44. Raven Press, New York.

Suckow, R. F. (1983). *J. Liq. Chromatogr.* **6**, 2195–2208.

Sulman, F. G., Pfeifer, Y., and Superstine, E. (1977). *Headache* **17**, 203–207.

Svensson, L., and Ahlenius, S. (1983). *Psychopharmacology* **79**, 104–107.

Symoens, J. (1982). *In* "5-Hydroxytryptamine in Peripheral Reactions" (F. De Clerck and P. M. Vanhoutte, eds), pp. 199–212. Raven Press, New York.

Thiebot, M. H. (1986). *Pharmacol. Biochem. Behav.* **24**, 1471–1477.

Traber, J., Davies, M. A., Dompert, W. U., Glaser, T., Schuurman, T., and Seidel, P.-R. (1984). *Brain Res. Bull.* **12**, 741–744.

Tye, N. C., Everitt, B. J., and Iversen, S. D. (1977). *Nature* **268**, 741–743.

Vanhoutte, P. M. (1985). *J. Cardiovasc. Pharmacol.* **7** (Suppl. 7), S105–S109.

Wander, T. J., Nelson, A., Okazaki, H., and Richelson, E.. (1986). *Eur. J. Pharmacol.* **132**, 115–121.

Wenting, G. J., Man in 'T Veld, A. J., Woittiez, A. J., Boomsma, F., and Schalekamp, M. A. D. H. (1982). *Clin. Sci.* **63**, 435S–438S.

Wong, D. T., and Fuller, R. W. (1987). *Int. J. Obes.* **11**(Suppl. 3), 125–133.

Wouters, W., Janssen, C. G. M., Van Dun, J., Thijssen, J. B. A., and Laduron, P. M. (1986). *J. Med. Chem.* **29**, 1663–1668.

Wurtman, J. J., and Wurtman, R. J. (1979). *Life Sci.* **24**, 895–904.

Yagaloff, K. A., and Hartig, P. R. (1986). *Mol. Pharmacol.* **29**, 120–125.

Yarbrough, G. G., Singh, D. K., and Pettibone, D. J. (1984). *Neuropharmacology* **23**, 1271–1277.

Yocca, F. D., Smith, D. W., Hyslop, D. W., and Maayani, S. (1986a). *Soc. Neurosci. Abstr.* **12**, 422.

Yocca, F. D., Hyslop, D. K., Taylor, D. P., and Maayani, S. (1986b). *Fed. Proc.* **45**, 436.

Zabik, J. E., Binkerd, K., and Roache, J. D. (1985). *In* "Research Advances in New Psychopharmacological Treatments for Alcoholism" (C. A. Naranjo and E. M. Sellers, eds), pp. 87–101. Excerpta Medica, Amsterdam.

Recent Advances in GABA Agonists, Antagonists and Uptake Inhibitors: Structure–Activity Relationships and Therapeutic Potential

POVL KROGSGAARD-LARSEN, HANS HJEDS, ERIK FALCH, FLEMMING S. JØRGENSEN and LONE NIELSEN

Department of Chemistry BC, The Royal Danish School of Pharmacy, Copenhagen, Denmark

ADVANCES IN DRUG RESEARCH, VOL. 17
ISBN 0-12-013317-2

1 Introduction

The neutral amino acid, 4-aminobutanoic acid (**1**, GABA), is an inhibitory neurotransmitter which plays an important role in the control of neuronal activity in the mammalian central nervous system (CNS). GABA is involved in the regulation of many physiological mechanisms including the secretion of a number of hormones (Racagni and Donoso, 1986) such as prolactin (Müller *et al.*, 1983) and growth hormone (Enna, 1981). GABA also plays a role in the control of cardiovascular functions (Antonaccio and Taylor, 1977; DeFeudis, 1981; Gillis *et al.*, 1982; Brennan *et al.*, 1983; Mesdjian *et al.*, 1983; Thyagarajan *et al.*, 1983; DiMicco *et al.*, 1984) and is involved in the neuronal mechanisms underlying pain (Hill *et al.*, 1981; DeFeudis, 1982; Grognet *et al.*, 1983; Andree *et al.*, 1983; Hynes *et al.*, 1984; Hammond and Drower, 1984; Sivam and Ho, 1985; Moreau and Fields, 1986; Zorn *et al.*, 1986), and anxiety (Cananzi *et al.*, 1980; Hoehn-Saric, 1983; Biggio and Costa, 1986). Feeding (Blavet *et al.*, 1982) and aggressive behaviour (Mandel *et al.*, 1979; Simler *et al.*, 1982; Ciesielski *et al.*, 1985) in animals are also under GABA control. The growing interest in the pharmacology of GABA has been stimulated by the findings that GABA dysfunctions may play an important role in some neurological and psychiatric disorders. Analysis of brain tissue samples from sites near seizure foci in epileptic patients or in animals made epileptic have revealed severe impairments of the GABA system (Morselli *et al.*, 1981; Fariello *et al.*, 1984; Nistico *et al.*, 1986). The low levels of the GABA-synthesizing enzyme (*S*)-glutamate decarboxylase (GAD), and the reduced GABA uptake capacity measured in different models of epilepsy probably reflect more or less advanced stages of degeneration of GABA neurons (Ribak *et al.*, 1979; Ross and Craig, 1981; Ribak, 1985; Roberts *et al.*, 1985; Olsen *et al.*, 1985; Houser *et al.*, 1986; Löscher and Schwartz-Porsche, 1986; Piredda *et al.*, 1987). Indirect evidence derived from numerous animal studies strongly supports the view that impairments of the GABA-mediated neurotransmission are major factors underlying epileptic phenomena (Meldrum, 1975, 1982).

Low levels of GABA and GAD have been measured in post-mortem brain tissues from patients dying with Huntington's chorea (Enna *et al.*, 1976; Chase *et al.*, 1979; Hamel *et al.*, 1981), and neurochemical studies have disclosed abnormalities of GABA receptors in certain regions of brains of choreic patients (Olsen *et al.*, 1980; Van Ness *et al.*, 1982; Kish *et al.*, 1983). There is circumstantial evidence for GABA dysfunctions in schizophrenia (Bird *et al.*, 1979; Van Kammen *et al.*, 1982), and these observations have recently been supported by receptor binding studies demonstrating GABA receptor abnormalities in autopsied brains of chronic schizophrenics (Hanada *et al.*, 1987). A GABA-ergic contribution to the symptoms in parkinsonian (Lloyd *et al.*, 1975; McGeer and McGeer, 1976; Lloyd *et al.*, 1977; Rinne *et al.*, 1978; Marsden and Sheehy, 1981) and depressed (Petty and Coffman, 1984; Lloyd and Pilc, 1984) patients has been proposed. Remarkably low plasma GABA levels have been measured in alcoholics (Petty and Coffman, 1984), and accumulating evidence strongly supports the view that ethanol has severe effects on GABA receptors (Davidoff, 1973; Frye *et al.*, 1983; Rastogi *et al.*, 1986).

These aspects clearly focus attention on the various processes and mechanisms associated with GABA-mediated neurotransmission in the CNS as potential targets for clinically useful drugs (Krogsgaard-Larsen *et al.*, 1979b).

2 Multiplicity of GABA-Operated Synaptic Mechanisms

The biochemical pathways underlying the biosynthesis and catabolism of GABA have largely been mapped out and the key enzymes identified and characterized (Roberts *et al.*, 1976; Mandel and DeFeudis, 1979; Okada and Roberts, 1982; Hertz *et al.*, 1983). Although the relative importance of the various biosynthetic routes for GABA have not been determined precisely, it is generally accepted that the major pathway involves decarboxylation of (S)-glutamic acid (GLU) to GABA catalysed by the enzyme GAD (Fig. 1). The apparent multiplicity of GAD (Spink and Martin, 1983) and the fact that GLU has a variety of additional functions in the CNS (Hertz *et al.*, 1983), including a role as the major excitatory neurotransmitter (Roberts *et al.*, 1986), do, however, make quantitative studies difficult.

GABA is released from the presynaptic terminals via a specific release system (Hertz *et al.*, 1983). This release system, which may be regulated by autoreceptors (Bowery, 1983; Fig. 1), is, at least partially, dependent on calcium ions (Arias and Tapia, 1986).

The initial step of the catabolism of GABA is transformation into succinic semialdehyde (SSA). This transamination reaction, which is catalysed by GABA:2-oxoglutarate aminotransferase (GABA-T) (Roberts *et al.*, 1976; Mandel and DeFeudis, 1979; Okada and Roberts, 1982; Hertz *et al.*, 1983), takes place within presynaptic GABA terminals as well as surrounding glia

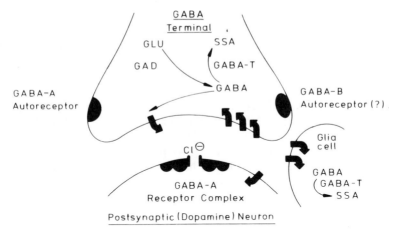

FIG. 1. A schematic illustration of an axo-somatic GABA-operated synapse containing GABA-A and GABA-B autoreceptors.

cells (Fig. 1). Extracellular enzymatic degradation does not seem to play any role in the inactivation of GABA.

Since the discovery of high-affinity GABA uptake systems in brain tissue preparations (Iversen and Neal, 1968; Iversen and Johnston, 1971), the physiological role of these membrane processes has been the subject of extensive studies. It is now generally accepted that these mechanisms are concerned with the removal of synaptically released GABA as part of the termination of the GABA neurotransmission process, but the precise mechanism of action, including the time course and capacity, of these mechanisms *in vivo* are not fully understood (Martin, 1976; Schousboe, 1981; Krogsgaard-Larsen *et al.*, 1987). The involvement of neuronal as well as glial cells in high-affinity GABA uptake has been demonstrated using a variety of different techniques and model systems (Martin, 1976; Schousboe, 1981). Studies of the uptake of GABA into isolated nerve endings (synaptosomes) have revealed the presence of both high- and low-affinity transport systems (Levi and Raiteri, 1973; Hitzemann and Loh, 1978). Recent GABA uptake data have been interpreted in terms of the existence of three rather than two transport systems for GABA in nerve terminals (Wood and Sidhu, 1986). GABA uptake data obtained from studies using cultured cells from the mammalian CNS are consistent with heterogeneity not only of neuronal, but also of glial transport mechanisms (Larsson *et al.*, 1983, 1985). It has recently been proposed that facilitated diffusion of GABA into the postsynaptic membrane rather than carrier-mediated transport into terminals and glia cells may constitute the primary event in the termination of the synaptic actions of GABA with subsequent transfer of GABA from the postsynaptic cell to nerve terminals and/or glia cells (Cupello and Hydén, 1985, 1986; Hydén et al., 1986). The amount of GABA accumulated in terminals, but not that taken up by glia cells, is partially re-used as neurotransmitter substance (Chase and Walters, 1976; Martin, 1976; Schousboe, 1981).

The synaptic release of GABA could possibly be enhanced by selectively augmenting the synthesis of this amino acid or, alternatively, via selective blockade of putative GABA autoreceptors (Fig. 1). While the former approach has not yet been the subject of systematic exploration (Chase and Walters, 1976), some pharmacological interest has been focused on GABA autoreceptors. Based on a simple synaptosomal model, assumed to reflect GABA autoreceptor activity, the pharmacological characteristics of such putative autoreceptors have been elucidated (see Section 5).

Electrophysiological and receptor binding studies have been used to detect GABA receptors and to identify subtypes of these receptors (Enna, 1983; Bowery, 1984). GABA receptors are now divided into two main classes: GABA-A receptors, which are blocked by the alkaloid bicuculline (**61**) (see Fig. 14) or bicuculline methochloride (**5**, BMC) (see Fig. 3) (Curtis et al., 1971; Curtis and Johnston, 1974), and bicuculline- or BMC-insensitive GABA receptors, including GABA-B receptors (Bowery, 1983). Both classes of GABA receptors probably are heterogeneous (Enna, 1983).

GABA-A receptors are coupled to a chloride ion channel (Fig. 1; Curtis and Johnston, 1974; Krnjevic, 1974), and activation of this receptor results in a net influx or efflux of chloride ions, depending on the prevailing concentration gradient. GABA-A receptors include postsynaptic (axo-somatic or axo-dendritic) as well as presynaptic (axo-axonic; Fig. 2) receptors. The postsynaptic GABA-A receptor, which actually is a receptor complex containing a number of subsynaptic receptors (see Fig. 3, Section 3), regulates the passage of chloride ions, in such a way that receptor activation causes hyperpolarization of the cell membrane and, thus, decreased sensitivity of the neuron to excitatory input. Activation of presynaptic GABA-A receptors normally leads to net efflux of chloride ions, causing partial depolarization (Curtis, 1978; Simmonds, 1984; see Section 4).

GABA-A receptors also include extrasynaptic receptors (Fig. 2; see Section 4), and there are reports supporting the view that GABA-A receptors can be further subdivided. Thus, the agonist profile and sensitivity to antagonists of GABA-A receptors in the mammalian spinal cord and cerebral cortex appear to be different (Krogsgaard-Larsen, 1983), and some pharmacological effects of GABA-A agonists have shown resistance to antagonism by BMC (**5**) (Krogsgaard-Larsen et al., 1986; Zorn et al., 1986).

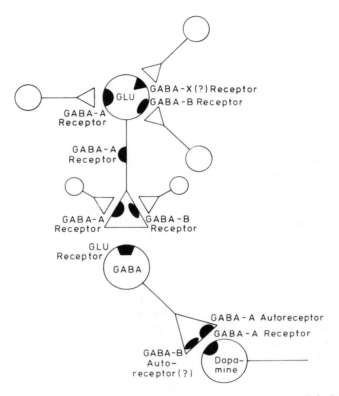

Fig. 2. A schematic illustration of the multiplicity of GABA receptors and the location of different types of GABA receptors.

Within the group of central bicuculline- and BMC-insensitive GABA receptors, the GABA-B receptors have been most extensively studied (Bowery, 1983, 1984). These receptors are activated by GABA and, in contrast to GABA-A receptors, also by the GABA analogue baclofen (see Fig. 23, Section 6.1). Although very little is known about the physiological role of GABA-B receptors, they seem to regulate the release of certain neurotransmitters, including (GLU), as exemplified in Figs 2 and 22. Accumulating evidence suggests that GABA-B receptors are predominantly located presynaptically and that they affect neurotransmitter release via regulation of a calcium ion channel (Bowery, 1983). In a recent report postsynaptically located GABA-B receptors linked to potassium channels have been described (Ogata *et al.*, 1987). GABA-B receptors have also been detected and characterized in a variety of tissue preparations of peripheral origin (Bowery *et al.*, 1984; Erdö and Bowery, 1986), and neurochemical data have been interpreted in terms of the presence of presynaptic GABA-B receptors on GABA terminals (Anderson and Mitchell, 1985; Fig. 2). Accumulating evidence derived from neurochemical and pharmacological studies suggests that GABA-operated receptors different from GABA-A and GABA-B receptor sub-types ("GABA-X receptors") exist in the mammalian CNS (Johnston and Allan, 1984; Johnston *et al.*, 1984; Krogsgaard-Larsen *et al.*, 1986; Zorn *et al.*, 1986).

3 Postsynaptic GABA-A Receptor Complex

Our present knowledge of the structure of the postsynaptic GABA-A receptor complex (Fig. 1) is summarized in Fig. 3 (Braestrup and Nielsen, 1983; Tallman, 1983; Haefely *et al.*, 1985; Olsen and Venter, 1986). Following the demonstration of saturable binding of ^{3}H-GABA to brain synaptic membranes (Peck *et al.*, 1973; Zukin *et al.*, 1974; Enna and Snyder, 1975), a number of radioactive ligands, including the tritiated forms of the specific GABA-A agonists isoguvacine (**2**) (Morin and Wasterlain, 1980), piperidine-4-sulphonic acid (**3**, P4S) (Krogsgaard-Larsen *et al.*, 1981a; Falch and Krogsgaard-Larsen, 1982) and 4,5,6,7-tetrahydroisoxazolo[5,4-*c*]pyridin-3-ol (**4**, THIP) (Falch and Krogsgaard-Larsen, 1982; Fig. 3), were introduced for GABA-A receptor binding studies. Furthermore, ^{3}H-BMC (**5**) (Möhler and Okada, 1977a; Olsen and Snowman, 1983) and ^{3}H-SR 95531 (**67**) (see Fig. 14; Heaulme *et al.*, 1986a), an analogue of the GABA-A antagonist SR 42641 (**6**) (Fig. 3), have been used as ligands for studies of GABA-A receptor sites.

Computer-aided analyses of such binding data are consistent with the presence of two or, perhaps more likely, three GABA receptor binding sites, as exemplified for GABA and THIP in Fig. 4. These receptor sites are not interconvertible under the assay conditions (Olsen and Venter, 1986). Normally, the affinity of ligands for the low-affinity binding site is too low for satisfactory characterization (Olsen *et al.*, 1981; Falch and Krogsgaard-Larsen, 1982).

The physiological relevance of these multiple binding sites is unknown. In general, low-affinity receptor sites for neurotransmitters are likely to correspond to functional receptors (Olsen and Venter, 1986). In the case of GABA, this view may be supported by the observation that the coupling between the GABA-A receptors and the benzodiazepine (BZD) sites (Fig. 3) seems to involve low-affinity GABA receptor sites (Olsen *et al.*, 1981; Olsen and Venter, 1986). It has been proposed that the different affinities may reflect anatomical, rather than functional, differences; thus, high-affinity GABA binding sites were proposed to relate to postsynaptic GABA-A receptors, whereas low-affinity sites were supposed to reflect presynaptic GABA-A receptors (Frere *et al.*, 1982; Nowak *et al.*, 1982).

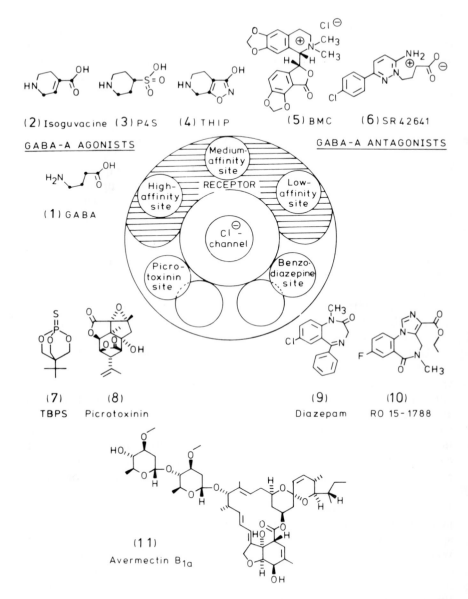

(2) Isoguvacine (3) P4S (4) THIP (5) BMC (6) SR 42641

GABA-A AGONISTS · GABA-A ANTAGONISTS

(1) GABA

(7) TBPS (8) Picrotoxinin (9) Diazepam (10) RO 15-1788

(11) Avermectin B₁ₐ

Fig. 3. A schematic illustration of the postsynaptic GABA-A receptor complex and the sites of action of some GABA-A agonists and antagonists and drugs acting at different subsynaptic receptors within this receptor complex.

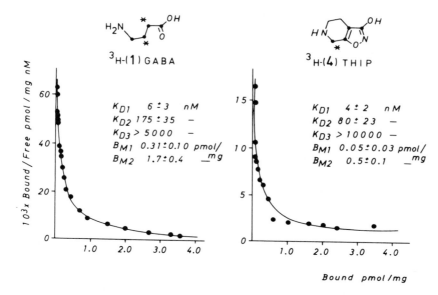

FIG. 4. Scatchard plots of the specific binding of radioactive GABA and THIP (**4**) to rat brain synaptic membranes. The binding parameters are derived from computer fitted non-linear regression analysis of the data.

The GABA receptor function is associated with (Sigel *et al.*, 1983; Schoch *et al.*, 1985; Olsen and Venter, 1986), and appears to be modulated by, various additional units (Bowery, 1984; Olsen and Venter, 1986; Mathers, 1987) which can be detected *in vitro* as distinct binding sites for the BZDs (Squires and Braestrup, 1977; Möhler and Okada, 1977b), such as diazepam (**9**) or the BZD antagonist RO 15-1788 (**10**) and for picrotoxinin (**8**) or the cage convulsant *tert*-butyl bicyclophosphothionate (**7**, TBPS) (Fig. 3; Squires *et al.*, 1983; Seifert and Casida, 1985). There is some evidence of heterogeneity for both of these binding sites (Olsen and Venter, 1986; Hebebrand *et al.*, 1986), and for the existence of a distinct binding site at the postsynaptic GABA-A receptor complex for the avermectines, including ivermectin and avermectin B_{1a} (Supavilai and Karobath, 1981; Pong and Wang, 1982; Williams and Risley, 1984; Fig. 3). There is strong evidence that the picrotoxinin/TBPS binding sites represent the pharmacological receptors for the barbiturates (Olsen, 1981; Squires *et al.*, 1983; Johnston, 1983; Maksay and Ticku, 1985; Wamsley *et al.*, 1986).

    The physiological role of these additional sites ("pharmacological recep-tors") at the GABA receptor complex, which can be co-solubilized to different extents depending on the nature of the detergent used (Olsen,

1981; Fischer and Olsen, 1986; Hammond and Martin, 1986), is unknown. The intimate contact and allosteric interactions between these units and the GABA-A receptor site *in vitro* may, however, reflect certain aspects of the dynamic properties of the GABA-A receptor complex (Olsen and Venter, 1986; see Section 3.3).

3.1 STRUCTURAL REQUIREMENTS FOR ACTIVATION OF GABA-A RECEPTORS

The development on a rational basis of compounds with specific effects on different GABA synaptic mechanisms implies information about the mechanism of interaction of GABA itself with the recognition sites concerned. A considerable degree of conformational flexibility is a trait of the molecule of GABA, and molecular orbital calculations have disclosed a relatively high degree of delocalization of the positive as well as the negative charges of GABA (Fig. 5; Steward *et al.*, 1975; Warner and Steward, 1975). These molecular characteristics apparently are essential for the synaptic activity of GABA, and there is strong evidence supporting the view that GABA adopts dissimilar active conformations at different synaptic recognition sites (Krogsgaard-Larsen, 1987). Although the molecule of GABA is achiral, the enantiotopic hydrogen atoms at each carbon atom of the GABA backbone become mutually distinct upon the interaction of GABA with the chiral biomolecules of the different GABA synaptic mechanisms. These aspects make GABA itself inherently unsuitable for molecular pharmacological studies. Synthesis and structure–activity studies of GABA analogues, in which the conformational and electronic parameters have been systemati-

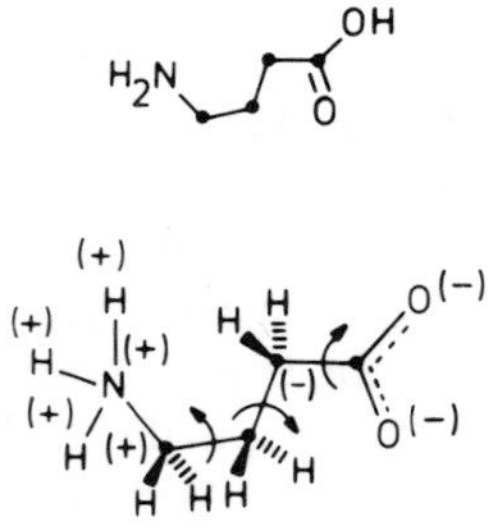

(1) GABA

GABA a complex molecule
with multiple functions

FIG. 5. The structure of GABA.

cally modified, and model compounds containing chiral centres with established absolute stereochemistry have, however, shed much light on the molecular pharmacology of the GABA synaptic mechanisms. As a result of such studies a variety of compounds with specific actions at different sites of GABA-operated synapses are now available (Allan and Johnston, 1983; Krogsgaard-Larsen *et al.*, 1985a; Krogsgaard-Larsen, 1987).

3.1.1 Muscimol and Related GABA-A Agonists

The observation that muscimol (12) is a very powerful neuronal depressant which acts through activation of the GABA-A receptors (Curtis *et al.*, 1971; Krogsgaard-Larsen *et al.*, 1975, 1979a), prompted the syntheses and structure–activity studies of a variety of aminoalkyl-substituted acidic heterocyclic compounds (Fig. 6). These studies have shown that the effects of such conformationally restricted analogues of GABA are strictly dependent on the structure of the heterocyclic rings. It must be emphasized that although these compounds are depicted in the un-ionized forms, all of them exist predominantly in the zwitterionic form, the degree of zwitterion formation being a function of the pK_a values of the compounds (see Section 3.4). Alterations of the carbon skeleton of muscimol along different lines result in pronounced, and frequently complete, loss of GABA-A agonist activity. Thus, 5-(1-aminoethyl)-3-isoxazolol is only a moderately potent GABA-A agonist (Krogsgaard-Larsen *et al.*, 1975; Krogsgaard-Larsen and Johnston, 1978), the (*S*)-isomer (13) being more potent than the (*R*)-isomer (14) (Krogsgaard-Larsen *et al.*, 1983a). The muscimol analogues (15) and (16) are very weak and inactive, respectively, as GABA-A agonists (Krogsgaard-Larsen *et al.*, 1975; Krogsgaard-Larsen and Johnston, 1978).

Whereas thiomuscimol (17) and 4,5-dihydromuscimol (DHM) are highly potent GABA-A agonists (Krogsgaard-Larsen *et al.*, 1979c), (*S*)-DHM (18) being the most powerful agonist at GABA-A receptors so far described (Krogsgaard-Larsen *et al.*, 1985b; Fig. 7), isomuscimol (20) is several orders of magnitude weaker than muscimol (12) (Krogsgaard-Larsen *et al.*, 1979c). Similarly, azamuscimol (21) is a very weak GABA-A agonist, and (22) and the triazole muscimol analogue (23) are inactive (Krogsgaard-Larsen *et al.*, 1979c; Armstrong *et al.*, 1982). Kojic amine (26) is a moderately potent but non-specific GABA-A agonist (Atkinson *et al.*, 1979; Yarbrough *et al.*, 1979), whereas its five-membered ring analogue, 5-aminomethyl-3-hydroxy-furan-2(5*H*)-one (24) (Allan *et al.*, 1983) as well as the aza-analogue (27) (Atkinson *et al.*, 1979) are totally inactive. Neither quisqualamine (25) (Evans *et al.*, 1978) nor compound (28) (Mann *et al.*, 1985) show significant GABA-A agonist activity.

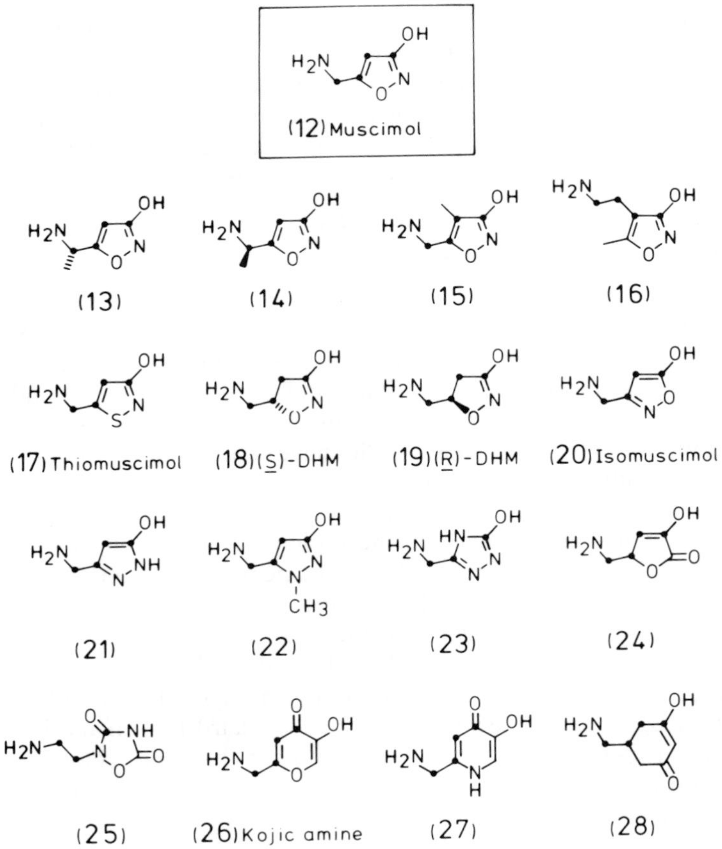

FIG. 6. Structures of the GABA-A agonist muscimol (12) and a number of related cyclic GABA analogues.

Although the structural parameters of importance for the effects, or lack of effects, on GABA-A receptors of the heterocyclic analogues of GABA illustrated in Fig. 6 have not yet been mapped out in detail, the degree of delocalization of the negative charges of these compounds seem to be a factor of major importance (Krogsgaard-Larsen *et al.*, 1979c, 1984b, 1985a; Krogsgaard-Larsen and Falch, 1981; Armstrong *et al.*, 1982). Thus, the negative charge of (20), and probably also those of (21) and (23), are delocalized to a much greater extent than that of muscimol (12) and those of thiomuscimol (17) and the isomers of DHM (18 and 19) (Krogsgaard-Larsen *et al.*, 1979c; Krogsgaard-Larsen and Falch, 1981).

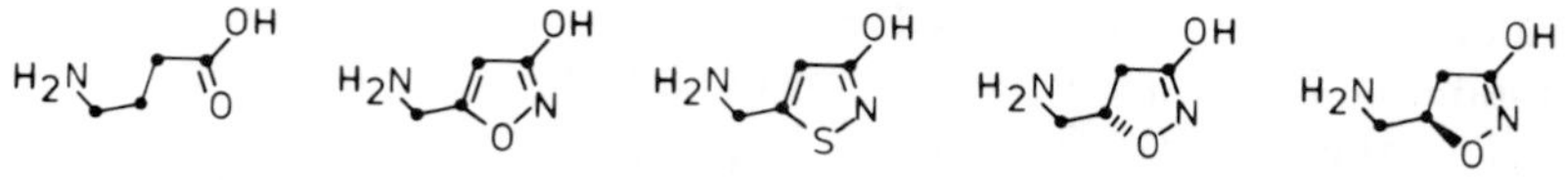

	(1)\nGABA	(12)\nMuscimol	(17)\nThiomuscimol	(18)\n(S)-DHM	(19)\n(R)-DHM
AG	– – –	– – – –	– – – –	– – – –	– – –
A-B	0.03	0.006	0.02	0.004	0.3
B-B	0.03	2.5	4 5	12.5	4.5
UPT-S	3	240	> 300	> 300	7 0
UPT-N	15	2500	>5000	>5000	800
UPT-G	35	2000	>5000	>5000	2000
GABA-T	1.92	1.27	ca.1	2.2	2.2
pK_a	4.0;10.7	4.8;8.4	6.1;8.9	5.8;9.3	5.8;9.3
I/U	800,000	900	15	600	600
BBB	N O	Yes	Yes	Yes	Yes

FIG. 7. Structure, biological and *in vitro* activity, and pharmacokinetic properties of GABA and some GABA analogues. AG, relative GABA-A agonist activity determined microelectrophoretically; A-B and B-B, inhibition of GABA-A and GABA-B receptor binding, respectively (IC_{50}, μM); UPT-S, UPT-N and UPT-G, inhibition of synaptosomal, neuronal and glial GABA uptake, respectively (IC_{50}, μM); GABA-T, effect on GABA-T (K_m, mM); I/U, ratio between ionized (zwitterionic) and un-ionized compound in aqueous solution; BBB, ability to permeate the blood–brain barrier.

These structure–activity studies indicate that the 3-isoxazolol, the 3-isothiazolol, and the 2-isoxazolin-3-ol heterocyclic systems are effective bioisosteres of the acid moiety of GABA. These findings make the respective GABA analogues muscimol (**12**), thiomuscimol (**17**), and the enantiomers of DHM (**18** and **19**) important tools for molecular pharmacological studies and leads for the design of new GABA-A agonists. In order to elucidate the pharmacological importance of these compounds, their effects on different GABA synaptic mechanisms have been studied (Fig. 7).

GABA itself obviously interacts with all GABA synaptic processes and functions, and, in contrast to the heterocyclic GABA analogues shown, GABA does not cross the blood–brain barrier (BBB) in agreement with the high I/U ratio (800,000) for this amino acid (see Section 3.4). Whereas muscimol (**12**) interacts more effectively with GABA-A receptors *in vivo* (AG) and *in vitro* (A-B) (Curtis *et al.*, 1971; Krogsgaard-Larsen *et al.*, 1975, 1979c), it binds much less tightly to GABA-B receptor sites (B-B) (Falch *et al.*, 1986) and to GABA transport mechanisms (Schousboe *et al.*, 1979;

Falch *et al.*, 1986). The IC_{50} values for the inhibition of synaptosomal GABA uptake (UPT-S) are generally lower than for the inhibition of neuronal (UPT-N) or glial (UPT-G) GABA uptake (Fig. 7). This difference reflects that synaptosomal uptake, which essentially is a measure of neuronal uptake, is determined at an external concentration of GABA much lower than that used for the determination of inhibitory effects on neuronal and glial GABA uptake, using brain slices and cultured astrocyte cells, respectively (Schousboe *et al.*, 1979; Larsson *et al.*, 1980, 1981, 1985; Schousboe *et al.*, 1985). Thiomuscimol (**17**) does not affect GABA uptake *in vitro*, but the K_m values for this GABA analogue and for muscimol (**12**) as substrates for GABA-T are lower than the K_m value of 1.92 for GABA (Fowler *et al.*, 1983; L. J. Fowler and P. Krogsgaard-Larsen, unpubl.). Thus, the fact that muscimol (**12**) (Maggi and Enna, 1979) and thiomuscimol (**17**) are metabolized *in vivo* by GABA-T reduces the value of these potent GABA-A agonists for pharmacological studies. The relatively weak GABA uptake affinity of racemic DHM resides exclusively in the (*R*)-isomer (**19**) (Krogsgaard-Larsen *et al.*, 1985b; Falch *et al.*, 1986), and (*R*)-DHM (**19**) is slightly more potent than the (*S*)-isomer (**18**) as an inhibitor of GABA-B binding (Falch *et al.*, 1986). Interestingly, however, (**18**) and (**19**) show very similar affinity for GABA-T, the K_m values being slightly higher than that of GABA (L. J. Fowler and P. Krogsgaard-Larsen, unpubl.; Fig. 7). Although (*S*)-DHM (**18**) appears to be only a relatively poor substrate for GABA-T, metabolic decomposition *in vivo* is likely to limit the pharmacological importance of this GABA-A agonist.

In Fig. 8 the effects of (*S*)-DHM (**18**) and (*R*)-DHM (**19**) on GABA-A

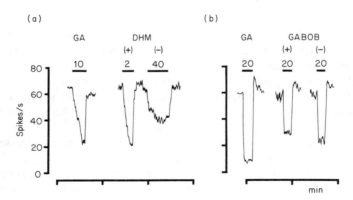

FIG. 8. Effects of GABA (GA), (*S*)-(+)-DHM (**18**), (*R*)-(−)-DHM (**19**), (*S*)-(+)-GABOB (**29**), and (*R*)-(−)-GABOB (**30**) on the firing of two spinal interneurons (a and b). The sensitivity of these neuronal depressant effects to BMC (**5**) is not indicated (for details see Krogsgaard-Larsen *et al.*, 1985b). Reproduced with permission.

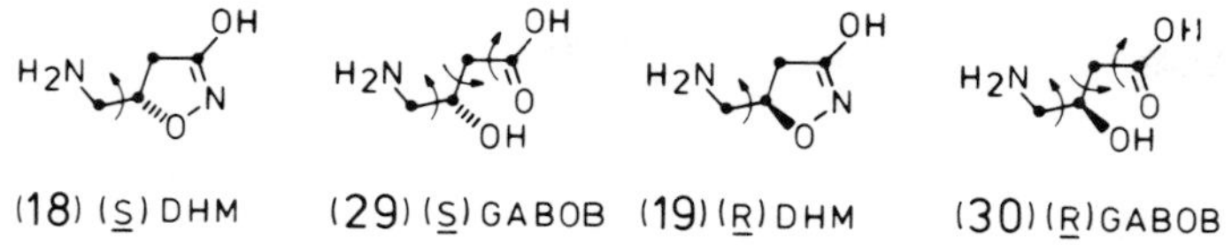

(18) (S) DHM   (29) (S) GABOB   (19) (R) DHM   (30) (R) GABOB

FIG. 9. An illustration of the conformational mobility of the enantiomers of DHM and GABOB.

receptors on cat spinal neurons are illustrated, and the relative potencies of these compounds as GABA-A agonists are compared with those of the structurally related but much more flexible GABA analogues, (S)- (**29**) and (R)-3-hydroxy-4-aminobutanoic acid (GABOB) (**30**). In agreement with the relative potencies of these GABA analogues as inhibitors of GABA-A receptor binding, (S)-$(+)$- and (R)-$(-)$-GABOB are virtually equipotent as GABA-A agonists, whereas (S)-$(+)$-DHM is much more potent than its (R)-$(-)$-isomer (see also Fig. 7; Krogsgaard-Larsen et al., 1985b).

These comparative studies illustrate that the degree of stereoselectivity of GABA-A agonists depends on the structure of the asymmetric GABA analogues, being a function of the conformational flexibility of the compounds. Thus, the (S)- and (R)-isomers of conformationally flexible GABA-A agonists as well as GABA uptake inhibitors (see Section 7.1) are generally almost equipotent, whereas the optical isomers of structurally related but less flexible GABA analogues typically show a much higher degree of stereoselectivity (Krogsgaard-Larsen and Arnt, 1980; Krogsgaard-Larsen, 1981, 1987; Krogsgaard-Larsen and Falch, 1981; Krogsgaard-Larsen et al., 1986). In Fig. 9 the conformational flexibilities of (S)- (**29**) and (R)-GABOB (**30**) are compared with those of the respective heterocyclic bioisosteres, (S)-DHM (**18**) and (R)-DHM (**19**).

3.1.2 Imidazole-4-acetic Acid and Related GABA-A Agonists

The heterocyclic GABA analogue, imidazole-4-acetic acid (**31**, IAA; Fig. 10) is a relatively potent depressant of the firing of cat cortical neurons (Godfraind et al., 1973). IAA is present in the mammalian CNS, being a metabolite of histamine (Snyder et al., 1964), and, consequently, it may play a role in regulating the central GABA system. It affects the level of GLU, the precursor for GABA, in the brain, but has not yet been shown to alter the steady-state concentrations of GABA (Clifford et al., 1973). The pharmacological profile of IAA includes both hypnotic and analgesic effects (Roberts and Simonsen, 1966; Marcus et al., 1971). In these studies the

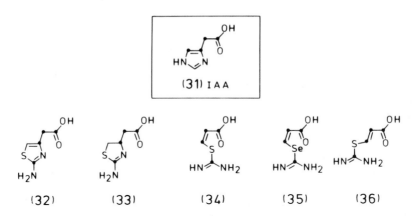

Fig. 10. Structures of the GABA-A agonist, imidazole-4-acetic acid (**31**, IAA) and a number of related GABA analogues.

correlation between blood and CNS levels of IAA was not studied in detail, but since IAA is a naturally occurring metabolite in the brain, it may be rapidly excreted from the CNS. In any case, IAA is an interesting GABAergic compound, the pharmacological and clinical potential of which has not yet been exhaustively studied.

The degree of charge delocalization of the imidazole unit of IAA is different from that of the amino group of GABA (Fig. 5), indicating that the GABA-A receptors show some tolerance with respect to this structural parameter, although an increasing degree of delocalization of the positive charge seems to be tantamount to reduced GABA-A agonist activity (Krogsgaard-Larsen *et al.*, 1983a).

Even minor structural modifications of IAA result in compounds with lower activity as GABA-A agonists (Krogsgaard-Larsen *et al.*, 1985a). A number of IAA analogues containing basic groups with protolytic properties similar to that of the imidazole nucleus of IAA have been synthesized and tested as GABA-A agonists (Fig. 10). Whereas 2-aminothiazole-4-acetic acid (**32**) shows very low affinity for GABA-A receptor sites (Breckenridge *et al.*, 1981), its unsaturated analogue, (*RS*)-2-aminothiazoline-4-acetic acid (**33**) is a potent GABA-A agonist (Bristow *et al.*, 1985). Similarly, the structurally related aliphatic compound, *cis*-3-[(aminoiminomethyl)thio]-propenoic acid (**34**), has properties reflecting effective interaction with GABA-A receptors, in particular with low-affinity GABA receptor sites (Allan *et al.*, 1986b). The seleno-analogue (**35**) shows an *in vitro* pharmacological profile similar to that of (**34**), but it is slightly weaker than (**34**). The *trans*-isomer (**36**) is inactive (Allan *et al.*, 1986b).

The structure–activity relationships discussed in this and the previous section illustrate that certain bioisosteric modifications of different structure elements of GABA are tolerated by the GABA-A receptors, and that some heterocyclic bioisosteres of GABA actually show higher affinity for and efficacy at such receptors than GABA itself. These observations represent a challenge to medicinal chemists interested in designing GABA agonists of therapeutic potential.

3.1.3 THIP and Related GABA-A Agonists

A number of analogues of the specific GABA-A agonist THIP (**4**) have been synthesized and tested (Fig. 11; Krogsgaard-Larsen *et al.*, 1977, 1979b). These structure–activity studies include analogues such as (**42**)–(**46**), in

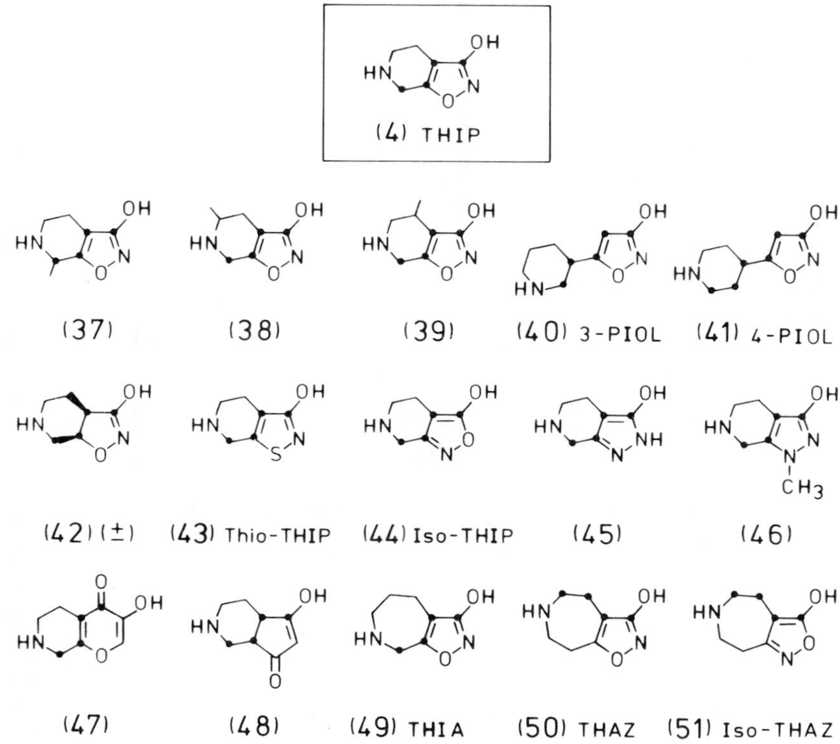

Fig. 11. Structures of the GABA-A agonist THIP (**4**) and a number of related bicyclic GABA analogues.

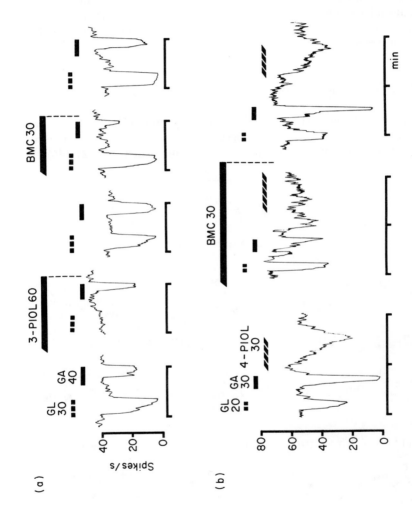

Fig. 12. a. Effects of GABA (GA), glycine (GL), 3-PIOL (**40**), and 4-PIOL (**41**) on the firing of two spinal interneurons. b. The sensitivity of the depressant effects of GABA and 4-PIOL to the GABA-A antagonist BMC (**5**) and the sensitivity of glycine-induced neuronal depression to 3-PIOL are illustrated (for details see Byberg *et al.*, 1987). Reproduced with permission.

which the 3-isoxazolol unit of THIP has been replaced by other heterocyclic systems. With the exception of thio-THIP (**43**), which is a very weak GABA-A agonist (Krogsgaard-Larsen *et al.*, 1983c), none of these THIP analogues show significant GABA-A receptor affinities (Krogsgaard-Larsen and Christiansen, 1979; Nordmann *et al.*, 1985). The *C*-alkylated analogues (**37**)–(**39**) are virtually devoid of affinity for GABA-A receptors (Haefliger *et al.*, 1984; Krogsgaard-Larsen *et al.*, 1985a), suggesting that the GABA-A receptors do not recognize and bind a limited part of the molecule of THIP, but rather the entire molecule. Neither the bicyclic GABA analogue (**47**) (Haefliger *et al.*, 1984), combining the structural characteristics of THIP and kojic amine (**26**) (see Fig. 6), nor compound (**18**) (Allan and Fong, 1983) interact significantly with GABA-A receptors. The ring homologues of THIP, THIA (**49**) and THAZ (**50**), have very little affinity for GABA-A receptors (Krogsgaard-Larsen *et al.*, 1975; Krogsgaard-Larsen and Johnston, 1978), but these compounds are antagonists for glycine receptors (Krogsgaard-Larsen *et al.*, 1982b; Brehm *et al.*, 1986). Similarly, iso-THAZ (**51**) is a glycine antagonist (Krogsgaard-Larsen *et al.*, 1982b; Brehm *et al.*, 1986), but, like iso-THIP (**44**), this 5-isoxazolol zwitterion also blocks GABA receptors in rat brains (Arnt and Krogsgaard-Larsen, 1979; see also Section 3.2).

The non-fused bicyclic THIP analogues (*RS*)-5-(3-piperidyl)-3-isoxazolol (**40**, 3-PIOL) and 5-(4-piperidyl)-3-isoxazolol (**41**, 4-PIOL) have recently been synthesized and tested (Byberg *et al.*, 1987). In spite of the fact that 4-PIOL (**41**) (Fig. 11) is not a GABA analogue in the strict sense of the word, it is a moderately potent agonist at GABA-A receptors in the cat spinal cord (Fig. 12) and it inhibits the binding of GABA to GABA-A receptor sites in rat brains (Byberg *et al.*, 1987). 4-PIOL is, however, the first example of a GABA-A agonist without stimulatory effect on the binding of BZD (see Fig. 16, Section 3.3).

As mentioned above, minor structural modifications of GABA-A agonists often lead to glycine antagonists (Krogsgaard-Larsen *et al.*, 1982b, 1983b; Brehm *et al.*, 1986). In view of these observations, it may not be surprising that 3-PIOL (**40**) (Fig. 11) is an antagonist at glycine receptors (Fig. 12) without detectable affinity for GABA-A receptors (Byberg *et al.*, 1987). Interestingly, the (*S*)- and (*R*)-forms of 3-PIOL are equipotent as glycine antagonists (Byberg *et al.*, 1987).

3.1.4 Isoguvacine and Related GABA-A Agonists

The development of THIP (**4**) (Krogsgaard-Larsen, 1977) and the demonstration of its potency and specificity as a GABA-A agonist (Krogsgaard-

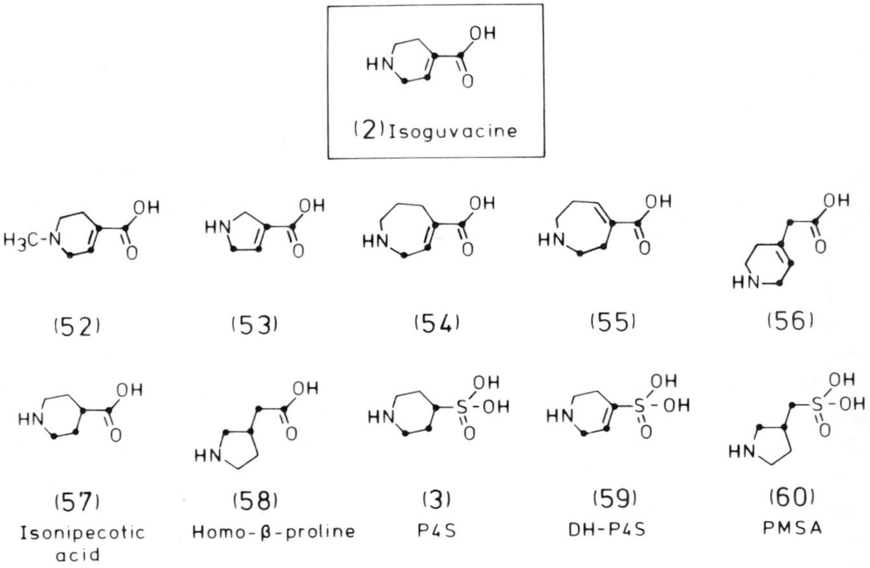

Fig. 13. Structures of the GABA-A agonist isoguvacine (2) and a number of related cyclic GABA analogues.

Larsen *et al.*, 1977, 1979b) prompted the synthesis (Krogsgaard-Larsen and Johnston, 1978; Krogsgaard-Larsen and Christiansen, 1979) and testing (Krogsgaard-Larsen *et al.*, 1977, 1979a) of the structurally related mono-cyclic amino acid, isoguvacine (2) (Fig. 13). Isoguvacine proved to be a very powerful GABA-A agonist showing a degree of specificity identical with that of THIP (Krogsgaard-Larsen *et al.*, 1977, 1979c; Schousboe *et al.*, 1985). The affinity of the lower ring homologue of isoguvacine, 3-pyrroline-3-carboxylic acid (53) for GABA-A receptor sites is some two orders of magnitude lower than that of isoguvacine (Schousboe *et al.*, 1979), and, whereas isoguvacine has no affinity for neuronal or glial GABA uptake (see Fig. 18), (53) interacts with both of these transport systems (Schousboe *et al.*, 1979). The higher ring homologues of isoguvacine, (54) and (55), do not affect GABA uptake *in vitro*, and these compounds are even weaker than (53) as inhibitors of GABA-A receptor binding (Krogsgaard-Larsen and Christiansen, 1979). In agreement with the findings for the 3-isoxazolol bioisosteres of (54) and (55), THIA (49) and THAZ (50) respectively, (54) and (55) block glycine-induced depressant effects on cat spinal neurons (Krogsgaard-Larsen *et al.*, 1982b). N-Methylisoguvacine (52) and 1,2,3,6-tetrahydropyridine-4-acetic acid (56) are very weak inhibitors of GABA-A receptor binding (Krogsgaard-Larsen and Johnston, 1978; Labouta *et al.*, 1982).

Isonipecotic acid (**57**) is a specific GABA-A agonist slightly weaker than isoguvacine (**2**) (Krogsgaard-Larsen *et al.*, 1977, 1979c), whereas the isomeric amino acid, homo-β-proline is a potent inhibitor of neuronal as well as glial GABA uptake in addition to its effect on GABA-A receptors, which is equipotent with that of isonipecotic acid (**57**) (Larsson *et al.*, 1981; Falch *et al.*, 1985a, 1986). Neither isonipecotic acid nor isoguvacine (Fig. 13) nor THIP (Fig. 11) show any affinity for GABA-B receptors (Bowery *et al.*, 1980b), supporting the view that these compounds reflect the active conformation of GABA at GABA-A receptors and, furthermore, that GABA adopts different conformations during its interaction with GABA-A and GABA-B receptors (Krogsgaard-Larsen *et al.*, 1986; Krogsgaard-Larsen, 1987). The sulphonic acid analogue (**3**, P4S) of isonipecotic acid, the corresponding unsaturated analogue (**59**, DH-P4S), and the sulphonic acid analogue of homo-β-proline, PMSA (**60**, Fig. 13) are very active GABA-A agonists with no, or, in the case of PMSA, very little effect on GABA uptake mechanisms (Krogsgaard-Larsen *et al.*, 1980; Falch *et al.*, 1985a). The mechanisms underlying the interaction of these amino sulphonic acid GABA agonists with the GABA-A receptor complex do, however, seem to be different from that of the corresponding amino acid GABA agonists (see Section 3.3).

3.2 STRUCTURAL REQUIREMENTS FOR BLOCKADE OF GABA-A RECEPTORS

As illustrated in Fig. 3, the classical GABA-A antagonists BMC (**5**) and picrotoxinin (**8**) have different sites of action at the postsynaptic GABA receptor complex, and both BMC and the parent alkaloid (1*S*,9*R*)-bicuculline (**61**) (Fig. 14) appear to interact directly with the GABA-A receptor (Frere *et al.*, 1982; Nowak *et al.*, 1982; Olsen *et al.*, 1984), possibly with an antagonist conformational state of this receptor (Möhler and Okada, 1977a). It has been shown that BMC selectively binds to low-affinity sites at the GABA-A receptor (Olsen *et al.*, 1984).

In agreement with the stereoselectivity of the activation of the GABA-A receptors in the CNS (Krogsgaard-Larsen, 1987; see Section 3.1.1), these receptors are blocked in a stereoselective manner (Enna *et al.*, 1977; Möhler and Okada, 1977a; Bowery *et al.*, 1979); thus, the (1*R*,9*S*)-isomer of bicuculline has only weak GABA-A antagonist properties, and it does not significantly affect the binding of radioactive BMC. Although narcotine (**62**) has the same absolute stereochemistry as bicuculline (**61**) (Fig. 14), it is ten times weaker than bicuculline as a GABA-A antagonist (Enna *et al.*, 1977),

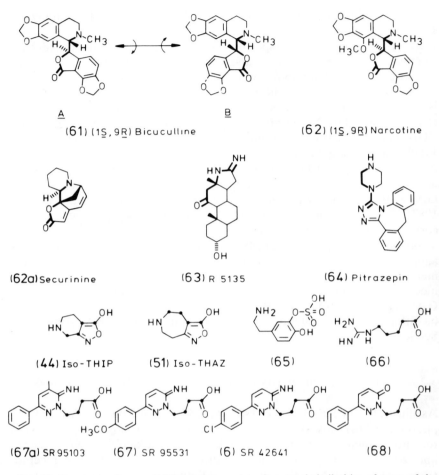

FIG. 14. Structures of some GABA-A antagonists. Structural similarities of some of the compounds are emphasized by heavy lines.

suggesting that the methoxy group on the tetrahydroisoquinoline ring of narcotine somehow disturbs the binding of this bicuculline analogue to the GABA-A receptors (for discussion see below). The $(1R,9S)$- and $(1S,9S)$-isomers of narcotine have negligible GABA-A antagonist properties (Enna *et al.*, 1977; Bowery *et al.*, 1979). The relatively strict structural constraints imposed on antagonists for the GABA-A receptors have been emphasized by structure–activity studies on a comprehensive series of synthetic analogues of bicuculline (**61**) (Kardos *et al.*, 1984).

In recent years, a number of GABA-A antagonists with structures more or less different from that of bicuculline (**61**) have been discovered. The alkaloid securinine (**62a**) is somewhat weaker than bicuculline in displacing GABA from its receptor sites, but the molecular pharmacology of securinine is similar to that of bicuculline (Beutler *et al.*, 1985). The steroid derivative R 5135 (**63**) is a GABA-A antagonist, which also interacts with the BZD receptor site (see Fig. 3) as well as with glycine receptors (Hunt and Clements-Jewery, 1981). A similar pharmacological profile is shown by the polycyclic 5-piperazinyl-1,2,4-triazole derivative, pitrazepin (**64**) (Gähwiler *et al.*, 1984; Braestrup and Nielsen, 1985; Curtis and Gynther, 1986).

Although the GABA-A antagonists (**61**)–(**64**) have quite different structures, certain parts of these molecules have comparable structural features, as emphasized in Fig. 14 by heavy lines. A comparison of these structure elements of the conformationally immobilized compounds securinine and R 5135 with the comparable parts of the molecule of bicuculline suggests that bicuculline adopts conformation *A* rather than conformation *B* during its binding to the low-affinity site of the GABA-A receptor. A similar conformation may be adopted by narcotine during its interaction with the GABA-A receptor, suggesting that the lower receptor affinity of narcotine is the result of direct steric hindrance for binding to the receptor by the methoxy group. This group is likely to stabilize the conformation of narcotine depicted in Fig. 14, which is similar to conformation *A* of bicuculline. The different relative potencies of the compounds (**61**)–(**64**) as GABA-A and glycine antagonists is difficult to rationalize on the basis of structural considerations.

In agreement with the findings for R 5135 (**63**) and pitrazepin (**64**), iso-THAZ (**51**), which is more potent than iso-THIP (**44**) (Arnt and Krogsgaard-Larsen, 1979), is an antagonist at GABA-A as well as at glycine receptors (Krogsgaard-Larsen *et al.*, 1982b). Dopamine-3-*O*-sulphate (**65**) and its 4-*O*-isomer, both of which are dopamine metabolites, have been shown to possess GABA-A antagonist profiles (Buu *et al.*, 1984). Evidence derived from electroencephalographic studies suggests that 5-guanidinopentanoic acid (**66**) is an endogenous GABA antagonist (Yokoi *et al.*, 1987).

In contrast to R 5135 (**63**) and pitrazepin (**64**), the aminopyridazine GABA-A antagonist SR 95103 (**67a**) does not interact directly with BZD binding sites but, like BMC (**5**), it antagonizes the GABA-induced enhancement of BZDs via blockade of the BZD-coupled GABA-A receptors (Chambon *et al.*, 1985; see Fig. 3). On the other hand, like R 5135 (**63**) and pitrazepin (**64**), SR 95103 (**67a**) also is an antagonist at central glycine receptors (Gynther and Curtis, 1986; Michaud *et al.*, 1986), but other pyridazinyl GABA analogues closely related to SR 95103, notably SR 42641 (**6**) and the corresponding 4-methoxyphenyl analogue, SR 95531 (**67**), are more selective GABA-A antagonists (Michaud *et al.*, 1986; Curtis and Gynther, 1987). The binding characteristics of these novel GABA-A antagonists, which contain a GABA structure element (Fig. 14), suggest that these compounds bind (Heaulme *et al.*, 1986a,b) to an antagonist conformational state of the high-affinity GABA-A receptor sites (Heaulme *et al.*, 1986a), making this class of GABA analogues valuable tools for studies of the GABA-A receptors. The inactivity of compound (**68**) emphasizes the importance of the aminopyridazine structure element, and thus the zwitterionic character, of the "SR-series" of GABA analogues for GABA-A antagonist activity (Wermuth *et al.*, 1987).

In general, the availability of antagonists with specific or highly selective effects on receptors is essential for elucidation of the physiological role and pharmacological importance of the receptors concerned, and in many areas of neuropharmacology, antagonists have proved to be extremely useful therapeutic agents. The fact that all GABA-A antagonists that have been studied pharmacologically are convulsants makes it unlikely that such compounds are going to play an important role in future psychotherapy. On the other hand, GABA-A agonists have been shown to aggravate symptoms in certain neurological diseases (Marsden and Sheehy, 1981; Krogsgaard-Larsen *et al.*, 1984a, 1985a; see also Section 3.6), and in such cases GABA-A antagonist therapies may, at least theoretically, be beneficial.

3.3 MOLECULAR PHARMACOLOGY OF THE GABA-A AGONIST–BENZODIAZEPINE INTERACTIONS

The demonstration of enhancing effects of GABA-A agonists on the binding of BZDs *in vitro* (Martin and Candy, 1978; Tallman *et al.*, 1978; Braestrup *et al.*, 1979; Karobath *et al.*, 1979) prompted extensive studies of the mechanisms underlying the GABA–BZD interactions. Although these mechanisms have not yet been elucidated (Olsen and Venter, 1986), the GABA-A agonists have proved useful tools for studies of the molecular mechanisms of the postsynaptic GABA-A receptor complex (Fig. 3).

Studies *in vitro* have revealed striking differences between the effects on BZD binding of different structural classes of GABA-A agonists (Braestrup *et al.*, 1979; Karobath *et al.*, 1979; Krogsgaard-Larsen *et al.*, 1984b; Falch *et al.*, 1985a,b). GABA and the GABA-A agonists (*S*)-DHM (**18**), muscimol (**12**), and thiomuscimol (**17**) (see Figs 6 and 7) are very effective activators of BZD binding in the absence of chloride ions and at 0°C (Fig. 15). Other GABA-A agonists such as THIP are much weaker, and P4S is a deactivator of BZD binding under these conditions (Braestrup *et al.*, 1979; Krogsgaard-Larsen *et al.*, 1984b; Fig. 16). This conspicuous lack of correlation between the potent GABA-A agonist effects of these latter compounds *in vivo* and *in*

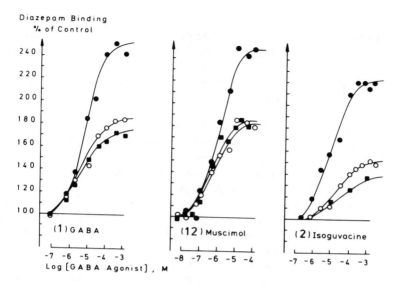

FIG. 15. Effects of GABA, muscimol (**12**), and isoguvacine (**2**) on the binding of radioactive diazepam at 0°C and in the absence of chloride (■) or at 30°C in the presence (●) or absence (○) of 150 mM sodium chloride. The experiments were performed in analogy with published procedures (Braestrup *et al.*, 1979; Falch *et al.*, 1985a).

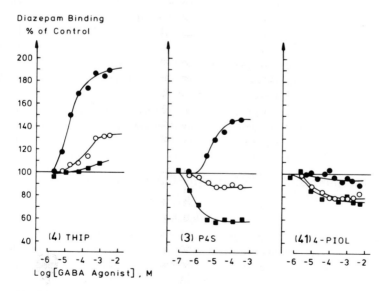

FIG. 16. Effects of THIP (**4**), P4S (**3**), and 4-PIOL (**41**) on the binding of radioactive diazepam under different conditions (for legend see Fig. 15).

vitro (see Figs 7 and 18) and their effects on BZD binding, at 0°C and in the absence of chloride ions, prompted the proposals of various hypotheses on the mechanisms involved in the GABA–BZD interactions. The effects were explained in terms of partial GABA agonist/antagonist properties of THIP and P4S (Braestrup *et al.*, 1979), or in terms of the existence of a distinct type of GABA-A receptors coupled to the BZD receptors (Karobath *et al.*, 1979).

It is now generally accepted that the effects concerned are initiated by activation of the physiological GABA-A receptor (Bowery, 1984; Olsen and Venter, 1986). The fact that substantially higher concentrations of the GABA-A agonists are required for activation of BZD binding (EC_{50} values), than for inhibition of GABA-A receptor binding (IC_{50} values), EC_{50} values being typically two orders of magnitude higher than the corresponding IC_{50} values, lends support to the proposal that the BZD site is coupled to a low-affinity site of the GABA-A receptor (Fig. 3; Olsen, 1981; Bowery, 1984; Olsen and Venter, 1986). The results of studies on the reverse effect, i.e. the stimulatory effects of BZDs on GABA-A agonist binding *in vivo* (Ferrero *et al.*, 1984) and *in vitro* (Skerritt *et al.*, 1982; Biggio *et al.*, 1984; Kardos *et al.*, 1986; Corda *et al.*, 1986) are in agreement with this view (Browner *et al.*, 1981).

The effects of GABA-A agonists on BZD binding *in vitro* are strongly dependent on the experimental conditions. Thus, elevation of the temperature to 30°C and, in particular, addition of appropriate concentrations of chloride to the incubation medium, have pronounced effects (Supavilai and Karobath, 1980; Figs 15 and 16). Under these conditions, both P4S and DH-P4S are converted from deactivators into activators of BZD binding (Falch *et al.*, 1985a,b; Wong and Iversen, 1985). In general, the maximal levels of BZD stimulation attainable by GABA-A agonists are increased in the presence of chloride ions, reflecting the close association between the GABA-A and BZD receptors and the chloride channel in the GABA receptor complex (Fig. 3). The efficacy of GABA agonists as stimulators of BZD binding appears to be determined by at least two structural parameters of the GABA-A agonists (Fig. 17):

(1) the conformational mobility of the GABA analogue; and
(2) the structure of the acid moiety of the GABA analogue.

Although the aminosulphonic acids PMSA (**60**), P4S (**3**), and DH-P4S (**59**) (Fig. 13) are very active GABA-A agonists (Falch *et al.*, 1985a), these compounds are remarkably ineffective as stimulators of BZD binding even under optimal binding conditions (Falch *et al.*, 1985a; Fig. 16). In the light of these observations, it is interesting to compare the pharmacological profiles of isonipecotic acid and P4S with those of their respective unsaturated

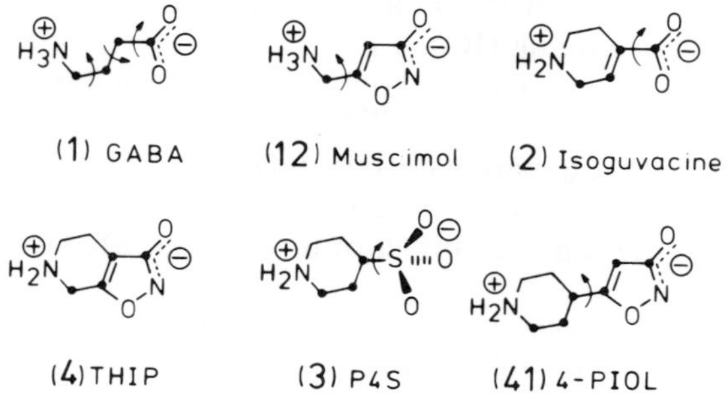

FIG. 17. An illustration of the charged structures and conformational flexibilities of GABA and some GABA-A agonists.

analogues, isoguvacine and DH-P4S (Fig. 13). While isoguvacine is substantially more effective than isonipecotic acid as a GABA-A agonist (Krogsgaard-Larsen et al., 1977), DH-P4S is proportionally weaker than P4S (Falch et al., 1985a). Under certain experimental conditions the binding of P4S was more sensitive than the binding of GABA to stimulation by barbiturates (Fischer and Olsen, 1986), and P4S has been shown to be virtually inactive at certain invertebrate receptors, which otherwise have agonist specificities similar to those of GABA-A receptors in the mammalian CNS (Roberts et al., 1981). Although the binding characteristics of ^{3}H-P4S and ^{3}H-GABA are very similar (Krogsgaard-Larsen et al., 1981a; Falch and Krogsgaard-Larsen, 1982), the above structure–activity discussion suggests that the mechanisms underlying the effects of GABA-A agonists containing the tetrahedrally orientated sulphonate group are somehow different from those of GABA-A agonists containing planar carboxylate groups or 3-isoxazolol or 3-isothiazolol anionic groups.

The non-fused THIP analogue, 4-PIOL (41) (Fig. 17), has a unique molecular pharmacological profile. As illustrated in Fig. 12, 4-PIOL is a moderately potent agonist at GABA-A receptors in the spinal cord (Byberg et al., 1987). The slow ceasing of this BMC-sensitive neuronal depressant effect as compared with that of GABA (Fig. 12) suggests that 4-PIOL does not interact with GABA uptake (Byberg et al., 1987) and, thus, is not readily removed from the synaptic cleft. In spite of the GABA-A agonist effect of 4-PIOL, it does not significantly affect the binding of BZD under different experimental conditions (Fig. 16). The apparent deactivation of BZD binding by 4-PIOL seen at low temperature and in the absence of chloride ions, probably reflects blockade of the stimulatory effects of the very low concentrations of GABA present in the brain synaptic membranes used. These effects of 4-PIOL actually are observed at surprisingly low concentrations as compared with the relatively weak effects of 4-PIOL as an inhibitor of GABA binding (IC_{50} 6 μM). The effects of 4-PIOL on BZD binding are, qualitatively and quantitatively, very similar to those of the GABA-A antagonist bicuculline (**61**) (Braestrup *et al.*, 1979). In this regard it is noteworthy that the apparent deactivating effect of P4S on BZD binding at low temperature and in the absence of chloride (Fig. 16) is even more pronounced than the reported effect of bicuculline (**61**) (Braestrup *et al.*, 1979).

This unique profile may reflect that 4-PIOL is an agonist at spinal GABA-A receptors, whereas an antagonist profile of 4-PIOL is expressed by supraspinal GABA-A receptors. Alternatively, 4-PIOL may interact with a subpopulation of GABA-A receptors, which are not coupled to BZD receptors. Such receptors are proposed to exist (Haefely *et al.*, 1985; Olsen and Venter, 1986), and 4-PIOL may prove to be a useful tool for studies of these aspects, which may have considerable therapeutic interest.

3.4 PHARMACOKINETIC ASPECTS OF GABA-A AGONISTS AND GABA UPTAKE INHIBITORS

All compounds so far known with specific actions on GABA receptors have zwitterionic structures, and the early stage of the pharmacology of GABA-A agonists reflects the difficulties in developing such compounds with satisfactory pharmacokinetic properties. Small, and frequently negligible, fractions of amino acids exist as un-ionized molecules in solution, the ratio between the concentrations of ionized (zwitterionic) and un-ionized molecules (I/U ratio, zwitterionic constant) being a function of the difference between the pK_a I and II values (Edsall and Wyman, 1958; Krogsgaard-Larsen, 1981; Krogsgaard-Larsen and Falch, 1981; Krogsgaard-Larsen *et al.*, 1981c, 1982a). A great difference between the pK_a values of neutral amino acids is tantamount to high I/U ratios for the compounds.

Since amino acids are likely to cross the BBB in the un-ionized form, it is of pharmacological interest to develop analogues of GABA with small differences in the pK_a values, and thus lower I/U ratios, compared to GABA (Krogsgaard-Larsen *et al.*, 1982a). Like GABA, isoguvacine and, in particular, P4S have high I/U ratios (Fig. 18), and none of these compounds permeate the BBB (Krogsgaard-Larsen, 1981, 1984; Krogsgaard-Larsen *et al.*, 1981c). THIP (Fig. 18) and muscimol (Fig. 7), on the other hand, have much lower I/U ratios, and approximately 0.1 and 0.2%, respectively, of doses of THIP or muscimol exist as un-ionized molecules in aqueous solution, and these values can explain why THIP and muscimol enter the brain very easily after peripheral administration in mice, rats (Krogsgaard-

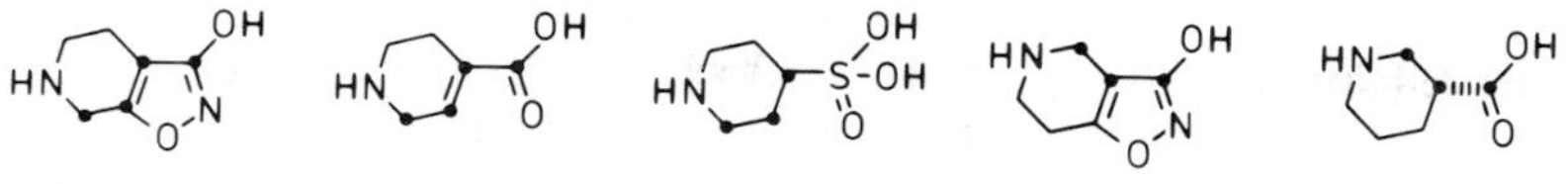

	(4) THIP	(2) Isoguvacine	(3) P4S	(69) THPO	(70) (R)Nipecotic acid
AG	— — — (−)	— — — —	— — — —	0	0
A-B	0.1	0.04	0.03	100	>100
B-B	>100	>100	>100	>100	>100
UPT-S	>300	>300	>300	160	4
UPT-N	>5000	>5000	>5000	5000	70
UPT-G	>5000	>5000	>5000	300	30
GABA-T	N.e.	N.e.	N.e.	N.e.	N.e.
pK_a	4.4;8.5	3.6;9.8	1;10.3	4.3;9.1	3.9;10.3
I/U	1,500	200,000	>1,000,000	2,500	250,000
BBB	Yes	No	No	Yes/No	No

FIG. 18. Structure, biological and *in vitro* activity, and pharmacokinetic properties of the GABA-A agonists THIP (**4**), isoguvacine (**2**), and P4S (**3**) and the GABA uptake inhibitors THPO (**69**) and (*R*)-nipecotic acid (**70**) (for legend see Fig. 7). N.e., no effect.

Larsen *et al.*, 1981c; Moroni *et al.*, 1982), and humans (Krogsgaard-Larsen *et al.*, 1984a).

The acid strength of the 3-isothiazolol nucleus is much less pronounced than that of the 3-isoxazolol unit, and as a result of the small difference in the pK_a values of the 3-isothiazolol zwitterion thiomuscimol, this compound has a very low I/U ratio (Fig. 7). Since thiomuscimol is approximately equipotent with muscimol as a GABA agonist (Krogsgaard-Larsen *et al.*, 1979c) and in view of its low I/U ratio, behavioural pharmacological studies of thio-muscimol obviously are of great interest, although thiomuscimol is a substrate for GABA-T (Fig. 7).

In addition to its lack of specificity as a GABA agonist (Krogsgaard-Larsen *et al.*, 1979c; Fig. 7) muscimol is relatively toxic (Christensen *et al.*, 1982) and, as mentioned earlier, it is rapidly metabolized after peripheral administration (Maggi and Enna, 1979; Moroni *et al.*, 1982). THIP, on the other hand, is well tolerated by various animal species (Christensen *et al.*, 1982; Krogsgaard-Larsen and Christensen, 1980; Krogsgaard-Larsen *et al.*, 1984a, 1985a), it is active after oral administration, and it is excreted unchanged and to some extent in a conjugated form in the urine from animals and humans (Schultz *et al.*, 1981). THIP has been the subject of investigations in the human clinic (see Section 3.6).

In Fig. 18 the *in vivo* and *in vitro* pharmacological effects and pharmacokinetic properties of THIP (**4**), isoguvacine (**2**), and P4S (**3**) are compared
with those of the GABA uptake inhibitors THPO (**69**) and (*R*)-nipecotic
acid (**70**) (see Section 7). None of these compounds containing secondary
amino groups interact detectably with GABA-T (Krogsgaard-Larsen and
Johnston, 1978). In contrast to the amino acid (*R*)-nipecotic acid, its
structurally related 3-isoxazolol bioisostere THPO is, to some extent,
capable of crossing the BBB. Thus, in young animals, in which the BBB is
not yet fully developed, THPO is capable of entering the brain after systemic
administration, whereas the BBB in adult animals is relatively impermeable
to THPO (Wood *et al.*, 1980; Schousboe *et al.*, 1986; Krogsgaard-Larsen *et
al.*, 1987).

3.5 PRODRUGS OF GABA AND GABA-A AGONISTS

As discussed in the previous sections, a variety of heterocyclic bioisosteres
of GABA have been synthesized and tested for GABAergic activities. So
far, these comprehensive drug design programmes have provided a variety
of GABA analogues with specific or highly selective actions at different
GABA synaptic mechanisms. Structure–activity analyses of these conformationally restricted bioisosteres, in which the structural parameters of
GABA (Fig. 5) have been systematically changed, have provided much
insight into the molecular mechanisms underlying the synaptic effects of
GABA. Some of these GABA bioisosteres have pharmacokinetic (see
Figs 7 and 18) and toxicological properties making pharmacological and, in
a few cases, clinical studies possible (see below).

Like GABA itself (Fig. 7) most of the specific GABA-A agonists, notably
isonipecotic acid (**57**), isoguvacine (**2**) and P4S (**3**) (Figs 13 and 18), do not
easily permeate the BBB. The pharmacological interest in GABA and these
GABA analogues has prompted the development and pharmacological
testing of a variety of prodrugs of these compounds. This approach may, in
principle, be particularly attractive in the central amino acid neurotransmitter field. Ideally, the active amino acids would be "trapped" within the
brain following cleavage of the lipophilic transport-facilitating group(s).
Most prodrugs of these amino acids are esters (Figs 19 and 20), and the
reduced basic character of amino acid esters as compared with the amino
groups of the corresponding amino acids (Edsall and Wyman, 1958;
Krogsgaard-Larsen, 1981; Krogsgaard-Larsen *et al.*, 1981c) facilitates the
passage of amino acid ester prodrugs through the BBB. An ideal prodrug is
a derivative without pharmacological effects *per se* that is converted in the
brain tissue into the active compound without formation of toxic byproducts.

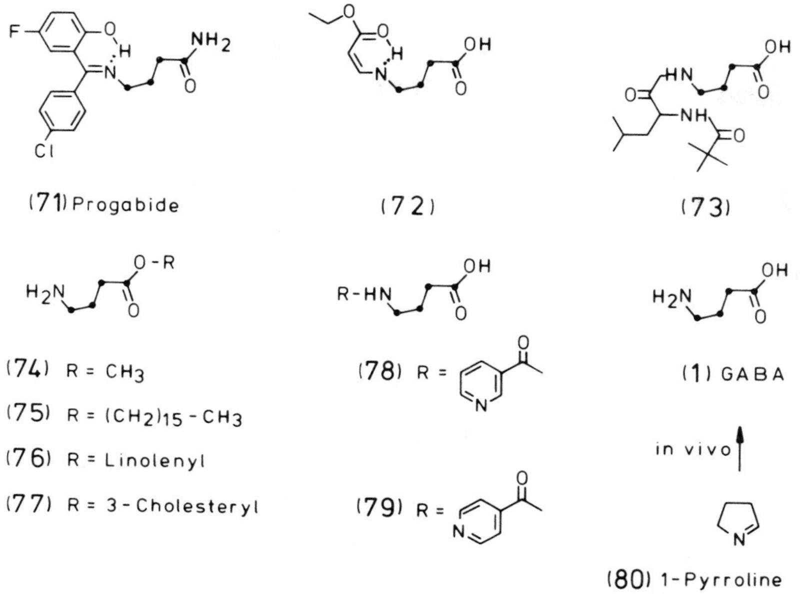

(71) Progabide

(72)

(73)

(74) R = CH$_3$

(75) R = (CH$_2$)$_{15}$ - CH$_3$

(76) R = Linolenyl

(77) R = 3 - Cholesteryl

(78) R =

(79) R =

(1) GABA

in vivo

(80) 1-Pyrroline

FIG. 19. Structures of a number of prodrugs of GABA.

In Fig. 19 a variety of prodrugs and potential prodrugs of GABA are shown. The most exhaustively studied GABA prodrug is progabide (71), in which the amino group of GABA-amide forms an imino group with a benzophenone derivative (Kaplan *et al.*, 1980). The spectroscopic data for progabide (Kaplan *et al.*, 1980) indicate that the imino structure element of this molecule is stabilized by a hydrogen bond, and in aqueous solution progabide probably is in equilibrium with the hydrolysis products GABA-amide and the substituted benzophenone (Krogsgaard-Larsen *et al.*, 1986). *In vivo*, progabide appears to be partially converted into the corresponding carboxylic acid (SL 75.102), which has GABA agonist properties, whereas GABA-amide is hydrolysed to give GABA (Worms *et al.*, 1982). These aspects make a detailed analysis of the mechanisms underlying the pharmacological and clinical effects of progabide difficult (Lloyd *et al.*, 1982). At rather high doses progabide has a broad spectrum of anticonvulsant activities in a variety of experimental models of epilepsy, and progabide shows anticonvulsant activity in different types of epilepsy (for reviews see Morselli *et al.*, 1981; Nistico *et al.*, 1986). So far, there are no reports on the potential toxicity of the benzophenone moiety of progabide.

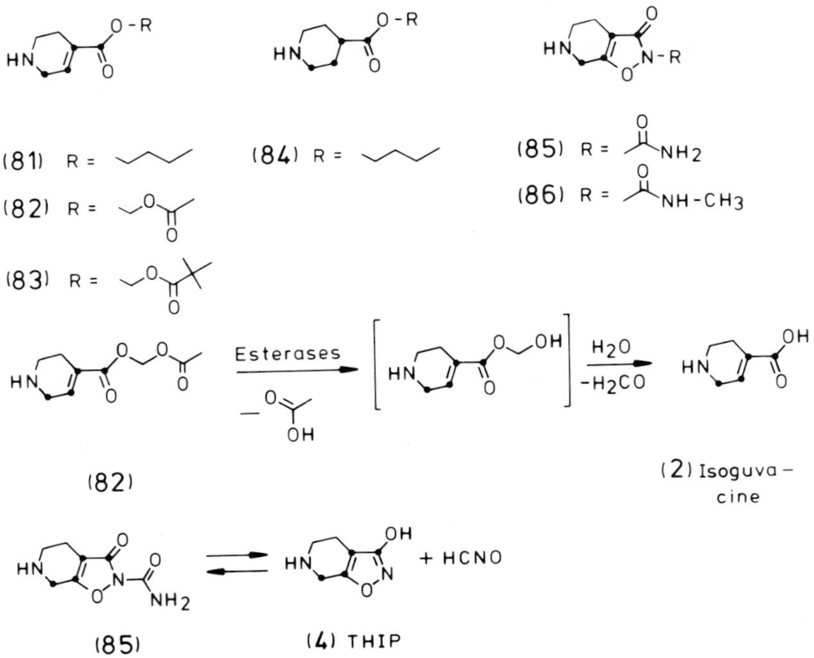

FIG. 20. Structures of some prodrugs of the GABA-A agonists isoguvacine (**2**), isonipecotic acid (**57**), and THIP (**4**).

In the potential GABA prodrug (**72**) the amino group of GABA is incorporated into an enamine structure stabilized by a hydrogen bond involving the ester carbonyl group (Larsen and Bundgaard, 1986). The rate of hydrolysis *in vitro* of (**72**) and a number of related potential prodrugs has been determined (Larsen and Bundgaard, 1986), but pharmacological data have not been reported. The *N*-pivaloyl-leucyl-GABA derivative (**73**) is capable of crossing the BBB in rats with subsequent increases of central GABA levels (Galzigna *et al.*, 1984). Compound (**73**) shows persistent anticonvulsant effects in rats, probably as a result of decomposition in the brain to give GABA, although (**73**) itself and/or partially hydrolysed products from (**73**) seem to be pharmacologically active (Galzigna *et al.*, 1984). A number of simple esters of GABA, including (**74**), have been tested as potential prodrugs of GABA (Galzigna *et al.*, 1978; Bianchi *et al.*, 1983). The fact that these derivatives undergo rapid cyclization in addition to their hydro-lysis to give GABA makes interpretation of the pharmacological data com-plex. GABA cetyl ester (**75**) is pharmacologically active in a variety of ani-mal models, primarily as a result of decomposition of (**75**) *in vivo* to give GABA (Delini-Stula, 1979). Similarly, the linolenyl (**76**) and the 3-choles-teryl (**77**) esters are pharmacologically active in different animal models as a result of their entry into the CNS and subsequent enzymatic hydrolysis to GABA (Shashoua *et al.*, 1984). The *N*-protected GABA analogues (**78**) and (**79**) have been evaluated as GABA prodrugs (Matsuyama *et al.*, 1984), and 1-pyrroline (**80**) and substituted 1-pyrrolines represent potential therapeutically useful "prodrugs" of GABA and substituted GABA analogues, respectively (Callery *et al.*, 1982; Fig. 19).

The potency and specificity of isoguvacine (**2**) as a GABA-A agonist (Fig. 18) have made prodrugs of this compound pharmacologically interest-ing. A number of simple esters of isoguvacine such as (**81**) (Fig. 20) and a series of double esters including the acetyloxymethyl (**82**) and pivaloyloxymethyl (**83**) esters of isoguvacine have been synthesized and tested (Falch *et al.*, 1981). While (**81**) hydrolysed very slowly under approxi-mately physiological conditions, the acyloxymethyl esters (**82**) and (**83**) were much more labile, the half-lives being strongly dependent on the structure of the acyloxy moieties in the ester groups (Falch *et al.*, 1981), and a certain degree of correlation of the half-lives of these double esters and their anticonvulsant effects was observed (Falch *et al.*, 1981). It is assumed that the rate-limiting step in the cleavage of acyloxymethyl esters is the hydrolysis of the acyloxy group to give the corresponding hydroxymethyl esters, which then decompose spontaneously to furnish the parent (amino) acids and formaldehyde (Falch *et al.*, 1981; Krogsgaard-Larsen *et al.*, 1982a; Fig. 20). A series of esters of isonipecotic acid (**57**), including the butyl ester (**84**), have been synthesized and evaluated as prodrugs for the parent GABA-A agonist (**57**) (Crider *et al.*, 1982). In contrast to the corresponding 4-nit-rophenyl ester of (**57**), (**84**) showed only marginal pharmacological effects in different seizure tests (Crider *et al.*, 1982), probably reflecting very low rates of hydrolysis to produce the active amino acid *in vivo*. A number of 2-substituted analogues of THIP (**4**) such as (**85**) and (**86**) have been synthesized (Haefliger *et al.*, 1984; N. Lassen and P. Krogsgaard-Larsen, unpubl.). The pharmacological profiles of these *N*-carbamoyl analogues in different test systems are similar to that of the parent compound, THIP (**4**), reflecting that in aqueous solution, these analogues are in equilibrium with THIP, as exemplified for (**85**) in Fig. 20. A similar equilibrium has been determined for a 2-carbamoyl analogue of DHM (Fig. 7) (Krogsgaard-Larsen *et al.*, 1982a, 1985a).

3.6 BEHAVIOURAL AND CLINICAL PHARMACOLOGY OF GABA-A AGONISTS

The very effective GABA-A agonist, muscimol (12) (Fig. 7), has been extensively used as a neurochemical and pharmacological tool, and muscimol has been administered to patients suffering from certain neurological and psychiatric disorders in short-term clinical trials (Krogsgaard-Larsen *et al.*, 1979b, 1985a; Enna, 1981; Marsden and Sheehy, 1981). However, the toxicity and rapid metabolism of muscimol (see Section 3.1.1) make interpretation of such pharmacological and clinical data difficult, and these aspects may explain the conflicting pharmacological observations, which, in some cases, have been reported for muscimol.

The potency and specificity of THIP (4) as a GABA-A agonist and its favourable pharmacokinetic and animal toxicological properties (Krogsgaard-Larsen *et al.*, 1984a, 1985a) have made THIP (Fig. 18) the "classical" GABA-A agonist for pharmacological and clinical studies, and, together with isoguvacine (2) and P4S (3), THIP has become the standard GABA-A agonist for *in vitro* pharmacological studies. In the following sections a major part of the available pharmacological and clinical data is summarized.

3.6.1 Effects on Seizures and Ethanol Withdrawal Symptoms

There is overwhelming indirect evidence, derived from experimental models of epilepsy, supporting the view that pharmacological stimulation of the GABA neurotransmission may have therapeutic interest in epilepsy (Meldrum, 1975, 1982). The anticonvulsant effects of THIP (4) and muscimol (12) have been compared in a variety of animal models. THIP typically is 2–5 times weaker than muscimol in suppressing seizure activities. In mice (Löscher, 1982) and in gerbils with genetically determined epilepsy (Löscher *et al.*, 1983), systemically administered THIP has proved very effective in suppressing seizure activity, and THIP is capable of reducing audiogenic seizures in DBA/2 mice (Meldrum and Horton, 1980). However, THIP failed to protect baboons with photosensitive epilepsy against photically induced myoclonic responses (Meldrum and Horton, 1980). An analysis of the effects of THIP on pento-geniculo-occipital (PGO) activity in cats (Neal and Bond, 1983) seems to indicate an as yet unclarified involvement of the serotonin system. THIP has been subjected to a single-blind controlled trial in patients with epilepsy, in which THIP was added to the concomitant antiepileptic treatment (Petersen *et al.*, 1983). Under these conditions no significant effects of THIP were detected, although a trend was observed for lower seizure frequency during a period of submaximal doses of THIP (for further discussion see Section 3.7).

The effects of THIP on ethanol withdrawal symptoms in rats have been studied (Frye *et al.*, 1983). While intracisternally administered THIP proved effective in reducing audiogenic clonictonic seizures, no effects on forelimb tremor were observed. These selective effects may have clinical interest.

3.6.2 Analgesic and Anxiolytic Effects

The involvement of the central GABA system in pain mechanisms has been the subject of intensive studies (DeFeudis, 1982; Andree *et al.*, 1983). The demonstration of very potent analgesic effects of THIP in different animal models (Hill *et al.*, 1981; Christensen and Larsen, 1982) has made studies of the clinical prospects of GABA-mediated analgesia possible. THIP-induced analgesia is insensitive to naloxone (Hill *et al.*, 1981; Kendall *et al.*, 1982; Grognet *et al.*, 1983), indicating that the effect is not mediated by the opiate receptors. Quite surprisingly, THIP analgesia cannot be reversed by bicuculline (Hill *et al.*, 1981; DeFeudis, 1982; Kendall *et al.*, 1982), which may reflect the involvement of a distinct class of GABA receptor ("GABA-X receptor"; Fig. 2; Krogsgaard-Larsen *et al.*, 1986; Zorn *et al.*, 1986). On the other hand, THIP-induced analgesia can be reduced by atropine (Kendall *et al.*, 1982; Grognet *et al.*, 1983), and potentiated by cholinergics such as physostigmine, reflecting as yet unclarified functional interactions between GABA and acetylcholine neurons and the central opiate systems rather than a direct action of THIP on muscarinic receptors.

THIP and morphine are approximately equipotent as analgesics, although their relative potencies are dependent on the animal species and experimental models used (Christensen and Larsen, 1982; Grognet *et al.*, 1983). Acute injection of THIP potentiates morphine-induced analgesia, and chronic administration of THIP produces a certain degree of functional tolerance to its analgesic effects (Andree *et al.*, 1983). In contrast to earlier findings (Christensen and Larsen, 1982), the results of recent studies have been interpreted in terms of some cross-tolerance between THIP and morphine (Andree *et al.*, 1983). In contrast to morphine, THIP does not cause respiratory depression (Lindeburg *et al.*, 1983). Clinical studies on postoperation patients, and patients with chronic pain of malignant origin (Kjaer and Nielsen, 1983) have disclosed potent analgesic effects of THIP, in the latter group of patients at doses of 5–30 mg (i.m.) of THIP.

In these cancer patients and also in patients with chronic anxiety (Hoehn-Saric, 1983) the desired effects of THIP were accompanied by side effects, notably sedation, nausea, and in a few cases euphoria. The side effects of THIP have been described as mild and similar in quality to those of other GABA-mimetics (Hoehn-Saric, 1983). These undesirable effects of THIP may to a certain extent be ascribed to the non-optimal pharmacokinetics of THIP (Hoehn-Saric, 1983), emphasizing the need for a sustained release preparation of THIP.

It is assumed that the postsynaptic GABA receptor complex mediates the anxiolytic effects of the BZDs (Paul *et al.*, 1981), and, consequently, it is of interest to see whether GABA agonists have anxiolytic effects. Muscimol has proved effective in conflict tests, though with a pharmacological profile different from that of diazepam (Cuomo *et al.*, 1981), and in humans muscimol in low doses was found to sedate and calm schizophrenic patients (Tamminga *et al.*, 1979). In a number of patients with chronic anxiety the effects of THIP were assessed on several measures of anxiety (Hoehn-Saric, 1983). Although these effects were accompanied by side effects (Hoehn-Saric, 1983), the combination of analgesic and anxiolytic effects of THIP would seem to have therapeutic prospects.

The neuronal and synaptic mechanisms underlying THIP- and, in general, GABA-induced analgesia have been studied in some detail. The insensitivity of THIP-induced analgesia to naloxone (Hill *et al.*, 1981; Kendall *et al.*, 1982; Grognet *et al.*, 1983) is consistently demonstrated (Murray *et al.*, 1983; Hynes *et al.*, 1984). The earlier reported antagonism of THIP analgesia to atropine could not be reproduced in a series of animal experiments (Hynes *et al.*, 1984), whereas a sensitivity of this effect to a serotonin agonist (Murray *et al.*, 1983) seems to support the interaction mentioned earlier (Section 3.6.1) between central GABA and serotonin systems. In apparent contrast to earlier findings (Christensen and Larsen, 1982), GABA-induced analgesia does not seem to be mediated primarily by spinal GABA receptors (Hammond and Drower, 1984), but rather by GABA mechanisms in the forebrain (Lim *et al.*, 1985) and it appears also to involve neurons in the midbrain (Moreau and Fields, 1986). Although these mechanisms are far from being fully elucidated, the naloxone-insensitivity and apparent lack of dependence liability of GABA-mediated analgesia (Sivam and Ho, 1985) suggest that GABAergic drugs may play a role in future treatment of pain. Furthermore, it has been suggested that pharmacological manipulation of GABA mechanisms may have some relevance for future treatment of opiate drug addicts (DeFeudis, 1984).

3.6.3 Cardiovascular Effects

There is very strong evidence that GABA is involved in the regulation of cardiovascular mechanisms (Antonaccio and Taylor, 1977; DeFeudis,

1981). While intracerebroventricularly (i.c.v.) administered THIP reduced blood pressure as well as heart rate, systemically administered THIP did not affect these functions significantly (Mesdjian *et al.*, 1983; Persson, 1981). On the other hand, systemically administered GABA and isoguvacine had significant cardiovascular effects, which could be blocked by BMC (Mesdjian *et al.*, 1983). Since THIP, but not GABA and isoguvacine, are capable of crossing the BBB (Schultz *et al.*, 1981; Krogsgaard-Larsen *et al.*, 1982a), these results seem to indicate that peripheral GABA receptors are involved in the regulation of cardiovascular functions (Mesdjian *et al.*, 1983). It is interesting to note that GABA and a number of GABA agonists produce a dose-dependent dilation of isolated cat and dog artery segments, apparently by activation of GABA receptors with pharmacological characteristics similar to those of central postsynaptic GABA receptors (Edvinsson and Krause, 1979).

3.6.4 Effects on Spasticity

The results of pharmacological studies on the spastic mouse are consistent with a role of GABA in spasticity (Biscoe and Fry, 1982). Systemic administration of the GABA agonists muscimol, THIP, and isoguvacine to cat affected spinal cord activities (Polc, 1979). Since isoguvacine does not readily penetrate the BBB, its pharmacological effects in this animal model (Polc, 1979) may suggest that some parts of the spinal cord are not effectively protected by a BBB. THIP has been studied in spastic patients (Mondrup and Pedersen, 1983). At oral doses of 15–25 mg, THIP clearly reduced the monosynaptic T-reflexes without affecting the flexor threshold significantly (Mondrup and Pedersen, 1983).

3.6.5 Interactions of THIP with Dopaminergic and Cholinergic Systems in the CNS

Studies in recent years have disclosed very complex interactions between different neurotransmitter systems in the basal ganglia, notably the dopamine (DA), GABA, and cholinergic systems (Chase and Walters, 1976; Di Chiara and Gessa, 1981; Christensen *et al.*, 1982). These interactions have been extensively studied with the intention of gaining better insight into the mechanisms underlying schizophrenia, Parkinson's disease, and different dyskinetic syndromes and, furthermore, of developing new strategies for the treatment of these severe diseases. Much interest has been focused on the nigrostriatal DA neurons, which form part of the nigrostriatal "feedback" pathway, of which the striatonigral GABA neurons terminate within the substantia nigra (SN) pars reticulata, possibly on cholinergic neurons. The DA neurons of this system originating in SN pars compacta as well as the mesolimbic DA neurons involved in an analogous "feedback" loop are assumed to be under inhibitory GABA control (Chase and Walters, 1976; Di Chiara and Gessa, 1981; Christensen *et al.*, 1982). These aspects have opened up the prospects of using GABA-stimulating therapies in the treatment of schizophrenia, and, consequently, THIP has been quite extensively studied in different animal models.

While activation of GABA receptors in SN pars reticulata of rats has dramatic behavioural consequences (Arnt *et al.*, 1979), the DA neurons in SN pars compacta and the mesolimbic DA neurons are much less sensitive. Direct application of THIP in the respective brain areas has weak inhibitory effects on both types of DA neurons, whereas systemically administered THIP weakly stimulates these DA neurons (Waszczak and Walters, 1980; Waszczak *et al.*, 1980). No simple explanation of these apparently contradictory observations has been forwarded. The behavioural effects of acute and chronic administration of THIP have been studied (Christensen *et al.*, 1982). DA agonist-induced locomotor activity and stereotypies are altered by simultaneous treatment with GABA agonists, the former activity being depressed and the latter intensified (Christensen *et al.*, 1979). From a clinical point of view the interactions between THIP and neuroleptics may be particularly interesting. Most neuroleptic drugs inhibit DA-induced stereotypy and induce catalepsy in animals, the former effect being related to clinical antipsychotic effects and the latter to extrapyramidal side effects of neuroleptics (Arnt and Christensen, 1981). Since THIP, and also scopolamine, antagonize the antistereotypic effects of some neuroleptics, it has been tentatively concluded that GABA agonists such as THIP would probably not potentiate the antipsychotic effect of neuroleptics but rather antagonize it (Arnt and Christensen, 1981).

The interactions between THIP and the central DA systems have also been studied in monkeys (Bjoerndal *et al.*, 1983). Analyses of the complex pharmacological profile in this animal of THIP, which to some extent was similar to that of diazepam, led to the conclusion that THIP would probably have a limited therapeutic effect in different kinds of dyskinesia, and THIP has proved ineffective in reducing the symptoms of dyskinetic patients (Korsgaard *et al.*, 1982).

3.7 GABA-GLYCINE INTERACTIONS

It is generally accepted that the inhibitory neurotransmitters GABA and glycine operate through distinct receptor systems (Curtis and Johnston,

1974; Krnjevic, 1974). Both of these transmitter systems are involved in the control of neuronal mechanisms in the brain and the spinal cord, but whereas GABA is the major inhibitory neurotransmitter in supraspinal regions of the CNS, glycine has a similar dominating role in the spinal cord (Curtis and Johnston, 1974; Krnjevic, 1974). There are, however, several reports describing apparent functional interactions between GABA and glycine, in particular in certain brain regions (Braestrup and Nielsen, 1980), and there is electrophysiological evidence supporting the view that GABA and glycine may share the same chloride conductance channel (Barker and McBurney, 1979).

As discussed in previous sections, there are also many examples of "pharmacological similarities" between GABA and glycine receptor mechanisms. Thus, a number of compounds are almost equally effective as GABA and glycine antagonists (see Section 3.2), and minor alterations of GABA-A agonists frequently result in compounds with glycine antagonist properties (see Sections 3.1.3 and 3.1.4).

In recent years a number of observations of pharmacological interactions between the GABA and glycine neurotransmitter systems have been reported. Thus, synergistic anticonvulsant effects of GABA-T inhibitors and glycine have been described (Sarhan et al., 1984) and, similarly, glycine amplifies the protective effect of the GABA-A agonist, muscimol (12), against seizures caused by impairment of the GABA-mediated neuro-transmission (Seiler and Sarhan, 1984). Glycine, administered concomit-antly with the GABA uptake inhibitor THPO (Figs 18 and 21), also greatly enhanced the anticonvulsant effects of this latter compound (Seiler et al., 1985). Even the epileptiform EEG activities of the GABA-A antagonist SR 95103 (67a) (Fig. 14), was facilitated by glycine (Santucci et al., 1985).

The mechanism(s) underlying these synergistic effects of systemically administered glycine on different types of GABAergic drugs, also adminis-tered systemically, are unknown. Pharmacokinetic factors can hardly

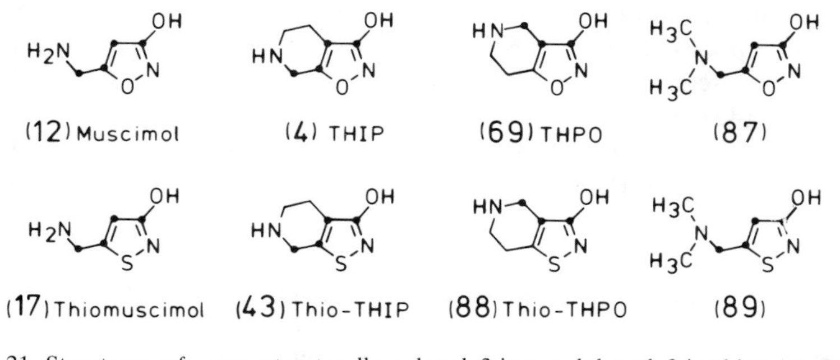

FIG. 21. Structures of some structurally related 3-isoxazolol and 3-isothiazolol GABA analogues.

explain these pronounced effects, which may be the results of interactions between the activated glycine and GABA-A receptors, perhaps through the chloride channel, which may be shared by these receptors (Barker and McBurney, 1979).

In the case of THPO, which in addition to its effect on GABA uptake (see Sections 7.1 and 7.2) has very weak glycine antagonist properties (Krogsgaard-Larsen *et al.*, 1975, 1983c), it is possible that abolition of this weak profile by glycine is sufficient to explain the enhanced anticonvulsant effect of THPO resulting from its inhibition of glial GABA uptake. THIP also binds very weakly to glycine receptors (Braestrup *et al.*, 1986), possibly as an antagonist, and it is tempting to assume that its surprisingly weak antiepileptic effect (see Section 3.6.1) may be partly explained by a weak antiglycine effect, which reduces the inhibitory effect resulting from its activation of GABA-A receptors. The weak antiepileptic effect of THIP may alternatively reflect that the prolonged hyperpolarization of neuronal membranes by effective and sustained activation by GABA-A agonists is too "unphysiological" to cause the expected inhibitory effect, which may be partially abolished by compensatory mechanisms of unknown character.

The possibility that the 3-isoxazolol nucleus of the GABAergic compounds muscimol (12), THIP (4), and THPO (69) (Fig. 21) is responsible for the weak affinity of these compounds for glycine receptors prompted us to develop the corresponding 3-isothiazolol analogues, thiomuscimol (17), thio-THIP (43), and thio-THPO (88) (Fig. 21). This approach to the design of heterocyclic GABAergic agents devoid of glycine receptor affinities was stimulated by the observation that *N,N*-dimethylmuscimol (87), which does not affect GABA synaptic mechanisms, is a glycine antagonist (Krogsgaard-Larsen *et al.*, 1982b), whereas the corresponding 3-isothiazolol compound (89) is totally inactive (Krogsgaard-Larsen *et al.*, 1982b). Thio-THPO (88) is weaker than THPO (69) as an inhibitor of GABA uptake *in vitro*, but it does not reduce glycine-induced neuronal inhibition (Krogsgaard-Larsen *et al.*, 1983c). Perhaps as a result of this lack of glycine antagonist effect, it is approximately equipotent with THPO in enhancing GABA-induced neuronal depression *in vivo* (Krogsgaard-Larsen *et al.*, 1983c; see Fig. 33). While thiomuscimol (17) is a potent GABA-A agonist (see Section 3.1.1), thio-THIP (43) proved to be a very weak agonist at GABA-A receptors (Krogsgaard-Larsen *et al.*, 1983c). This approach to designing a GABA-A agonist related to THIP but with more potent antiepileptic properties has, so far, been unsuccessful.

4 Presynaptic and Extrasynaptic GABA-A Receptors

Relatively little is known about the physiological function and the pharmacological characteristics of extrasynaptic GABA-A receptors (Figs 2 and

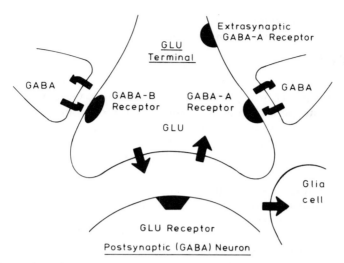

Fig. 22. A schematic illustration of an axo-somatic glutamic acid (GLU)-operated synapse containing extrasynaptic GABA-A receptors and presynaptic GABA-A and GABA-B receptors.

22). Such receptors, which are sensitive to the GABA-A antagonists, BMC (**5**) (Fig. 3) and bicuculline (**61**) (Fig. 14), apparently have agonist specificities somewhat different from those of synaptic GABA-A receptors (Curtis, 1978; Brown, 1979; Alger and Nicoll, 1982). The depolarizing effect of GABA on extrasynaptic GABA receptors on myelinated axons in amphibian peripheral nerves was blocked by BMC in a competitive manner, whereas picrotoxinin (**8**) (Fig. 3) showed a more complex antagonist profile (Barolet *et al.*, 1985).

GABA nerve terminals impinge on 1a primary afferent fibres, where GABA decreases the evoked release of sensory transmitter(s), and a presynaptic depolarizing inhibitory process mediated by GABA may be confined to terminals of such primary afferent fibres (Curtis and Malik, 1984). The lack of direct electrophysiological evidence for different pharmacological profiles of these presynaptic GABA receptors (Fig. 22) and the GABA-A receptors in the postsynaptic receptor complex (Figs 1 and 3) has hampered progress in establishing GABA as the transmitter at presynaptic sites (Curtis, 1978). It has, however, recently been shown that the terminal axonal arborizations in the spinal cord of neurons in the red nucleus have GABA receptors different from those on the cell bodies as illustrated by the lack of sensitivity to BMC (**5**) of the depressant actions of GABA and the GABA-A agonist P4S (**3**) at the former type of receptors (Curtis and Malik, 1984).

There is circumstantial evidence for the existence of presynaptically located GABA-A receptors in the brain located on GABA nerve terminals (Bowery, 1983) and, in particular, on terminals of neurons utilizing other neurotransmitter substances. Thus, GABA enhances the potassium-evoked release of transmitter from cerebellar cortex slices in a bicuculline (**61**)-sensitive manner (Bowery *et al.*, 1980b). Similarly, GABA is capable of facilitating the potassium-evoked release of DA from slices of corpus striatum, but antagonism by bicuculline is not always apparent (Stoof and Mulder, 1977; Giorguieff *et al.*, 1978; Starr, 1979; Ennis and Cox, 1981). A facilitation by GABA of potassium-stimulated release of GLU (Fig. 22) from striatal tissue has been reported (Mitchell, 1982); this effect appears to be mediated by GABA receptors sensitive to BMC (**5**) but showing a profile of agonist sensitivity different from that characterizing the GABA-A receptors in the postsynaptic receptor complex (Fig. 3). The physiological significance of this observation, which has interesting therapeutic prospects, is, however, not clear (Bowery, 1983). On the other hand, the evoked release of GLU from cultured cerebellar granule cells has been shown to be under inhibitory control by GABA receptors sensitive to BMC (Meier *et al.*, 1984). These receptors showed an agonist profile typical for GABA-A receptors, THIP (**4**) and muscimol (**12**) being active, whereas no effect of the GABA-B agonist, baclofen (**90**), could be demonstrated. Interestingly, these effects of GABA-A agonists proved to be mediated by low- rather than high-affinity GABA-A receptors (Meier *et al.*, 1984; see Fig. 3 and Section 3.3).

5 GABA-A Autoreceptors

Although the existence of GABA autoreceptors (Fig. 1) has not yet been supported by studies employing electrophysiological techniques, neurochemical data are consistent with the existence of such receptors (Mitchell and Martin, 1978; Snodgrass, 1978; Arbilla *et al.*, 1979; Brennan and Cantrill, 1979). Studies on the effects of GABA itself on the depolarization-induced release of labelled GABA from preloaded slices or synaptosomes prepared from brain tissue are hampered by homoexchange phenomena. Thus, uptake of GABA applied to the exterior surface of the tissue preparations produces an apparent efflux of the labelled transmitter because of 1:1 exchange.

The most convincing pieces of evidence for the existence of GABA autoreceptors are derived from *in vitro* studies on GABA release using GABA agonists such as isoguvacine (**2**), P4S (**3**), and THIP (**4**) (Fig. 3), which are not substrates for the GABA uptake mechanisms (Krogsgaard-Larsen, 1980; Krogsgaard-Larsen *et al.*, 1980; Schousboe *et al.*, 1985). The sensitivity of the receptors mediating this phenomenon to GABA-A agonists and GABA-A antagonists, such as BMC (**5**), appears to be very similar to that of the postsynaptic GABA-A receptors, and, furthermore, the GABA-B agonist baclofen is inactive at the receptors concerned (Lockerbie and Gordon-Weeks, 1985). On the other hand, the GABA homologue δ-aminolaevulinic acid apparently is a relatively selective agonist at GABA-A autoreceptors (Brennan and Cantrill, 1979), and, in contrast to postsynaptic GABA-A receptors, autoreceptors do not seem to be coupled to BZD receptor sites (Brennan, 1982; Fig. 3).

6 GABA-B Receptors

In 1974 two groups independently demonstrated that the depressant effects of baclofen, the (R)-form (**90**) being the active one (Fig. 23), on mammalian central neurons could not be blocked by the GABA-A antagonists bicuculline (**61**) or BMC (**5**) (Curtis *et al.*, 1974; Davies and Watkins, 1974). Subsequently, it was demonstrated that neither bicuculline nor picrotoxinin (**8**) blocked the depressant action of GABA on the evoked release of noradrenaline from sympathetic nerve terminals (Bowery and Hudson, 1979). In this preparation, the GABA-A agonists isoguvacine (**2**) and P4S (**3**) were inactive and muscimol (**12**) was much weaker than GABA, whereas the particular effect of GABA was mimicked by baclofen (Bowery *et al.*, 1981). Similarly, GABA and baclofen have been shown to decrease neuro-transmitter release in the CNS by activation of receptors at which BMC or bicuculline are not antagonists (Bowery *et al.*, 1980a,b). On the basis of these observations the existence of a subclass of GABA receptors, the GABA-B receptors, distinctly different from the "classical" GABA-A receptors, was proposed (Bowery *et al.*, 1980a,b). The GABA-B receptor sites can be readily demonstrated in brain synaptic membranes using binding techniques with either radioactive baclofen or GABA, in the latter case under conditions where GABA-A receptor sites are blocked by isoguvacine (**2**) (Hill and Bowery, 1981; Bowery, 1983). Since these original obser-vations, GABA-B receptors have been detected and described in a variety of tissue preparations of central or peripheral origin (Bowery, 1983; Bowery *et al.*, 1984).

In addition to the different pharmacological profiles of the GABA-A and GABA-B receptors, major differences between these receptor systems have been disclosed (Enna, 1983; Bowery, 1984). While pre- as well as postsynaptic GABA-A receptors are coupled to chloride channels, GABA-B recep-tors are coupled to calcium channels, and, in contrast to GABA-A receptors, GABA-B receptors appear to be associated with a second messenger

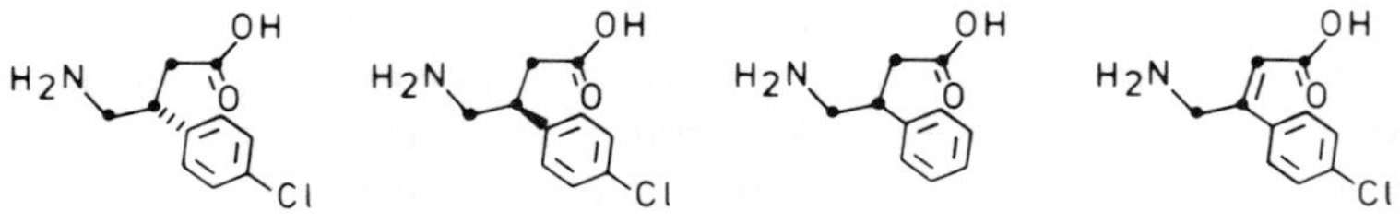

(90) (R) Baclofen   (91) (S) Baclofen   (92)   (93)

FIG. 23. Structures of (R)-baclofen (90) and some related compounds.

system. Thus, GABA as well as (R)-baclofen (90), but not (S)-baclofen (91), (Fig. 23) are capable of potentiating the response to stimulation of adenyl cyclase by catecholamines, whereas neither compound has any significant effect on basal adenyl cyclase activity in brain slices or membranes (Enna and Karbon, 1984; Hill *et al.*, 1984; Watling and Bristow, 1986). On the other hand, GABA (90), but not (91), were shown to inhibit forskolin-induced cAMP production (Enna and Karbon, 1984; Hill *et al.*, 1984; Watling and Bristow, 1986).

While an association between a large population of postsynaptic GABA-A receptors and BZD receptor sites is well documented (Enna, 1983; Bowery, 1984; Fig. 3), it seems unlikely that GABA-B receptors are linked to BZD receptor sites (Bowery, 1983; Bowery *et al.*, 1984). Finally, the regional distributions of GABA-A and GABA-B receptors in the CNS are different; in the cerebellum, GABA-B sites are confined to the molecular layer, whereas GABA-A sites predominate in the granule cell layer (Wilkin *et al.*, 1981; Palacios *et al.*, 1981). In the spinal cord the largest density of GABA-B sites are detected in the dorsal horn laminae I, II, and III, whereas the GABA-A sites seem to be more uniformly distributed throughout the dorsal and ventral horns (Bowery, 1983; Bowery *et al.*, 1984).

6.1 GABA-B AGONISTS

Baclofen is clinically effective in certain types of spasticity (Burke *et al.*, 1971; Bowery, 1982). Furthermore, baclofen has non-opioid analgesic effects, showing a pharmacological profile in different test systems different from that of the GABA-A agonist, THIP (4) (see Section 3.6.2; Hill *et al.*, 1981; Sawynok and LaBella, 1981, 1982; DeFeudis, 1982; Sivam and Ho, 1985; Zorn *et al.*, 1986), and baclofen has anticonvulsant properties, which are not identical with those of THIP or the BZDs in terms of antiseizure effects and profile of side effects (Krogsgaard-Larsen *et al.*, 1986). These aspects have prompted the synthesis of a variety of analogues of baclofen as exemplified in Fig. 23 and an intense search for GABA-B agonists with structures different from that of baclofen, and for GABA-B antagonists (Section 6.2). The latter group of agents are essential as tools for basic studies of GABA-B receptor functions and for studies of the mechanisms underlying the pharmacological effects of baclofen, some of which may not be mediated by GABA-B receptors (Bowery, 1982). The pharmacological profiles of a variety of baclofen analogues, including (92) (Fig. 23), have been assessed on the basis of microelectrophoretic experiments on single neurons and pharmacological studies on reflexes in the cat (Olpe *et al.*, 1980). Alterations of the amino acid as well as the aromatic moiety of baclofen have resulted in substantial or complete loss of pharmacological effects. Replacement of the chloro atom of baclofen by a trifluoromethyl group led to complete loss of activity, and compound (92), containing an unsubstituted phenyl group, was much weaker than baclofen in terms of reflex-inhibiting properties, and somewhat weaker as a depressant of the spontaneous firing of single neurons (Olpe *et al.*, 1980). Shortening or extension of the amino acid backbone of baclofen also gave much weaker compounds. Unsaturated analogues of baclofen such as *trans*-4-amino-3-(4-chlorophenyl)but-2-enoic (93) have been synthesized (Allan and Tran, 1981) and shown to be inactive.

A number of simple GABA analogues have been studied as inhibitors of GABA-B binding, including the enantiomers of GABOB and a variety of structurally related hydroxylated GABA analogues (Falch *et al.*, 1986). In Fig. 24 the effects of these compounds on GABA-B receptor binding are compared with their effects on GABA-A receptor binding and synaptosomal GABA uptake. Among these compounds, (R)-GABOB is the most potent inhibitor of GABA-B binding. With the exception of 2-hydroxy-5-aminopentanoic acid (95, 2-OH-DAVA) these analogues of GABOB did not affect GABA-B binding (Falch *et al.*, 1986). Surprisingly, replacement of the hydroxy group of GABOB by the less polar methoxy group resulted in complete loss of GABA-B receptor affinity (Fig. 24).

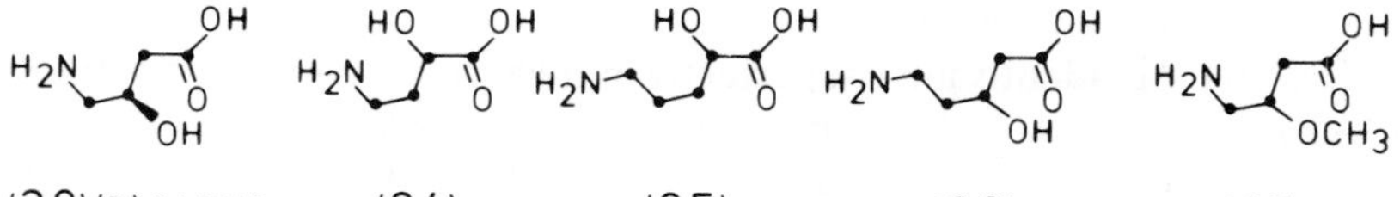

	(30)(R)GABOB	(94)	(95)	(96)	(97)
A-B	1	15	51	15	25
B-B	0.4	>100	23	>100	>100
UPT-S	67	5	>300	>300	>300

FIG. 24. Structures and *in vitro* biological effects of (R)-GABOB (30) and some related amino acids (for legend see Fig. 7).

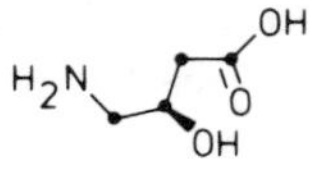

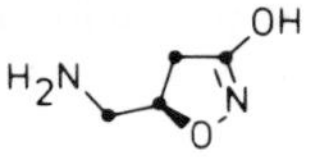

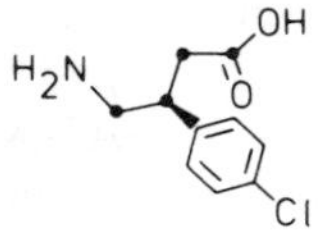

	(30) (*R*) GABOB	(19) (*R*) DHM	(91) (*S*) Baclofen
A-B	1	0.3	>100
B-B	0.4	5	25
UPT-S	67	70	>300

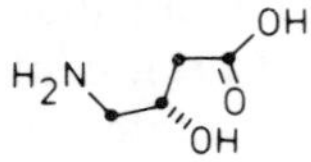

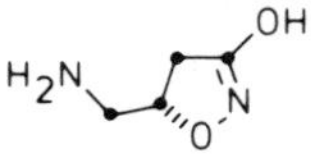

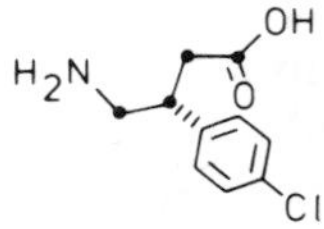

	(29) (*S*) GABOB	(18) (*S*) DHM	(90) (*R*) Baclofen
A-B	0.4	0.004	>100
B-B	2.5	13	0.08
UPT-S	30	>300	300

FIG. 25. Structures and *in vitro* biological effects of the optical isomers of GABOB, DHM, and baclofen (for legend see Fig. 7).

Comparative stereostructure–activity studies using the (*R*)- and (*S*)-isomers of GABOB, DHM, and baclofen have disclosed that GABA-A and GABA-B receptor sites exhibit opposite stereoselectivity (Falch *et al.*, 1986; Krogsgaard-Larsen, 1987; Fig. 25). (*R*)-GABOB is a potent inhibitor of GABA-B binding, showing about one-fifth of the affinity of (*R*)-baclofen (**90**) for GABA-B sites (Falch *et al.*, 1986). Furthermore, (*R*)-DHM (**19**) is somewhat more potent as an inhibitor of GABA-B binding than (*S*)-DHM (**18**), the most powerful GABA-A agonist so far described (Fig. 7).

(*S*)-DHM evidently almost perfectly mimics the active conformation(s) of GABA at the GABA-A receptors, whereas (*R*)-GABOB and (*R*)-baclofen seem to reflect the conformation(s) adopted by GABA during its binding to GABA-B receptor sites. Due to the considerable conformational mobility of both of these compounds (Fig. 26), it is not possible to deduce the active conformation(s) of GABA at the GABA-B receptors from these structure–activity studies. (*R*)-GABOB and (*R*)-baclofen have opposite stereochemical orientations of the hydroxy and 4-chlorophenyl groups, respectively (Fig. 26). This observation strongly suggests that the polar hydroxy group in

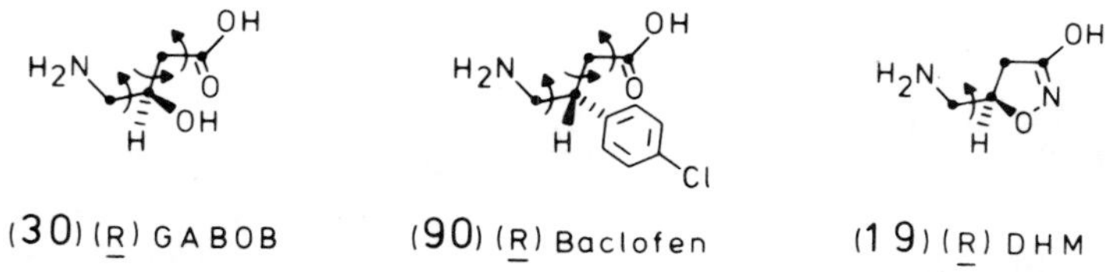

FIG. 26. Structures and conformational flexibilities of (R)-GABOB (30), (R)-baclofen (90), and (R)-DHM (19).

the former GABA analogue interacts with a structure element of the GABA-B receptor site different from that, which binds the lipophilic 4-chlorophenyl group of (90) during its interaction with GABA-B receptor sites.

The recent observation that baclofen apparently activates two distinct GABA-B receptors (Sawynok, 1986) complicates structure–activity studies on compounds interacting with these receptor sites.

Evidence derived from different lines of research strongly suggests that hyperactivity of the central excitatory neurotransmitter GLU is a major causal factor in certain neurodegenerative disorders (Roberts et al., 1986; Hicks et al., 1987). The results of numerous neurochemical studies have demonstrated that the release of GLU (Figs 2 and 22) may be regulated by GABA-B receptors located on terminals of GLU-utilizing neurons (Bowery, 1983). Such findings have focused much pharmacological and therapeutic interest on these presynaptic receptors (Bowery, 1982), which may represent a subclass of GABA-B receptors (Sawynok, 1986). Selective activation of presynaptic GABA-B receptors may represent a flexible way of reducing excessive activation of neurons in the brain by GLU. Although recent studies have demonstrated that baclofen stimulates rather than reduces the in vivo release of GLU in the rat hippocampus (Nielsen et al., 1987), this GABA-B receptor-directed approach may lead to the development of new drugs in the highly complex field of neurodegenerative disorders.

There also is a pharmacological and therapeutic interest in GABA-B receptor antagonists. Thus, extensive neurochemical studies indicate that the in vitro release of monoamine neurotransmitters, such as DA, serotonin, and noradrenaline, may also be regulated by presynaptically located GABA-B receptors (Bowery, 1983; Bowery et al., 1984; see Section 4), and, in principle, administration of GABA-B antagonists would stimulate the release of such neurotransmitters, which may have therapeutic prospects in certain psychiatric diseases.

6.2 GABA-B ANTAGONISTS

The GABA homologue, 5-aminopentanoic acid (**99**, DAVA) (Fig. 27), which is an endogenous amino acid (Callery and Geelhaar, 1984), has been shown to possess a weak antagonist profile at peripheral GABA-B receptors (Muhyaddin *et al.*, 1982). Furthermore, DAVA, as well as (*S*)-baclofen (**91**) (Fig. 27), inhibited the antinociceptive effect of (*R*)-baclofen (Fig. 23) after intrathecal injection (Sawynok, 1986). Under these conditions 3-amino-propanesulphonic acid (**101**, 3-APS), which has GABA-B antagonist properties on peripheral GABA-B receptors (Giotti *et al.*, 1983), did not significantly antagonize (*R*)-baclofen-induced antinociception (Sawynok, 1986). On the other hand, DAVA and 3-APS, but not (*S*)-baclofen, antagonized the inhibitory effect of (*R*)-baclofen on a guinea-pig muscle preparation (Sawynok, 1986). Neither DAVA nor 3-APS interact selectively with GABA-B receptors. DAVA shows affinity for all GABA-A synaptic mechanisms (Allan and Johnston, 1983; Falch *et al.*, 1986) and 3-APS is a very potent agonist at GABA-A receptors in the mammalian CNS (Krogsgaard-Larsen *et al.*, 1980, 1981a, 1985a; Falch *et al.*, 1985a,b). There is evidence suggesting that the antagonism by DAVA at GABA-B receptors in the guinea-pig ileum may be due to an interaction between GABA-A and GABA-B receptors (Allan and Dickenson, 1986). In any case, lack of selectivity reduces the value of DAVA and 3-APS as tools for studies of GABA-B receptor mechanisms.

It has recently been demonstrated that compound (**100**) (Fig. 27) has weak GABA-B antagonist properties in a guinea-pig muscle preparation (Luzzi *et al.*, 1986), and the phosphonic acid analogue of baclofen, phaclofen (**98**), shows antagonist effects on central as well as peripheral GABA-B receptors (Kerr *et al.*, 1987). These observations are likely to accelerate the studies of the physiological role of GABA-B receptors and may stimulate the development of therapeutically useful GABA-B antagonists.

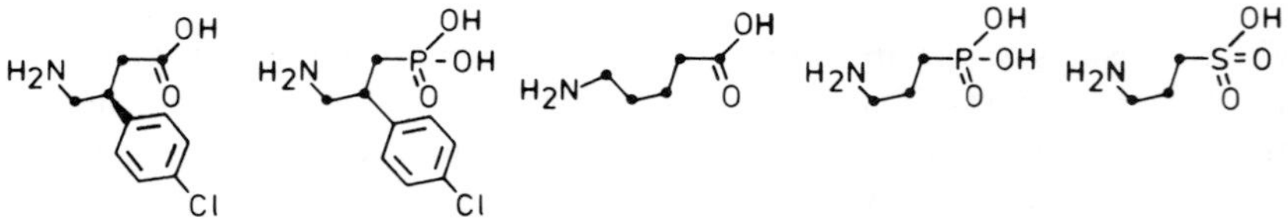

FIG. 27. Structures of some compounds with GABA-B antagonist properties.

7 GABA Uptake Mechanisms as Pharmacological Targets

Inhibition of GABA transport (uptake) mechanisms may represent a flexible way of stimulating GABA-mediated neurotransmission (Krogsgaard-Larsen, 1980; Krogsgaard-Larsen et al., 1981b, 1987). In view of the limited knowledge of the relative importance of the processes underlying the termination of the synaptic action of GABA, it is not possible at present to single out with certainty the transport mechanisms most susceptible to pharmacological intervention (see Fig. 1). It has been established that neuronal and glial GABA uptake mechanisms have dissimilar inhibitor/substrate specificities (Schousboe et al., 1979; Krogsgaard-Larsen, 1980; Krogsgaard-Larsen et al., 1981b, 1987), and the most logical and realistic strategies for pharmacological interventions into these systems with the purpose of stimulating GABA neurotransmission seem to be (Krogsgaard-Larsen et al., 1981b, 1987):

(1) effective blockade of both neuronal and glial GABA uptake in order to enhance the inhibitory effect of synaptically released GABA or
(2) selective blockade of glial GABA uptake in order to increase the amount of GABA taken up by the neuronal carrier with subsequent elevation of the GABA concentration in nerve terminals.

While substrates/inhibitors of neuronal GABA uptake appear to be proconvulsants or convulsants (Horton et al., 1979; Krogsgaard-Larsen et al., 1981b, 1987), compounds acting as selective substrates/inhibitors for the glial uptake system have anticonvulsant effects (Krogsgaard-Larsen, 1980; Krogsgaard-Larsen et al., 1981b, 1987; Croucher et al., 1983). There is a pharmacological interest in selective inhibitors of glial uptake, which do not act as substrates for the transport carrier (Krogsgaard-Larsen et al., 1987) (see below).

7.1 SEPARATION OF GABA-A RECEPTOR AND GABA UPTAKE AFFINITIES

While replacement of the ring oxygen atom of the key lead structure, muscimol (12), by sulphur to give thiomuscimol (17) and the conversion of muscimol into (S)-DHM (18) resulted in *elimination* of the GABA uptake affinity of muscimol without significant loss of GABA-A agonist activity (Krogsgaard-Larsen et al., 1979c, 1985b; Fig. 7), another approach led to a complete *separation* of the GABA-A receptor and GABA uptake affinity of muscimol (Krogsgaard-Larsen et al., 1977, 1984b; Krogsgaard-Larsen, 1987). This separation was accomplished through incorporation of the

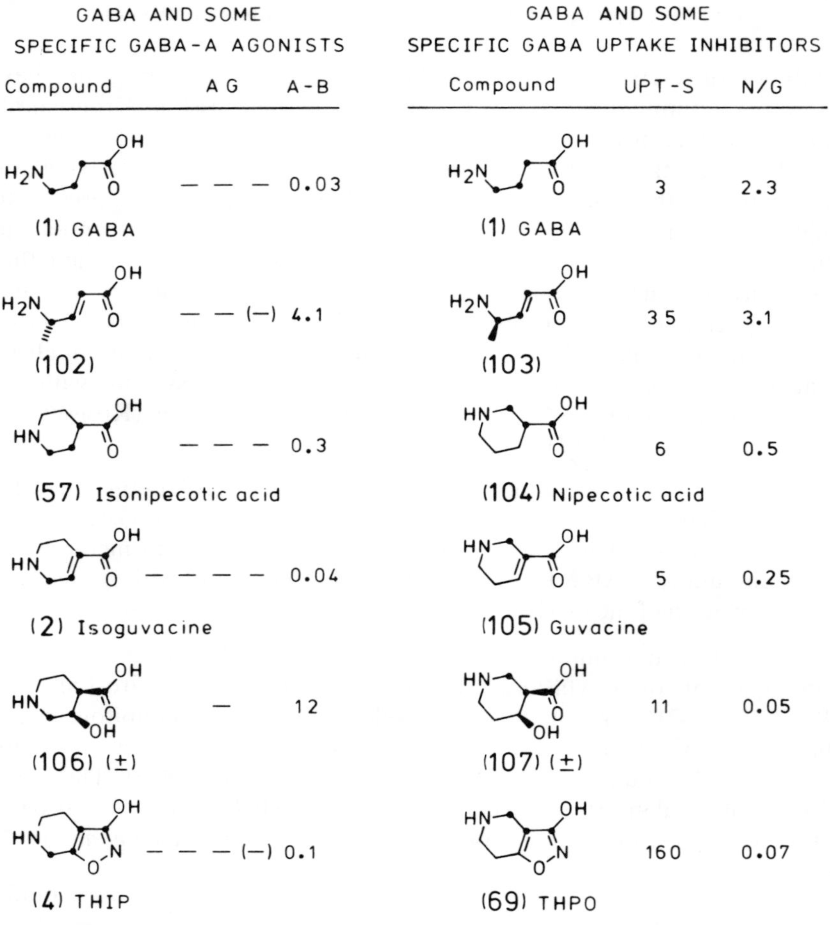

GABA AND SOME
SPECIFIC GABA-A AGONISTS

Compound	A G	A-B

OH
H₂N O
(1) GABA — — — 0.03

OH
H₂N O
(102) — — (−) 4.1

OH
HN O
(57) Isonipecotic acid — — — 0.3

OH
HN O
(2) Isoguvacine — — — — 0.04

OH
HN O OH
(106) (±) — 12

OH
HN N O
(4) THIP — — — (−) 0.1

GABA AND SOME
SPECIFIC GABA UPTAKE INHIBITORS

Compound	UPT-S	N/G

OH
H₂N O
(1) GABA 3 2.3

OH
H₂N O
(103) 3 5 3.1

OH
HN O
(104) Nipecotic acid 6 0.5

OH
HN O
(105) Guvacine 5 0.25

OH
HN O OH
(107) (±) 11 0.05

OH
HN N O
(69) THPO 160 0.07

FIG. 28. Comparative structure–activity studies of some GABA analogues. N/G indicates the ratio between the affinity of GABA uptake inhibitors for neuronal (N) and glial (G) GABA uptake, a high value indicating selectivity for neuronal and a low value selectivity for glial uptake (for legend see Fig. 7).

amino group of muscimol into additional ring structures to give the conformationally immobilized analogues THIP (**4**) and THPO (**69**) (Krogsgaard-Larsen *et al.*, 1977, 1985a; Krogsgaard-Larsen and Falch, 1981) and subsequent "conversion" of these bicyclic compounds into the corresponding monocyclic amino acids as illustrated in Fig. 28 (see also Fig. 18). A comparison of the structures of the compounds in these two series of mutually isomeric amino acids illustrates the similar but distinctly different structural specificities of the GABA-A receptors and GABA uptake systems.

It is evident that the GABA structure elements of isonipecotic acid (**57**), isoguvacine (**2**), and THIP (**4**), perhaps of the low-energy conformations of these compounds, reflect the active conformation(s) of GABA at the GABA-A receptors. Since no parts of the molecules of the cyclic GABA uptake inhibitors shown in Fig. 28 unequivocally reflect the molecule of GABA, these analogues are of limited value as model compounds for studies of the conformation(s) in which GABA interacts with the GABA transport carriers. Nevertheless, the comparative structure–activity studies illustrated in Fig. 28 suggest that GABA adopts different conformations during its binding to GABA-A receptors and to GABA transport carriers.

In agreement with the discussion in Section 3.1.1, the *in vivo* and *in vitro* pharmacological data for the enantiomers of *trans*-4-aminopent-2-enoic acid (**102** and **103**) (Fig. 28) illustrate that GABA-A receptors and GABA uptake systems have opposite stereochemical requirements, the (*S*)-form (**102**) being a specific GABA-A agonist and the (*R*)-form (**103**) a specific uptake inhibitor (Krogsgaard-Larsen, 1981; Krogsgaard-Larsen *et al.*, 1983b). This observation is emphasized by stereostructure–activity studies on the aminocyclopentane- and aminocyclopentenecarboxylic acids depicted in Fig. 29 (Allan *et al.*, 1986a).

These studies on conformationally immobilized and/or chiral GABA analogues with established absolute stereochemistry do not necessarily support the view that the GABA-A receptors and the GABA transport carriers recognize and bind different conformations of GABA. They do, however, demonstrate that the biomolecules of the GABA-A receptors are different from those of the transport carriers. All of the model compounds illustrated in Figs 28 and 29 contain groups or ring residues in addition to the GABA or GABA-like structure elements. The specificity of the model compounds concerned may simply reflect that the biomolecules of the binding sites of the GABA-operated mechanisms under study have distinctly different capabilities to accommodate these additional structure elements of

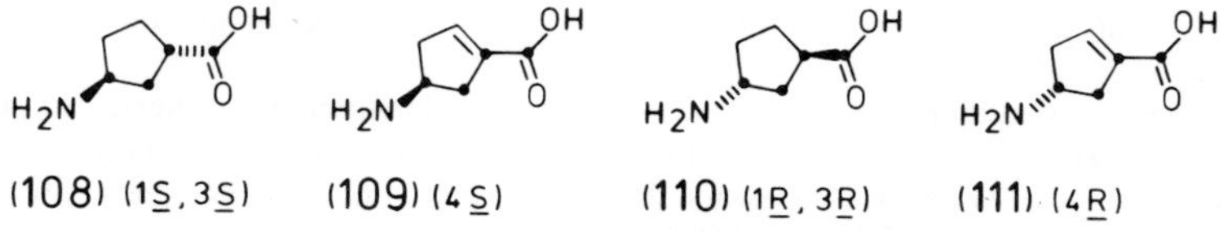

(**108**) (1S̲,3S̲)   (**109**) (4 S̲)   (**110**) (1R̲,3R̲)   (**111**) (4R̲)

GABA-A AGONISTS   GABA UPTAKE INHIBITORS

FIG. 29. The structures of some cyclic GABA-A agonists and uptake inhibitors.

the model compounds. Plates 1a–d and 2a–d illustrate the three-dimensional structural features of some of the model compounds shown in Figs 28 and 29 emphasizing the ranges of conformations accessible to some of the relatively flexible compounds and the degree of structural similarity or differences between key model compounds.

7.2 SUBSTRATE AND INHIBITOR CHARACTERISTICS OF NEURONAL AND GLIAL GABA UPTAKE SYSTEMS

As discussed earlier (see Figs 18 and 28), nipecotic acid (**104**) is an effective inhibitor of neuronal (N) as well as glial (G) uptake, being slightly more potent at the latter system as indicated by an N/G ratio of 0.5 (Fig. 28) (Krogsgaard-Larsen and Johnston, 1975; Schousboe *et al.*, 1979; Larsson *et al.*, 1981; Krogsgaard-Larsen *et al.*, 1987). Furthermore, nipecotic acid has been shown to be a substrate for both neuronal (Johnston *et al.*, 1976a; Larsson *et al.*, 1985) and glial (Larsson *et al.*, 1980, 1985) GABA transport carriers, and nipecotic acid appears to provide a retrograde tracer specific to neurons whose terminals exhibit preferential GABA uptake (Ryan and Schwartz, 1986). Guvacine (**105**) shows an *in vitro* pharmacological profile very similar to that of nipecotic acid (**104**) being, perhaps, a slightly more selective inhibitor of the glial GABA uptake system (N/G 0.25, Fig. 28) (Schousboe *et al.*, 1979), and based on kinetic data guvacine seems to be a substrate for the neuronal GABA transport carrier (Johnston *et al.*, 1975). The observations that guvacine has a slightly lower N/G ratio than nipecotic acid and the conformationally restricted analogue, THPO (**69**), a much lower N/G ratio than nipecotic acid do seem to indicate that a certain degree of rotational freedom of the acid functions is a factor of importance for the binding of these compounds to the neuronal GABA transport carrier.

Like *cis*-4-OH-nipecotic acid (**107**) (Krogsgaard-Larsen, 1978; Krogsgaard-Larsen *et al.*, 1978), THPO has an oxygen function in the

---

PLATE 1a–d. a. Stereo representation of the GABA-A agonist (**102**) (Fig. 28) in a conformation fitted to a preferred conformation of THIP (**4**). The green vectors show the possible orientations of the C–N bond. The blue vectors show the possible orientations of the C–O bonds.

b. Stereo representation of muscimol (**12**) in a conformation fitted to a preferred conformation of THIP (**4**). The green vectors show the possible orientations of the C–N bond.

c. Stereo representation of isoguvacine (**2**) (green) and muscimol (**12**) (blue) fitted to a preferred conformation of THIP (**4**) (red).

d. Stereo representation of THIP (**4**), muscimol (**12**), and isoguvacine (**2**) (all in red) and (**102**) (green). The blue volume is the extra volume of (**102**) relative to THIP, muscimol, and isoguvacine.

a)

b)

c)

d)

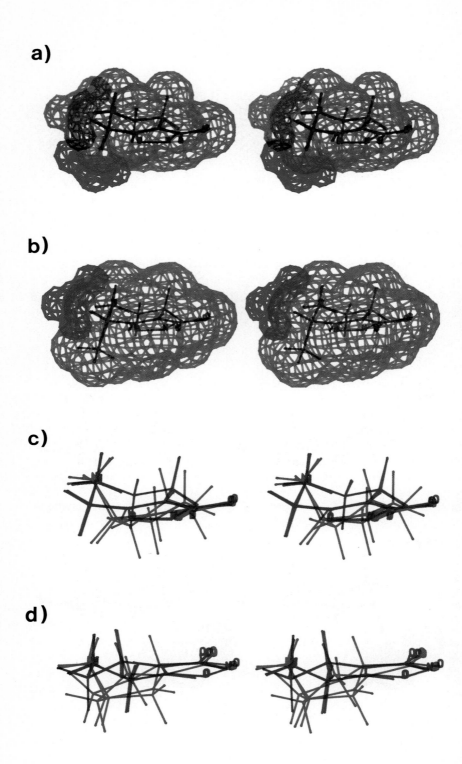

4-position of the piperidine ring, which for unknown reasons may contribute to the selectivity of these compounds for the glial GABA uptake system (Fig. 28). In contrast to cis-4-OH-nipecotic acid (107), which is a substrate for neuronal as well as glial GABA transport mechanisms, THPO does not seem to be a substrate for the glial transport carrier (Larsson et al., 1985). Thus, a prerequisite for transport by, but not for binding to, the glial uptake system by GABA analogues appears to be a certain degree of rotational freedom of the acid functionalities.

The depressant action of microelectrophoretically applied GABA on spinal (Krogsgaard-Larsen et al., 1975; Curtis et al., 1976), cerebellar (Curtis et al., 1976), and cortical (Curtis et al., 1976; Yarbrough, 1978) neurons was reversibly enhanced by simultaneously administered nipecotic acid. (R)-Nipecotic acid (70) was more potent than its (S)-isomer (113) in enhancing the depressant action of GABA on spinal neurons (Curtis et al., 1976; Fig. 30), in agreement with the relative potency of these optical isomers as uptake inhibitors in vitro (see Fig. 32; Johnston et al., 1976a; Schousboe et al., 1979). Using the same technique, guvacine (105) has been shown to enhance the depressant action of exogenous GABA on single cat spinal neurons (Lodge et al., 1977). An analysis of such single cell pharmacological data indicates that the GABA-enhancing effects of these GABA uptake inhibitors really are the results of inhibition of the GABA transport processes in vivo rather than of heteroexchange phenomena between the uptake inhibitors and endogenous GABA in nerve terminals (Krogsgaard-Larsen et al., 1981b, 1987).

Electrophoretically applied cis-4-OH-nipecotic acid (107) or THPO (69) (Fig. 31), selective inhibitors of glial GABA uptake (see Fig. 28), also enhance the action of similarly administered GABA on cat spinal neurons (Krogsgaard-Larsen et al., 1975, 1983c). These effects compared with those of nipecotic acid and a number of other GABA uptake inhibitors are consistent with both glial and neuronal GABA transport systems playing a role in the termination of GABA-mediated neurotransmission (Martin, 1976; Schousboe, 1981; Krogsgaard-Larsen et al., 1987).

PLATE 2a–d. a. Stereo representation of the volumes of THIP (4), muscimol (12), and isoguvacine (2) (green). The extra volume of the GABA-A agonist (102) is shown in blue and that of the GABA uptake inhibitor (103) (Fig. 28) in brown. The framework of the molecules are depicted inside the volumes: THIP (4) (red), (102) (blue), and (103) (brown).

b. Stereo representation of the common volume for the GABA-A agonists THIP (4), muscimol (12), isoguvacine (2), (102), (108), and (109) (green) and the extra volume for the GABA uptake inhibitor (103) (blue).

c and d. Stereo representation of (108) and (109) (blue) fitted to a preferred conformation of THIP (4) (red). The structures of muscimol (12) and isoguvacine (2) are also drawn in red. The two sets of pictures represent different views.

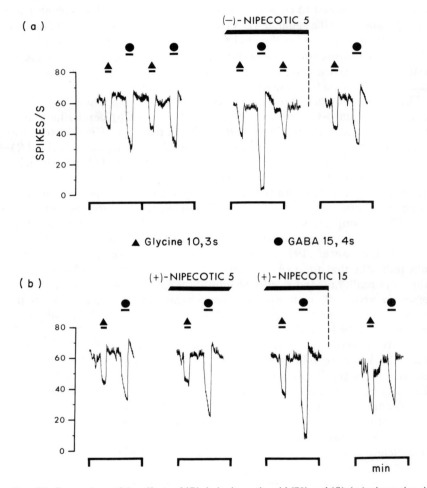

FIG. 30. Comparison of the effects of (R)-$(-)$-nipecotic acid (**70**) and (S)-$(+)$-nipecotic acid (**113**) on the depressant actions of glycine or GABA on a cat spinal Renshaw cell (for details see Curtis *et al.*, 1976). Reproduced with permission.

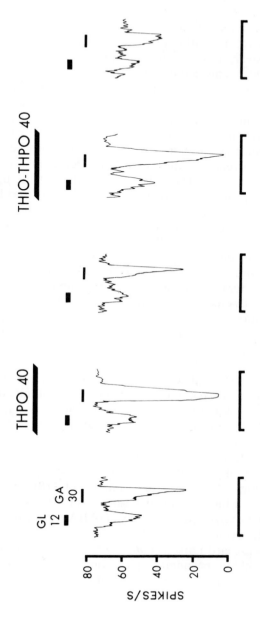

Fig. 31. Comparison of the effects of THPO (**69**) and thio-THPO (**88**) on the depressant actions of glycine (GL) or GABA (GA) on a cat spinal interneuron (for details see Krogsgaard-Larsen *et al.*, 1983c). Reproduced with permission.

In contrast to the described enhancement of the depressant effects of exogenous GABA by uptake inhibitors, electrophoretic application of (*R*)-nipecotic acid near Purkinje cells in cat cerebellum failed to prolong the GABA-mediated basket cell inhibition of these cells (Curtis *et al.*, 1976; Lodge *et al.*, 1977). However, studies on the rat hippocampal dentate gyrus demonstrated pronounced enhancement of the duration of recurrent inhibition of granule cells by electrophoretically applied guvacine (**105**) (Matthews *et al.*, 1981). Similar effects on GABA-mediated inhibition in the hippocampus by GABA uptake inhibitors have recently been demonstrated *in situ* (Rovira *et al.*, 1984) and using slice preparations (Korn and Dingledine, 1986). In the latter studies *cis*-4-OH-nipecotic acid (**107**) proved to be particularly potent, possibly reflecting the preferential effect of this inhibitor on glial GABA uptake (Fig. 28). The predominant effect of the uptake inhibitors was a marked prolongation of the falling phase of the IPSPs (Rovira *et al.*, 1984; Korn and Dingledine, 1986), an effect which may become of major importance during repetitive activation of GABA-mediated inhibitory processes (Krnjevic, 1984). Nipecotic acid was shown to abolish the fading of the inhibitory action of GABA in the stratum pyramidale of CA1 (Rovira *et al.*, 1984; Krnjevic, 1984), suggesting that GABA-fading to a large extent may be caused by GABA uptake rather than true desensitization of GABA receptors (Krnjevic, 1984). The lack of fading phenomena after application of GABA at the dendritic level in the stratum radiatum and of enhancement of GABA responses by uptake inhibitors in this region (Rovira *et al.*, 1984) are consistent with a low density of GABAergic nerve endings on the dendrites (Krnjevic, 1984).

Introduction of small substituents on the amino groups of guvacine or nipecotic acid normally results in compounds with decreased affinity for the GABA transport carriers (Wood *et al.*, 1979; Krogsgaard-Larsen, 1980; Krogsgaard-Larsen *et al.*, 1985a), consistent with a high degree of inhibitor/ substrate specificity of these uptake mechanisms. In view of these observations, the very potent effects on synaptosomal GABA uptake of a series of amino acids containing bulky substituents on the amino groups is remarkable (Ali *et al.*, 1985; Fig. 32). These compounds (**114–118**) have been prepared by introduction of the 4,4-diphenyl-3-butenyl (DPB) substituent on the nitrogen atoms of GABA and the classical GABA uptake inhibitors such as nipecotic acid, guvacine, *cis*-4-OH-nipecotic acid, and, more recently, THPO (P. Krogsgaard-Larsen *et al.*, 1987). The DPB analogues of these GABA uptake inhibitors containing a secondary amino group are typically at least an order of magnitude more potent than the parent amino acids as inhibitors of synaptosomal GABA uptake (Ali *et al.*, 1985; Yunger *et al.*, 1984; Fig. 32).

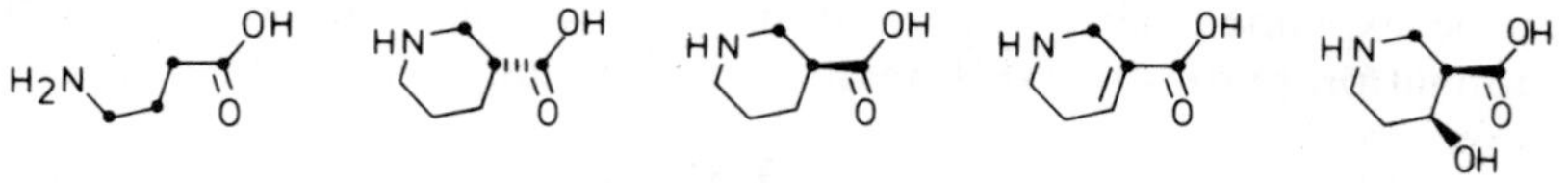

| | (1) | (70) (R)- | (113) (S)- | (105) | (107) |
| | GABA | Nipecotic acid | Nipecotic acid | Guvacine | |

PARENT AMINO ACIDS

UPT-S 2.6   1.7   9.9   4.9   4.6

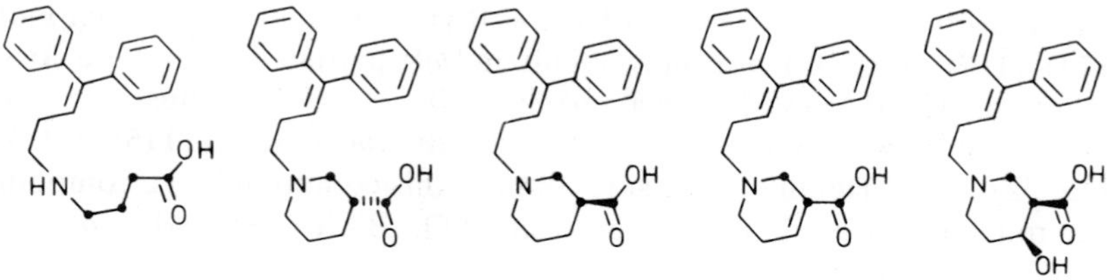

| | (114) | (115) | (116) | (117) | (118) |

UPT-S 17   0.11   1.9   0.20   0.26

FIG. 32. Comparative structure–activity studies of some GABA uptake inhibitors and their 4,4-diphenyl-3-butenyl (DPB) analogues (for legend see Fig. 7).

The precise mechanisms underlying the interaction of this series of analogues with GABA uptake systems are still unknown. The relative potencies of these DPB analogues and of the respective classical amino acid uptake inhibitors (Johnston *et al.*, 1976b) are, however, very similar (Fig. 32). This structure–activity relationship strongly suggests that the amino acid moieties of these DPB analogues are recognized and bound by the GABA transport carriers, with which the parent amino acids interact. However, introduction of the DPB substituent on the amino groups of GABA and other GABA uptake inhibitors containing primary amino groups did not lead to analogues with increased affinity for GABA uptake mechanisms in synaptosomes. These DPB analogues containing secondary amino groups, as exemplified by compound (**114**), proved to be weaker than the parent amino acids (Ali *et al.*, 1985; Fig. 32). This conspicuous difference may indicate that the mechanism of action for the DPB analogue of for example GABA is different from that of the DPB analogues of the rest of the GABA uptake inhibitors listed in Fig. 32. It is possible that this difference can be explained partly on the basis of different protolytic and conformational properties of DPB analogues containing secondary and tertiary amino groups.

It has recently been demonstrated that the DPB analogue of nipecotic acid, in contrast to nipecotic acid itself (Johnston *et al.*, 1976a; Larsson *et al.*, 1980, 1985), is acting as a simple competitive inhibitor of neuronal as well as glial GABA uptake and is not transported by the uptake carriers concerned, and, furthermore, the DPB analogues of glia-selective GABA uptake inhibitors (see Fig. 28) seem to be approximately equipotent as inhibitors of neuronal and glial GABA uptake (O. M. Larsson, E. Falch, P. Krogsgaard-Larsen, and A. Schousboe, unpubl.).

Alterations of the structure of the DPB substituent of the compounds (**114**)–(**118**) (Fig. 32) normally result in substantial or complete loss of affinity for GABA uptake mechanisms (Ali *et al.*, 1985). Thus, removal of the double bond of *N*-DPB-nipecotic acid, the racemate of (**115**) and (**116**) (Fig. 32), or shortening of the side chain of this compound give compounds with much lower affinity for synaptosomal GABA uptake (Ali *et al.*, 1985; Krogsgaard-Larsen *et al.*, 1987).

7.3 PRODRUGS OF GABA UPTAKE INHIBITORS

In agreement with the high I/U ratios (see Section 3.4) for nipecotic acid (**104**) (pK_a 3.9, 10.3; I/U 250,000), guvacine (**105**) (pK_a 3.5, 9.9; I/U 150,000), and *cis*-4-OH-nipecotic acid (**107**) (pK_a 3.4, 10.0; I/U 300,000) (Krogsgaard-Larsen *et al.*, 1981b, 1987), these GABA uptake inhibitors show very weak pharmacological effects after systemic administration, reflecting the fact that the BBB effectively prevents these compounds from entering the brain from the bloodstream. The relatively low I/U ratio for THPO (**69**) (2500) is consistent with the observation that THPO, to some extent, is capable of penetrating the BBB (Schousboe *et al.*, 1986; see Section 3.4). These aspects have prompted the development of prodrugs of nipecotic acid, guvacine, and *cis*-4-OH-nipecotic acid for studies of the pharmacology of these GABA uptake inhibitors.

A number of simple esters of these GABA uptake inhibitors (Fig. 33) have been tested as potential prodrugs. The ethyl esters of nipecotic acid and guvacine, (**119**) and (**123**) respectively, have been studied pharmacologically, but muscarinic cholinergic effects of these esters limit their utility as prodrugs (Frey *et al.*, 1979; Zorn *et al.*, 1987). It was, however, demonstrated that systemically administered (**119**) is capable of crossing the BBB with subsequent complete hydrolysis of the ester to the free amino acid in the

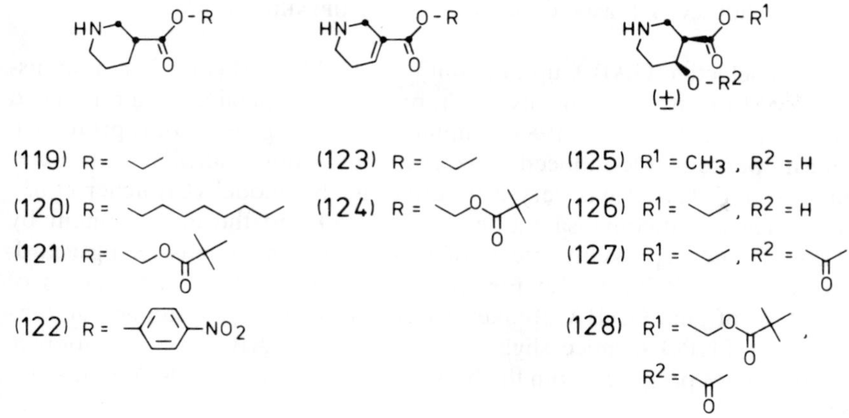

(119) R = ⌄

(120) R = ⌄⌄⌄⌄

(121) R = ⌄O⌄⊣<

(122) R = —⟨ ⟩—NO₂

(123) R = ⌄

(124) R = ⌄O⌄⊣<

(125) R¹ = CH₃ , R² = H

(126) R¹ = ⌄ , R² = H

(127) R¹ = ⌄ , R² = ⊣<

(128) R¹ = ⌄O⌄⊣< ,

R² = ⊣<

FIG. 33. Structures of some prodrugs of the GABA uptake inhibitors nipecotic acid (104), guvacine (105), and cis-4-OH-nipecotic acid (107).

brain tissue within 30 min (Frey et al., 1979). The ethyl ester of (R)-nipecotic acid (70), the more potent isomer of nipecotic acid (see Fig. 32), showed more potent anticonvulsant effects than (S)-ethyl nipecotate, the free amino acids formed after hydrolysis of these ethyl esters being responsible for the pharmacological effects observed (Frey et al., 1979). The octyl (120) and the 4-nitrophenyl (122) esters of nipecotic acid have been shown to protect mice against seizures induced by the GABA-A antagonist bicuculline (61) (Crider et al., 1982, 1984). The methyl (125) and ethyl (126) esters of cis-4-OH-nipecotic acid (107) have also been used as potential prodrugs (Frey et al., 1979; Croucher et al., 1983). The former compound (125) proved to be more effective than (126) in protecting animals against audiogenic seizures (Croucher et al., 1983) and electroconvulsions (Frey et al., 1979). Dissimilar pharmacokinetic properties of (125) and (126) may explain this difference.

Whereas simple esters of nipecotic acid or guvacine such as (119) and (123) show muscarinic cholinergic effect per se (see above), the methyl (125) or ethyl (126) esters of cis-4-OH-nipecotic acid (Fig. 33) do not affect cholinergic mechanisms (Frey et al., 1979; Croucher et al., 1983). More complex esters of nipecotic acid or guvacine such as the pivaloyloxymethyl esters (121) and (124), on the other hand, do not show detectable cholinergic side effects (Croucher et al., 1983; Falch et al., 1987), whereas the double ester derivatives (127) and (128) of cis-4-OH-nipecotic acid (Fig. 33) have pronounced muscarinic cholinergic effects (Falch et al., 1987; for discussion see Section 7.4).

7.4 BEHAVIOURAL PHARMACOLOGY OF GABA UPTAKE INHIBITORS

The glia-selective GABA uptake inhibitor THPO (**69**) (Fig. 28), administered i.c.v. or intraperitoneally (i.p.), protects mice against sound-induced seizures (Croucher *et al.*, 1983). Similarly, THPO, given i.p., is protective against pentetrazole-induced seizures, but, quite surprisingly, i.c.v. administered THPO has very little effect in this model (Croucher *et al.*, 1983). These anticonvulsant effects of THPO and the enhancement by THPO of the depressant effects of GABA on single cells (Krogsgaard-Larsen *et al.*, 1975, 1983c; Fig. 31) are probably the consequences of inhibition of glial GABA uptake *in vivo*. Accordingly, systemic administration of THPO in mice slightly increases the GABA concentration in synaptosomes prepared from the brains of the treated animals (Wood *et al.*, 1980).

The pivaloyloxymethyl esters of nipecotic acid and guvacine, (**121**) and (**124**), (Figs 33 and 34) have been studied pharmacologically (Croucher *et al.*, 1983; Falch *et al.*, 1987). As mentioned in the previous section, neither compound shows cholinergic side effects, and studies *in vitro* under approximate physiological conditions demonstrate that the hydrolysis products of (**121**) and (**124**) are nipecotic acid and guvacine, respectively (Falch *et al.*, 1987). Consequently, these compounds are assumed also to be hydrolysed to the parent amino acids in brain tissues *in vivo* and, thus, that the pharmacological profiles of (**121**) and (**124**) are purely GABAergic. As expected from the similar pharmacological effects *in vitro* (Fig. 28) and on single cells *in vivo* of nipecotic acid and guvacine (see Section 7.2), the pharmacological profiles of (**121**) and (**124**) in intact animals are very similar.

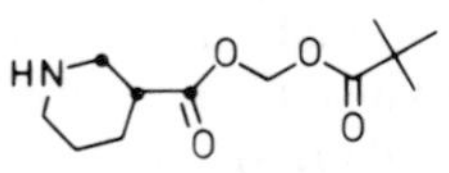

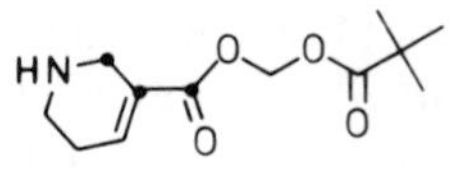

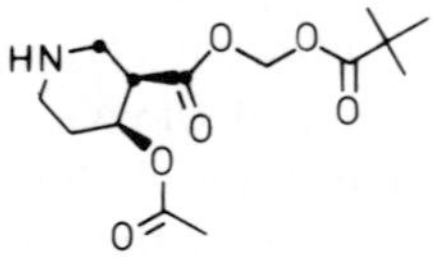

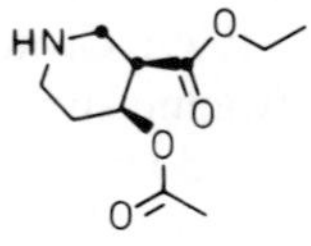

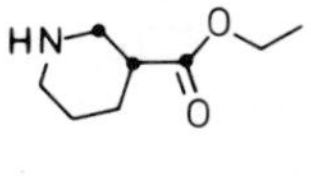

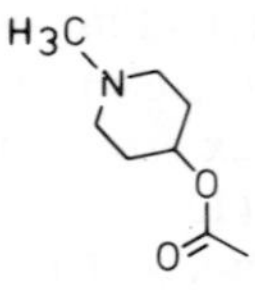

FIG. 34. Structures of some prodrugs of nipecotic acid (**104**), guvacine (**105**), and *cis*-4-OH-nipecotic acid (**107**) and the structure of the muscarinic cholinergic agonist (**129**).

At doses of (121) and (124) above 2.0 mmol/kg i.p., virtually all phases of the audiogenic seizure responses of mice were suppressed (Croucher *et al.*, 1983; Falch *et al.*, 1987). The relatively mild side effects of these compounds, notably sedation and impairment of motor activity, accompanying these anticonvulsant effects probably also result from activation of GABAergic systems. The hypothermic effects of (121) and (124) are also consequences of activation of GABAergic mechanisms (Croucher *et al.*, 1983).

The pharmacological profiles of the ethyl (127) and the pivaloyloxymethyl (128) esters of *cis*-4-acetoxynipecotic acid (Fig. 34) were similar, but strikingly different from those of (121) and (124). Neither (127) nor (128) showed marked anticonvulsant effects. Their pharmacological profiles were dominated by unwanted effects resulting from activation of muscarinic cholinergic mechanisms, such as tremors, salivation, and seizures (Falch *et al.*, 1987).

A structure–activity analysis of (127) and (128) may explain their apparent effects on muscarinic receptors. A comparison of the structures of (127) and (128) with that of the potent muscarinic agonist, 1-methyl-4-acetoxy-piperidine (129) (Höltje *et al.*, 1978) suggests that the 4-acetoxypiperidine "moieties" of (127) and (128) may be recognized by muscarinic receptors (Fig. 34). Furthermore, the structural similarity of (127) and the muscarinic agonist nipecotic acid ethyl ester (119) (Frey *et al.*, 1979; Zorn *et al.*, 1987) may contribute to the ability of (127) to activate muscarinic receptors. Since compound (121) does not affect significantly muscarinic receptor mechanisms (Croucher *et al.*, 1983; Falch *et al.*, 1987), the pivaloyl-oxymethyl ester group of (128) is unlikely to contribute to the cholinergic effects of (128). This structure–activity analysis implies that the acetoxy groups of (127) and (128) are not readily hydrolysed *in vivo*. The rates of hydrolysis of the ethyl and pivaloyloxymethyl ester groups of (127) and (128), respectively, have not been studied.

In conclusion, the "double" ester derivatives (127) and (128) have been shown not to be useful prodrugs of the glia-selective GABA uptake inhibitor *cis*-4-OH-nipecotic acid (107). On the other hand, the pivaloyloxymethyl esters of nipecotic acid and guvacine, (121) and (124) respectively, may have therapeutic interest as anticonvulsant agents. Clarification of these prospects does, however, imply more detailed pharmacological and toxicological studies.

Based on the highly lipophilic character of the DPB group, the GABA uptake inhibitors containing this substituent, (114)–(118) (Fig. 32), cross the BBB. The presence of this substituent also reduces the basic character of the amino groups as compared with the parent amino acids (Ali *et al.*, 1985). Consequently, the I/U ratios for the *N*-DPB analogues are lower than those of the parent amino acids (see Section 7.3), and this factor also makes the BBB more permeable for the *N*-DPB analogues. These pharmacokinetic properties of the DPB-compounds have made studies of their pharmacological effect after systemic administration in animals possible.

The compounds (117) and *N*-DPB-nipecotic acid, the racemate of (115) and (116) (Fig. 32), have been shown to be potent inhibitors of pentetrazole-induced convulsions in rats (Yunger *et al.*, 1984). The former compound also protected rats against maximal electroshock seizures (MES), but neither compound affected MES or electroshock seizure thresholds in mice (Yunger *et al.*, 1984). Since inhibition of MES and pentetrazole-induced seizures in rats or mice are considered indicative of anticonvulsant efficacy in man (Yunger *et al.*, 1984), it is difficult to predict the potential antiepileptic effects of these compounds. Systemically administered *N*-DPB-nipecotic acid and (117) have anticonvulsant effects in epileptic gerbils more potent than those of the ethyl ester prodrug of nipecotic acid (Löscher, 1985). These compounds produced dose-dependent anticonvulsant effects on all seizure parameters in amygdaloid kindled rats, and, in contrast to diazepam, these compounds did not produce significant sedative effects at anticonvulsant doses (Schwark and Löscher, 1985). The anticonvulsant profiles of *N*-DPB-nipecotic acid (Löscher, 1986a) and (117) (Löscher, 1986b) have been summarized and their prospects as future antiepileptic drugs discussed. The anticonvulsant and antinociceptive effects of *N*-DPB-nipecotic acid have been studied and compared with the effects of other GABAergic drugs. It was demonstrated that this GABA uptake inhibitor generally shows higher efficacy than for example the GABA-A agonist, THIP (Zorn *et al.*, 1986).

8 Conclusions

As a result of medicinal chemical research during the past 10–15 years a number of compounds with specific actions at different GABA synaptic mechanisms have been designed and developed. The conformationally restricted GABA analogues isoguvacine (2), P4S (3), and THIP (4) are specific GABA-A agonists, and (*S*)-DHM (18) is the most potent GABA-A agonist so far described. THIP has been the subject of extensive pharmacological studies, and in the human clinic, THIP has shown interesting effects, notably non-opioid analgesic effects, and it shows anxiolytic and antispastic profiles. THIP does, however, only show very weak antiepileptic properties, and unwanted effects such as sedation may make THIP unacceptable for human therapy. There is a need for new types of GABA-A agonists, perhaps partial GABA-A agonists, showing the above pharmacological profile devoid of the sedative component. Work along such lines is in progress, and in this regard 4-PIOL (41), showing a novel GABA-A agonist profile with no effect on the GABA-BZD coupling mechanism, is a very interesting compound. The development of new types of GABA-A antagonists, such as the aminopyridazines (6) and (67), is an important achievement, and comparative studies of these compounds, which interact with high-affinity states of GABA-A receptors, and the classical GABA-A antagonists, BMC (5) and bicuculline (61), which preferentially bind to low-affinity receptor sites, is likely to provide new insight into GABA-A receptor mechanisms.

(R)-Baclofen (90) is still the most potent GABA-A agonist known. However, the demonstration of opposite stereochemical requirements of GABA-A and GABA-B receptor sites is likely to stimulate the design and development of novel types of GABA-B agonists. Such agents, and also GABA-B antagonists, have considerable pharmacological and therapeutic interest. The development of the new GABA-B antagonist phaclofen (98) is of major importance and is likely to stimulate research in the GABA-B field.

The recent developments in the field of GABA uptake inhibitors have greatly stimulated the therapeutic interest in compounds with effects on GABA transport mechanisms. Since the GABA-A agonist THIP has only very weak antiepileptic properties, and in view of the high doses of the GABA prodrug, progabide (71), required for significant reductions of symptoms in epileptic patients, the potent anticonvulsant effects in animals of a new type of GABA uptake inhibitors, as exemplified by (117), is very interesting. The observation that the anticonvulsant properties of (117) are not accompanied by sedative effects to the same degree as those of diazepam is promising. It is likely that compounds with selective effects on glial GABA uptake have primary interest as anticonvulsants, making the glia-selective uptake inhibitor THPO (69) an important lead structure for further drug design in this area.

It is to be anticipated that some of the discoveries in the GABA field will greatly stimulate drug design programmes in this area.

Acknowledgements

This work was supported by grants from the Danish Medical and Technical Research Councils. The secretarial and technical assistance of Mrs B. Hare and Mr S. Stilling are gratefully acknowledged.

Appendix: List of Abbreviations

The following abbreviations are used in this article:

A-B	inhibition of GABA-A receptor binding *in vitro*
AG	relative GABA-A agonist activity determined microelectrophoretically *in vivo*

3-APS	3-aminopropanesulphonic acid
B-B	inhibition of GABA-B receptor binding *in vitro*
BBB	blood–brain barrier
BMC	bicuculline methochloride
BZD	benzodiazepine
CA1	area of hippocampus
cAMP	cyclic AMP (adenosine 3′,5′-cyclic monophosphate)
CNS	central nervous system
DA	dopamine
DAVA	δ-aminovaleric acid (5-aminopentanoic acid)
DBA/2	sound-sensitive mouse strain
DHM	4,5-dihydromuscimol
DH-P4S	dehydropiperidine-4-sulphonic acid (1,2,3,6-tetrahydropyridine-4-sulphonic acid)
DPB	4,4-diphenyl-3-butenyl-
EC_{50}	concentration producing a 50% effect
GABA	γ-aminobutyric acid (4-aminobutanoic acid)
GABA-T	GABA:2-oxoglutarate aminotransferase
GABOB	γ-amino-β-oxybutyric acid (3-hydroxy-4-aminobutanoic acid)
GAD	glutamic acid decarboxylase
GLU	glutamic acid
IAA	imidazole-4-acetic acid
IC_{50}	concentration producing a 50% inhibition
i.c.v.	intracerebroventricular(ly)
i.m.	intramuscular(ly)
i.p.	intraperitoneal(ly)
IPSP	inhibitory postsynaptic potential
iso-THAZ	5,6,7,8-tetrahydro-4H-isoxazolo[3,4-d]azepin-3-ol
iso-THIP	4,5,6,7-tetrahydroisoxazolo[3,4-c]pyridin-3-ol
I/U	ionized/un-ionized
K_m	Michaelis–Menten constant
MES	maximal electroshock seizure
N/G	neuronal/glial
2-OH-DAVA	2-hydroxy-DAVA
P4S	piperidine-4-sulphonic acid
PGO	pento-geniculo-occipetal
3-PIOL	5-(3-piperidyl)-3-isoxazole
4-PIOL	5-(4-piperidyl)-3-isoxazole
PMSA	3-pyrrolidylmethyl sulphonic acid
SN	substantia nigra
SSA	succinic semialdehyde

TBPS	*tert*-butyl bicyclophosphothionate
THAZ	5,6,7,8-tetrahydro-4*H*-isoxazolo[4,5-*d*]azepin-3-ol
THIA	5,6,7,8-tetrahydro-4*H*-isoxazolo[5,4-*c*]azepin-3-ol
thio-THIP	4,5,6,7-tetrahydroisothiazolo[5,4-*c*]pyridin-3-ol
thio-THPO	4,5,6,7-tetrahydroisothiazolo[4,5-*c*]pyridin-3-ol
THIP	4,5,6,7-tetrahydroisoxazolo[5,4-*c*]pyridin-3-ol
THPO	4,5,6,7-tetrahydroisoxazolo[4,5-*c*]pyridin-3-ol
UPT-G	glial uptake
UPT-N	neuronal uptake
UPT-S	synaptosomal uptake

References

Alger, B. E., and Nicoll, R. A. (1982). *J. Physiol. (London)* **328**, 125–141.

Ali, F. E., Bondinell, W. E., Dandridge, P. A., Frazee, J. S., Garvey, E., Girard, G. R., Kaiser, C., Ku, T. W., Lafferty, J. J., Moonsammy, G. I., Oh, H.-J., Rush, J. A., Setler, P. E., Stringer, O. D., Venslavsky, J. W., Volpe, B. W., Yunger, L. M., and Zirkle, C. L. (1985). *J. Med. Chem.* **28**, 653–660.

Allan, R. D., and Dickenson, H. W. (1986). *Eur. J. Pharmacol.* **120**, 119–122.

Allan, R. D., and Fong, J. (1983). *Aust. J. Chem.* **36**, 1221–1226.

Allan, R. D., and Johnston, G. A. R. (1983). *Med. Res. Rev.* **3**, 91–118.

Allan, R. D., and Tran, H. (1981). *Aust. J. Chem.* **34**, 2641–2645.

Allan, R. D., Johnston, G. A. R., Kazlauskas, R., and Tran, H. (1983). *Aust. J. Chem.* **36**, 977–981.

Allan, R. D., Dickenson, H. W., and Fong, J. (1986a). *Eur. J. Pharmacol.* **122**, 339–348.

Allan, R. D., Dickenson, H. W., Hiern, B. P., Johnston, G. A. R., and Kazlauskas, R. (1986b). *Br. J. Pharmacol.* **88**, 379–387.

Anderson, R. A., and Mitchell, R. (1985). *Eur. J. Pharmacol.* **118**, 355–358.

Andree, T., Kendall, D. A., and Enna, S. J. (1983). *Life Sci.* **32**, 2265–2272.

Antonaccio, M. J., and Taylor, D. G. (1977). *Eur. J. Pharmacol.* **46**, 283–287.

Arbilla, S., Kamal, L., and Langer, S. Z. (1979). *Eur. J. Pharmacol.* **57**, 211–217.

Arias, C., and Tapia, R. (1986). *J. Neurochem.* **47**, 396–404.

Armstrong, D. R., Breckenridge, R. J., and Suckling, C. J. (1982). *J. Theor. Biol.* **97**, 267–276.

Arnt, J., and Christensen, A. V. (1981). *Eur. J. Pharmacol.* **69**, 107–111.

Arnt, J., and Krogsgaard-Larsen, P. (1979). *Brain Res.* **177**, 395–400.

Arnt, J., Scheel-Krüger, J., Magelund, G., and Krogsgaard-Larsen, P. (1979). *J. Pharm. Pharmacol.* **31**, 306–313.

Atkinson, J. G., Girard, Y., Rokach, J., Rooney, C. S., McFarlane, C. S., Rackham, A., and Share, N. N. (1979). *J. Med. Chem.* **22**, 99–106.

Barker, J. L., and McBurney, R. N. (1979). *Nature (London)* **277**, 234–236.

Barolet, A. W., Li, A., Liske, S., and Morris, M. E. (1985). *Can. J. Physiol. Pharmacol.* **63**, 1465–1470.

Beutler, J. A., Karbon, E. W., Brubaker, A. N., Malik, R., Curtis, D. R., and Enna, S. J. (1985). *Brain Res.* **330**, 135–140.

Bianchi, M., Deana, R., Quadro, G., Mourier, G., and Galzigna, L. (1983). *Biochem. Pharmacol.* **32**, 1093–1096.

Biggio, G., and Costa, E. (eds) (1986). "GABAergic Transmission and Anxiety." Raven Press, New York.

Biggio, G., Concas, A., Serra, M., Salis, M., Corda, M. G., Nurchi, V., Crisponi, G., and Gessa, G. L. (1984). *Brain Res.* **305**, 13–18.

Bird, E. D., Spokes, E. G. S., and Iversen, L. L. (1979). *Brain* **102**, 347–360.

Biscoe, T. J., and Fry, J. P. (1982). *Br. J. Pharmacol.* **75**, 23–25.

Bjoerndal, N., Gerlach, J., Casey, D. E., and Christensson, E. (1983). *Psychopharmacology* **79**, 220–225.

Blavet, N., DeFeudis, F. V., and Clostre, F. (1982). *Psychopharmacology* **76**, 75–78.

Bowery, N. G. (1982). *Trends Pharmacol. Sci.* **3**, 400–403.

Bowery, N. G. (1983). *In* "The GABA Receptors" (S. J. Enna, ed.), pp. 177–213. The Humana Press, Clifton, NJ.

Bowery, N. G. (ed.) (1984). "Actions and Interactions of GABA and Benzodiazepines". Raven Press, New York.

Bowery, N. G., and Hudson, A. L. (1979). *Br. J. Pharmacol.* **66**, 108P.

Bowery, N. G., Collins, J. F., Cryer, G., Inch, T. D., and McLaughlin, N. J. (1979). *In* "GABA-Biochemistry and CNS Functions" (P. Mandel and F. V. DeFeudis, eds), pp. 339–353. Plenum Press, New York.

Bowery, N. G., Doble, A., Hill, D. R., Hudson, A. L., and Turnbull, M. J. (1980a). *Br. J. Pharmacol.* **70**, 77P.

Bowery, N. G., Hill, D. R., Hudson, A. L., Doble, A., Middlemiss, D. N., Shaw, J., and Turnbull, M. (1980b). *Nature (London)* **283**, 92–94.

Bowery, N. G., Doble, A., Hill, D. R., Hudson, A. L., Shaw, J. S., Turnbull, M. J., and Warrington, R. (1981). *Eur. J. Pharmacol.* **71**, 53–70.

Bowery, N. G., Hill, D. R., Hudson, A. L., Price, G. W., Turnbull, M. J., and Wilkin, G. P. (1984). *In* "Actions and Interactions of GABA and Benzodiazepines" (N. G. Bowery, ed.), pp. 81–108. Raven Press, New York.

Braestrup, C., and Nielsen, M. (1980). *Brain Res. Bull.* **5** (Suppl. 2), 681–684.

Braestrup, C., and Nielsen, M. (1983). *In* "Handbook of Psychopharmacology" (L. L. Iversen, S. D. Iversen and S. H. Snyder, eds), Vol. 17, pp. 285–384. Plenum Press, New York.

Braestrup, C., and Nielsen, M. (1985). *Eur. J. Pharmacol.* **118**, 115–121.

Braestrup, C., Nielsen, M., Krogsgaard-Larsen, P., and Falch, E. (1979). *Nature (London)* **280**, 331–333.

Braestrup, C., Nielsen, M., and Krogsgaard-Larsen, P. (1986). *J. Neurochem.* **47**, 691–696.

Breckenridge, R. J., Nicholson, S. H., Nicol, A. J., Suckling, C. J., Leigh, B., and Iversen, L. L. (1981). *J. Neurochem.* **37**, 837–844.

Brehm, L., Krogsgaard-Larsen, P., Schaumburg, K., Johansen, J. S., Falch, E., and Curtis, D. R. (1986). *J. Med. Chem.* **29**, 224–229.

Brennan, M. J. W. (1982). *J. Neurochem.* **38**, 264–266.

Brennan, M. J. W., and Cantrill, R. C. (1979). *Nature (London)* **280**, 514–515.

Brennan, T. J., Haywood, J. R., and Ticku, M. K. (1983). *Life Sci.* **33**, 701–709.

Bristow, D. R., Campbell, M. M., Iversen, L. L., Kemp, J. A., Marshall, G. R., Watling, K. J., and Wong, E. H. F. (1985). *Proc. Br. Pharmacol. Soc.* April.

Brown, D. A. (1979). *Trends Neurosci.* **2**, 271–273.

Browner, M., Ferkany, J. W., and Enna, S. J. (1981). *J. Neurosci.* **1**, 514–518.

Burke, D., Andrews, C. J., and Knowles, L. (1971). *J. Neurol. Sci.* **14**, 199–208.

Buu, N. T., Duhaime, J., and Kuchel, O. (1984). *Life Sci.* **35**, 1083–1090.

Byberg, J. R., Labouta, I. M., Falch, E., Hjeds, H., Krogsgaard-Larsen, P., Curtis, D. R., and Gynther, B. D. (1987). *Drug Design and Delivery* **1**, 261–274.

Callery, P. S., and Geelhaar, L. A. (1984). *J. Neurochem.* **43**, 1631–1634.

Callery, P. S., Geelhaar, L. A., Nayar, M. S. B., Stogniew, M., and Rao, K. G. (1982). *J. Neurochem.* **38**, 1063–1067.

Cananzi, A. R., Costa, E., and Guidotti, A. (1980). *Brain Res.* **196**, 447–453.

Chambon, J.-P., Feltz, P., Heaulme, M., Restle, S., Schlichter, R., Biziere, K., and Wermuth, C. G. (1985). *Proc. Natl. Acad. Sci. USA* **82**, 1832–1836.

Chase, T. N., and Walters, J. R. (1976). *In* "GABA in Nervous System Function" (E. Roberts, T. N. Chase and D. B. Tower, eds), pp. 497–513. Raven Press, New York.

Chase, T. N., Wexler, N. S., and Barbeau, A. (eds) (1979). "Huntington's Disease". Raven Press, New York.

Christensen, A. V., and Larsen, J. J. (1982). *Pol. J. Pharmacol. Pharm.* **34**, 127–134.

Christensen, A. V., Arnt, J., and Scheel-Krüger, J. (1979). *Life Sci.* **24**, 1395–1402.

Christensen, A. V., Svendsen, O., and Krogsgaard-Larsen, P. (1982). *Pharm. Week. Sci. Ed.* **4**, 145–153.

Ciesielski, L., Simler, S., Clement, J., and Mandel, P. (1985). *J. Neurochem.* **45**, 244–248.

Clifford, J. M., Taberner, P. V., Tunnicliff, G., Rick, J. T., and Kerkut, G. A. (1973). *Biochem. Pharmacol.* **22**, 535–542.

Corda, M. G., Sanna, E., Concas, A., Giorgi, O., Ongini, E., Nurchi, V., Pintori, T., Crisponi, G., and Biggio, G. (1986). *J. Neurochem.* **47**, 370–374.

Crider, A. M., Tita, T. T., Wood, J. D., and Hinko, C. N. (1982). *J. Pharm. Sci.* **71**, 1214–1219.

Crider, A. M., Wood, J. D., Tschappat, K. D., Hinko, C. N., and Seibert, K. (1984). *J. Pharm. Sci.* **73**, 1612–1616.

Croucher, M. J., Meldrum, B. S., and Krogsgaard-Larsen, P. (1983). *Eur. J. Pharmacol.* **89**, 217–228.

Cuomo, V., Cortese, I., and Siro-Brigiani, G. (1981). *Arzneim.-Forsch.* **31**, 1724–1726.

Cupello, A., and Hydén, H. (1985). *Brain Res.* **358**, 364–366.

Cupello, A., and Hydén, H. (1986). *Cell. Mol. Neurobiol.* **6**, 1–16.

Curtis, D. R. (1978). *In* "Amino Acids as Chemical Transmitters" (F. Fonnum, ed.), pp. 55–86. Plenum Press, New York.

Curtis, D. R., and Gynther, B. D. (1986). *Eur. J. Pharmacol.* **131**, 311–313.

Curtis, D. R., and Gynther, B. D. (1987). *Trends Pharmacol. Sci.* **8**, 90.

Curtis, D. R., and Johnston, G. A. R. (1974). *Ergebn. Physiol.* **69**, 97–188.

Curtis, D. R., and Malik, R. (1984). *Proc. Roy. Soc. Lond. B* **223**, 25–33.

Curtis, D. R., Duggan, A. W., Felix, D., and Johnston, G. A. R. (1971). *Brain Res.* **32**, 69–96.

Curtis, D. R., Game, C. J. A., Johnston, G. A. R., and McCulloch, R. M. (1974). *Brain Res.* **70**, 493–499.

Curtis, D. R., Game, C. J. A., and Lodge, D. (1976). *Exp. Brain Res.* **25**, 413–428.

Davidoff, R. S. (1973). *Arch. Neurol.* **28**, 60–63.

Davies, J., and Watkins, J. C. (1974). *Brain Res.* **70**, 501–505.

DeFeudis, F. V. (1981). *Neurochem. Int.* **3**, 113–122.

DeFeudis, F. V. (1982). *Trends Pharmacol. Sci.* **3**, 444–446.

DeFeudis, F. V. (1984). *Drug Alcohol Depend.* **14**, 101–111.

Delini-Stula, A. (1979). *In* "GABA-Neurotransmitters. Pharmacochemical, Biochemical and Pharmacological Aspects" (P. Krogsgaard-Larsen, J. Scheel-Krüger and H. Kofod, eds), pp. 482–499. Munksgaard, Copenhagen.

Di Chiara, G., and Gessa, G. L. (eds) (1981). "GABA and the Basal Ganglia". Raven Press, New York.

DiMicco, J. A., Alsip, N. L., and Wible, J. H. (1984). *Neuropharmacology* **23**, 819–820.

Edsall, J. T., and Wyman, J. (1958). *In* "Biophysical Chemistry", Vol. 1, pp. 485–486. Academic Press, New York.

Edvinsson, L., and Krause, D. N. (1979). *Brain Res.* **173**, 89–97.

Enna, S. J. (1981). *Biochem. Pharmacol.* **30**, 907–913.

Enna, S. J. (ed.) (1983). "The GABA Receptors". The Humana Press, Clifton, NJ.

Enna, S. J., and Karbon, E. W. (1984). *Neuropharmacology* **23**, 821–822.

Enna, S. J., and Snyder, S. H. (1975). *Brain Res.* **100**, 81–97.

Enna, S. J., Bird, E. D., Bennett, J. P., Bylund, D. B., Yamamura, H. I., Iversen, L. L., and Snyder, S. H. (1976). *New Engl. J. Med.* **294**, 1305–1309.

Enna, S. J., Collins, J. F., and Snyder,, S. H. (1977). *Brain Res.* **124**, 185–190.

Ennis, C., and Cox, B. (1981). *Eur. J. Pharmacol.* **70**, 417–420.

Erdö, S. L., and Bowery, N. G. (eds) (1986). "GABAergic Mechanisms in Mammalian Periphery". Raven Press, New York.

Evans, R. H., Francis, A. A., Hunt, K., Martin, M. R., and Watkins, J. C. (1978). *J. Pharm. Pharmacol.* **30**, 364–367.

Falch, E., and Krogsgaard-Larsen, P. (1982). *J. Neurochem.* **38**, 1123–1129.

Falch, E., Krogsgaard-Larsen, P., and Christensen, A. V. (1981). *J. Med. Chem.* **24**, 285–289.

Falch, E., Jacobsen, P., Krogsgaard-Larsen, P., and Curtis, D. R. (1985a). *J. Neurochem.* **44**, 68–75.

Falch, E., Krogsgaard-Larsen, P., Jacobsen, P., Engesgaard, A., Braestrup, C., and Curtis, D. R. (1985b). *Eur. J. Med. Chem.* **20**, 447–453.

Falch, E., Hedegaard, A., Nielsen, L., Jensen, B. R., Hjeds, H., and Krogsgaard-Larsen, P. (1986). *J. Neurochem.* **47**, 898–903.

Falch, E., Meldrum, B. S., and Krogsgaard-Larsen, P. (1987). *Drug Design and Delivery* **2**, 9–21.

Fariello, R. G., Morselli, P. L., Lloyd, K. G., Quesney, L. F., and Engel, J. (eds) (1984). "Neurotransmitters, Seizures, and Epilepsy II". Raven Press, New York.

Ferrero, P., Guidotti, A., and Costa, E. (1984). *Proc. Natl. Acad. Sci. USA* **81**, 2247–2251.

Fischer, J. B., and Olsen, R. W. (1986). *In* "Benzodiazepine-GABA Receptors and Chloride Channels: Structural and Functional Properties" (R. W. Olsen and J. C. Venter, eds), pp. 241–259. Alan R. Liss, New York.

Fowler, L. J., Lovell, D. H., and John, R. A. (1983). *J. Neurochem.* **41**, 1751–1754.

Frere, R. C., Macdonald, R. L., and Young, A. B. (1982). *Brain Res.* **244**, 145–153.

Frey, H.-H., and Löscher, W. (1980). *Neuropharmacology* **19**, 217–220.

Frey, H.-H., Popp, C., and Löscher, W. (1979). *Neuropharmacology* **18**, 581–590.

Frye, G. D., McCown, T. J., and Breese, G. R. (1983). *J. Pharmacol. Exp. Ther.* **226**, 720–725.

Galzigna, L., Garbin, L., Bianchi, M., and Marzotto, A. (1978). *Arch. Int. Pharmacodyn. Ther.* **235**, 73–85.

Galzigna, L., Bianchi, M., Bertazzon, A., Barthez, A., Quadro, G., and Coletti-Previero, M. A. (1984). *J. Neurochem.* **42**, 1762–1766.

Gähwiler, B. H., Maurer, R., and Wüthrich, H. J. (1984). *Neurosci. Lett.* **45**, 311–316.

Gillis, R. A., Williford, D. J., Dias Souza, J., and Quest, J. A. (1982). *Neuropharmacology* **21**, 545–547.

Giorguieff, M. F., Kemel, M. L., Glowinski, J., and Besson, M. J. (1978). *Brain Res.* **139**, 115–130.

Giotti, A., Luzzi, S., Spagnesi, S., and Zilletti, L. (1983). *Br. J. Pharmacol.* **79**, 855–862.

Godfraind, J. M., Krnjevic, K., Maretic, H., and Pumain, R. (1973). *Can. J. Physiol. Pharmacol.* **51**, 790–797.

Grandison, L., and Guidotti, A. (1979). *Endocrinology* **105**, 754–759.

Grognet, A., Hertz, F., and DeFeudis, F. V. (1983). *Gen. Pharmacol.* **14**, 585–589.

Gynther, B. D., and Curtis, D. R. (1986). *Neurosci. Lett.* **68**, 211–215.

Haefely, W., Kyburz, E., Gerecke, M., and Möhler, H. (1985). *Adv. Drug Res.* **14**, 165–322.

Haefliger, W., Révész, L., Maurer, R., Römer, D., and Büscher, H.-H. (1984). *Eur. J. Med. Chem.* **19**, 149–156.

Hamel, E., Goetz, I. E., and Roberts, E. (1981). *J. Neurochem.* **37**, 1032–1038.
Hammond, D. L., and Drower, E. J. (1984). *Eur. J. Pharmacol.* **103**, 121–125.
Hammond, J. R., and Martin, I. L. (1986). *J. Neurochem.* **47**, 1161–1171.
Hanada, S., Mita, T., Nishino, N., and Tanaka, C. (1987). *Life Sci.* **40**, 259–266.
Heaulme, M., Chambon, J.-P., Leyris, R., Molimard, J.-C., Wermuth, C. G., and Biziere, K. (1986a). *Brain Res.* **384**, 224–231.
Heaulme, M., Chambon, J.-P., Leyris, R., Wermuth, C. G., and Biziere, K. (1986b). *Neuropharmacology* **25**, 1279–1283.
Hebebrand, J., Friedl, W., Unverzagt, B., and Propping, P. (1986). *J. Neurochem.* **47**, 790–793.
Hertz, L., Kvamme, E., McGeer, E. G., and Schousboe, A. (eds) (1983). "Glutamine, Glutamate, and GABA in the Central Nervous System". Alan R. Liss, New York.
Hicks, T. P., Lodge, D., and McLennan, H. (eds) (1987). "Excitatory Amino Acid Transmission". Alan R. Liss, New York.
Hill, D. R., and Bowery, N. G. (1981). *Nature (London)* **290**, 149–152.
Hill, D. R., Bowery, N. G., and Hudson, A. L. (1984). *J. Neurochem.* **42**, 652–657.
Hill, R. C., Maurer, R., Buescher, H. H., and Roemer, D. (1981). *Eur. J. Pharmacol.* **69**, 221–224.
Hitzemann, R. J., and Loh, H. H. (1978). *J. Neurochem.* **30**, 471–477.
Hoehn-Saric, R. (1983). *Psychopharmacology* **80**, 338–341.
Horton, R. W., Collins, J. F., Anlezark, G. M., and Meldrum, B. S. (1979). *Eur. J. Pharmacol.* **59**, 75–83.
Houser, C. R., Harris, A. B., and Vaughn, J. E. (1986). *Brain Res.* **383**, 129–145.
Hunt, P., and Clements-Jewery, S. (1981). *Neuropharmacology* **20**, 357–361.
Hydén, H., Cupello, A., and Palm, A. (1986). *Neurochem. Res.* **11**, 695–706.
Hynes, M. D., Leander, J. D., Frederickson, R. C. A., Ho, P. P. K., Johnson, D. W., and Archer, R. A. (1984). *Drug Dev. Res.* **4**, 405–419.
Höltje, H.-D., Jensen, B., and Lambrecht, G. (1978). *Eur. J. Med. Chem.* **13**, 453–463.
Iversen, L. L., and Johnston, G. A. R. (1971). *J. Neurochem.* **18**, 1939–1950.
Iversen, L. L., and Neal, M. J. (1968). *J. Neurochem.* **15**, 1141–1149.
Johnston, G. A. R. (1983). *In* "The GABA Receptors" (S. J. Enna, ed.), pp. 107–128. The Humana Press, Clifton, NJ.
Johnston, G. A. R., and Allan, R. D. (1984). *Neuropharmacology* **23**, 831–832.
Johnston, G. A. R., Krogsgaard-Larsen, P., and Stephanson, A. L. (1975). *Nature (London)* **258**, 627–628.
Johnston, G. A. R., Stephanson, A. L., and Twitchin, B. (1976a). *J. Neurochem.* **26**, 83–87.
Johnston, G. A. R., Krogsgaard-Larsen, P., Stephanson, A. L., and Twitchin, B. (1976b). *J. Neurochem.* **26**, 1029–1032.
Johnston, G. A. R., Allan, R. D., Andrews, P. R., Kennedy, S. M. E., and Twitchin, B. (1978). *In* "Advances in Pharmacology and Therapeutics" (P. Simon, ed.), Vol. 2, pp. 11–18. Pergamon Press, Oxford.
Johnston, G. A. R., Allan, R. D., Kennedy, S. M. E., and Twitchin, B. (1979). *In* "GABA-Neurotransmitters. Pharmacochemical, Biochemical and Pharmacological Aspects" (P. Krogsgaard-Larsen, J. Scheel-Krüger and H. Kofod, eds), pp. 149–164. Munksgaard, Copenhagen.
Johnston, G. A. R., Allan, R. D., Benton, A. D., Chen Chow, S., Drew, C. A., Hiern, B. P., Holan, G., Kazlauskas, H., and Weatherby, R. P. (1984). *Proc. 9th Int. Con. Pharmacol., London* **3**, 179–183.
Kaplan, J.-P., Raizon, B. M., Desarmenien, M., Feltz, P., Headley, P. M., Worms, P., Lloyd, K. G., and Bartholini, G. (1980). *J. Med. Chem.* **23**, 702–704.

450 P. KROGSGAARD-LARSEN *et al.*

Kardos, J., Blasko, G., Kerekes, P., Kovacs, I., and Simonyi, M. (1984). *Biochem. Pharmacol.* **33**, 3537–3545.

Kardos, J., Blasko, G., and Simonyi, M. (1986). *Arzneim.-Forsch.* **36**, 939–940.

Karobath, M., Placheta, P., Lippitsch, M., and Krogsgaard-Larsen, P. (1979). *Nature (London)* **278**, 748–749.

Kendall, D. A., Browner, M., and Enna, S. J. (1982). *J. Pharmacol. Exp. Ther.* **220**, 482–487.

Kerr, D. I. B., Ong, J., Prager, R. H., Gynther, B. D., and Curtis, D. R. (1987). *Brain Res.* **405**, 150–154.

Kish, S. J., Shannak, K. S., Perry, T. L., and Hornykiewicz, O. (1983). *J. Neurochem.* **41**, 1495–1497.

Kjaer, M., and Nielsen, H. (1983). *Br. J. Clin. Pharmacol.* **16**, 477–485.

Korn, S. J., and Dingledine, R. (1986). *Brain Res.* **368**, 247–255.

Korsgaard, S., Casey, D. E., Gerlach, J., Hetmar, O., Kaldan, B., and Mikkelsen, L. B. (1982). *Arch. Gen. Psychiatry* **39**, 1017–1021.

Krnjevic, K. (1974). *Physiol. Rev.* **54**, 418–540.

Krnjevic, K. (1984). *Neurosci. Lett.* **47**, 283–287.

Krogsgaard-Larsen, P. (1977). *Acta Chem. Scand.* **B31**, 584–588.

Krogsgaard-Larsen, P. (1978). *In* "Amino Acids as Chemical Transmitters" (F. Fonnum, ed.), pp. 305–321. Plenum Press, New York.

Krogsgaard-Larsen, P. (1980). *Mol. Cell. Biochem.* **31**, 105–121.

Krogsgaard-Larsen, P. (1981). *J. Med. Chem.* **24**, 1377–1383.

Krogsgaard-Larsen, P. (1983). *In* "Glutamine, Glutamate and GABA in the Central Nervous System" (L. Hertz, E. Kvamme, E. G. McGeer, and A. Schousboe, eds), pp. 537–557. Alan R. Liss, New York.

Krogsgaard-Larsen, P. (1984). *Neuropharmacology* **23**, 837–838.

Krogsgaard-Larsen, P. (1988). *Med. Res. Rev.* **8**, 27–56.

Krogsgaard-Larsen, P., and Arnt, J. (1980). *Brain Res. Bull.* **5** (Suppl. 2), 867–872.

Krogsgaard-Larsen, P., and Christensen, A. V. (1980). *Ann. Rep. Med. Chem.* **15**, 41–50.

Krogsgaard-Larsen, P., and Christiansen, T. R. (1979). *Eur. J. Med. Chem.* **14**, 157–164.

Krogsgaard-Larsen, P., and Falch, E. (1981). *Mol. Cell. Biochem.* **38**, 129–146.

Krogsgaard-Larsen, P., and Johnston, G. A. R. (1975). *J. Neurochem.* **25**, 797–802.

Krogsgaard-Larsen, P., and Johnston, G. A. R. (1978). *J. Neurochem.* **30**, 1377–1382.

Krogsgaard-Larsen, P., Johnston, G. A. R., Curtis, D. R., Game, C. J. A., and McCulloch, R. M. (1975). *J. Neurochem.* **25**, 803–809.

Krogsgaard-Larsen, P., Johnston, G. A. R., Lodge, D., and Curtis, D. R. (1977). *Nature (London)* **268**, 53–55.

Krogsgaard-Larsen, P., Thyssen, K., and Schaumburg, K. (1978). *Acta Chem. Scand.* **B32**, 327–334.

Krogsgaard-Larsen, P., Honoré, T., and Thyssen, K. (1979a). *In* "GABA-Neurotransmitters. Pharmacochemical, Biochemical and Pharmacological Aspects" (P. Krogsgaard-Larsen, J. Scheel-Krüger and H. Kofod, eds), pp. 201–216. Munksgaard, Copenhagen.

Krogsgaard-Larsen, P., Scheel-Krüger, J., and Kofod, H. (eds) (1979b). "GABA-Neurotransmitters. Pharmacochemical, Biochemical and Pharmacological Aspects". Munksgaard, Copenhagen.

Krogsgaard-Larsen, P., Hjeds, H., Curtis, D. R., Lodge, D., and Johnston, G. A. R. (1979c). *J. Neurochem.* **32**, 1717–1724.

Krogsgaard-Larsen, P., Falch, E., Schousboe, A., Curtis, D. R., and Lodge, D. (1980). *J. Neurochem.* **34**, 756–759.

Krogsgaard-Larsen, P., Snowman, A., Lummis, S. C., and Olsen, R. W. (1981a). *J. Neurochem.* **37**, 401–409.

Krogsgaard-Larsen, P., Labouta, I.M., Meldrum, B., Croucher, M., and Schousboe, A. (1981b). *In* "Neurotransmitters, Seizures, and Epilepsy" (P. L. Morselli, K. G. Lloyd, W. Löscher, B. Meldrum and E. H. Reynolds, eds), pp. 23–33. Raven Press, New York.

Krogsgaard-Larsen, P., Schultz, B., Mikkelsen, H., Aaes-Jørgensen, T., and Bøgesø, K. P. (1981c). *In* "Amino Acid Neurotransmitters" (F. V. DeFeudis and P. Mandel, eds), pp. 69–76. Raven Press, New York.

Krogsgaard-Larsen, P., Falch, E., Mikkelsen, H., and Jacobsen, P. (1982a). *In* "Optimization of Drug Delivery" (H. Bundgaard, A. B. Hansen and H. Kofod, eds), pp. 225–234. Munksgaard, Copenhagen.

Krogsgaard-Larsen, P., Hjeds, H., Curtis, D. R., Leah, J. D., and Peet, M. J. (1982b). *J. Neurochem.* **39**, 1319–1324.

Krogsgaard-Larsen, P., Jacobsen, P., and Falch, E. (1983a). *In* "The GABA Receptors" (S. J. Enna, ed.), pp. 149–176. The Humana Press, Clifton, NJ.

Krogsgaard-Larsen, P., Falch, E., Peet, M. J., Leah, J. D., and Curtis, D. R. (1983b). *In* "CNS Receptors—From Molecular Pharmacology to Behaviour" (P. Mandel and F. V. DeFeudis, eds), pp. 1–13. Raven Press, New York.

Krogsgaard-Larsen, P., Mikkelsen, H., Jacobsen, P., Falch, E., Curtis, D. R., Peet, M. J., and Leah, J. D. (1983c). *J. Med. Chem.* **26**, 895–900.

Krogsgaard-Larsen, P., Falch, E., and Christensen, A. V. (1984a). *Drugs of the Future* **9**, 597–618.

Krogsgaard-Larsen, P., Falch, E., and Jacobsen, P. (1984b). *In* "Actions and Interactions of GABA and Benzodiazepines" (N. G. Bowery, ed.), pp. 109–132. Raven Press, New York.

Krogsgaard-Larsen, P., Lenicque, P., and Jacobsen, P. (1984c). *In* "Handbook of Stereoisomers: Drugs in Psychopharmacology" (D. F. Smith, ed.), pp. 369–399. CRC Press, Boca Raton, FL.

Krogsgaard-Larsen, P., Falch, E., and Hjeds, H. (1985a). *Prog. Med. Chem.* **22**, 67–120.

Krogsgaard-Larsen, P., Nielsen, L., Falch, E., and Curtis, D. R. (1985b). *J. Med. Chem.* **28**, 1612–1617.

Krogsgaard-Larsen, P., Falch, E., Schousboe, A., and Curtis, D. R. (1986). *In* "Neurotransmitters, Seizures, and Epilepsy" (G. Nistico, P. L. Morselli, K. G. Lloyd, R. G. Fariello and J. Engel, eds), Vol. III, pp. 135–150. Raven Press, New York.

Krogsgaard-Larsen, P., Falch, E., Larsson, O. M., and Schousboe, A. (1987). *Epilepsy Res.* **1**, 77–93.

Labouta, I. M., Falch, E., Hjeds, H., and Krogsgaard-Larsen, P. (1982). *Eur. J. Med. Chem.* **17**, 531–535.

Larsen, J. D., and Bundgaard, H. (1986). *Arch. Pharm. Chem. Sci. Ed.* **14**, 52–63.

Larsson, O. M., Krogsgaard-Larsen, P., and Schousboe, A. (1980). *J. Neurochem.* **34**, 970–977.

Larsson, O. M., Thorbek, P., Krogsgaard-Larsen, P., and Schousboe, A. (1981). *J. Neurochem.* **37**, 1509–1516.

Larsson, O. M., Johnston, G. A. R., and Schousboe, A. (1983). *Brain Res.* **260**, 279–285.

Larsson, O. M., Krogsgaard-Larsen, P., and Schousboe, A. (1985). *Neurochem. Int.* **7**, 853–860.

Levi, G., and Raiteri, M. (1973). *Life Sci.* **12**, 81–88.

Lim, C. R., Garant, D. S., and Gale, K. (1985). *Eur. J. Pharmacol.* **107**, 91–94.

Lindeburg, T., Foelsgaard, S., Sillesen, H., Jacobsen, E., and Kehlet, H. (1983). *Acta Anaesthesiol. Scand.* **27**, 10–12.

Lloyd, K. G., and Pilc, A. (1984). *Neuropharmacology* **23**, 841–842.

Lloyd, K. G., Möhler, H., Heitz, P., and Bartholini, G. (1975). *J. Neurochem.* **25**, 789–795.

Lloyd, K. G., Shemen, L., and Hornykiewicz, O. (1977). *Brain Res.* **127**, 269–278.

Lloyd, K. G., Arbilla, S., Beaumont, K., Briley, M., De Montis, G., Scatton, B., Langer, S. Z., and Bartholini, G. (1982). *J. Pharmacol. Exp. Ther.* **220**, 672–677.

Lockerbie, R. O., and Gordon-Weeks, P. R. (1985). *Neurosci. Lett.* **55**, 273–277.

Lodge, D., Johnston, G. A. R., Curtis, D. R., and Brand, S. J. (1977). *Brain Res.* **136**, 513–522.

Luzzi, S., Franchi-Micheli, S., Ciuffi, M., Pajani, A., and Zilletti, L. (1986). *J. Auton. Pharmacol.* **6**, 163–169.

Löscher, W. (1982). *Neuropharmacology* **21**, 803–810.

Löscher, W. (1985). *Eur. J. Pharmacol.* **110**, 103–108.

Löscher, W. (1986a). *Drugs of the Future* **11**, 36–38.

Löscher, W. (1986b). *Drugs of the Future* **11**, 39–41.

Löscher, W., and Schwartz-Porsche, D. (1986). *J. Neurochem.* **46**, 1322–1325.

Löscher, W., and Siemes, H. (1985). *Epilepsia* **26**, 314–319.

Löscher, W., Frey, H.-H., Reiche, R., and Schultz, D. (1983). *J. Pharmacol. Exp. Ther.* **226**, 839–844.

Maggi, A., and Enna, S. J. (1979). *Neuropharmacology* **18**, 361–366.

Maksay, G., and Ticku, M. K. (1985). *J. Neurochem.* **44**, 480–486.

Mandel, P., and DeFeudis, F. V. (eds) (1979). "GABA—Biochemistry and CNS Functions". Plenum Press, New York.

Mandel, P., Ciesielski, L., Maitre, M., Simler, S., Mack, G., and Kempf, E. (1979). *In* "GABA—Biochemistry and CNS Functions" (P. Mandel and F. V. DeFeudis, eds), pp. 475–492. Plenum Press, New York.

Mann, A., Humblet, C., Chambon, J.-P., Schlichter, R., Desarmenien, M., Feltz, P., and Wermuth, C.-G. (1985). *J. Med. Chem.* **28**, 1440–1446.

Marcus, R. J., Winters, W. D., Roberts, E., and Simonsen, D. G. (1971). *Neuropharmacology* **10**, 203–215.

Marsden, C. D., and Sheehy, M. P. (1981). *In* "GABA and the Basal Ganglia" (G. DiChiara and G. L. Gessa, eds), pp. 225–234. Raven Press, New York.

Martin, D. L. (1976). *In* "GABA in Nervous System Function" (E. Roberts, T. N. Chase and D. B. Tower, eds), pp. 347–386. Raven Press, New York.

Martin, I. L., and Candy, J. M. (1978). *Neuropharmacology* **17**, 993–998.

Mathers, D. A. (1987). *Synapse* **1**, 96–101.

Matsuyama, K., Yamashita, C., Noda, A., Goto, S., Noda, H., Ichimura, Y., and Gomita, Y. (1984). *Chem. Pharm. Bull.* **32**, 4089–4095.

Matthews, W. D., McCafferty, G. P., and Setler, P. E. (1981). *Neuropharmacology* **20**, 561–565.

McGeer, P. L., and McGeer, E. G. (1976). *J. Neurochem.* **26**, 65–76.

Meier, E., Drejer, J., and Schousboe, A. (1984). *J. Neurochem.* **43**, 1737–1744.

Meldrum, B. S. (1975). *Int. Rev. Neurobiol.* **17**, 1–36.

Meldrum, B. (1982). *Clin. Neuropharmacol.* **5**, 293–316.

Meldrum, B., and Horton, R. (1980). *Eur. J. Pharmacol.* **61**, 231–237.

Mesdjian, E., DeFeudis, F. V., Jadot, G., Valli, M., Brugerolle, B., and Bouyard, P. (1983). *Drug Dev. Res.* **3**, 311–318.

Michaud, J. C., Mienville, J. M., Chambon, J.-P., and Biziere, K. (1986). *Neuropharmacology* **25**, 1197–1203.

Minchin, M. C. W., and Nutt, D. J. (1983). *Proc. Br. Pharmacol. Soc., Cambridge*, 6–8 April, p. 11.

Mitchell, R. (1982). *Biochem. Pharmacol.* **31**, 2684–2686.

Mitchell, R., and Martin, I. L. (1978). *Nature (London)* **274**, 904–905.

Mondrup, K., and Pedersen, E. (1983). *Acta Neurol. Scand.* **67**, 48–54.

Moreau, J.-L., and Fields, H. L. (1986). *Brain Res.* **397**, 37–46.

Morin, A. M., and Wasterlain, C. (1980). *Life Sci.* **26**, 1239–1245.

Moroni, F., Forchetti, M. C., Krogsgaard-Larsen, P., and Guidotti, A. (1982). *J. Pharm. Pharmacol.* **34**, 676–678.

Morselli, P. L., Löscher, W., Lloyd, K. G., Meldrum, B., and Reynolds, E. H. (eds) (1981). "Neurotransmitters, Seizures, and Epilepsy". Raven Press, New York.

Muhyaddin, M., Roberts, P. J., and Woodruff, G. N. (1982). *Br. J. Pharmacol.* **77**, 163–168.

Murray, T. F., McGill, W., and Cheney, D. L. (1983). *Eur. J. Pharmacol.* **90**, 179–184.

Müller, E. E., Cocchi, D., Locatelli, V., Apud, J. A., Tappaz, M. L., Masotto, C., Novelli, A., and Racagni, G. (1983). *In* "The GABA Receptors" (S. J. Enna, ed.), pp. 257–304. The Humana Press, Clifton, NJ.

Möhler, H., and Okada, T. (1977a). *Nature (London)* **267**, 65–67.

Möhler, H., and Okada, T. (1977b). *Science* **198**, 849–851.

Neal, H., and Bond, A. (1983). *Neuropharmacology* **22**, 881–886.

Nielsen, E. Ø., Aarslew-Jensen, M., Diemer, N. H., Krogsgaard-Larsen, P., and Schousboe, A. (1987). *J. Neurochem.* (in press).

Nistico, G., Morselli, P. L., Lloyd, K. G., Fariello, R. G., and Engel, J. (eds) (1986). "Neurotransmitters, Seizures, and Epilepsy", Vol. III. Raven Press, New York.

Nordmann, R., Graff, P., Maurer, R., and Gähwiler, B. H. (1985). *J. Med. Chem.* **28**, 1109–1111.

Nowak, L. M., Young, A. B., and Macdonald, R. L. (1982). *Brain Res.* **244**, 155–164.

Ogata, N., Inoue, M., and Matsuo, T. (1987). *Synapse* **1**, 62–69.

Okada, Y., and Roberts, E. (eds) (1982). "Problems in GABA Research from Brain to Bacteria". Excerpta Medica, Amsterdam.

Olpe, H.-R., Glatt, A., and Bencze, W. (1980). *Brain Res. Bull.* **5** (Suppl. 2), 507–511.

Olsen, R. W. (1981). *J. Neurochem.* **37**, 1–13.

Olsen, R. W., and Snowman, A. M. (1983). *J. Neurochem.* **41**, 1653–1663.

Olsen, R. W., and Venter, J. C. (eds) (1986). "Benzodiazepine/GABA Receptors and Chloride Channels. Structural and Functional Properties". Alan R. Liss, New York.

Olsen, R. W., Ticku, M. K., Greenlee, D., and Van Ness, P. (1979). *In* "GABA-Neuro-transmitters. Pharmacochemical, Biochemical and Pharmacological Aspects" (P. Krogsgaard-Larsen, J. Scheel-Krüger and H. Kofod, eds), pp. 165–178. Munksgaard, Copenhagen.

Olsen, R. W., Van Ness, P., Napias, C., Bergman, O., and Tourtellotte, W. W. (1980). *In* "Receptors for Neurotransmitters and Peptide Hormones" (G. Pepeu, M. J. Kuhar and S. J. Enna, eds), pp. 451–460. Raven Press, New York.

Olsen, R. W., Bergman, O., Van Ness, P. C., Lummis, S. C., Watkins, A. E., Napias, C., and Greenlee, D. V. (1981). *Mol. Pharmacol.* **19**, 217–227.

Olsen, R. W., Snowhill, E. W., and Wamsley, J. K. (1984). *Eur. J. Pharmacol.* **99**, 247–248.

Olsen, R. W., Wamsley, J. K., McCabe, R. T., Randall, J. L., and Lomax, P. (1985). *Proc. Natl. Acad. Sci. USA* **82**, 6701–6705.

Palacios, J. M., Wamsley, J. K., and Kuhar, M. J. (1981). *Brain Res.* **222**, 285–307.

Paul, S. M., Marangos, P. J., and Skolnick, P. (1981). *Biol. Psychiatry* **16**, 213–229.

Peck, E. J., Schaeffer, J. M., and Clark, J. H. (1973). *Biochem. Biophys. Res. Commun.* **52**, 394–400.

Persson, B. (1981). *J. Pharm. Pharmacol.* **35**, 759–761.

Petersen, H. R., Jensen, I., and Dam, M. (1983). *Acta Neurol. Scand.* **67**, 114–117.

Petty, F., and Coffman, J. A. (1984). *Neuropharmacology* **23**, 859–860.

Piredda, S., Pavlick, M., and Gale, K. (1987). *Epilepsy Res.* **1**, 102–106.

Polc, P. (1979). *Prog. Neuro-Psychopharmacol.* **3**, 345–352.

Pong, S. S., and Wang, C. C. (1982). *J. Neurochem.* **38**, 375–379.

454 P. KROGSGAARD-LARSEN *et al.*

Racagni, G., and Donoso, A. O. (eds) (1986). "GABA and Endocrine Function". Raven Press, New York.

Rastogi, S. K., Thyagarajan, R., Clothier, J., and Ticku, M. K. (1986). *Neuropharmacology* **25**, 1179–1184.

Ribak, C. E. (1985). *Brain Res.* **326**, 251–260.

Ribak, C. E., Harris, A. B., Anderson, L., Vaughn, J. E., and Roberts, E. (1979). *Science* **205**, 211–214.

Rinne, U. K., Koskinen, V., Laaksonen, H., Lönnberg, P., and Sonninen, V. (1978). *Life Sci.* **22**, 2225–2228.

Roberts, C. J., Krogsgaard-Larsen, P., and Walker, R. J. (1981). *Comp. Biochem. Physiol.* **69C**, 7–11.

Roberts, E., and Simonsen, D. G. (1966). *Biochem. Pharmacol.* **15**, 1875–1877.

Roberts, E., Chase, T. N., and Tower, D. B. (eds) (1976). "GABA in Nervous System Function". Raven Press, New York.

Roberts, P. J., Storm-Mathisen, J., and Bradford, H. F. (eds) (1986). "Excitatory Amino Acids". The Macmillan Press, London.

Roberts, R. C., Ribak, C. E., and Oertel, W. H. (1985). *Brain Res.* **361**, 324–338.

Ross, S. M., and Craig, C. R. (1981). *J. Neurochem.* **36**, 1006–1011.

Rovira, C., Ben-Ari, Y., and Cherubini, E. (1984). *Neuroscience* **12**, 543–555.

Ryan, A. F., and Schwartz, I. R. (1986). *Brain Res.* **399**, 399–403.

Santucci, V., Fournier, M., Chambon, J.-P., and Biziere, K. (1985). *Eur. J. Pharmacol.* **114**, 219–222.

Sarhan, S., Kolb, M., and Seiler, N. (1984). *Drug Res.* **34**, 687–690.

Sawynok, J. (1986). *Neuropharmacology* **25**, 795–798.

Sawynok, J., and LaBella, F. S. (1981). *Eur. J. Pharmacol.* **70**, 103–110.

Sawynok, J., and LaBella, F. S. (1982). *Neuropharmacology* **21**, 397–403.

Schoch, P., Richards, J. G., Häring, P., Takacs, B., Stähli, C., Staehelin, T., Haefely, W., and Möhler, H. (1985). *Nature (London)* **314**, 168–171.

Schousboe, A. (1981). *Int. Rev. Neurobiol.* **22**, 1–45.

Schousboe, A., Thorbek, P., Hertz, L., and Krogsgaard-Larsen, P. (1979). *J. Neurochem.* **33**, 181–189.

Schousboe, A., Larsson, O. M., and Krogsgaard-Larsen, P. (1985). *Neurochem. Int.* **7**, 505–508.

Schousboe, A., Hjeds, H., Engler, J., Krogsgaard-Larsen, P., and Wood, J. D. (1986). *J. Neurochem.* **47**, 758–763.

Schultz, B., Aaes-Jørgensen, T., Bøgesø, K. P., and Jørgensen, A. (1981). *Acta Pharmacol. Toxicol.* **49**, 116–124.

Schwark, W. S., and Löscher, W. (1985). *Naunyn-Schmiedeberg's Arch. Exp. Path. Pharmak.* **329**, 367–371.

Seifert, J., and Casida, J. E. (1985). *J. Neurochem.* **44**, 110–116.

Seiler, N., and Sarhan, S. (1984). *Gen. Pharmacol.* **15**, 367–369.

Seiler, N., Sarhan, S., Krogsgaard-Larsen, P., Hjeds, H., and Schousboe, A. (1985). *Gen. Pharmacol.* **16**, 509–511.

Shashoua, V. E., Jacob, J. N., Ridge, R., Campbell, A., and Baldessarini, R. J. (1984). *J. Med. Chem.* **27**, 659–664.

Sigel, E., Stephenson, F. A., Mamalaki, C., and Barnard, E. A. (1983). *J. Biol. Chem.* **258**, 6965–6971.

Simler, S., Puglisi-Allegra, S., and Mandel, P. (1982). *Pharmacol. Biochem. Behav.* **16**, 57–61.

Simmonds, M. A. (1984). *In* "Actions and Interactions of GABA and Benzodiazepines" (N. G. Bowery, ed.), pp. 27–41. Raven Press, New York.

Sivam, S. P., and Ho, I. K. (1985). *Life Sci.* **37**, 199–208.

Skerritt, J. H., Willow, M., and Johnston, G. A. R. (1982). *Neurosci. Lett.* **29**, 63–66.

Snodgrass, S. R. (1978). *Nature (London)* **274**, 392–394.

Snyder, S. H., Axelrod, J., and Rauer, H. (1964). *J. Pharmacol. Exp. Ther.* **144**, 373–379.

Spink, D. C., and Martin, D. L. (1983). *In* "Glutamine, Glutamate, and GABA in the Central Nervous System" (L. Hertz, E. Kvamme, E. G. McGeer and A. Schousboe, eds), pp. 129–143. Alan R. Liss, New York.

Squires, R. F., and Braestrup, C. (1977). *Nature (London)* **266**, 732–734.

Squires, R. F., Casida, J. E., Richardson, M., and Saederup, E. (1983). *Mol. Pharmacol.* **23**, 326–336.

Starr, M. S. (1979). *Eur. J. Pharmacol.* **53**, 215–226.

Steward, E. G., Borthwick, P. W., Clarke, G. R., and Warner, D. (1975). *Nature (London)* **256**, 600–602.

Stoof, J. C., and Mulder, A.H. (1977). *Eur. J. Pharmacol.* **46**, 177–180.

Supavilai, P., and Karobath, M. (1980). *Neurosci. Lett.* **19**, 337–341.

Supavilai, P., and Karobath, M. (1981). *J. Neurochem.* **36**, 798–803.

Tallman, J. F. (1983). *In* "The GABA Receptors" (S. J. Enna, ed.), pp. 93–106. The Humana Press, Clifton, NJ.

Tallman, J. F., Thomas, J. W., and Gallager, D. W. (1978). *Nature (London)* **274**, 383–385.

Tamminga, C. A., Crayton, J. W., and Chase, T. N. (1979). *Arch. Gen. Psychiatry* **36**, 595–598.

Thyagarajan, R., Brennan, T. J., and Ticku, M. K. (1983). *Eur. J. Pharmacol.* **93**, 127–136.

Van Kammen, D. P., Sternberg, D. E., Hare, T. A., and Waters, R. N. (1982). *Arch. Gen. Psychiatry* **39**, 91–97.

Van Ness, P. C., Watkins, A. E., Bergman, M. O., Tourtellotte, W. W., and Olsen, R. W. (1982). *Neurology (Ny)* **32**, 63–68.

Wamsley, J. K., Gehlert, D. R., and Olsen, R. W. (1986). *In* "Benzodiazepine-GABA Receptors and Chloride Channels: Structural and Functional Properties" (R. W. Olsen and J. C. Venter, eds), pp. 299–313. Alan R. Liss, New York.

Warner, D., and Steward, E. G. (1975). *J. Mol. Struct.* **25**, 403–411.

Waszczak, B. L., and Walters, J. R. (1980). *Brain Res. Bull.* **5** (Suppl. 2), 465–470.

Waszczak, B. L., Hruska, R. E., and Walters, J. R. (1980). *Eur. J. Pharmacol.* **65**, 21–29.

Watling, K. J., and Bristow, D. R. (1986). *J. Neurochem.* **46**, 1755–1762.

Wermuth, C.-G., Bourguignon, J.-J., Schlewer, G., Gies, J.-P., Schoenfelder, A., Melikian, A., Bouchet, M.-J., Chantreux, D., Molimard, J.-C., Heaulme, M., Chambon, J.-P., and Biziere, K. (1987). *J. Med. Chem.* **30**, 239–249.

Wilkin, G. P., Hudson, A. L., Hill, D. R., and Bowery, N. G. (1981). *Nature (London)* **274**, 584–587.

Williams, M., and Risley, E. A. (1984). *J. Neurochem.* **42**, 745–753.

Wong, E. H. F., and Iversen, L. L. (1985). *J. Neurochem.* **44**, 1162–1167.

Wood, J. D., and Sidhu, H. S. (1986). *J. Neurochem.* **46**, 739–744.

Wood, J. D., Tsui, D., and Phillis, J. W. (1979). *Can. J. Physiol. Pharmacol.* **57**, 581–585.

Wood, J. D., Schousboe, A., and Krogsgaard-Larsen, P. (1980). *Neuropharmacology* **19**, 1149–1152.

Worms, P., Depoortere, H., Durand, A., Morselli, P. L., Lloyd, K. G., and Bartholini, G. (1982). *J. Pharmacol. Exp. Ther.* **220**, 660–671.

Yarbrough, G. G. (1978). *Can. J. Physiol. Pharmacol.* **56**, 443–446.

Yarbrough, G. G., Williams, M., and Haubrich, D. R. (1979). *Arch. Int. Pharmacodyn.* **241**, 266–279.

Yokoi, I., Tsuruta, K., Shigara, H., and Mori, A. (1987). *Epilepsy Res.* **1**, 114–120.

Yunger, L. M., Fowler, P. J., Zarevics, P., and Setler, P. E. (1984). *J. Pharmacol. Exp. Ther.* **228**, 109–115.

Zorn, S. H., Willmore, L. J., Bailey, C. M., and Enna, S. J. (1986). *In* "Neurotransmitters, Seizures, and Epilepsy" (G. Nistico, P. L. Morselli, K. G. Lloyd, R. G. Fariello and J. Engel, eds), Vol. III, pp. 123–133. Raven Press, New York.

Zorn, S. H., Duman, R. S., Giachetti, A., Micheletti, R., Giraldo, E., Krogsgaard-Larsen, P., and Enna, S. J. (1987). *J. Pharmacol. Exp. Ther.* **242**, 173–178.

Zukin, S. R., Young, A. B., and Snyder, S. H. (1974). *Proc. Natl. Acad. Sci. USA* **71**, 4802–4807.

Note: The full chemical names of drugs better known by their common/approved/ abbreviated names have generally been omitted.

A

AC-1370, *see* Cefpimizole
7-ACA, *see* 7-Aminocephalosporanic acid
3'-Acetoxy group of cephems, displacement, 105
1-Acetoxyethyl prodrug esters, primary metabolites, 198
3-Acetoxymethyl cephem derivatives, 109
Acetylcholine release, regulation, 247–248
ACV *see* Acyclovir
Acycloguanosine, *see* Acyclovir
Acyclovir (acycloguanosine; zovirax), 2, 4, 6–12
  actions, mechanisms, 7–8
  derivatives, 8–12
  disadvantages, 8
  uses, 2
    indications, 6
    prophylactic, 6
Acyclovir triphosphate, 7, 11, 12
7-Acyl side chain of cephalosporins, variations at the, 146–162
7-Acylamido side chain of cephalosporins, importance, 146
N-Acylated (phenylglycyl) cephalosporins, 160, 161, 183–185
Acylimine, 7α-methoxylation of cephalosporins via, 122
7-ADCA, *see* 7-Amino-deacetoxycephalosporanic acid
Adenine arabinoside, *see* Vidarabine
(*RS*)-3-Adenin-9-yl-2-hydroxy-propanoic acid = (*RS*)-AHPA, 28, 30

Adenosine
  actions and receptors of, 321–325 *passim*
  analogues, acyclic and cyclic, 27–32
Adenosine diphosphate receptors, 321, 323
Adenosine monophosphate, cyclic, *see* cAMP
Adenosine triphosphate
  cardiovascular effects, 323–325 *passim*
  as a neurotransmitter, 320–321
Adenosine triphosphate receptors, 321, 323
S-Adenosylhomocysteine hydrolase inhibitors, 28–30
Adenylate cyclase
  prostacyclin-activated, 303
  purinergic receptor interactions with, 321–322
α-Adrenoceptors, 239–280
  central medullary, 239–245, 278
  extrajunctional, 252–253
  myocardial, 273–274
  occupancy (by agonist) and response/activation of, 254, 265–266, 272–273
  peripheral, 245–278, 278–280
  postsynaptic, *see* Postsynaptic α-adrenoceptors
  presynaptic, *see* Presynaptic α-adrenoceptors
  renal, 274–278
  reserves in arteries *vs.* veins, 269–270
  vascular, 248–273
α-Adrenoceptor agonists, 239–245
  actions, 239–245, 278
  central, 239–245, 278
  neurotransmitter release and the effects of, 246
  withdrawal effects, 245

CUMULATIVE INDEX OF AUTHORS

CUMULATIVE INDEX OF TITLES